CAWSON'S ESSENTIALS OF
ORAL PATHOLOGY AND ORAL MEDICINE

Commissioning Editor: Michael Parkinson
Project Development Editors: Jim Killgore, Hannah Kenner
Design Direction: George Ajayi
Project Manager: Frances Affleck

CAWSON'S ESSENTIALS OF
ORAL PATHOLOGY AND ORAL MEDICINE

SEVENTH EDITION

R. A. CAWSON MD FDSRCS FDSRCPS(Glas) FRCPath

Emeritus Professor of Oral Medicine and Pathology, Guy's, King's and St Thomas' Dental Institute, London.
Honorary Consultant, Eastman Dental Institute for Oral Health Care Sciences, University College, London.
Visiting Professor in Oral Pathology, Baylor College of Dentistry, Texas A & M University System, Dallas, Texas

and

E. W. ODELL BDS FDSRCS MSc PhD FRCPath

Reader in Oral Pathology and Oral Medicine, Guy's, King's and St Thomas' Dental Institute, London.
Honorary Consultant, Guy's and St Thomas' Hospitals, London

with the assistance of

S. PORTER MD PhD FDSRCS FDSRCSE

Professor of Oral Medicine, Head of Oral Medicine and Special Needs Dentistry,
Eastman Dental Institute for Oral Health Care Sciences, University College, London.
Honorary Consultant, University College London Hospital, London

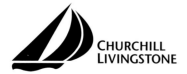

CHURCHILL
LIVINGSTONE

EDINBURGH LONDON NEW YORK OXFORD PHILADELPHIA ST LOUIS SYDNEY TORONTO 2002

CHURCHILL LIVINGSTONE
An imprint of Elsevier Limited

First edition 1962
Second edition 1968
Third edition 1978
Fourth edition 1984
Fifth edition 1991
Sixth edition 1998
Seventh edition 2002

Standard Edition ISBN 0 443 071063
Reprinted 2005, 2006

International Student Edition ISBN 0 443 071055
Reprinted 2003 (twice), 2005, 2006

Formerly published as *Essentials of Dental Surgery and Pathology*

British Library Cataloguing in Publication Data
A catalogue record for this book is available from the British Library

Library of Congress Cataloging in Publication Data
A catalog record for this book is available from the Library of Congress

ELSEVIER your source for books,
journals and multimedia
in the health sciences
www.elsevierhealth.com

Working together to grow
libraries in developing countries

www.elsevier.com | www.bookaid.org | www.sabre.org

ELSEVIER BOOK AID International Sabre Foundation

The
Publisher's
policy is to use
**paper manufactured
from sustainable forests**

Printed in Spain

Preface

It may perhaps be a surprise to many that *Essentials* has been in continuous publication for forty years. It was the first short book on dental surgery and pathology and published in hard cover by the old-established firm of Churchill. Since then it has survived, among other hazards, successive publishers' take-overs from Churchill, to Churchill Livingstone, to Harcourt Brace and, most recently, to Elsevier Science.

The text has been updated, but please remember that by the time you read this (does anyone read Prefaces?) some of it will inevitably be out of date as a result of the rapidity of medical progress.

We are flattered that the previous edition was adopted as a standard text for the MFDS and hope that the present edition will help to bring success to even more candidates sitting this examination.

Under the valued supervision of Mike Parkinson, the Publishing Editor, and Jim Killgore and Hannah Kenner, the Project Development Managers, the text illustrations are now in colour throughout. The few exceptions are mostly pictures taken before the advent of colour photography of conditions that are unlikely to be seen now. However, they should still be of interest to compare with similar conditions which might be seen now and may suggest that some progress may have been made.

We are immensely pleased that the colour reproductions of both clinical pictures and photomicrographs are of quite outstanding quality and are deeply grateful to our publishers for the trouble they have taken.

London, 2002

R. A. C.
E. W. O

Contents

Principles of investigation and diagnosis

The principles of patient investigation and diagnosis are summarised in Table 1.1.

Taking a history

History-taking needs to be tailored to suit the individual patient but it is sometimes difficult to get a clear idea of the complaint. Many patients are nervous, some are inarticulate, others are confused.

Rapport is critical for eliciting useful information. Initial questions should allow patients to speak at some length and to gain confidence. It is usually best to start with an 'open' question. Medical jargon should be avoided and even regular hospital attenders who appear to understand medical terminology may use it wrongly and misunderstand. Leading questions, which suggest a particular answer, should be avoided because patients may feel compelled to agree with the clinician.

It is sometimes difficult to avoid interrupting patients when trying to structure the history for the records. Structure can only be given after the patient has had time to give the information. Constant note-taking while patients are speaking is undesirable.

Questioning technique is most critical when eliciting any relevant social or psychological history or dealing with embarrassing medical conditions. It may be appropriate to delay asking such questions until after rapport has been gained. Some patients do not consider medical questions to be the concern of the dentist and it is important to give reasons for such questions when necessary (Table 1.2).

During history-taking, the mental and emotional state of the patient should be assessed. This may have a bearing on psychosomatic disease and will also suggest what the patient expects to gain from the consultation and treatment. If the patient's expectations are unreasonable it is important to try to modify them during the consultation, otherwise no treatment may be satisfactory.

Table 1.1 Principles of investigation and diagnosis

- A detailed history
- Clinical examination
    Extraoral
    Intraoral
- Special investigations (as appropriate)
    Radiography or other imaging techniques
    Biosy for histopathology (including immunofluorescence,
       immunocytochemistry, electron microscopy, molecular
       biological tests)
    Specimen for microbial culture
    Haematological or biochemical tests

Type of question	Example
Open	Tell me about the pain?
Closed	What does the pain feel like?
Leading	Does the pain feel like an electric shock?

Type of question	Advantages	Disadvantages
Open	Allows patients to use their own words and summarise their view of the problem	Clinicians must listen carefully and avoid interruptions to extract the relevant information
	Allows patients to partly direct the history-taking, gives them confidence and quickly generates rapport	Patients tend to decide what information is relevant
Closed	Elicits specific information quickly. Useful to fill gaps in the information given in response to open questions	Patients may infer that the clinician is not really interested in their problem if only closed questions are asked
	Prevents vague patients from rambling away from the complaint	Important information may be lost if not specifically requested
		Restricts the patient's opportunities to talk

Table 1.2 Essential principles of history-taking technique

- Introduce yourself and greet the patient by name
- Put patients at their ease
- Start with an open question
- Mix open and closed questions
- Avoid leading questions
- Avoid jargon
- Explain the need for specific questions
- Assess the patient's mental state
- Assess the patient's expectations from treatment

Demographic details

The age, gender, ethnic group and occupation of the patient should be noted. Such information is occasionally critical. For instance, an elderly woman with arthritis and a dry mouth is likely to have Sjögren's syndrome (Ch. 18), but, a young man with a parotid swelling due to similar lymphoproliferation is far more likely to have HIV infection (Ch. 24). Some diseases such as oral submucous fibrosis (Ch. 11) have a restricted ethnic distribution.

History of the present complaint

Frequently a complaint, such as toothache, suggests the diagnosis. In many cases a detailed history (Table 1.3) is required and sometimes, as in aphthous ulceration, the diagnosis can be made on the history without examination or investigation.

If earlier treatment has been ineffective, the diagnosis should be reconsidered. Many patients' lives have been shortened by having malignant tumours treated with repeated courses of antibiotics.

Pain is completely subjective and when physical signs are absent special care must be taken to detail all its features (Table 1.4). Especially important are features suggesting a dental cause. A fractured tooth or cusp, dentinal hypersensitivity or occlusal pain are easily misdiagnosed.

Factors triggering different causes of pain are discussed in detail in Chapter 34.

Table 1.3 History of the present complaint

- Record the description of the complaint *in the patient's own words*
- Elicit the exact meaning of those words
- Record the duration and the time course of any changes in symptoms or signs
- Include any relevant facts in the patient's medical history
- Note any temporal relationship between them and the present complaint
- Consider any previous treatments and their effectiveness

Table 1.4 Taking a pain history

Characteristic	Informative features
Type	Ache, tenderness, dull pain, throbbing, stabbing, electric shock. These terms are of limited use and the constancy of pain is more useful
Severity	Mild — managed with mild analgesics (e.g. aspirin/paracetamol) Moderate — unresponsive to mild analgesics Severe — disturbs sleep
Duration	Time since onset. Duration of pain or attacks.
Nature	Continuous, periodic or paroxysmal. *sudden onset* If not continuous, is pain present between attacks?
Initiating factors	Any potential initiating factors. Association with dental treatment or lack of it is especially important in eliminating dental causes
Exacerbating and relieving factors	Record all and note especially hot and cold sensitivity or pain on eating which suggest a dental cause.
Localisation	The patient should map out the distribution of pain if possible. Is it well or poorly defined?
Referral	Try to determine whether the pain could be referred.

The medical history

A medical history is important as it aids the diagnosis of oral manifestations of systemic disease. It also ensures that medical conditions and medication which affect dental or surgical treatment are identified.

To ensure that nothing significant is forgotten, a printed questionnaire for patients to complete is valuable and saves time. It also helps to avoid medicolegal problems by providing a written record that the patient's medical background has been considered.

A suggested medical history questionnaire is shown in Table 1.5.

If the history suggests, or examination reveals, any condition beyond the scope of the dentist's experience or clinical knowledge, referral for specialist medical examination may be necessary.

Medical warning cards may indicate that the patient is, for example, a haemophiliac, on long-term corticosteroid therapy or is allergic to penicillin. It is also worthwhile to leave a final section open for patients to supply any other information that they think might be relevant.

A questionnaire does *not* constitute a medical history and the information must be checked verbally, verified, and augmented as necessary. It is important to assess whether the patient's reading ability and understanding are sufficient to provide valid answers to the questionnaire.

A detailed drug history is essential. Drugs can have oral effects or complicate dental management in important ways (Chs 13 & 35).

Table 1.5 An example of a medical history questionnaire

SURNAME .... Address ....

Other names ....

Date of birth .... Telephone number ....

The following questions are asked in the interests of your safety and any particular precautions that may need to be taken as a result of thorough knowledge of any previous illnesses or medications. Please, therefore, answer these questions as accurately as you can.
   If you are in any doubt about how to answer them, please do not hesitate to ask.

1. Are you undergoing any medical treatment at present?	Yes	No
2. Do you have, or have you had any of the following:		
a. Heart disease?	Yes	No
b. Rheumatic fever?	Yes	No
c. Hepatitis?	Yes	No
d. Jaundice?	Yes	Np
e. Epilepsy	Yes	No
f. Diabetes?	Yes	No
g. Raised blood pressure?	Yes	No
h. Anaemia?	Yes	No
i. Asthma, hay fever or other allergies?	Yes	No
j. Familial or acquired bleeding tendencies?	Yes	No
k. Any other serious illnesses	Yes	No
3. Have you suffered allergy or other reactions (rash, itchiness etc) to:		
a. Penicillin?	Yes	No
b. Other medicines or tablets?	Yes	No
c. Substances or chemicals?	Yes	No
4. Have you ever had any adverse effects from local anaesthetics?	Yes	No
5. Have you ever experienced unusually prolonged bleeding after injury or tooth extraction?	Yes	No
6. Have you ever been given penicillin?	Yes	No
7. Are you taking any medicines, tablets, injections (etc.) at present?	Yes	No
If YES can you please indicate the nature of this medication?		
8. Have you been treated with any of the following in the past 5 years:		
a. Cortisone (hydrocortisone, prednisone etc)?	Yes	No
b. Blood-thinning medication?	Yes	No
c. Antidepressants?	Yes	No
9. Have you ever received radiotherapy?	Yes	No
10. Do you smoke?	Yes	No
If YES how much on average per day?		
11. For female patients — are you pregnant?	Yes	No

PLEASE ADD ANY OTHER INFORMATION OR COMMENTS ON YOUR MEDICAL HISTORY, BELOW

....

Signature .... Date ....

Address (if not the patient) ....

In some ethnic groups, enquiry should be made about habits such as betel quid (pan) or smokeless tobacco use.

The dental history

A dental history and examination are obviously essential for the diagnosis of dental pain or to exclude teeth as cause of symptoms in the head and neck region.

Symptoms of toothache are very variable and may masquerade as a variety of conditions from trivial to sinister. The relationship between symptoms and any dental treatment, or lack of it, should be noted.

The family and social history

Whenever a symptom or sign suggests an inherited disorder, such as haemophilia, the family history should be elicited. Ideally, this is recorded as a pedigree diagram noting the proband (presenting case) and all family members for at least three gen-

erations. Even when no familial disease is suspected, questions about other family members often usefully lead naturally into questions about home circumstances, relatives and social history which can be revealing if, for example, psychosomatic factors are suspected.

Consent

It is imperative to obtain patients' consent for any procedure. At the very least, the procedure to be used should be explained to the patient and verbal consent obtained. If no more than this is done, the patients' consent should be noted in their records. However, it is better to obtain written consent.

Patients frequently ask for particular types of treatment, such as fillings or extractions. This implies consent and usually no written agreement is expected. However, with the growing risk of litigation, many dental hospitals now require clinicians to give precise descriptions of treatment plans, however routine, and to obtain written consent.

Patients have a legal right to refuse treatment. Any such refusals may sometimes be due to failure of the clinician to explain the need for a particular procedure, or failure to soothe the patient's fears about possible complications. Some of these fears may be irrational, such as the idea of an inherited allergy to local anaesthetics. In such cases even prolonged explanations and persuasion may be unsuccessful.

When a biopsy is necessary, its purpose should be explained and that the biopsied area may be sore after the local anaesthetic has worn off. Also, it seems likely that when the patient's tissue is to be retained, even in a block for histological examination, it should be explained that this has to be done in case future reference to it is needed and consent obtained accordingly.

In the case of more major surgery a consent form should state the nature of the operation and also the likelihood of any significant complications or risks. In the case of an ameloblastoma, for example, it would be necessary to point out that a further operation may be unavoidable and that the alternative might be a relatively massive excision. Also, in such circumstances or when sedation or a general anaesthetic is indicated, patients should be encouraged to ask whatever questions or express any concerns about the procedure, and to have it explained fully.

Even greater difficulties may arise in the matter of consent for parotid gland surgery. Explanation of the possibility of permanently disfiguring facial palsy has to be balanced against the need for complete eradication of a tumour. Also, in the case of older patients it may seem probable that a benign tumour may not cause significant trouble within the patient's lifetime and that the operative risks are not justified. On the other hand, such a patient may find the idea of living with a tumour emotionally unacceptable so that surgery with its possible complications has to be accepted.

For consent to be legally valid, patients should be given sufficient information, in understandable terms, about the proposed treatment for them to make their own decisions. It is not enough to get a patient, due to have major oral surgery, to sign a blanket consent form without any explanations. Though this has happened many times, the patient may later claim for assault, particularly if there have been unexpected complications.

A Consent Form should therefore be used and should state:

1. The type of operation or investigation.
2. Possible risks and complications
3. A signed and dated statement by the clinician that he or she has explained these matters and any options that may be available in terms understandable to the patient, parent or guardian.
4. A section for the patient, parent or guardian to confirm;
   a. that the information was understandable.
   b. that the person signing the form has a legal right to do so, i.e. is the patient, parent or guardian
   c. that the procedure has been explained and agreed
   d. that there are certain additional procedures that would be completely unacceptable and should not be carried out.

The form should be signed and dated by the clinician and patient, parent or guardian.

Clinical examination — extraoral

First, *look* at the patient, before looking into the patient's mouth. Anaemia, thyroid disease, long-term corticosteroid treatment, parotid swellings, or significantly enlarged cervical nodes are a few conditions that can affect the facial appearance.

The parotid glands, temporomandibular joints (for clicks, crepitus or deviation), cervical and submandibular lymph nodes and thyroid gland should be palpated. Lymphadenopathy (Ch. 26) is a common manifestation of infection but may also signify malignancy — the cervical lymph nodes are often the first affected by lymphomas. Note the character (site, shape, size, surface texture and consistency) of any enlargement. Press on the maxilla and frontal bone over the sinuses to elicit tenderness if sinusitis is suspected.

Oral examination

Examination of the oral cavity can only be performed adequately with good light, mirrors and compressed air or other means of drying the teeth. If viscid saliva prevents visualisation of the tissues and teeth, a rinse with sodium bicarbonate mouthwash will help.

Soft tissues

The soft tissues of the mouth should usually be inspected first. Examination should be systematic to include all areas of the mouth. Care should be taken that mirrors or retractors do not obscure lesions. To ensure complete examination of the lateral tongue and posterior floor of mouth the tongue must be held in gauze and gently extended from side to side.

Abnormal-looking areas of mucosa should be palpated for scarring or induration indicating previous ulceration, inflammation or malignancy. Examination should include deeper tissues accessible to palpation, including the submandibular glands.

If lesions extend close to the gingiva the gingival crevice or pockets should be probed for any communication. Mucosal nodules, especially those on the gingiva or alveolar mucosa, which suggest sinus openings should be probed to identify any sinus or fistula. Check the openings of the salivary ducts while expressing saliva by gentle pressure. Check that saliva flows freely and equally from all glands and is clear in colour. Do not mistake anatomical variations (Table 1.6) for disease.

After examination of the oral mucosa try to visualise the oropharynx and tonsils.

Teeth

As a minimum, the standing teeth with a summary of their periodontal health, caries and restorative state, should be recorded. Tooth wear should be checked for 'parafunction'. Dental examination should be thorough both for the patient's

Table 1.6 Some anatomical variants and normal structures often misdiagnosed as lesions

Structure	Description
Fordyce spots	Sebaceous glands lying superficially in the mucosa are visible as white or cream coloured spots up to 0.5 mm across. Usually labial mucosa and buccal mucosa. Occasionally prominent and very numerous (Fig. 15.4)
Lingual tonsils	Enlarge with viral infection and occasionally noted by patients. Sometimes large or ectopic and then mistaken for disease (Figs 1.1 and 1.2)
Circumvallate papillae	Readily identifiable but sometimes prominent and misinterpreted by patients or health care workers.
Retrocuspid papilla	Firm pink nodule 0.5–4 mm diameter on the attached gingiva lingual to the lower canine and lateral incisor, usually bilaterally but sometimes unilateral. Prominent in children but regress with age.
Dorsal tongue fur	Furring of the dorsal tongue mucosa is very variable and is heavier when the diet is soft. Even light furring is regarded as pathological by many patients. When pigmented black by bacteria the condition is called black hairy tongue (Ch. 14).
Leukoedema	A milky white translucent whitening of the oral mucosa which disappears or fades on stretching. Commoner in black races (Ch. 15).
Tori	Exostoses in the midline of the palate or in the lingual alveolus in the premolar region are termed tori (Ch. 9).

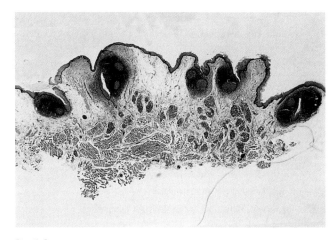

Fig. 1.2 Section showing the nodular surface and lymphoid follicles in a foliate papilla.

Table 1.7 Precautions for electric pulp testing

- Isolate individual teeth with a small portion of rubber dam if necessary
- Always record electric pulp test values in the notes — a progressive change in reading over time may indicate declining vitality
- If results remain uncertain, cut a test cavity or remove suspect restorations without local anaesthetic
- Poorly localised pulp pain from teeth of dubious vitality can be difficult to ascribe to an individual tooth. In such circumstances a diagnostic local anaesthetic injection on a suspect tooth may stop the pain and indicate its source
- Other sources of referred pain may sometimes be identified by the same means

sake and for medicolegal reasons. When dental pain is a possibility, full charting, assessment of mobility and percussion of teeth are necessary and further dental investigations will probably be required. However, before any investigations are begun, *the patient's consent must be obtained* (see below).

Testing vitality of teeth

The vitality of teeth must be checked if they appear to be causing symptoms. It is also essential to determine the vitality of teeth in the region of cysts and other radiolucent lesions in the jaws at presentation. The information may be essential for diagnosis.

To be absolutely certain, several methods may have to be used. Checking hot and cold sensitivity and electric pulp testing are relatively easily performed (Table 1.7).

Unfortunately it may not be apparent that a pulp test result is misleading. Care must always be taken to avoid causes of false positive or false negative results (Table 1.8).

Medical examination

In practice it is usual for dental investigations to be performed first, but the dentist should be capable of performing simple medical examinations of the head and neck. Examination of the

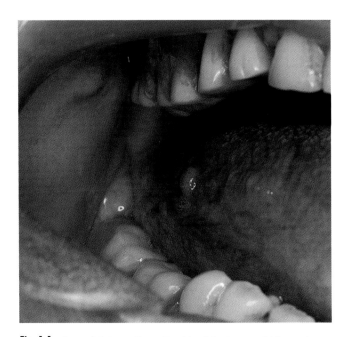

Fig. 1.1 Large foliate papilla on the side of the tongue which may be mistaken for a lesion.

Table 1.8 Possible causes of misleading electric pulp test results

Problem	Causes to consider
Pulp bypassed by electric current	Electrical contact with next tooth by touching amalgam restorations
	Electrical contact with gingival margin by amalgam restoration or saliva film
Electrical insulation of the pulp	Large composite or non-conducting restorations
Falsely low reading	Incompletely formed root apex
Partially vital pulps	Multiple canals
No check on validity of results	No normal teeth for comparison
Patient fails to report accurately	Failure to differentiate pulpal from soft tissue sensation

Table 1.9 Useful diagnostic information from examination of the hands

Site	Signs
Flexor surface of wrist	Rash (or history of rash) consisting of purplish papules suggests lichen planus, especially if itchy
Finger morphology	Clubbing may be associated with some chronic respiratory and cardiac conditions (including infective endocarditis) and sometimes remote malignancy
	Joint changes may suggest rheumatoid arthritis (joint swelling, ulnar drift) or osteoarthritis (Heberden's nodes)
Abnormal nails	Koilonychia suggests long-standing anaemia. Hypoplastic nails may be associated with several inherited epithelial disorders of oral significance including ectodermal dysplasia and dyskeratosis congenita (see also Ch. 15)
Skin of fingers	May be thin, shiny and white in Raynaud's phenomenon (periodic ischaemia resulting from exposure to cold — often associated with autoimmune conditions particularly systemic sclerosis (Fig. 1.3) or Sjögren's syndrome)
	Note any tobacco staining. Is the degree commensurate with the patient's reported tobacco use?
Palmar-plantar keratosis	Associated with several syndromes including Papillon-Lefèvre syndrome (includes juvenile periodontitis)

skin of the face, hair, scalp and neck may reveal unexpected foci of infection to account for cervical lymphadenopathy or even malignant neoplasms. The eye can readily be inspected for conjunctivitis or signs of mucous membrane pemphigoid, anaemia or jaundice. Examination of the hands may also reveal relevant information (Table 1.9). Dentists should be able to examine cranial nerve function but more extensive medical examination by dentists is usually done in hospital.

Making a clinical differential diagnosis and investigation plan

The diagnosis and appropriate treatment may be obvious from the history and examination. More frequently there are various possible diagnoses and a clinical differential diagnosis and plan of investigation should be worked out. Possible diagnoses should be recorded in order of probability, based on their prevalence and likelihood of causing the symptoms and signs. Even if only one diagnosis seems appropriate it is worthwhile noting the next most likely possibility and any other causes which can be excluded. This ensures that all appropriate investigations are remembered and reduces the possibility of the patient having to return for further investigations. Drawing up such a written differential diagnosis helps even experienced clinicians to organise their thoughts. The list also forms the basis on which special investigations are selected. Precise diagnosis may depend on histological findings so that a preliminary generic diagnosis, such as 'benign neoplasm' or 'odontogenic tumour', often has to be made.

Special investigations

Innumerable types of investigation are possible, and it may be difficult to refrain from asking for every conceivable investigation in the anxiety not to miss something unsuspected and to avoid medicolegal complications. Though it may be tempting to explore every possibility, however remote, this approach may prove counterproductive in that it can produce a plethora of

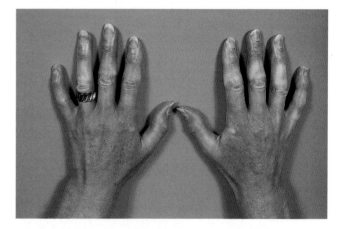

Fig. 1.3 Hands with taut shiny pale skin on the tapering fingers, a result of Raynaud's phenomenon, in this case in systemic sclerosis.

reports that confuse rather than inform. Laboratory staff soon also become aware of, and may become less helpful to, those who overburden them.

Special investigations should only be requested to answer specific questions about a possible diagnosis, not as a routine. Some investigations have a high specificity and sensitivity for particular diseases, but few investigations provide a specific diagnosis. A few diseases, such as mumps, may be diagnosed on the basis of a single test, but others, such as Sjögren's syndrome, may require many tests. Therefore, the usefulness of each investigation must be borne in mind when interpreting the results.

Table 1.10 Imaging techniques for lesions of the head and neck

Techniques	Advantages	Disadvantages
Conventional radiography	Simple, widely available, many common lesions may be identified with a high degree of accuracy	Difficult to interpret in some areas of the jaws because of the complex anatomy
	Panoramic radiographs can show unsuspected lesions	X-ray dose unavoidable
		Little information about soft tissue lesions
Computerised tomography	Provides tomographic (sectional) images of high clarity in any plane without superimposition	Expensive and not always available
		Higher X-ray dose than plain radiographs
	Very useful where complex anatomy hinders interpretation of plain radiographs	Radiopaque dental restorations cause artefactual shadows which can obscure part of the image
		Less information on soft tissue lesions than MRI
Use of contrast media with plain radiography or computerised tomography	Useful for outlining the extent of duct systems (e.g. the salivary gland ducts in sialography), hollow lesions such as cysts or blood vessels (angiography)	Requires more expertise than plain radiography
	Can be used to outline lesions in soft tissues	
Magnetic resonance imaging	No X-ray dose	Expensive and limited availability
	Produces clear tomograms without superimposition	Does not image bone
	Particularly good for soft tissue lesions	
Ultrasound	No X-ray dose	Requires expertise in interpretation
	Shows soft tissue masses and cysts well	Overlying bone obscures soft tissue lesions
	Useful for salivary gland cysts, Sjögren's syndrome and stones, and to detect lesions in the thyroid gland and neck	
Technetium scan	Provides an assessment of function in each salivary gland	Equipment not always available
	Can be used if sialography is not possible	Radiation dose

Imaging

The most informative imaging techniques in the head and neck are radiography and computerised tomography (CT), magnetic resonance imaging (MRI) and ultrasound. Their advantages and disadvantages are shown in Table 1.10.

Plain radiography is widely available but the value of additional techniques should be understood (Table 1.11). Even simple manoeuvres such as introducing a gutta percha point or probe into a sinus to trace its origins may provide critical infor-

Table 1.11 Requirements for useful radiographic information

- Always take bitewings when dental pain is suspected. Small carious lesions may be missed in periapical films and poorly localised pain may originate in the opposing arch
- When imaging bony swellings always take two views at right angles
- Panoramic tomograms cannot provide high definition of bony lesions. Only a cross-section of the lesion is in the focal trough and if the bone is greatly expanded only a small portion will be in focus. For more information, oblique lateral views of the mandible or oblique occlusal films should be taken
- Radiography of soft tissues is occasionally useful, for instance to detect a foreign body or calcification in lymph nodes

mation. It is also advisable to request a formal radiologist's report on radiographic films, whenever the radiographic features appear unusual or beyond the experience of the clinician.

Histopathology

Value and limitations

Removal of a biopsy specimen for histopathological examination is the mainstay of diagnosis for diseases of the mucosa, soft tissues and bone. In the few conditions in which a biopsy is not helpful, it may still be valuable to exclude other possible causes (Table 1.12).

As with all other investigations, biopsy must address a specific question. For instance recurrent aphthae lack specific microscopic features and biopsy is rarely justified. Conversely a major aphtha may mimic a carcinoma which only microscopy will exclude.

Biopsy

Biopsy is the removal and examination of a part or the whole of a lesion. There are several types of biopsy technique (Table 1.13).

The most important technique is surgical biopsy. The only important contraindication is incisional biopsy of parotid gland

Table 1.12 Possible reasons for failures in histological diagnosis

- Specimen poorly fixed or damaged during removal (Figs 1.4 and 1.5)
- Specimen is unrepresentative of the lesion or too small
- Plane of histological section does not include critical features
- The condition does not have diagnostic histological features, e.g. aphthous ulcers
- The histological features have several possible causes, e.g. granulomas (Chs 28 and 29)
- The histological features are difficult to interpret, e.g. malignant tumours may be so poorly differentiated that their type cannot be determined
- Inflammation may mask the correct diagnosis

Table 1.13 Types of biopsy

- Surgical biopsy (incisional or excisional)
  Fixed specimen for paraffin blocks
  Frozen sections
- Fine needle aspiration biopsy
- Thick needle/core biopsy

Table 1.14 Essential biopsy principles

- Choose most suspicious area, e.g. red area when premalignancy is suspected
- Avoid sloughs or necrotic areas
- Give regional or local anaesthetic — *not* into the lesion
- Include normal tissue margin
- Specimen should preferably be at least 1 × 0.6 cm by 2 mm deep
- Specimen edges should be vertical not bevelled
- Pass a suture through the specimen to control it and prevent it being swallowed or aspirated by the suction
- For large lesions, several areas may need to be sampled
- Include every fragment for histological examination
- Label specimen bottle with patient's name and clinical details
- Suture and control any bleeding
- Warn patient of possible soreness afterwards. Give an analgesic
- Check the findings are consistent with the clinical diagnosis and investigations
- Discuss with pathologist or repeat biopsy if diagnosis is unclear or not understood

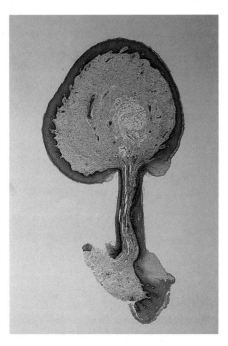

Fig. 1.4 An artefactual polyp produced by grasping normal mucosa with forceps to steady it during biopsy.

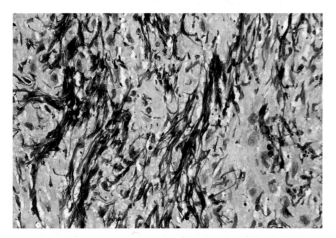

Fig. 1.5 Stringy artefact. This appearance is due to breakage of cells and their nuclei when the specimen is stretched or crushed. It is particularly common in lymphoma and some types of carcinoma.

tumours. The most common type (pleomorphic adenoma) has an unusual tendency to seed its cells and recur in the incision wound. Such tumours should therefore be examined microscopically only *after* excision with a margin of surrounding normal tissue.

Surgical biopsy

Incisional biopsy (removal of part of a lesion) is used to determine the diagnosis before treatment. Excisional biopsy (removal of the whole lesion such as a mucocele) is used to confirm a clinical diagnosis. It is a simple procedure but certain precautions must be observed (Table 1.14).

Occasionally general anaesthesia is required for children or problem patients. For those that gag a short-acting benzodiazepine is usually effective. The request form should contain all the clinical information used to reach the clinical diagnosis. The purpose is to ensure an accurate diagnosis — not (as some clinicians seem to think) to see if the pathologist can guess it without the relevant information. If appropriate, give the vitality of teeth associated with the lesion.

Frozen sections (Table 1.15)

Frozen section technique allows a stained slide to be examined within 10 minutes of taking the specimen. The tissue is sent fresh to the laboratory to be quickly frozen, preferably to about −70°C by, for example, immersion in liquid nitrogen or dry ice. A section is then cut on a refrigerated microtome and stained.

Table 1.15   Advantages and limitations of frozen sections

- Can establish, at operation, whether or not a tumour is malignant and whether excision needs to be extended
- Can confirm, at operation, that excision margins are free of tumour
- Appearances differ from those in fixed material
- Freezing artefacts due to poor technique can distort the cellular picture
- Definitive diagnosis sometimes impossible

The theatre suite often includes equipment for frozen sections to speed the process even further.

Frozen sections can only be justified if the rapidity of the result will make an immediate difference to the operation in progress. If a rapid diagnosis is required in other circumstances other techniques such as fine needle aspiration biopsy may be used.

Fine needle (FNA) aspiration biopsy (Table 1.16)

Even if not completely conclusive, the information from fine needle aspiration (FNA) is often sufficient to distinguish benign from malignant neoplasms, to initiate treatment, or to indicate a need for further investigations.

Table 1.16   Principles and uses of fine needle aspiration biopsy

- A 21 gauge needle is inserted into the lesion and cells aspirated and smeared on a slide
- Rapid and usually effective aid to diagnosis of swellings in lymph nodes and parotid tumours especially
- Cells can be fixed, stained and examined within minutes
- Valuable when surgical biopsy could spread tumour cells (e.g. pleomorphic adenomas)
- For deep lesions ultrasound or radiological guidance may be used to ensure that the needle enters the lesion
- No significant complications
- Small size of the needle avoids damage to vital structures in the head and neck
- Disadvantages
  Experience required for interpretation
  Small specimen may be unrepresentative
  Definitive diagnosis not always possible

Needle/core biopsy (Table 1.17)

Table 1.17   Advantages and limitations of needle/core biopsy

- Needle up to 2 mm diameter used to remove a core of tissue
- Specimen processed as for a surgical biopsy
- Larger sample than FNA, preserves tissue architecture in the specimen
- Definitive diagnosis more likely than with FNA
- Risk of seeding some types of neoplasms into the tissues
- Risk of damaging adjacent anatomical structures
- Useful for inaccessible tumours, e.g. in the pharynx
- Less used in the head and neck now that FNA is more widely available

Table 1.18   Uses and limitations of exfoliative cytology

- Quick, easy
- Local anaesthetic not required
- Special techniques such as immunostaining can be applied
- Most useful for detecting virally-damaged cells, acantholytic cells of pemphigus or candidal hyphae
- Unreliable for diagnosing cancer. Frequent false-positive or false-negative results

Exfoliative cytology

Exfoliative cytology is examination of cells scraped from the surface of a lesion or occasionally of material in aspirates of a cyst (Table 1.18).

Biopsy is always more reliable and can be so readily carried out in the mouth that it is mandatory when cancer or premalignancy is suspected. Exfoliative cytology samples only surface cells and provides no information on deeper tissues.

Brush biopsy

This technique uses a round stiff bristle brush to collect cells from the surface and subsurface layers of a lesion by vigorous abrasion and is discussed more fully in Chapter 17.

Laboratory procedures

Although a clinician does not need to understand the details of laboratory procedures it is necessary to understand the principles to enable the optimal results to be obtained.

Fixation

In the absence of proper fixative it is better to delay the biopsy and obtain the correct solution. Specimens placed in alcohols, saline or other materials commonly available in dental surgeries are frequently useless for diagnosis (Table 1.19).

Special types of fixative are required for electron microscopy and for urgent specimens. Whenever microbiological culture is

Table 1.19   Essential points about specimen fixation

- Fixation is necessary to prevent autolysis and destruction of microscopic features of the specimen
- The usual, routine fixative is 10% formal saline (formaldehyde solution in normal saline or a neutral pH buffer)
- Fixation must be complete before the specimen can be processed
- Fixative must diffuse into the specimen — a slow process
- Small surgical specimens fix overnight but large specimens take 24 hours or longer
- The centre of large specimens can autolyse before being fixed but the pathologist can incise them to allow fixative to penetrate
- Chemical reaction with the tissue causes the fixative to become weaker as fixation proceeds. Therefore specimens should generally be put in at least ten times their own volume of fixative

required the specimen should be sent fresh to the laboratory or a separate specimen taken because fixation will kill any microorganisms.

Tissue processing

The fixed tissue is dehydrated by immersion in a series of solvents, and impregnated with paraffin wax. The wax block is mounted on a microtome and sections, usually 4 μm thick, are cut and mounted on glass microscope slides for staining. It takes 24–48 hours to fix, process, section and stain a specimen before the pathologist can report on it.

Some common stains used for microscopy

The combination of haematoxylin and eosin (H & E) is the most common routine histological stain. Haematoxylin is a blue-black basic dye, eosin is a red acid dye. Their typical staining patterns are shown in Table 1.20.

Table 1.20 Examples of haematoxylin and eosin staining of various tissues

Eosin (acidic)	Haematoxylin (basic)
Cytoplasm of most cells*	Nuclei (DNA and RNA)
Keratin	Mucopolysaccharide-rich ground substance
Muscle cytoplasm	
Bone (decalcified only)	Reversal lines in decalcified bone
Collagen	

*The cytoplasm of some cells (as in some salivary gland tumours) is intensely eosinophilic. In others such as plasma cells it is basophilic or intermediate (amphophilic).

Periodic acid–Schiff (PAS) stain is probably the second most frequently used stain. It stains carbohydrates and mucinous substances pink. This is useful to identify salivary and other mucins, glycogen and candidal hyphae in sections. Silver staining is also useful for identifying fungi in sections but gram-staining is quicker and more useful for smears.

Silver stains also stain reticulin fibres black.

Decalcified and ground (undecalcified) sections

Specimens containing bone and teeth need to be softened by decalcifying in acid to enable a thin section to be cut. This delays the diagnosis by days or weeks according to the size of the specimen.

Decalcification must be avoided if examination of dental enamel is required, for instance to aid diagnosis of amelogenesis imperfecta, because the heavily mineralised enamel is almost completely dissolved. In such cases a ground section is prepared by sawing and grinding using special saws and abrasives.

Table 1.21 Important uses of immunostaining techniques

Disease	Molecule detected	Significance
Pemphigus	Autoantibody bound to the epithelial prickle cells	Indicates pemphigus
Pemphigoid	Autoantibody and/or complement C3 bound to the basement membrane	Indicates pemphigoid
Suspected lymphoma	Kappa and lambda light chains of immunoglobulin expressed by B lymphocytes or plasma cells	Normal inflammatory infiltrates contain B lymphocytes secreting antibody with both kappa and lambda light chain. If all cells in an infiltrate express only one type of light chain the infiltrate is monoclonal and therefore neoplastic
Lymphoma	Cell surface markers specific for T or B lymphocytes	Indicate whether a lymphoma is of B or T cell origin
Undifferentiated malignant neoplasms	Intermediate filaments (components of the cytoskeleton), including keratins (in epithelial cells), vimentin (in mesenchymal tissues), or desmin (in muscle)	Indicate the type of tumour in an undifferentiated malignancy

Immunofluorescent and immunohistochemical staining

Immunostaining methods make use of the highly specific binding between antibodies and antigens to stain specific molecules within the tissues. Fresh (unfixed) tissue is sometimes required.

Immunostaining has revolutionised histological diagnosis and has made some more complex techniques such as electron microscopy almost redundant. It is time-consuming and must be meticulously carried out with adequate controls to avoid both false-positive and false-negative results.

The main circumstances where diagnosis depends on immunostaining are shown in Table 1.21.

Antibodies, often monoclonal, can be purchased. They react with the target molecule and the combination is labelled, either by being coupled to a fluorescein or an enzyme such as peroxidase. The antibody is incubated on the section where it binds specifically to the target molecule. Surplus reagent is washed off and any binding (a positive reaction) is visible by its fluorescence in an ultraviolet light microscope or by reacting the enzyme with synthetic substrate to produce a coloured product (Figs 1.6–1.8).

Molecular biological tests

Molecular biological diagnostic tests have revolutionised diagnosis, particularly in screening for and identification of genetic abnormalities and rapid identification of bacteria and viruses. Some malignant neoplasms have characteristic genetic

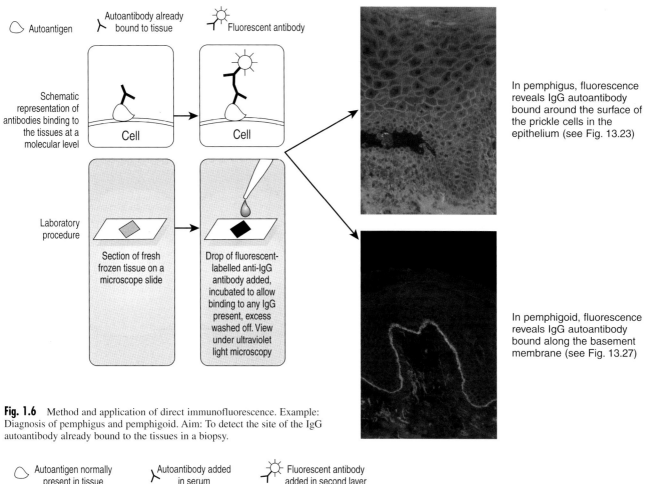

Autoantigen · Autoantibody already bound to tissue · Fluorescent antibody

Schematic representation of antibodies binding to the tissues at a molecular level

Laboratory procedure

Section of fresh frozen tissue on a microscope slide

Drop of fluorescent-labelled anti-IgG antibody added, incubated to allow binding to any IgG present, excess washed off. View under ultraviolet light microscopy

In pemphigus, fluorescence reveals IgG autoantibody bound around the surface of the prickle cells in the epithelium (see Fig. 13.23)

In pemphigoid, fluorescence reveals IgG autoantibody bound along the basement membrane (see Fig. 13.27)

Fig. 1.6 Method and application of direct immunofluorescence. Example: Diagnosis of pemphigus and pemphigoid. Aim: To detect the site of the IgG autoantibody already bound to the tissues in a biopsy.

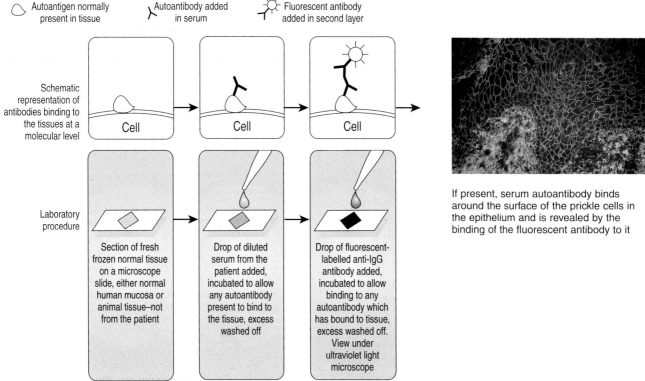

Autoantigen normally present in tissue · Autoantibody added in serum · Fluorescent antibody added in second layer

Schematic representation of antibodies binding to the tissues at a molecular level

Laboratory procedure

Section of fresh frozen normal tissue on a microscope slide, either normal human mucosa or animal tissue–not from the patient

Drop of diluted serum from the patient added, incubated to allow any autoantibody present to bind to the tissue, excess washed off

Drop of fluorescent-labelled anti-IgG antibody added, incubated to allow binding to any autoantibody which has bound to tissue, excess washed off. View under ultraviolet light microscope

If present, serum autoantibody binds around the surface of the prickle cells in the epithelium and is revealed by the binding of the fluorescent antibody to it

Fig. 1.7 Method and application of indirect immunofluorescence. Example: Control of treatment for pemphigus. Aim: To detect circulating autoantibody in the serum of patients with pemphigus.

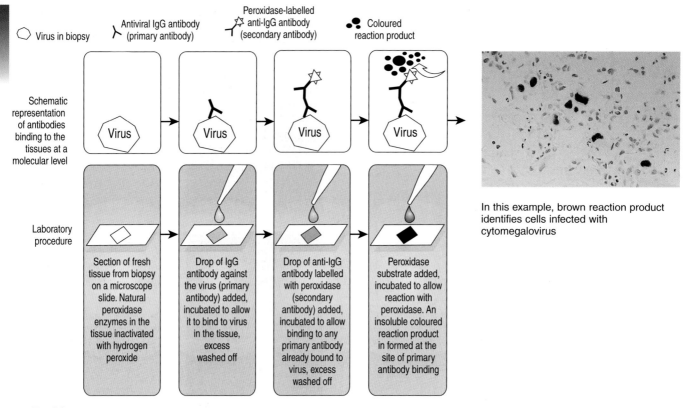

In this example, brown reaction product identifies cells infected with cytomegalovirus

Fig. 1.8 Method and application of immunocytochemistry. Example: Diagnosis of viral infection. Aim: To detect viral antigens in infected cells.

abnormalities, mostly chromosomal translocations, which can be detected by cytogenetics, polymerase chain reaction (PCR) or fluorescent in situ hybridisation. Molecular techniques are also the method of choice for the diagnosis of some lymphomas which cannot be accurately categorised by routine histological methods.

Identification of many bacteria and viruses is now often undertaken using PCR. In this test the clinical sample is solubilised and the nucleic acids hybridised with complementary probes which are specific for known pathogens. If the pathogen is present in the sample, PCR will copy the nucleic acid repeatedly until enough is synthesised to be seen in an electrophoresis gel (Fig. 1.9). If no pathogen is present no nucleic acid is synthesised. Identification of mycobacteria is a good example of the value of this type of test. Previously, identification of mycobacterial infection required approximately 6 weeks to culture the sample. PCR can be performed in 48 hours, is more sensitive and differentiates different types of mycobacteria with a high degree of precision. This test is therefore ideal for investigation of enlarged lymph nodes in the neck. A more recent application of PCR to detect micrometastases of tumours is potentially also of enormous value.

Such methods have yet to become widespread in dentistry, even in hospital specialities. However, when confronted with a difficult diagnosis it is sensible to discuss the case with the pathologist or microbiologist before biopsy, to ensure that appropriate samples are available for these specialised tests.

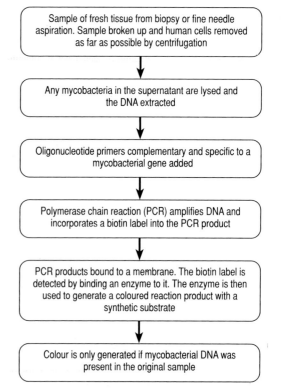

Fig. 1.9 Example application for the technique of polymerase chain reaction for identification of mycobacterial infection.

Haematology, clinical chemistry and serology

Blood investigations are clearly essential for the diagnosis of diseases such as leukaemias, myelomas, or leukopenias which have oral manifestations, or for defects of haemostasis which can greatly affect management. Blood investigations are also helpful in the diagnosis of other conditions such as some infections, and sore tongues or recurrent aphthae which are sometimes associated with anaemia.

Table 1.22 Types of blood test useful in oral diagnosis (see also Appendix 1.1)

Test	Main uses
'Full blood picture' usually includes erythrocyte number, size and haemoglobin indices and differential white cell count	Anaemia and the effects of sideropaenia and vitamin B_{12} deficiency associated with several common oral disorders. Leukaemias
Blood film	Leukaemias, infectious mononucleosis, anaemias
Erythrocyte sedimentation rate	Raised in systemic inflammatory and autoimmune disorders. Particularly important in giant cell arteritis and Wegener's granulomatosis
Serum iron and total iron binding capacity	Iron deficiency associated with several common oral disorders
Serum ferritin	A more sensitive indicator of body stores of iron than serum iron and total iron binding capacity but not available in all laboratories
Red cell folate level	Folic acid deficiency is sometimes associated with recurrent aphthous ulceration and recurrent candidosis
Vitamin B_{12} level	Vitamin B_{12} deficiency is sometimes associated with recurrent aphthous ulceration and recurrent candidosis
Autoantibodies (e.g. rheumatoid factor, antinuclear factor, DNA binding antibodies, SS-A, SS-B)	Raised in autoimmune diseases. Specific autoantibody levels suggest certain diseases
Viral antibody titres (e.g. herpes simplex, varicella zoster, mumps virus)	A rising titre of specific antibody indicates active infection by the virus
Paul–Bunnell or monospot test	Infectious mononucleosis
Syphilis serology	Syphilis
Complement tests	Occasionally useful in diagnosis of SLE or familial angio-oedema.
Serum angiotensin converting enzyme	Sarcoidosis
Serum calcium, phosphate, and parathormone levels	Paget's disease and hyperparathyroidism
HIV test	HIV infection (testing only possible under particular circumstances)
Skeletal serum alkaline phosphatase	Raised in conditions with increased bone turnover, e.g. Paget's disease and hyperparathyroidism. Lowered in hypophosphatasia

There are many different types of haematological examinations but despite the frequent use of the term 'routine blood test', no test should ever be requested as a routine, only to answer a specific question (Table 1.22). The request form should always be completed with sufficient clinical detail to allow the haematologist or clinical chemist to check that the appropriate tests have been ordered and to allow the interpretation of the results. It is important to include details of any drug treatment on blood test request forms. Always put the blood into the appropriate tube because some anticoagulants are incompatible with certain tests. A haematologist will not be impressed with a request for assessment of clotting function on a specimen of coagulated blood.

Microbiology

Despite the fact that the most common oral diseases are infective, microbiology is surprisingly rarely of practical diagnostic value in dentistry (Table 1.23). Direct Gram-stained smears will quickly confirm the diagnosis of thrush or acute ulcerative gingivitis, and H & E-stained smears can show the distorted, virally infected epithelial cells in herpetic infections more easily than microbiological tests for the organisms themselves.

A key microbiological investigation is culture and sensitivity of pus organisms. Whenever pus is obtained from a soft tissue or bone infection it should be sent for culture and determination of antibiotic sensitivity of the causative microbes. Those of osteomyelitis, cellulitis, acute parotitis, systemic mycoses (frequently mistaken for tumours), or other severe infections need to be identified if appropriate antimicrobial treatment is to be given. However, such treatment has usually to be started empirically without this information but the sensitivity test may dictate a change.

Table 1.23 Microbiological tests useful in oral diagnosis

Test	Main uses
Culture and antibiotic sensitivity	Detect unusual pathogens, e.g. actinomycosis in soft tissue infection. Antibiotic sensitivity for all infections, particularly osteomyelitis and acute facial soft tissue infection.
Smear for candida	Candidosis
Viral culture or antigen screen	Viral culture identifies many viruses but requires considerable time. Screening for viral antigen is faster but of more limited diagnostic value

Viral identification is rarely required for oral diseases as many oral viral infections are clinically typical and indicate the causative virus. A smear alone may show the nuclear changes of herpetic infection in epithelial cells from the margins of mucosal ulcers. A more sensitive and almost as rapid result may be obtained by sending a swab for virus detection using ELISA (enzyme-linked immunosorbent assay).

CHAPTER 1

> **Practical point** Always take a sample of pus for culture and antibiotic sensitivity from bone and soft tissue infections before giving an antibiotic

> **Practical point** Always take the temperature of any patient with a swollen face, enlarged lymph nodes, malaise or other symptom or sign which might indicate infection

Other clinical tests

Several simple clinical tests may be valuable in diagnosis of oral disease. Urine tests are valuable for the diagnosis of diabetes (suggested by repeated candidal or periodontal infection), auto-immune conditions which damage the kidneys, for instance Wegener's granulomatosis, and for the detection of Bence-Jones protein in myeloma.

Taking the patient's temperature is an easily forgotten investigation. The temperature should be noted whenever bone or soft tissue infections are suspected. It helps distinguish facial inflammatory oedema from cellulitis and indicates systemic effects of infections and the need for more aggressive therapy.

Interpreting special investigations and making a diagnosis and treatment plan

The history, examination and results of special investigations should provide the material for a diagnosis and treatment plan. Check that the results of each investigation are compatible with the preliminary diagnosis and do not indicate any need to avoid a particular treatment.

If a result appears at odds with other information take into account the normal variation, perhaps with age or diurnal variation, and consider the possibility of false-positive and false-negative results. A common cause of unusual blood test results is a delay in taking blood samples to the laboratory.

Further advice and specialised tests may be appropriate. General medical, ear, nose and throat, neurological and psychiatric referral are among the specialities to whom patients may be referred. In referrals, it is important to state whether the dentist is requesting the medical specialist to exclude a condition and refer the patient back, or to take over investigation. If the latter, it is essential that dental causes have been completely eliminated as the cause of the problem.

> **Practical point** Good clinical record keeping is essential for good patient management as well as for medicolegal reasons

Finally, ensure that the patient's notes include a complete record of the consultation and investigation results. This must be correctly dated, legible, limited to relevant facts and include a clear complaint history, list of clinical findings, test results and plan of treatment organised in a suitable form for quick reappraisal. It must be signed by the clinician and in addition, the name should be printed below if the signature is anything less than perfectly legible. It should be possible for another person to continue to investigate or treat the patient without difficulty on the basis of the clinical record.

Photograhy or computerised video imaging is a very valuable adjunct to the clinical record. Pictures are especially useful in monitoring lesions which may vary in the course of a long follow-up, for instance white patches. It is useful to include teeth or a scale in the frame to allow accurate assessment of small changes in size. Photographs may also be helpful in explaining to patients about their condition and to show the effects of treatment.

SUGGESTED FURTHER READING

Arends M J, Bird C C 1992 Recombinant DNA technology and its diagnostic applications. Histopathology 21:303–313

Ghossein R A, Rosai J 1996 Polymerase chain reaction in the detection of micrometastases and circulating tumor cells. Cancer 78:10–16

Heatley M K 1996 Cytokeratins and cytokeratin staining in diagnostic histopathology. Histopathology 28:479–483

Kabala J, Goddard P, Cook P 1992 Magnetic resonance imaging of extracranial head and neck tumours. Br J Radiol 65:375–383

Komoroski R A, Pappas A, Hough A 1992 Nuclear magnetic resonance imaging in pathology. I. Principles and general aspects. Hum Pathol 22:1077–1084

Layton S, Korsen J 1994 Informed consent in oral and maxillofacial surgery: a study of the value of written warnings. Br J Oral Maxillofac Surg 32:34–36

Minden N J, Fast T B 1994 Evaluation of health history forms used in U.S. dental schools. Oral Surg Oral Med Oral Pathol 77:105–109

Nathan A W, Havard C W H 1979 The face in diagnosis. Br J Hosp Med 21:104–111

O'Connor N 1995 Laboratory diagnosis in haematology. Medicine UK 23:489–494

Stanley M W 1995 False-positive diagnoses in exfoliative cytology (editorial). Am J Clin Pathol 104:117–119

Thibodeau E A, Rossomondo K J 1992 Survey of the medical history questionnaire. Oral Surg Oral Med Oral Pathol 74:400–403

Whaites E 1996 Essentials of dental radiography and radiology. 2nd edn. Churchill Livingstone, Edinburgh

Normal haematological values

Red cells

Haemoglobin	Males 13–17 g/dl. Females 11.5–16 g/dl (adults)
Haematocrit (packed cell volume – PCV)	Males 40–50 l/l. Females 34–47 l/l
Mean corpuscular volume (MCV)	78–98 fl
Mean corpuscular haemoglobin concentration (MCHC)	30–35 g/dl
Red cell count	Males $4–6 \times 10^{12}$ l. Females $4–5 \times 10^{12}$ l
Erythrocyte sedimentation rate (ESR)	0–15 mm/h

White cells

Total count	$4–10 \times 10^9$/l
Neutrophils	$2–7.5 \times 10^9$/l
Lymphocytes	$1–3 \times 10^9$/l
Monocytes	$0.15–0.8 \times 10^9$/l
Eosinophils	$0.05–0.4 \times 10^9$/l
Platelets	$150–400 \times 10^9$/l

Note. These are average values and may vary slightly between laboratories. Also, approximtely 5% of normal persons have values outside the figures quoted above.

HARD-TISSUE PATHOLOGY

Disorders of development of the teeth and related tissues

Development of an ideal dentition depends on many factors (Table 2.1).

Table 2.1 Requirements for development of an ideal dentition
● Formation of a full complement of teeth ● Normal structural development of the dental tissues ● Eruption of each group of teeth at the appropriate time into an adequate space ● Eruption of teeth into correct relationship to occlude with their opposite numbers

Significant structural defects of teeth are uncommon but disorders of occlusion due to irregularities of the teeth in the arch or abnormal relationship of the arches to each other are so common that their treatment has become a specialty in its own right. The main groups of disorders affecting development of the dentition are summarised in Table 2.2.

Table 2.2 Disorders of development of the teeth

● Abnormalities in number
  Anodontia or hypodontia
  Additional teeth (hyperdontia)
● Disorders of eruption
● Defects of structure
  Enamel defects
  Dentine defects
● Developmental anomalies of several dental tissues
  Odontomas

ABNORMALITIES IN THE NUMBER OF TEETH

Isolated hypodontia or anodontia

Failure of development of one or two teeth is relatively common and often hereditary. The teeth most frequently missing are third molars, second premolars, or maxillary second incisors (Fig. 2.1). Absence of third molars can be a disadvantage if first or second molars, or both, have been lost. The absence of lower premolars worsens malocclusion if there is already disparity between an underdeveloped mandible and a normal upper

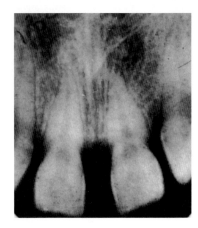

Fig. 2.1 Congenital absence of lateral incisors with spacing of the anterior teeth.

arch. Otherwise absence of these teeth may have little or no noticeable effect.

Absence of lateral incisors can sometimes be conspicuous because the large, pointed canines erupt in the front of the mouth beside the central incisors. It is usually impossible to prevent the canine from erupting into this empty space, even if the patient is seen early. It is also very difficult to make room between the centrals and canines by orthodontic means to replace the laterals. An attempt has often therefore to be made to disguise the shape of the canines.

Total failure of development of a complete dentition (anodontia) is exceedingly rare. If the permanent dentition fails to form, the deciduous dentition is retained for many years, but when these deciduous teeth become excessively worn or too much damaged by caries then they must be replaced by dentures or implants.

Hypodontia or anodontia with systemic defects
Anhidrotic (hereditary) ectodermal dysplasia

The main features are summarised in Table 2.3. In severe cases no teeth form. More often, most of the deciduous teeth form but there are few or no permanent teeth. The teeth are usually peg-shaped or conical (Fig. 2.2).

Table 2.3 Major features of anhidrotic ectodermal dyplasia

- Usually a sex-linked recessive trait
- Hypodontia
- Hypotrichosis (scanty hair)
- Anhidrosis (inability to sweat)

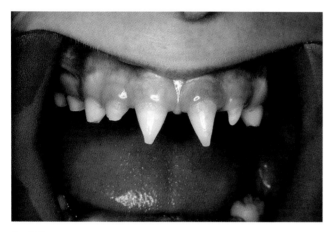

Fig. 2.2 Anhidrotic ectodermal dysplasia showing conical teeth, giving an undesirable, Dracula-like appearance.

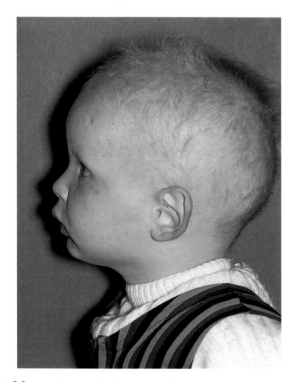

Fig. 2.3 Another case showing typical fine and scanty hair and loss of support for the facial soft tissues.

When there is anodontia, the alveolar process, without teeth to support, fails to develop and has too little bone to support implants. The profile then resembles that of an elderly person because of the gross loss of vertical dimension. The hair is fine and sparse (Fig. 2.3), particularly in the tonsural region. The

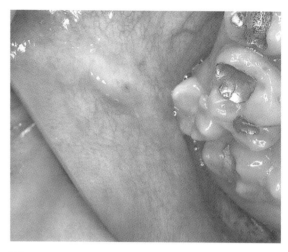

Fig. 2.4 A paramolar, a buccally placed supernumerary molar tooth.

skin is smooth, shiny and dry due to absence of sweat glands. Heat is therefore poorly tolerated. The finger nails are usually also defective. All that can be done to improve the patient's appearance and mastication is to fit dentures, which are usually well tolerated by children.

Other conditions associated with hypodontia

There are many rare syndromes where hypodontia is a feature, but the only common one is Down's syndrome (Ch. 33). One or more third molars are absent in over 90% of these patients, while absence of individual teeth scattered about the arch is also common. Anodontia is rare. Palatal clefts may be associated.

Additional teeth: hyperdontia

Additional teeth are relatively common. They are usually of simple conical shape (*supernumerary teeth*) but less frequently resemble teeth of the normal series (*supplemental teeth*). These are the results of excessive but organised growth of the dental lamina of unknown cause.

Supernumerary teeth. Conical or more seriously malformed additional teeth most frequently form in the incisor or molar region (Fig. 2.4) and very occasionally, in the midline (mesiodens).

Supplemental teeth. Occasionally an additional maxillary incisor (Fig. 2.5), premolar or, rarely, a fourth molar develops.

Effects and treatment

Additional teeth usually erupt in abnormal positions, labial or buccal to the arch, creating stagnation areas and increasing susceptibility to caries. Alternatively, a supernumerary tooth may prevent a normal tooth from erupting. These additional teeth should usually be extracted.

19

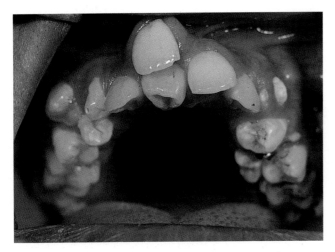

Fig. 2.5 Maleruption of a midline tuberculate supernumerary and two supplemental premolars.

Syndromes associated with hyperdontia

These syndromes are all rare but probably the best known is cleidocranial dysplasia (Ch. 10) where many additional teeth develop but fail to erupt.

DISORDERS OF ERUPTION

Eighteenth century parish registers are replete with the names of infants who had died as a result of teething. Nevertheless the idea that teething, the normal eruption of infants' teeth, can cause systemic symptoms or serious illness is of course a myth. The time of teething coincides with a period of naturally low resistance to infection and declining maternal passive immunity so that infection during the period of teething is merely coincidental. As might be expected, several studies have shown that teething does not cause systemic disorders. Nevertheless, so resistant is this traditional belief to rational explanation, that yet another study was carried out in 2000, confirming yet again that teething was harmless.

However, an ingenious neuropathologist has suggested that the minute wounds left by the shedding of deciduous teeth could provide a means of entry for the BSE ('mad cow disease') prion to cause variant CJD. In view of an incubation period of many years, this suggestion is consistent with the onset of the disease in adolescence. However, this theory is as yet unproven.

Eruption of deciduous teeth starts at about 6 months, usually with the appearance of the lower incisors, and is complete by about 2 years. Mass failure of eruption is very rare. More often eruption of a single tooth is prevented by local obstruction. In the permanent dentition, delay in eruption of a tooth or, more frequently, too early loss of a deciduous predecessor tends to cause irregularities because movement of adjacent teeth closes the available space.

Delayed eruption associated with skeletal disorders

Metabolic diseases particularly *cretinism* and *rickets* are now uncommon causes of delayed eruption of teeth. *Cleidocranial dysplasia*, in which there are typically many additional teeth but failure of most of them to erupt, has been mentioned earlier. In severe *hereditary gingival fibromatosis*, eruption may apparently fail merely because the teeth are buried in the excessive fibrous gingival tissue and only their tips show in the mouth (*pseudoanodontia*). In *cherubism* (Ch. 10) several teeth may be displaced by the proliferating connective tissue masses containing giant cells and are prevented from erupting.

Local factors affecting eruption of deciduous teeth

Having no predecessors, deciduous teeth usually erupt unobstructed. Occasionally an eruption cyst may overlie a tooth but is unlikely to block eruption.

Local factors affecting eruption of permanent teeth

A permanent tooth may be prevented from erupting or misplaced by various causes (Table 2.4).

Table 2.4 Local causes of failure of eruption of permanent teeth

- Loss of space
- Abnormal position of the crypt
- Overcrowding
- Supernumerary and supplemental teeth
- Displacement in a dentigerous cyst
- Rentention of a deciduous predecessor

Treatment depends on the circumstances, but room may be made for the unerupted tooth by orthodontic means or extractions. A retained deciduous tooth should be extracted if radiographs show a normal permanent successor. If a buried tooth partially erupts and becomes infected, it may have to be removed — mandibular third molars are the main source of this complication.

Changes affecting buried teeth

Teeth may occasionally remain buried in the jaws for many years without complications. The roots of these teeth may undergo varying degrees of hypercementosis or resorption. Alternatively the teeth may become enveloped in dentigerous cysts, as in cleidocranial dysplasia for example.

DEFECTS OF STRUCTURE: HYPOPLASIA AND HYPOCALCIFICATION

Minor structural defects of the teeth, such as pitting or discolouration, or, occasionally, more serious defects may be markers of past disease, but only rarely is the disease still active. Hypoplasia of the teeth is not an important contributory cause of dental caries; indeed, hypoplasia due to fluorosis is associated with enhanced resistance. The main clinical requirement is usually cosmetic improvement.

Defects of deciduous teeth

Calcification of deciduous teeth begins about the fourth month of intrauterine life. Disturbances of metabolism or infections that effect the fetus at this early stage without causing abortion are rare. Defective structure of the deciduous teeth is therefore uncommon, but in a few places such as parts of India, where the fluoride content of the water is excessively high, the deciduous teeth may be mottled.

The deciduous teeth may be discoloured by abnormal pigments circulating in the blood. Severe neonatal jaundice may cause the teeth to become yellow, or there may be bands of greenish discolouration. In congenital porphyria, a rare disorder of haemoglobin metabolism, the teeth are red or purple. Tetracycline given during dental development is the main cause of permanent discolouration.

Defects of permanent teeth

Single permanent teeth may be malformed as a result of local causes such as periapical infection of a predecessor (Turner teeth — Fig. 2.6) or damage by intubation, for instance (Fig. 2.7) or multiple teeth by systemic diseases as summarised in Table 2.5.

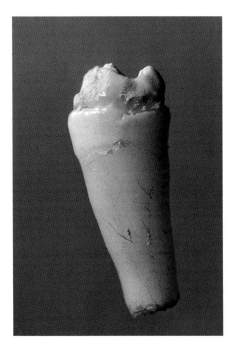

Fig. 2.6 Turner tooth, a hypoplastic tooth resulting from periapical infection, usually of the deciduous predecessor.

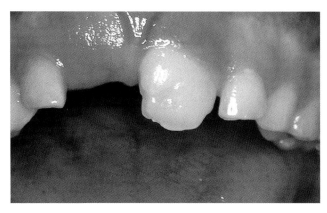

Fig. 2.7 Localised dental disturbance caused by prolonged intubation during tooth development. The upper left central incisor shows enamel pitting incisally and the upper right central incisor is deformed and has failed to erupt.

Table 2.5 Important causes of multiple malformed permanent teeth

- Genetic
    Amelogenesis imperfecta
        Hypoplastic (type 1)
        Hypomaturation (type 2)
        Hypocalcified (type 3)
    Dentinogenesis imperfecta
        Shell teeth
    Dentinal dysplasia
    Regional odontodysplasia
    Multisystem disorders with associated dental defects
- Infective
    Congenital syphilis
- Metabolic
    Childhood infections, rickets, hypoparathyroidism
- Drugs
    Tetracycline pigmentation
    Cytotoxic chemotherapy
- Fluorosis
- Other acquired developmental anomalies
    Fetal alcohol syndrome

Amelogenesis imperfecta

Amelogenesis imperfecta is a group of conditions caused by defects in the genes encoding enamel matrix proteins. Classification is complex and based on pattern of inheritance, enamel hypoplasia, hypomineralisation or hypomaturation and appearance; smooth, rough or pitted. At least 16 forms are recognised.

Inheritance can be autosomal dominant, recessive or X-linked. However, the most common types have an autosomal inheritance and are thought to be caused by mutations in the AMEL X gene, which codes for ameloblastin (C4), enamelin (C4) or tuftelin (C1). In the case of the autosomal dominant type of amelogenesis imperfecta, the locus of the defective gene is on chromosome 4q21 to which enamelin maps.

The less common X-linked types are caused by a variety of defects in the amelogenin genes and, confusingly, it seems the same mutation can sometimes cause hypoplastic, hypomineralisation or hypomaturation forms in different patients.

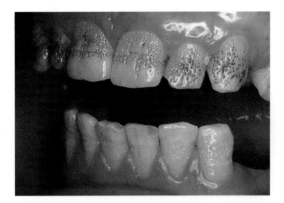

Fig. 2.8 Amelogenesis imperfecta, hypoplastic pitted type.

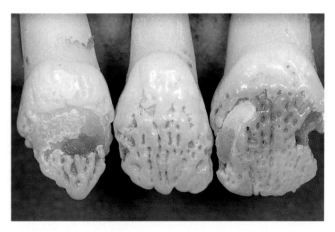

Fig. 2.9 Close-up of X-linked hypoplastic type amelogenesis imperfecta. These teeth from an affected female show the typical vertical ridged pattern of normal and abnormal enamel as a result of Lyonisation.

Genetic factors act throughout the whole duration of amelogenesis. Characteristically therefore, all teeth are affected and defects involve the whole, or are randomly distributed in the enamel. By contrast, exogenous factors affecting enamel formation (with the important exception of fluorosis) tend to act for a relatively brief period and produce defects related to that period of enamel formation.

Hypoplastic amelogenesis imperfecta

The main defect is in formation of the matrix. The enamel is randomly pitted, grooved or very thin, but hard and translucent (Fig. 2.8). The defects tend to become stained, but the teeth are not especially susceptible to caries unless the enamel is scanty and easily damaged.

The main patterns of inheritance are autosomal dominant and recessive, X-linked, and (a genetic rarity) an X-linked dominant type. In the last there is almost complete failure of enamel formation in affected males, while in females the enamel is ridged (Figs 2.9–2.11). Occasionally cases are difficult to classify (Fig. 2.12).

Hypomaturation amelogenesis imperfecta

The enamel is normal in form on eruption but opaque, white to brownish-yellow. The teeth appear similar to mottled fluoride effects (Figs 2.14 and 2.15). However, they are soft and vulnerable to attrition, though not as severely as the hypocalcified type.

There are several variants of hypomaturation defects such as a more severe, autosomal dominant (type 4) of hypomaturation combined with hypoplasia.

Hypocalcified amelogenesis imperfecta

Enamel matrix is formed in normal quantity but poorly calcified. When newly erupted, the enamel is normal in thickness and form, but weak and opaque or chalky in appearance.

The teeth tend to become stained and relatively rapidly worn

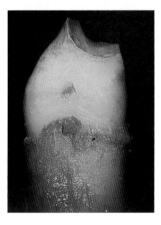

Fig. 2.10 Amelogenesis imperfecta X-linked hypoplastic form in a male. This premolar has a cap of enamel so thin that the shape of the tooth is virtually that of the dentine core.

away. The upper incisors may acquire a shouldered form due to the chipping away of the thin, soft enamel of the incisal edge (Fig. 2.13). There are dominant and recessive patterns of inheritance.

Dentinogenesis (odontogenesis) imperfecta

This uncommon defect of collagen formation is transmitted as an autosomal dominant trait. The gene is closely related to that of osteogenesis imperfecta (Ch. 10) particularly Type IV. Defects in the genes COL1A1 and COL1A2, for the procollagen alpha helix, prevent polymerisation into normal type 1 collagen.

In types III and IV osteogenesis imperfecta, dentinogenesis imperfecta is present in over 80% in the primary dentition. Tooth discolouration and attrition is less severe in the permanent teeth. Class III malocclusion is associated in over 70%. In type III disease, dental development is delayed in 20%, but type IV disease it is accelerated in over 20%. The dentine is soft and has an abnormally high water content.

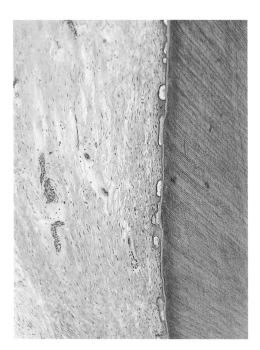

Fig. 2.11 Amelogenesis imperfecta X-linked hypoplastic type in a male showing a thin translucent layer of defective enamel on the dentine surface.

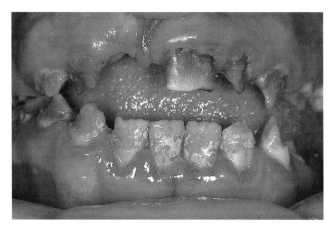

Fig. 2.12 Amelogenesis imperfecta, indeterminate type. Some cases, such as this, are difficult to classify but are clearly inherited, as shown by their long family history.

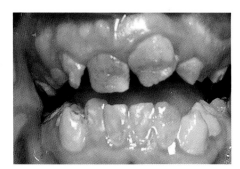

Fig. 2.13 Amelogenesis imperfecta, hypocalcified type. The soft chalky enamel was virtually of normal thickness and form but has chipped away during mastication.

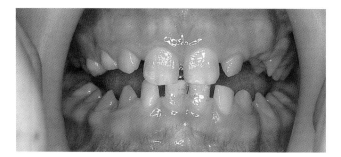

Fig. 2.14 Amelogenesis imperfecta, hypomaturation type. Tooth morphology is normal but there are opaque white and discoloured patches.

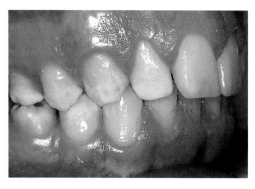

Fig. 2.15 Amelogenesis imperfecta, one of the several hypomaturation types. In this form there are opaque white flecks and patches affecting the occlusal half of the tooth surface.

Clinical features

The enamel appears normal but uniformly brownish or purplish and abnormally translucent (Fig. 2.16). The form of the teeth is essentially normal, but the crowns of the molars tend to be bulbous and the roots are usually short. Enamel is weakly attached and tends to chip away from the dentine abnormally easily. In severe cases the teeth become rapidly worn down to the gingivae (Fig. 2.17). Early fitting of full dentures then becomes inevitable, as the relatively soft dentine and short roots make crowning impractical.

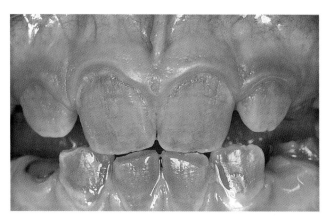

Fig. 2.16 Dentinogenesis imperfecta showing the translucent appearance of the teeth which are of normal morphology.

23

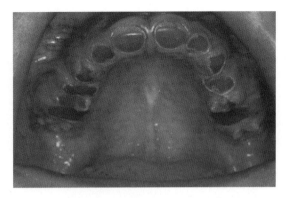

Fig. 2.17 Dentinogenesis imperfecta. In this 14-year-old, the teeth have worn down to gingival level but the pulp chambers have become obliterated as part of the disease process. Some enamel remains around the necks of the posterior teeth.

In some patients only a few teeth are severely affected, while the remainder appear normal. Radiographically the main features are obliterated pulp chambers and stunted roots.

Pathology

The earliest-formed dentine under the amelodentine junction usually appears normal. The deeper tissue is more defective, tubules become few, calcification is incomplete and the matrix is imperfectly formed. The pulp chamber becomes obliterated early and odontoblasts degenerate, but cellular inclusions in the dentine are common (Fig. 2.18). Scalloping of the amelodentinal junction is sometimes absent. The enamel tends to split from the dentine, but is otherwise normal in typical cases.

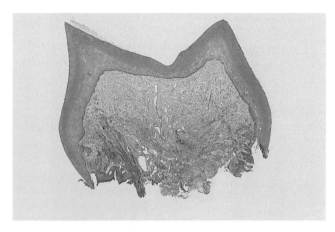

Fig. 2.19 Shell tooth. In this severe form of dentinogenesis imperfecta only a thin mantle of dentine is formed and no root develops.

Shell teeth (dentinogenesis imperfecta type 3)

This rare anomaly is so called because only a thin shell of hard dental tissue surrounds overlarge pulp chambers. Like other types of dentinogenesis imperfecta there is normal, but thin, mantle dentine which covers irregular dentine (Fig. 2.19). The pulp lacks a normal odontoblast layer and consists of coarse connective tissue which becomes incorporated into the deep surface of the dentine.

Dentinal dysplasia ('rootless' teeth)

In dentinal dysplasia, the roots are very short and conical. The pulp chambers are obliterated by multiple nodules of poorly organised dentine containing sheaves of tubules. Inevitably, these teeth tend to be lost early in life (Fig. 2.20).

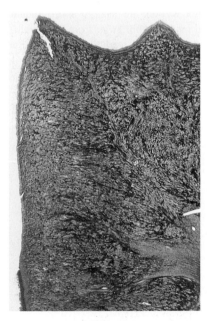

Fig. 2.18 Microscopic appearance of dentinogenesis imperfecta showing the grossly disorganised tubular structure with inclusions of pulp in the dentine and obliteration of the pulp cavity.

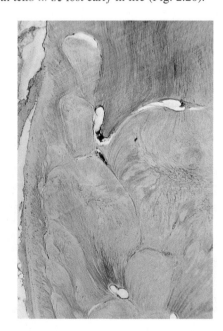

Fig. 2.20 Dentinal dysplasia. The pulp chamber is obliterated by nodules of dentine.

Regional odontodysplasia (ghost teeth)

This is a localised disorder of development affecting a group of teeth in which there are severe abnormalities of enamel, dentine and pulp.

The disorder is not hereditary and the aetiology is unknown. A few cases have been associated with facial vascular naevi or abnormalities such as hydrocephalus. There is no sex or racial predeliction.

Clinically, regional odontodysplasia may be recognisable at the time of eruption of the deciduous teeth (2 to 4 years) or of the permanent teeth (7 to 11 years). The maxillary teeth are most frequently affected. Either or both dentitions, and one or, at most, two quadrants may be affected. The abnormal teeth frequently fail to erupt, but if they do so, show yellowish deformed crowns, often with a rough surface.

Affected teeth have very thin enamel and dentine surrounding a greatly enlarged pulp chamber (Figs 2.21 and 2.22). In radiographs, the teeth appear crumpled and abnormally radiolucent or hazy, due to the paucity of dental hard tissues, to justify the term 'ghost teeth' (Fig. 2.23).

Histologically, the enamel thickness is highly irregular and lacks a well-defined prismatic structure. The dentine, which has a disorganised tubular structure, contains clefts and interglobular dentine mixed with amorphous tissue. The surrounding follicular tissue may contain small calcifications.

If they erupt, the teeth are susceptible to caries and fracture, and their complications. If they can be preserved and restored, crown and root dentine continue to form and the teeth may survive long enough to allow normal development of the alveolar ridge and occlusion. However, extraction is often required, but

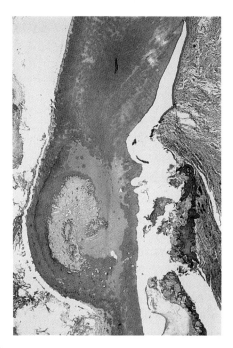

Fig. 2.22 Regional odontodysplasia showing dysplastic dentine with a disorganised tubule structure, an irregular enamel space and mineralised enamel epithelium.

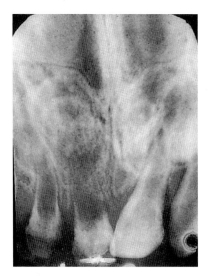

Fig. 2.23 Radiographic appearance of regional odontodysplasia. On one side of the midline the deciduous incisors have poor root formation with thin radicular dentine and enamel. A poorly organised spotty calcification is present at the site of the permanent successors.

this should not be done until it is certain that eruption has completely failed or the defects are too severe to be treatable, to allow for their replacement with a prothesis.

Multisystem disorders affecting the teeth

Ehlers–Danlos (floppy joint) syndromes

This group of collagen disorders is characterised (in varying degree), by hypermobile joints, loose hyperextensible skin,

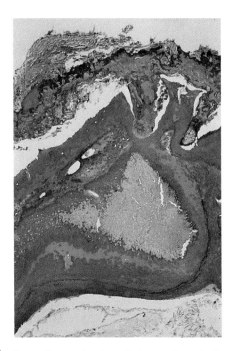

Fig. 2.21 Regional odontodysplasia. Both enamel and dentine are deformed and there is calcification of the reduced enamel epithelium.

CHAPTER
2

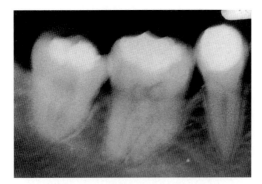

Fig. 2.24 Multiple pulp stones in a case of Ehlers–Danlos syndrome.

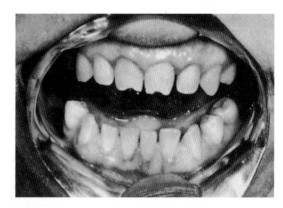

Fig. 2.25 Congenital syphilis; Hutchinson's teeth. The characteristics are the notched incisal edge and the peg shape tapering from neck to tip. (Taken before the advent of colour photography.)

fragile oral mucosa and, in type VIII, early onset periodontitis. There may also be temporomandibular joint symptoms such as recurrent dislocation.

The main dental abnormalities are small teeth with short roots and multiple pulp stones (Fig. 2.24).

Gardner's syndrome (familial adenomatous polyposis)

Gardner's syndrome is characterised by multiple osteomas, especially of the jaws (Ch. 8), colonic polyps and skin tumours. The majority of patients have dental abnormalities. These include impacted teeth other than third molars, supernumerary or missing teeth and abnormal root formation. Both familial adenomatous polyposis and Gardner's syndrome are caused by mutations in the same gene, the APC tumour suppressor gene, but only some patients develop the extra-colonic manifestations such as the dental anomalies.

The colonic polyps have a 100% frequency of malignant change by middle age, and the mortality is high. The dental abnormalities can be detected in childhood or adolescence and recognition of this syndrome may be life-saving by suggesting the need for colectomy.

Epidermolyis bullosa

Epidermolysis bullosa is a blistering disease of skin and mucosae (Ch. 13). Dental abnormalities include fine or coarse pitting defects, or thin and uneven enamel which may also lack prismatic structure. The amelodentinal junction may be smooth. Dental defects vary in the different subtypes of the disease but are most frequent in the autosomal recessive, scarring type of epidermolysis bullosa in which there may be delayed, or failure of, eruption.

Infection

Congenital syphilis

Prenatal syphilis, the result of maternal infection, can cause a characteristic dental deformity, described by Hutchinson in 1858.

If the fetus becomes infected at a very early stage, abortion follows. Infants born with stigmata of congenital syphilis result from later fetal infection, and the permanent teeth are affected. The characteristic defects are usually seen in the upper central incisors.

The incisors (Hutchinson's incisors) are small, barrel-shaped, and taper towards the tip (Fig. 2.25). The incisal edge sometimes shows a crescentic notch or deep fissure which forms before eruption and can be seen radiographically. An anterior open bite is also characteristic. The first molars may be dome-shaped (Moon's molars) or may have a rough pitted occlusal surface with compressed nodules instead of cusps (mulberry molars). These defects are now largely of historical interest.

Pathology

The effects are due to infection of the dental follicle by *Treponema pallidum*. The postulated consequences are chronic inflammation, fibrosis of the tooth sac, compression of the developing tooth and distortion of the ameloblast layer. *T. pallidum* causes proliferation of the odontogenic epithelium which bulges into the dentine papilla causing the characteristic central notch.

Metabolic disturbances

General disturbances of metabolism affecting the development of the teeth may be caused by the childhood fevers or severe infantile gastroenteritis.

Unlike inherited forms of hypoplasia, only a restricted area of enamel is defective, corresponding to the state of development at the time of the metabolic disturbance. Measles with severe secondary bacterial infection was the most common cause of this limited type of dental defect, but such defects have become uncommon because of more effective treatment.

Clinically, the typical effect is one or more rows of horizontally disposed pits or grooves across the crown of the incisors. These are usually in the incisal third, suggesting that

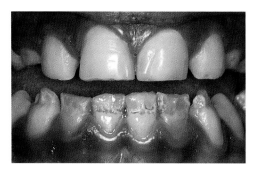

Fig. 2.26 Chronological hypoplasia due to metabolic upset. Unlike the hereditary types of amelogenesis imperfecta, defects are linear and thought to correspond to a short period of amelogenesis disturbed by a concurrent severe illness.

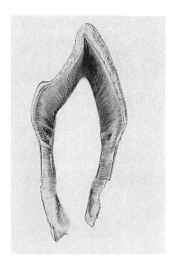

Fig. 2.28 Tooth in hypophosphatasia showing the enlarged pulp chamber and absence of cementum.

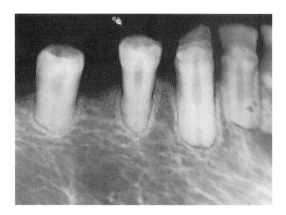

Fig. 2.27 Teeth in childhood hypoparathyroidism with short blunt roots, open apices and large pulp chambers.

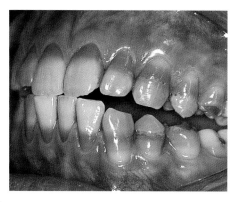

Fig. 2.29 Tetracycline staining. Note the chronological distribution of the dark-brown intrinsic stain.

the disorder had its effect during the first year or two of life, when such infections are most dangerous (Fig. 2.26).

Rickets can cause hypocalcification of the teeth but only if unusually severe (see Ch. 10).

Early onset idiopathic hypoparathyroidism is rare. Ectodermal effects are associated. The teeth may therefore be hypoplastic with ridged enamel, short blunt roots and persistently open apices (Fig. 2.27). The nails may be defective and there may be complete absence of hair. Patients with early onset idiopathic hypoparathyroidism may later develop other endocrine deficiencies (polyendocrinopathy syndrome) but chronic candidosis may be the first sign (Ch. 15).

Hypophosphatasia. This rare genetic disorder can have severe skeletal effects as a result of failure of development of mature bone. There may also be failure of cementum formation causing loosening or early loss of teeth (Fig. 2.28).

Drugs

Tetracycline pigmentation

Tetracycline is taken up by calcifying tissues, and the band of tetracycline-stained bone or tooth substance fluoresces bright yellow under ultraviolet light.

The teeth become stained only when tetracycline is given during their development, and it can cross the placenta to stain the developing teeth of the fetus. More frequently, permanent teeth are stained by tetracycline given during infancy. Tetracycline is deposited along the incremental lines of the dentine and, to lesser extent, of the enamel.

The more prolonged the course of treatment the broader the band of stain and the deeper the discolouration. The teeth are at first bright yellow, but become a dirty brown or grey (Fig. 2.29). The stain is permanent, and when the permanent incisors are affected the ugly appearance can only be disguised. When the history is vague the brownish colour of tetracycline-stained teeth must be distinguished from dentinogenesis imperfecta. In dentinogenesis imperfecta the teeth are obviously more translucent than normal and, in many cases, chipping of the enamel from the dentine can be seen. In tetracycline-induced defects the enamel is not abnormally translucent and is firmly attached to dentine. In very severe cases, intact teeth may fluoresce under ultraviolet light. Otherwise the diagnosis can

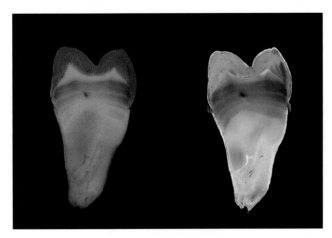

Fig. 2.30 Tetracycline pigmentation. Hard section (left) shows the broad bands of tetracycline deposited along the incremental lines of the dentine; (right) same tooth viewed under ultraviolet light shows fluorescence of the bands of tetracycline.

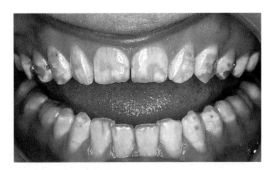

Fig. 2.31 Fluoride mottling. In this case, from an area of endemic fluorosis, there is generalised opaque white mottling with patchy enamel hypoplasia. Note the resemblance to the hypomaturation type of amelogenesis imperfecta.

only be confirmed after a tooth has been extracted. In an undecalcified section the yellow fluorescence of the tetracycline deposited along the incremental lines can be easily seen (Fig. 2.30).

It is no longer necessary to give tetracycline during dental development. There are equally effective alternatives and it should be avoided from approximately the fourth month to 12th year of childhood. Nevertheless tetracycline pigmentation is still seen.

Cytotoxic chemotherapy

Increasing numbers of children are surviving malignant disease, particularly acute leukaemia, as a result of cytotoxic chemotherapy.

Among survivors, teeth developing during treatment may have short roots, hypoplasia of the crowns and enamel defects. Microscopically, incremental lines may be more prominent, corresponding with the period of chemotherapy, but in extreme cases, tooth formation may be aborted.

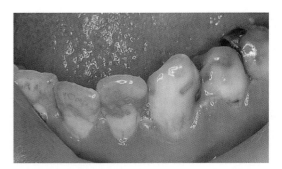

Fig. 2.32 Fluorosis. Moderate effects from an area of endemic fluorosis. Irregular patchy discolouration.

Fluorosis

Mottled enamel is the most frequently seen and most reliable sign of excess fluoride in the drinking water. It has distinctive features (Table 2.6).

Table 2.6 Distinctive features of dental fluorosis

- Mottling is endemic in areas where fluorides in the drinking water exceed about 2 parts per million, i.e. it has a geographical distribution
- Neighbouring communities with fluoride-free water do not suffer from the disorder
- Only those who have lived in a high-fluoride area during dental development show mottling. The defect is not acquired by older visitors to the area
- Permanent teeth are affected; mottling of deciduous teeth is rare
- Mottled teeth are less susceptible to caries than normal teeth from low-fluoride areas
- A typical effect is paper-white enamel opacities
- Brown staining of these patches may be acquired after eruption

Clinical features

Mottling ranges from paper-white patches to opaque, brown, pitted and brittle enamel. Clinically, it may be difficult to distinguish fluorotic defects from amelogenesis imperfecta when the degree of exposure to fluoride is unknown (Fig. 2.31).

There is considerable individual variation in the effects of fluorides. A few patients acquire mottling after exposure to relatively low concentrations, while others exposed to higher concentrations appear unaffected.

Changes due to mottling are graded as shown in Table 2.7.

Table 2.7 Grading of mottled enamel

- *Very mild*. Small paper-white areas involve less than 25% of surface
- *Mild*. Opaque areas involve up to 50% of surface
- *Moderate*. The whole of the enamel surface may be affected with paper-white or brownish areas or both (Fig. 2.32)
- *Severe*. The enamel is grossly defective, opaque, pitted, stained brown and brittle (Fig. 2.33)

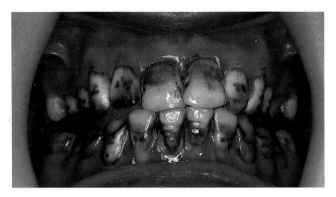

Fig. 2.33 Fluorosis. Severe effects from an area of endemic fluorosis. Closer view showing irregular depressions caused by hypoplasia and white opaque flecks and patches.

Table 2.8 Effects on enamel of raised fluoride levels

Fluoride concentration	Effects	Clinical appearance
Less than 0.5 ppm	Very mild or mild defects in up to 6% of patients	Inconspicuous
0.5 to 1.5 ppm	At the upper limit, 22% show very mild defects	
2.5 ppm	Very mild or mild defects in over 50%. Moderate or severe defects in nearly 10%	Noticeable
4.5 ppm	Nearly all patients affected in some degree; 46% have 'moderate' and 18% 'severe' defects.	Disfiguring
6.0 ppm and more	All patients affected; 50% severely disfiguring	

Pathology

Fluoride combines to form calcium fluorapatite in place of part of the hydroxyapatite. Damage to ameloblasts leading to defective matrix formation, is seen only when the concentrations of fluorides are exceptionally high. At intermediate levels (2 to 6 ppm) the matrix is normal in structure and quantity. The form of the tooth is unaffected, but there are patches of incomplete calcification beneath the surface layer. These appear as opacities because of high organic and water content. Where there are high concentrations of fluorides (over 6 ppm) the enamel is pitted and brittle, with severe and widespread staining. Deciduous teeth are rarely mottled because excess fluoride is taken up by the maternal skeleton. However, when fluoride levels are excessively high (over 8 ppm), as in parts of India, mottling of deciduous teeth may be seen.

With severe mottling of the enamel, other effects of excessive fluoride intake, especially sclerosis of the skeleton, may develop. Radiographically, increased density of the skeleton may be seen in areas where the fluoride content of the water exceeds 8 ppm.

The severity of defects in relation to fluoride concentrations is shown in Table 2.8 and its relationship to caries prevalence in Figure 2.34.

Mild dental fluorosis is not readily distinguishable from non-fluoride defects and non-specific defects are more common in areas where the water contains less than 1 ppm of fluorine.

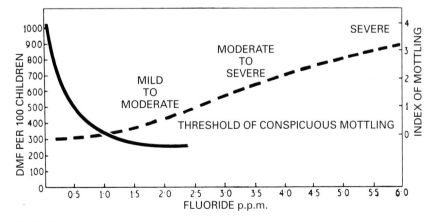

Fig. 2.34 Caries prevalence and mottling. The general relationship between the prevalence of caries (continuous line) and the severity of mottling (broken line) in persons continuously exposed to various levels of fluoride in the water during dental development. The optimum level of fluoride can be seen to be about 1 part per million. Higher concentrations of fluoride cause increasing incidence and severity of mottling without a comparable improvement in resistance to caries. The index of mottling is obtained by giving an arbitrary value for each degree of mottling and relating the numbers of patients with each grade to the total number examined.

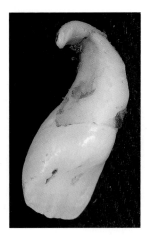

Fig. 2.35 A dilacerated upper central incisor. There has been an abrupt change in the direction of root growth after approximately one-third of the root was formed.

Other acquired developmental anomalies

Dilaceration

Trauma to a developing tooth can cause the root to form at an angle to the normal axis of the tooth — a rare deformity known as dilaceration. The sudden disturbance to odontogenesis may cause the formation of highly irregular dentine in the coronal part of the pulp chamber but the angulated root may consist of normal tubular dentine. The hook-shaped tooth is likely to be difficult to extract (Figs 2.35 and 36).

Fetal alcohol syndrome

Maternal alcoholism may cause developmental defects in the fetus. The eyes typically slant laterally, the lower half of the face is elongated and there is mental deficiency. Dental development may be delayed and there may be enamel defects such as mottled opacities in the enamel near the incisal margins but elsewhere abnormal enamel translucency.

Treatment of hypoplastic defects

Hypoplastic teeth can be disguised by restorative procedures such as veneers or jacket crowns. The latter should be delayed until adult life. The young pulp is large, is easily damaged during preparation of the tooth, and injuries are more frequent than in older persons.

ODONTOMAS

Odontomas result from aberrant development of the dental lamina. The most minor examples, though they are not usually called odontomas, are slight malformations such as an exaggerated cingulum or extra roots or cusps on otherwise normal teeth. All gradations exist between these anomalies and composite odontomas where the dental tissues have developed in a

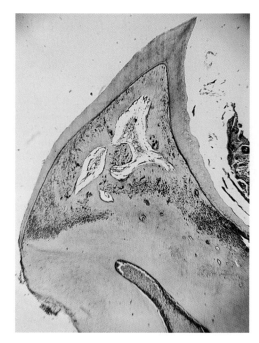

Fig. 2.36 Another dilacerated tooth showing, in addition to the deflected root, a change in enamel contour and disorganised coronal dentine formed after the causative trauma.

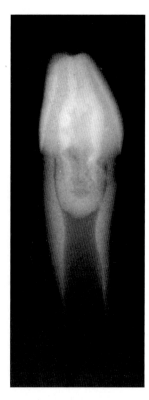

Fig. 2.37 Dens in dente or mild invaginated odontome. In this radiograph the enamel-lined invagination and its communication with the exterior at the incisal tip are clearly seen. The pulp is compressed to the periphery.

completely irregular and haphazard manner bearing no resemblance to a tooth and occasionally forming a large mass (Ch. 8).

Den invaginatus is an exaggeration of the process of formation of a cingular pit. Dentine and enamel-forming tissue invaginate the whole length of a tooth to appear radiographically as a tooth-within-a-tooth (*dens in dente* — Fig. 2.37). Extension of this process causes the formation of an invaginated odontome (Fig. 2.38). Food debris lodges in the

cavity to cause caries which rapidly penetrates the distorted pulp chamber.

Geminated teeth are most common in the maxillary incisor region. The pulp chambers may be entirely separate, joined in the middle of the tooth, or branched, with the pulp chambers of separated crowns sharing a common root canal. The crowns may be entirely separate or divided only by a shallow groove. The roots may be single or double.

These malformed teeth usually need to be removed before they obstruct the eruption of other teeth or become infected, or for cosmetic reasons.

Enamel pearls are uncommon, minor abnormalities, which are formed on otherwise normal teeth by displaced ameloblasts below the amelocemental junction. Enamel pearls may consist of only a nodule of enamel attached to the dentine, or may have a core of dentine containing a horn of the pulp. The pearls are usually round, a few millimetres in diameter, and often form at the bifurcation of upper permanent molars (Figs 2.39 and 2.40). They may cause a stagnation area at the gingival margin, but, if they contain pulp, this will be exposed when the pearl is removed.

GENETIC DISORDERS OF THE JAWS

Important developmental defects of the jaws are summarised in Table 2.9 and discussed more fully in subsequent chapters.

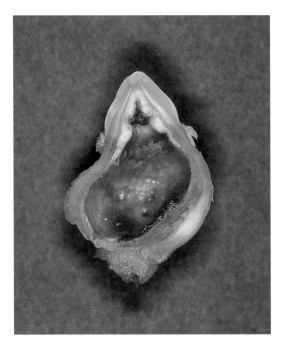

Fig. 2.38 A dilated and invaginated odontome in a lateral incisor, sectioned vertically. The central cavity communicates with the exterior through an invagination in the cusp tip.

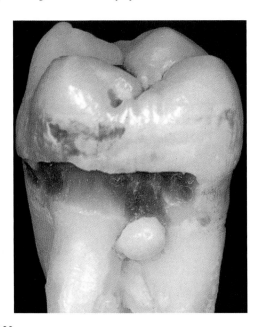

Fig. 2.39 Enamel pearl. There is a small mass of enamel at the root bifurcation.

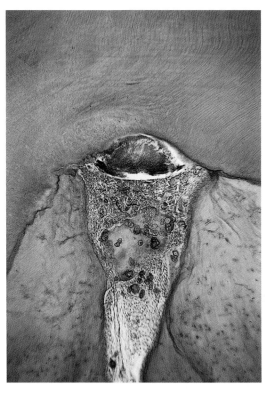

Fig. 2.40 Histological appearance of an enamel pearl showing a small isolated zone of enamel matrix on the root dentine.

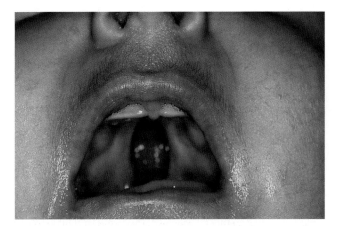

Fig. 2.41 Cleft palate. A broad midline defect is present. (By kind permission of Mrs E Horrocks.)

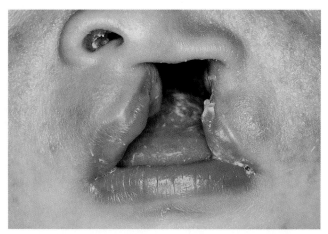

Fig. 2.42 Cleft lip and palate. Complete unilateral cleft of palate, alveolar bone and lip joining the oral and nasal cavities. (By kind permission of Mrs E Horrocks.)

Table 2.9 Developmental defects of the jaws

- Hereditary prognathism
- Clefts of the palate and/or lip
- Craniofacial anomalies
- Cleidocranial dysplasia (Ch. 10)
- Cherubism (Ch. 10)
- Basal cell naevus syndrome (Ch. 7)
- Gardner's syndrome (Ch. 9)
- Osteogenesis imperfecta (Ch. 10)

Hereditary prognathism

Historically, hereditary prognathism is best known in the Spanish branch of the Hapsburg royal family. The defect is seen in striking form in contemporaneous portraits and persisted for 300 years.

CLEFTS OF THE LIP AND PALATE

Clefts can form in the lip or palate alone or in both (Figs 2.41 and 2.42). The aetiology is unknown but there is a genetic component in approximately 40% of cases. The risk of having such defects is greatly increased if one, and particularly if both, of the parents are affected.

Cleft lip (with or without a palatal cleft) is more common in males, while cleft palate alone is approximately twice as common in females. The incidence of cleft lip is about 1 per 1000 live births, while that of isolated palatal clefts is about 1 per 2000 live births. In terms of relative frequencies, cleft lips form about 22%, combined defects of lip and palate form about 58% and isolated palatal clefts form about 20% of this group of defects. The reasons for the variations in the sites of clefts is that the lip and anterior palate (the primary palate) develop before the hard and soft palates (the secondary palate). Fusion of the secondary palate is from behind forwards. Isolated cleft lip is therefore the result of an early developmental disorder,

while isolated cleft palate results from influences acting later, after the primary palate has closed. By contrast, a prolonged disorder of development can prevent both primary and secondary palates from closing and leaves a severe combined defect.

Developmental disorders associated with clefting

In Down's syndrome, cleft lip or palate is present in approximately 1 in 200 patients (Ch. 33). In the less common trisomy 13 (Patau's syndrome) cleft lip or palate or both is present in up to 70% of cases, but multiple defects of the brain and other organs lead to early death. Clefts are also a feature of many other genetic craniofacial syndromes such as cleidocranial dysplasia.

Classification

The main types of cleft lip are summarised in Table 2.10.

Table 2.10 Clefts of lip and/or palate

- Cleft lip
  Unilateral (usually on the left side), with or without an anterior alveolar ridge cleft
  Bilateral, with or without alveolar ridge clefts, complete or incomplete
- Palatal clefts
  Bifid uvula
  Soft palate only
  Both hard and soft palate
- Combined lip and palatal defects
  Unilateral, complete or incomplete
  Cleft palate with bilateral cleft lip, complete or incomplete

In the worst cases there is complete separation of the anterior palate, which projects forward with the centre section of the lip and is attached only by the nasal septum.

Associated defects

1. *Local.* Teeth in the region of the defect are typically absent or malformed.
2. *Systemic.* Major congenital defects, particularly heart disease, limb defects, spina bifida or mental defects are associated in about 50% of these patients and can seriously affect their management. This is particularly so in the case of Down's syndrome.

Management

Important considerations are summarised in Table 2.11.

Table 2.11 **Important aspects of management of clefts**

- Provision for feeding in infancy when palatal clefts are severe
- Prevention of collapse of the two halves of the maxilla
- Measures to counteract speech defects
- Cosmetic repair of cleft lips

Repair of these clefts has traditionally been carried out at 15–18 months after birth. Nevertheless, early operation can severely inhibit growth both by damaging the delicate growing tissues and, particularly, by consequent scarring. Severe malocclusion can result, and re-operation may be necessary to lessen the deformity (Fig. 2.43).

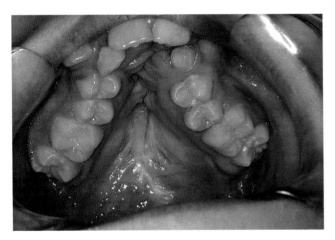

Fig. 2.43 Collapsed maxilla resulting from traditional surgical repair of cleft palate. Scarring and growth disturbance produce a distorted narrow maxilla. (By kind permission of Mrs E Horrocks.)

More recently, observation of untreated clefts has shown that the growth potential of these tissues is virtually normal. In some centres, therefore, a soft palate cleft is repaired early but hard palate repair is delayed until 8 or 9 years after temporary closure with an obturator. The results are good facial growth and occlusion, but speech may be impaired to some degree.

Submucous cleft palate

Submucous clefts are an abnormality of the attachment of the muscles of the soft palate beneath an intact mucosa. They are present in approximately 1 in 1200 births but frequently missed. The chief effects are slowness in feeding and nasal regurgitation. Middle ear infections and speech defects result from the defective muscle attachments as frequently as in those with overt clefts. Symptoms are absent in only 10% of cases.

Clinically, a submucous cleft is visible as a translucent area along the midline of the soft palate and frequently a bifid uvula. On palpation, a notched posterior nasal spine may be felt. The diagnosis can be confirmed by imaging techniques, such as videofluoroscopy. Operation to repair the muscle attachments is usually delayed for about 2.5 years, to enable the degree of the defect to be assessed.

DEVELOPMENTAL DEFECTS OF THE ORAL SOFT TISSUES

These defects (Table 2.12) are discussed in more detail in later chapters.

Table 2.12 **Important developmental defects of oral soft tissues**

- The gingivae and periodontium (Ch. 5)
  Hereditary gingival fibromatosis
  Ehlers–Danlos syndrome type VIII
- The oral mucosa (Ch. 15)
  White sponge naevus
  Epidermolysis bullosa
  Ehlers–Danlos syndrome

Other genetic diseases relevant to dentistry

There are many rare hereditary disorders which can affect the mouth or jaws, but from the practical clinical viewpoint, haemophilia is the most important (Ch. 26).

SUGGESTED FURTHER READING

Aine L, Mäki M, Collin P et al 1990 Dental enamel defects in celiac disease. J Oral Pathol Med 19:241–245

Aldred M J 1992 Unusual dentinal changes in dentinogenesis imperfecta associated with osteogenesis imperfecta. A case report. Oral Surg Oral Med Oral Pathol 73:461–464

Bhat M, Nelson K B, Cummins S K, Grether J K 1992 Prevalence of developmental enamel defects in children with cerebral palsy. J Oral Pathol Med 21:241–244

Chapple I L C 1993 Hypophosphatasia: dental aspects and mode of inheritance. J Clin Periodontol 20:615–622

Crawford P J M, Aldred M J 1989 Regional odontodysplasia: a bibliography. J Oral Pathol Med 18:251–263

Dong J, Gu T T, Simmons D et al 2000 Enamelin maps to human chromosome 4q21 within the autosomal dominant amelogenesis imperfecta locus. Eur J Oral Sci 108:353–359

Fanibunda K B, Soames J V 1996 Odontodysplasia, gingival manifestations, and accompanying abnormalities. Oral Surg Oral Med Oral Pathol Radiol Endod 81:84–88

Mäki M, Aine L, Lipsanen V et al 1991 Dental enamel defects in first-degree relatives of coeliac disease patients. Lancet 337:763–764

Markus A F, Smith W P, Delaire J 1993 Primary closure of cleft palate: a functional approach. Br J Oral Maxillofac Surg 31:71–77

O'Connell A C, Marini J C 1999 Evaluation of oral problems in an osteogenesis imperfecta population. Oral Surg Oral Med Oral Pathol Radiol Endod 87:189–196

Peyritz R E 2000 Ehlers–Danlos syndrome. N Engl J Med 342:730–732

Precious D S, Delaire J 1993 Clinical observations of cleft lip and palate. Oral Surg Oral Med Oral Pathol 75:141–151

Van der Wal J E, Rittersma J, Baart J A, van der Waal I 1993 Odontodysplasia: report of three cases. Int J Oral Maxillofac Surg 22:356–358

Wolff G, Wienker T F, Sander H 1993 On the genetics of mandibular prognathism: analysis of large European noble families. J Med Genet 30:112–116

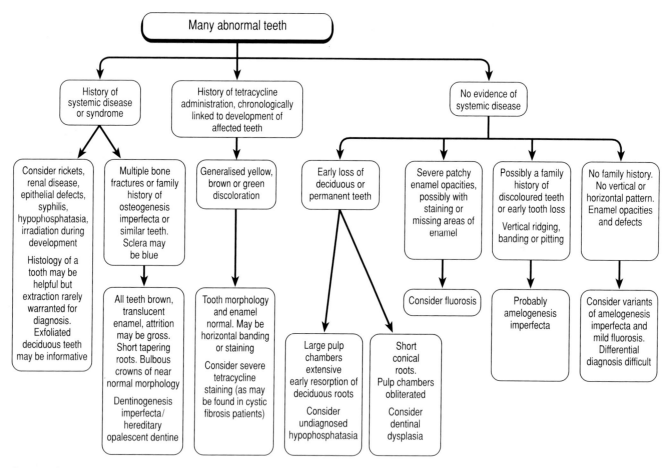

Summary 2.1 Differential diagnosis of developmental defects of the teeth.

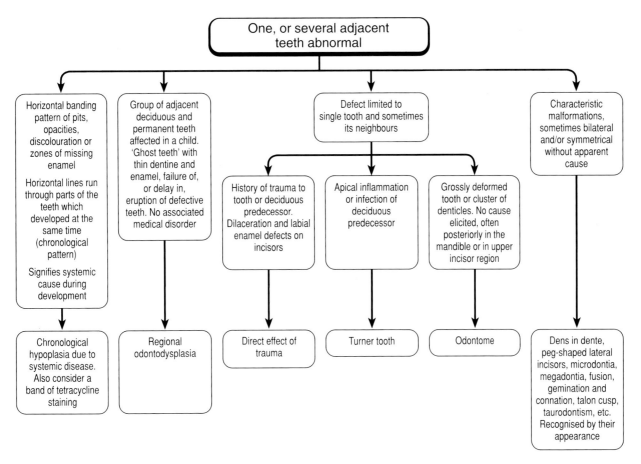

Summary 2.2 Differential diagnosis of developmental and acquired abnormalities of one or a group of teeth.

Dental caries

For sweetness and decay are of one root and sweetness ever riots to decay

Author, regrettably, unknown

Dental caries is progressive bacterial damage to teeth exposed to the saliva. Caries is one of the most common of all diseases and still a major cause of loss of teeth.

The ultimate effect of caries is to break down enamel and dentine and thus open a path for bacteria to reach the pulp. The consequences are inflammation of the pulp and, later, of the periapical tissues. Acute pulpitis and apical periodontitis caused in this way are the most common causes of toothache. Infection can spread from the periapical region to the jaw and beyond. Though this is rare in Britain, people in other countries occasionally die from this cause.

AETIOLOGY

In 1890, W. D. Miller showed that lesions similar to dental caries could be produced by incubating teeth in saliva when carbohydrates were added. Miller concluded that caries could result from decalcification caused by bacterial acid production followed by invasion and destruction of any remaining tissue. Though he took a laudably cautious view as to how these findings should be interpreted, Miller's basic hypothesis has been upheld, even though the infective nature of the disease was not confirmed until 1954 when Orland and his associates in the USA showed that caries did not develop in germ-free animals. However, dental caries develops only in the presence of several interacting variables (Fig. 3.1 and Table 3.1).

MICROBIOLOGY

Substantial evidence indicates that streptococci are essential for development of caries, particularly of smooth (interstitial) surfaces. These are viridans streptococci which are a heterogeneous group including *Streptococcus mutans*, *S. sobrinus*, *S. salivarius*, *S. mitior* and *S. sanguis*.

Possible interventions
Reduce intake of cariogenic sugars, particularly sucrose

Possible interventions
Reduce *Strep. mutans* numbers by:
• reduction in sugar intake
• active or passive immunisation

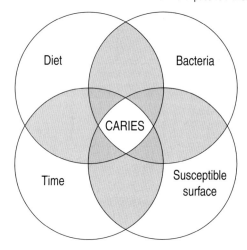

Possible interventions
Avoid frequent sucrose intake ('snacking')
Stimulate salivary flow and sugar clearance

Possible interventions
Water and other types of fluoridation
Prevention during post-eruptive maturation
Fissure sealing
Remineralising solutions
Properly contoured restorations

Fig. 3.1 The four major factors in the aetiology of dental caries.

Table 3.1 Essential requirements for development of dental caries

1. Cariogenic (acidogenic) bacteria
2. Bacterial plaque
3. Stagnation areas
4. Fermentable bacterial substrate (sugar)
5. Susceptible tooth surfaces

Viridans streptococci vary in their ability to attach to different types of tissues, their ability to ferment sugars (particularly sucrose), and the concentrations of acid thus produced. They also differ in the types of polysaccharides that they form.

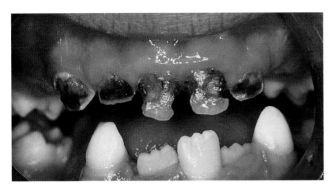

Fig. 3.2 Extensive caries of decidous incisors and canines. This pattern of caries is particularly associated with the use of sweetened dummies and sweetened infant drinks.

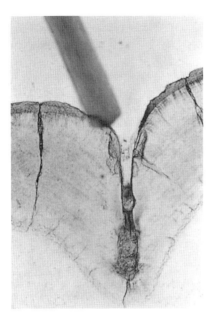

Fig. 3.3 The stagnation area in an occlusal pit. A ground section of a molar showing the size of the stagnation area in comparison with a toothbrush bristle placed above it. The complete inaccessibility of the stagnation area to cleaning is obvious.

Certain strains of *S. mutans* are strongly acidogenic and, at low pH, with freely available sucrose, also store an intracellular, glycogen-like, reserve polysaccharide. When the supply of substrate dries up, this reserve is metabolised to continue acid production for a time. Drastic reduction in dietary sucrose intake is followed by virtual elimination of *S. mutans* from plaque and reduces or abolishes caries activity. When sucrose is made freely available again *S. mutans* rapidly recolonises the plaque.

Germ-free animals do not develop dental caries when fed a sucrose-rich diet which causes caries in animals with a normal oral flora. Experiments using gnotobiotes have shown that the most potent causes of dental caries are a limited number of strains of the *S. mutans* group which are able to form cariogenic plaque.

S. mutans strains are a major component of plaque in human mouths, particularly in persons with a high dietary sucrose intake and high caries activity (Fig. 3.2). *S. mutans* isolated from such mouths are virulently cariogenic when introduced into the mouths of animals.

However, simple clinical observation of the sites (interstitially and in pits and fissures) where dental caries is active, shows that the bacteria responsible are not those floating free in the saliva. Dental caries develops only at the interface between tooth surface and dental plaque in stagnation areas (Fig. 3.3).

Bacterial polysaccharides

The ability of *S. mutans* to initiate smooth surface caries and form large amounts of adherent plaque depends on its ability to polymerise sucrose into high-molecular-weight, dextran-like, extracellular polysaccharides (*glucans*) (Table 3.2). The cariogenicity of *S. mutans* depends as much on its ability to form large amounts of insoluble extracellular glucans as on its ability to produce acid.

Table 3.2 Essential properties of cariogenic bacteria
● Acidogenic
● Able to produce a pH low enough (usually pH < 5) to decalcify tooth substance
● Able to survive and continue to produce acid at low levels of pH
● Possess attachment mechanisms for firm adhesion to smooth tooth surfaces
● Able to produce adhesive, insoluble plaque polysaccharides (glucans)

Glucans enable streptococci to adhere to one another and to the tooth surface, probably via specific receptors. In this way *S. mutans* and its glucans may initiate their attachment to the teeth and enable critical masses of plaque to be built up. Production of sticky, insoluble, extracellular glucan produced by strains of *S. mutans* is strongly related to their cariogenicity.

The importance of sucrose in this activity depends on the high energy of its glucose–fructose bond which allows the synthesis of polysaccharides by glucosyltransferase without any other source of energy. Sucrose is thus the main substrate for such polysaccharides. Other sugars are, to a variable degree, less cariogenic (in the absence of preformed plaque), partly because they are less readily formed into cariogenic glucans.

Plaque polysaccharides, synthesised by bacteria, play an essential role in the pathogenesis of dental caries. The proportions of the different types of polysaccharide, and the overall amounts formed, depend both on the kinds of bacteria present and the different sugars in the diet.

On a sucrose-rich diet the main extracellular polysaccharides are glucans. Fructans formed from fructose are produced in smaller amounts. They are more soluble than glucans and less important in caries. Acid-producing microorganisms that do not produce insoluble polysaccharides do not appear to be able to cause caries of smooth surfaces. Even mutant strains of *S. mutans* which produce more soluble polysaccharides seem not to be cariogenic. Polysaccharides thus contribute to the adhesiveness, bulk and resistance to solution of plaque.

In the past, lactobacilli were thought to be the main cause of dental caries because they are numerous in the saliva and can be isolated from carious cavities. They are also acidogenic. However, they are present only in relatively small numbers in dental plaque until after caries has developed.

In gnotobiotes, lactobacilli are weakly cariogenic but some can produce fissure caries where adherent plaque formation is less important. Overall there is little evidence that lactobacilli are clinically important in initiating dental caries but they may contribute to tooth destruction after the process has started.

Many other microorganisms can also be found in plaque. The role of the many filamentous forms is not known. Strains of actinomyces are also found, particularly when caries is rampant, but appear capable only of causing root surface lesions.

Though bacteria are responsible for acid production, *bacterial plaque* (Fig. 3.4) enables large concentrations of them to adhere to the teeth and, in stagnation areas, prevents effective buffering of bacterial acids by saliva. Important points about microbiological aspects of dental caries are summarised in Table 3.3.

The cariogenicity of *S. mutans* depends on properties summarised in Table 3.4.

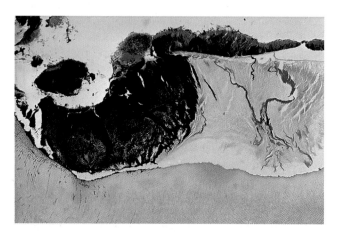

Fig. 3.4 Bacterial plaque. A decalcified section showing darkly staining plaque lying on enamel and within a carious cavity. The plaque has remained intact and adherent to the enamel throughout the processes to which the specimen was subjected in preparation for sectioning.

Table 3.3 **Microbiological aspects of dental caries**

- Dental caries is a bacterial disease
- The organisms mainly responsible are specific strains of *Streptococcus mutans*
- The cariogenicity of *S. mutans* has been established by inoculating it into the mouths of otherwise germfree animals (gnotobiotes)
- The presence of *S. mutans* in the human mouth is associated with caries activity
- Other bacteria including lactobacilli and other strains of streptococci are only weakly cariogenic or are non-cariogenic despite being able to produce acid

Table 3.4 **Cariogenic properties of *Streptococcus mutans***

- It produces lactic acid from sucrose
- It can live at a pH as low as 4.2
- It forms large amounts of extracellular, sticky and insoluble glucan plaque matrix
- It adheres to pellicle and contributes to plaque formation

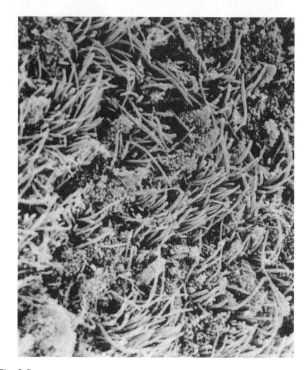

Fig. 3.5 This scanning electronmicrograph of plaque shows the large number of filamentous organisms and, in addition, many cocci clustered amongst them. (By kind permission of Dr Sheila J Jones.)

BACTERIAL PLAQUE

Plaque is a tenaciously adherent deposit that forms on tooth surfaces. It consists of an organic matrix containing a dense concentration of bacteria (Fig 3.4–3.6).

In microbiological terms, plaque is a *biofilm*. Biofilms consist of a hydrated viscous phase formed from bacteria and their extracellular polysaccharide matrices. In such a film, molecules and ions exist in concentrations that can be widely different from those of the surrounding fluid phase (saliva). Bacteria in biofilms can also exhibit cooperative activity and behave differently from the same species in isolation in a culture medium. As a consequence, a biofilm may be resistant to antimicrobials or to immunological defences to which the individual bacteria are normally sensitive. Bacterial plaque must therefore be regarded as a living entity and not as a mere collection of bacteria. In particular, the ability of dental plaque to concentrate and retain acid was recognised long before the special properties of biofilms were discovered.

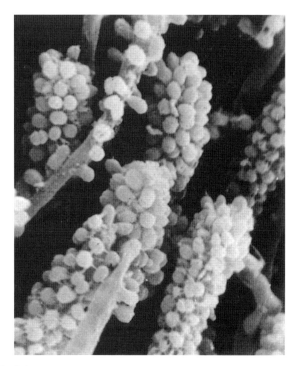

Fig. 3.6 This scanning electronmicrograph at higher power shows cocci attached to filamentous organisms to produce the corn-cob type of arrangement sometimes seen in plaque. (By kind permission of Dr Sheila J Jones.)

Clinically, bacterial plaque is a tenaciously adherent deposit on the teeth. It resists the friction of food during mastication, and can only be readily removed by toothbrushing. However, neither toothbrushing nor fibrous foods will remove plaque from inaccessible surfaces or pits (stagnation areas — see Fig. 3.3).

Plaque becomes visible, particularly on the labial surfaces of the incisors, when toothbrushing is stopped for 12–24 hours. It appears as a translucent film with a matt surface that dulls the otherwise smooth and shiny enamel. It can be made obvious when stained with disclosing agents. Little plaque forms under conditions of starvation but it forms rapidly and abundantly on a high-sucrose diet.

In stagnation areas where it is undisturbed, plaque bacteria can form acid from sugars over sufficiently long periods as to attack tooth surfaces.

Adhesion of bacteria to the teeth from which they would otherwise be washed away is an essential requirement for the colonisation of enamel. Attachment depends on complex mechanisms and depends on such molecules as glucans and/or glucosyltransferase. Components of plaque which act as adhesion receptors, include a group of *proline-rich proteins (PRPs)* from the saliva.

Stages of formation of bacterial plaque

If teeth are thoroughly cleaned by polishing with an abrasive, plaque quickly re-forms (Table 3.5).

Table 3.5 Stages of plaque formation

- Deposition of structureless cell-free, pellicle of salivary glycoprotein
- Further deposition of pellicle enhanced by bacterial action precipitating salivary proteins
- Colonisation of the cell-free layer by bacteria, particularly by *S. sanguis* and *S. mutans* strains within 24 hours
- Progressive build-up of plaque substance by bacterial polysaccharides
- Proliferation of filamentous and other bacteria as the plaque matures

Acid production in plaque

Sucrose diffuses rapidly into plaque, and acid production quickly follows. These changes have been measured directly in the human mouth using microelectrodes in direct contact with plaque. It has been shown by this means that, after rinsing the mouth with a 10% glucose solution, the pH falls within 2–5 minutes, often to a level sufficient to decalcify enamel. Even though no more sucrose may be taken and the surplus is washed away by the saliva, the pH level remains at a low level for about 15–20 minutes; it returns only gradually to the resting level after about an hour. These changes (the so-called Stephan curve) are shown diagrammatically in Figure 3.7. The rapidity with which the pH falls is a reflection of the speed with which sucrose can diffuse into plaque and the activity of the concentration of enzymes produced by the great numbers of bacteria in the plaque. The slow rate of recovery to the resting pH — a critical factor in

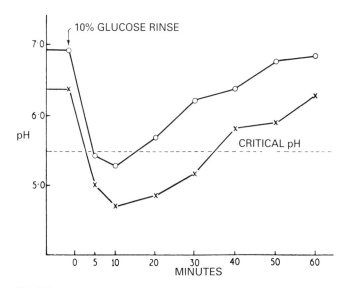

Fig. 3.7 Stephan curves. This is the usual form of curves obtained when changes in reaction to bacterial plaque are measured directly. When the pH falls below the critical level, enamel may become demineralised. Patients with active caries tend to show a lower fall in pH, as in the lower curve. Noteworthy features are the very rapid fall in pH and the slow recovery to the normal level in spite of the very short time the sugar is in the mouth. Carbohydrates which are retained on the teeth will have a more prolonged effect still.

Table 3.6 Factors contributing to maintenance of low plaque pH

- Rapid production of a high concentration of acid within the plaque, temporarily overcomes local buffering
- Escape of acid into the saliva, delayed by the diffusion-limiting properties of plaque and its thickness
- Diffusion of salivary buffers into plaque hampered by the diffusion-limiting properties of plaque and its thickness
- Continued sugar production from bacterial intracellular polysaccharides

caries production — depends mainly on factors summarised in Table 3.6.

As discussed in relation to the pathology of dental caries, it is clear that acid production is responsible for the carious attack. Lactic acid is mainly responsible. When plaque is sampled after exposure to sucrose, lactic acid is the quantitatively predominant acid during plaque activity, particularly during the trough of the Stephan curve. Lactic acid has a lower pK constant and causes a greater fall in pH than equimolar solutions of acetic or propionic acids that may also be detected in plaque.

Plaque minerals

In addition to bacteria and their polysaccharides, salivary components also contribute to the plaque matrix. Calcium, phosphorus and, often, fluorides are present in significant amounts. There is some evidence of an inverse relationship between calcium and phosphate levels in plaque and caries activity or sucrose intake. The ability of plaque to concentrate calcium and phosphorus is used in mineralising mouthwashes. The level of fluoride in plaque may be high, ranging from 15 to 75 ppm or more, and is largely dependent on the fluoride level in the drinking water and diet. This fluoride is probably mostly bound to organic material in the plaque but, at low pH levels, may become available and active in ionic form.

SUCROSE AS A PLAQUE SUBSTRATE

Direct measurement of pH changes in the mouth shows that there is intermittent acid production on the surface of the teeth and this follows the pattern shown earlier in the Stephan curves. Ingestion of sucrose leads to a burst of activity in the plaque so that the pH may fall low enough to attack enamel before slowly returning to the resting level. The frequency with which substrate is made available to the plaque is therefore important. When sucrose is taken as a sweet drink, any surplus, beyond the capacity of the organisms in the plaque to metabolise at the time, is washed away. If sucrose-containing drinks are taken repeatedly at short intervals, the supply of substrate to the bacteria can be sufficiently frequently renewed to cause acid in the plaque to remain persistently at a destructive level.

A similar effect may be caused by carbohydrate in sticky

form, such as a caramel, which clings to the teeth and is slowly dissolved, releasing substrate over a long period. The effects of maintaining plaque activity by repeated administration of small quantities of sucrose have been demonstrated by the use of animal feeding devices to dispense metered quantities of sucrose in diets at fixed intervals. These show that a given amount of sucrose is more cariogenic when fed in small increments, but at intervals to maintain maximal plaque activity, than the same amount fed as a single dose.

Effects of sucrose on plaque polysaccharide production

As discussed earlier, the cariogenicity of plaque depends on its ability to adhere to the teeth, to resist dissolution by saliva and its protection of bacterial acids from salivary buffering. These properties depend on the formation of insoluble polysaccharides produced particularly by cariogenic strains of *S. mutans*.

Effects of sucrose on the oral microbial flora

Colonisation by cariogenic bacteria, especially *S. mutans*, is highly dependent on the sucrose content of the diet. In the absence of sucrose, *S. mutans* cannot usually be made to colonise the mouths of experimental animals. In humans, the plaque counts of *S. mutans* also appear to depend on the sucrose content of the diet. Severe reduction in dietary sucrose causes *S. mutans* to decline in numbers or disappear from plaque.

Experimental evidence for the essential contribution of sucrose to caries activity is summarised in Table 3.7.

Table 3.7 Experimental evidence for the critical contribution of sucrose to caries activity

- In caries-susceptible animals a sucrose-rich diet promotes caries production
- Caries is not induced in susceptible animals if sucrose is fed only by stomach-tube — its effect is entirely local
- Sucrose in sticky form clings to the teeth and remains available to bacteria for a longer period and is more cariogenic
- Sucrose-containing fluids are quickly cleared from the mouth and less cariogenic
- Frequent feeds of small quantities of sucrose are more cariogenic than the same total amount fed on a single occasion
- Desalivation, by delaying clearance of sugars, enhances caries activity

The importance of sucrose in human caries depends mainly on epidemiological studies and a few interventional studies. The findings of epidemiological studies are summarised in Table 3.8.

Dental caries has been most prevalent in well-nourished, Westernised communities, such as Britain, the USA and others with similar lifestyles where large quantities of sucrose, particularly in the form of sweets or snack bars, are eaten. In the past particularly, there have been many studies of poor communities living on traditional diets with little or no sucrose con-

Table 3.8 Epidemiological evidence for sucrose as the cause of dental caries

- Low caries prevalence in populations with low sucrose intakes
- The decline in caries prevalence during wartime sucrose shortages
- The rise of caries prevalence with increasing availability of sucrose
- Archaeological evidence of low caries prevalence in eras before sucrose became freely available
- Low caries prevalence in disorders of sucrose metabolism (hereditary fructose intolerance)

tent. A low prevalence of caries has been shown (for example) in parts of China and of Africa, the Seychelles, Tristan da Cunha, Alaska and Greenland. Many studies were carried out on Eskimo races who were caries-free when consuming their traditional diet of seal or whale meat, and fish. Similarly in South African races, despite a high-starch carbohydrate diet, caries was found in fewer than 9% of those examined, but greatly increased when there was access to a modern diet.

In such studies no association has been found between malnutrition and caries. Generally the reverse is true, and, when nutrition is poor, caries is infrequent. These diets also vary widely in content, from rice as the staple in China or coarsely ground cereals in Africa to a mainly meat and fish diet among Eskimos. The common feature of these diets, and one differentiating them sharply from Westernised diets, is low or negligible consumption of sucrose.

Britain is an example of a country where consumption of sucrose is exceptionally high, and where the rest of the diet is more than adequate. A survey in England and Wales in 1973 showed, for example, that (in spite of the benefits of a National Health Service) 78% of 8-year-old children had active decay and many teeth which had been filled or lost from this cause. A survey in 1978 showed that dentate adults had on average only 13 sound and unfilled teeth.

In Britain and other countries, the incidence of caries has risen roughly parallel with rising consumption of sucrose. The incidence of caries has risen in spite of the much greater consumption of so-called 'protective' foods, namely dairy products, meat and fruit, in recent years. As a consequence of this more varied diet, carbohydrates overall have formed a smaller proportion of the diet. Nevertheless, sucrose forms a higher proportion of the carbohydrate component.

Where there has been a change from simple natural diets to a Westernised diet, as in Alaska, caries has increased sharply, and Eskimo children now have a caries incidence at least as high as other American children. A similar state of affairs is developing in Africa as sweet eating and sweet between-meals 'snacks' have become popular. In Nigeria many of the older adults are still totally caries-free but the prevalence of dental caries among children and young people who have picked up sweet-eating habits is rising rapidly. This effect has also been strikingly well documented in the population of Tristan da

Cunha who, up to the late 1930s, lived on a simple meat, fish and vegetable diet with a minimal sucrose content and had a very low caries prevalence. With the adoption of westernised diet, the caries prevalence had risen up to eight-fold in some age groups by the mid-1960s. Even in Europe, in the 1930s and 1940s there were isolated communities such as the Outer Hebrides or the Lötschental in Switzerland, where dental caries prevalence rose 20-fold or more when sucrose and sweets became widely consumed.

The effect of limiting sucrose consumption was shown on a vast scale in wartime. Those countries which suffered food shortages during the 1939–45 war had severe restrictions, mainly of meat, fats and sucrose. To maintain an adequate caloric intake, overall consumption of starchy carbohydrates rose considerably. In occupied Norway, where shortages were particularly severe, the pattern of dental caries during and after the war is shown diagrammatically in Figure 3.8. As sucrose became more plentiful at the end of the war, caries prevalence progressively rose.

In Japan also, rising caries prevalence has been associated with rising sucrose consumption. Towards the end of the Second World War sugar consumption and caries levels were very low. More recently, Japan is one of the few countries where sucrose consumption, from 16.5 kg per head in 1961, nearly doubled in 1970. Caries prevalence has risen in parallel. Unlike most other countries, this picture has not been significantly masked by use of fluoride toothpastes where the market share of fluoride toothpastes is only 15%.

Caries has become epidemic only in relatively recent years as sucrose became cheaper and widely available. In Britain there was a sudden, widespread rise in sucrose consumption in the middle of the 19th century. This resulted both from the falling cost of production and, in 1861, the abolition of a tax on sugar. Evidence from exhumed skulls confirms the low prevalence of caries before sucrose became widely available and the steady rise in prevalence thereafter.

Patients unable to metabolise fructose as a result of an enzyme deficiency cannot tolerate fructose-containing foods including disaccharides such as sucrose where fructose forms part of the molecule. These children therefore learn to avoid all sucrose-containing foods and have an unusually low incidence of caries.

Experimental studies on humans

In the Vipeholm study over 400 adult patients were studied in a closed institution. They received a basic low-carbohydrate diet to establish a baseline of caries activity for each group. They were then divided into seven groups which were each allocated different diets. A control group received the basic diet made up to an adequate calorie intake with margarine. Two groups received supplements of sucrose at mealtimes, either in solution or as sweetened bread. The four remaining groups received sweets (toffees, caramels, or chocolate) which were eaten between meals.

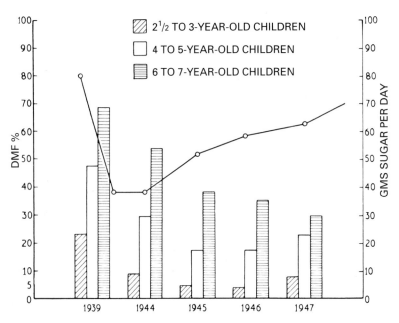

Fig. 3.8 The wartime restrictions on diet, and caries in Norway. The continuous line (above) shows an estimate of the individual daily sugar consumption during and after the war. The heights of the columns show the incidence of caries in children of various ages. Rationing of sugar started in 1938 but it is apparent that the incidence of caries declined slowly and continued for a short time after sugar became freely available. The greatest reduction in caries was in the youngest group of children whose teeth were exposed to the wartime diet for the shortest periods; the mothers of these children, on the other hand, had been exposed to the wartime diet throughout pregnancy and for a long period before this. (Mainly after Toverud G 1949 Journal of the American Dental Association 39:127.)

The effects of sucrose in different quantities and of different degrees of adhesiveness, and of eating sucrose at different times were thus tested over a period of 5 years. Caries activity was greatly enhanced by the eating, between meals, of sticky sweets (toffees and caramels) that were retained on the teeth. Sucrose at mealtimes only, had little effect (Fig. 3.9). The incidence of caries fell to its original low level when toffees or caramels were no longer given, and caries activity was very slight in the control group having the low carbohydrate diet.

In another large-scale clinical experiment in Turku (Finland) an experimental group was allowed a wide range of foods sweetened with xylitol (a sugar alcohol) but no sucrose. The control group was allowed as much sugary (sucrose-containing) foods as desired. After 2 years the experimental group showed 90% less caries than those who had been allowed sucrose.

Essential features of sucrose incriminating it as the most cariogenic substrate are summarised in Table 3.9.

Use of sugar substitutes (artificial sweeteners) in place of sucrose greatly reduces caries activity. The cariogenicity of sugars and artificial sweeteners are summarised in Table 3.10.

SUSCEPTIBILITY OF TEETH TO CARIES

Teeth may be resistant to decay because of factors affecting the structure of the tooth during formation. Serious efforts were made in the past to confirm the misguided belief that dental caries was due to hypocalcification of the teeth and was

THE EFFECTS ON DENTAL CARIES FREQUENCY OF SUPPLEMENTS OF SWEET FOODS DURING OR BETWEEN MEALS

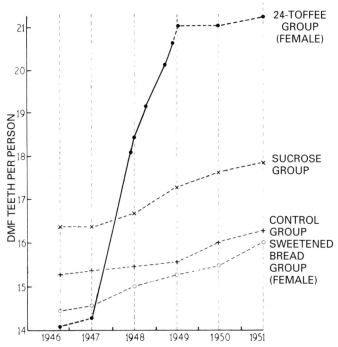

Fig. 3.9 The Vipeholm dental caries study. A simplified diagram showing the results in some of the groups of patients and in particular the striking effect on caries activity of sticky sweets eaten between meals when compared with the eating of sweet stuffs at mealtimes. The broken lines indicate those who consumed sugar only at meals, the continuous line shows those who consumed sugar both at and between meals. (After Gustafsson et al 1954 Acta Odontologica Scandinavica 11:232.)

Table 3.9 Factors determining the cariogenicity of sucrose

- Sucrose forms up to a third of the carbohydrate content of many persons' diets
- It promotes colonisation of teeth by *Streptococcus mutans*
- Its disaccharide bond alone contains enough energy to react with bacterial enzymes to form extracellular dextran matrix
- Its small molecule allows it to diffuse readily into plaque
- Bacterial metabolism of sucrose is rapid

Table 3.10 Sugars and non-sugar sweeteners

Compound	Nature and uses	Cariogenicity
Sucrose	A disaccharide sugar (β1–4-linked glucose–fructose)	Highest of all sugars
Glucose, fructose	Monosaccharide sugars	Less cariogenic than sucrose
Lactose and galactose	Monosaccharide (lactose) and disaccharide (galactose) sugars	Less cariogenic than sucrose
Glucose syrups and maltodextrins	Hydrolysis products of starch used as bulk sweeteners	Less cariogenic than sugars
Hydrogenated glucose syrup and lycasins	Hydrolysis products of starch which are then hydrogenated, used as bulk sweeteners	Less cariogenic than sugars
Isomalt	Mixture of two unusual 12-carbon sugars	Low cariogenicity
Xylitol, sorbitol, mannitol, lactitol etc.	Sugar alcohols (polyols) sometimes used as bulk sweeteners	Non-cariogenic
Saccharin, aspartame, thaumatin, acesulfame K and cyclamate	Non-sugar intense sweeteners	Non-cariogenic

essentially a vitamin deficiency disease. This simplistic view of course ignored the extensive epidemiological findings that the best-nourished populations had the worst record for dental disease while poverty-stricken communities on deficient diets had a low caries prevalence, as discussed earlier.

Hereditary hypoplasia or hypocalcification of the teeth in which there are severe disturbances of structure are also not particularly susceptible to caries and there is no evidence that the degree of calcification of the teeth affects their resistance to caries. However, newly erupted teeth are generally caries susceptible, apparently because of a hypomineralised enamel structure which is made progressively less vulnerable by deposition of materials from saliva.

Effects of fluorides

Fluorides from drinking water and other sources, are taken up by calcifying tissues during development. When the fluoride content of the water is 1 ppm or more the incidence of caries

Table 3.11 Actions of fluoride on dental caries

- Fluoride is incorporated into the teeth during development
- Fluoride acts mainly after eruption in early lesions by reducing enamel solubility and favouring remineralisation
- A constant supply of small amounts of fluoride is most effective in reducing dental caries
- Floride *may* reduce acid generation in plaque

declines substantially. Fluoride may affect caries activity by a variety of mechanisms (Table 3.11). Exposure to fluoride during dental development affects the structure of the developing teeth. This is shown by mottling of the enamel produced by excessive levels of fluoride. However, it is believed that the lower incidence of dental caries where water is fluoridated is due to its continued environmental effect on the teeth to reduce solubility of the enamel and promote remineralisation. These effects may be more important than the effect of fluoride on structure.

Fluoride is the only nutrient which has been proved to have this protective action. Despite the difficulties in distinguishing the degree of resistance of the teeth from the virulence of their cariogenic environment, it has become clear that fluorides have had a major impact on caries prevalence. There has undoubtedly been a significant decline in the prevalence of dental caries in countries where drinking water has been fluoridated. In Britain, as a result of widespread use of fluoridised dentifrices, there has also been so great a decrease in the disease as significantly to affect the nature of dental practice. These changes cannot be related to any comparable decline in sucrose consumption.

SALIVA AND DENTAL CARIES

The immediate environment of the teeth is bacterial plaque, but saliva is the medium in which plaque develops and works. Though saliva inevitably plays some part in the process of caries, it is a complex secretion whose rates of flow, composition and properties are not easy to determine.

Effects of desalivation

Salivary flow is highly important in clearing cariogenic foods from the mouth. In animals, removal or inactivation of major salivary glands leads to increased caries activity roughly in proportion to the reduction in saliva production. Dental caries may also become rampant in humans with xerostomia due to salivary gland disease (Ch. 18).

Rate of flow and buffering power

The buffering power of saliva depends mainly on its bicarbonate content and is increased at high rates of flow. The buffering power of the saliva affects the buffering power of dental plaque to some degree and helps to prevent the pH from falling to very low levels. A rapid flow rate, with greater salivary buffering power that is associated, has been found to be associated with low caries activity. In Down's syndrome, caries activity is low in spite of gross accumulation of plaque and immunodeficiencies possibly because of the high rate of salivation with greater buffering power. Whilst a rapid flow of saliva of low viscosity assists clearance of foodstuffs from the mouth, other physical properties of different salivas have not been shown to have a significant relationship to caries activity.

Other factors

Inorganic components and enamel maturation

Radioactive isotope studies suggest that there is some exchange of calcium and phosphate ions between enamel surface and saliva. In particular enamel undergoes post-eruptive changes. Clinical observations suggest that newly erupted teeth are more susceptible to caries than adult teeth and radioactive tracer studies show that newly erupted teeth can incorporate 10 to 20 times as much inorganic material in ionic form as adult teeth. More important is that saliva is a vehicle for fluoride which can enter plaque from the saliva and affect caries activity.

Enzymic activity

Salivary amylase breaks down polysaccharides such as starch. This contribution to digestion is small, and its main value is to make food residues on the teeth more soluble to assist their clearance. The breakdown of polysaccharides leads to production of sugars, but the amounts and their contribution to caries are small and are only likely to be seen with experimental sucrose-deficient diets. Usually, the amount of sucrose present in the diet overwhelms that produced by amylase activity. In general, therefore, amylase activity and caries prevalence are not closely related.

Antibacterial activities

Saliva contains thiocyanates, a lysozyme-like substance and other theoretically antibacterial substances. Nevertheless the mouth teems with bacteria, and there is no evidence that non-specific antibacterial substances in saliva have any significant effect on caries activity.

Immunological defences

IgA is secreted in saliva but small amounts of IgG enter the mouth from the gingival crevice. Persons who suffer from defects in non-specific host defences (complement and neutrophils) or specific immunological defences (IgA deficiency, Down's syndrome or AIDS) to not appear to suffer an excess of dental caries. Nevertheless, an immunological host resistance to dental

caries is detectable experimentally in man and appears to act by reducing the number of *S. mutans* in plaque. The effect does not appear to be very potent and is easily overwhelmed if the diet is high in sucrose or if low levels of the relevant antibody are produced.

Immunological defences against *S. mutans* could be mediated by salivary IgA or serum IgG from the crevicular fluid. Although salivary IgA is capable of preventing caries in experimental animals it appears to play no significant role in humans. Immunisation of monkeys against *S. mutans* generates specific serum IgG which protects them against caries. Serum IgG also appears to protect against *S. mutans* in humans but the response varies widely between individuals.

It has been shown that dripping a solution of monoclonal antibody against *S. mutans* onto the teeth prevents recolonisation by *S. mutans* in humans. However, plaque must be removed before treatment by using chlorhexidine and effective oral hygiene. This effect of antibody lasts for several months after applications and this 'passive immunisation' may reduce caries activity significantly.

Key facts about the effects of saliva on plaque activity are summarised in Table 3.12.

Table 3.12 Key facts about the effects of saliva on plaque activity

- Salivary components contribute to plaque formation
- Sucrose in saliva is taken up by plaque
- The buffering power of saliva may limit the fall in pH caused by acid formed in plaque
- The buffering power of saliva is related to the rate of secretion. High flow rates *may* be associated with lower caries activity
- Gross reduction in salivary secretion leads to increased caries activity when a cariogenic diet is eaten
- IgA is present in saliva but has little effect on caries activity

The main biochemical events in dental plaque in the development of dental caries are summarised diagrammatically in Figure 3.10.

PATHOLOGY OF ENAMEL CARIES

Enamel is the usual site of the initial lesion unless dentine or cementum becomes exposed by gingival recession. Enamel, the hardest and densest tissue in the body, consists almost entirely of calcium apatite with only a minute organic content. It therefore forms a formidable barrier to bacterial attack. However, once enamel has been breached, infection of dentine can spread with relatively little obstruction. Preventive measures must therefore be aimed primarily at stopping the attack or at making enamel more resistant.

The essential nature of the carious attack on enamel is permeation of acid into its substance. The crystalline lattice of calcium apatite crystals is relatively impermeable but part of the organic matrix of enamel which envelops the apatite

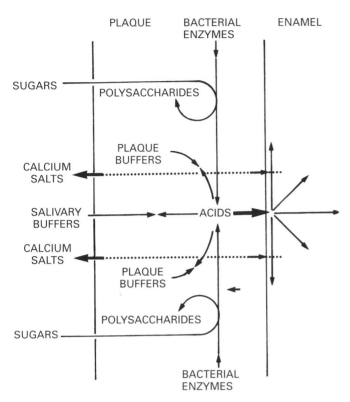

PLAQUE   BACTERIAL   ENAMEL
          ENZYMES

SUGARS

POLYSACCHARIDES

CALCIUM
SALTS

PLAQUE
BUFFERS

SALIVARY
BUFFERS

ACIDS

CALCIUM
SALTS

PLAQUE
BUFFERS

POLYSACCHARIDES

SUGARS

BACTERIAL
ENZYMES

Fig. 3.10 Diagrammatic representation of the main biochemical events in dental plaque, initiating caries. (From McCracken A W, Cawson R A 1983 Clinical and oral microbiology. McGraw-Hill.)

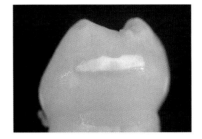

Fig. 3.11 Early enamel caries, a white spot lesion, in a deciduous molar. The lesion forms below the contact point and in consequence is much larger than an interproximal lesion in a permanent tooth (see Fig. 3.20).

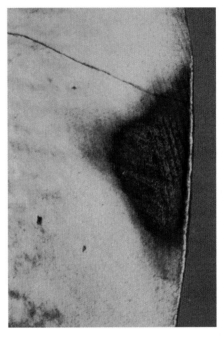

Fig. 3.12 Early interproximal caries. Ground section in water viewed by polarised light. The body of the lesion and the intact surface layer are visible. The translucent and dark zones are not seen until the section is viewed immersed in quinoline.

crystals, has a relatively high water content and is permeable to hydrogen ions. Permeation of enamel by acid causes a series of submicroscopic changes. This process of enamel caries is a dynamic one and, initially at least, consists of alternating phases of demineralisation and remineralisation, rather than a continuous process of dissolution.

Enamel caries develops in four main phases (Table 3.13). These stages of enamel caries are distinguishable microscopically and are also clinically significant. In particular, the early (white spot) lesion is potentially reversible, but cavity formation is irreversible and requires restorative measures to substitute for the lost tissue.

Table 3.13   Stages of enamel caries

- The early (submicroscopic) lesion
- Phase of nonbacterial enamel crystal destruction
- Cavity formation
- Bacterial invasion of enamel

The early lesion

The earliest visible changes are seen as a white opaque spot that forms just adjacent to a contact point. Despite the chalky appearance the enamel is hard and smooth to the probe (Fig. 3.11). The microscopic changes under this early white spot

lesion may be seen in undecalcified sections but more readily when polarised light is used. Microradiography indicates the degree of demineralisation seen in the different zones.

The initial lesion is conical in shape with its apex towards the dentine, and a series of four zones of differing translucency can be discerned. Working back from the deepest, advancing edge of the lesion, these zones consist first of a *translucent zone* most deeply; immediately within this is a second *dark zone*; the third consists of the *body of the lesion* and the fourth consists of the *surface zone* (Fig. 3.12).

These initial changes are not due to bacterial invasion, but due to bacterial lactic or other acids causing varying degrees of demineralisation and remineralisation in the enamel. The features of these zones are summarised in Table 3.14.

The *translucent zone* is the first observable change. The appearance of the translucent zone results from formation of submicroscopic spaces or pores apparently located at prism

Table 3.14 **Key features of the enamel zones preceding cavity formation**

Zone	Key features	Comments
Translucent zone	Earliest and deepest demineralisation. 1% mineral loss	Broader in progressing caries, narrow or absent in arrested or remineralised lesions
Dark zone	2–4% mineral loss overall but a zone of remineralisation just behind the advancing front	Broader in arrested or remineralised lesions, narrow in advancing lesions
Body	5–25% mineral loss	Broader in progressing caries, replaced by a broad dark zone in arrested or remineralised lesions
Surface zone	1% mineral loss. A zone of remineralisation resulting from the diffusion barrier and mineral content of plaque. Cavitation is loss of this layer, allowing bacteria to enter the lesion	Relatively constant width, a little thicker in arrested or remineralising lesions

boundaries and other junctional sites such as the striae of Retzius. When the section is mounted in quinoline, it fills the pores, and since it has the same refractive index as enamel the normal structural features disappear and the appearance of the pores is enhanced (Fig. 3.13). Microradiography confirms that the changes in the translucent zone are due to demineralisation.

The *dark zone* is fractionally superficial to the translucent zone. Polarised light microscopy shows that the volume of the pores in this zone has increased to 2–4% of the enamel volume. This change is due mainly to formation of additional small pores. Two different-size pores thus coexist in the dark zone. The small ones are so minute that molecules of quinoline are unable to enter and the tissue has become transformed into a molecular sieve. The small pores therefore remain filled with air — this appears to produce the zone's dark appearance.

Microradiography confirms that the dark zone has suffered a greater degree of demineralisation. However, when the lesion is exposed to saliva or synthetic calcifying solutions in vitro, the dark zone actually extends further. This may indicate that the formation of the dark zone may be due not merely to creation of new porosities but possibly also to remineralisation of the large pores of the translucent zone so that they become micropores impermeable to quinoline. It is widely believed therefore that these changes in the dark zone are evidence of remineralisation, as discussed later.

The *body of the lesion* forms the bulk of the lesion and extends from just beneath the surface zone to the dark zone. By transmitted light the body of the lesion is comparatively translucent compared with normal enamel and sharply demarcated from the dark zone. Within the body of the lesion the striae of

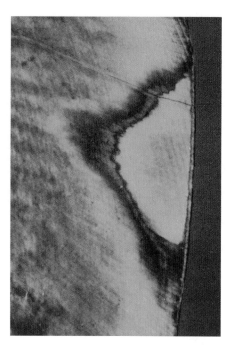

Fig. 3.13 Early interproximal caries. Ground section viewed by polarised light after immersion in quinoline. Quinoline has filled the larger pores, causing most of the fine detail in the body of the lesion to disappear (Fig. 3.12), but the dark zone with its smaller pores is accentuated.

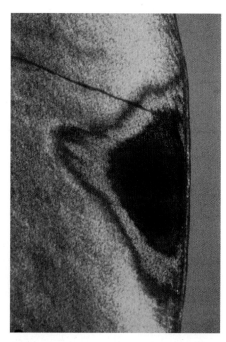

Fig. 3.14 The same lesion (Figs 3.12 and 3.13) viewed dry under polarised light to show the full extent of demineralisation. (Figs 3.12–3.14 by kind permission of Professor Leon Silverstone and the Editor of Dental Update 1989;10:262.)

Retzius appear enhanced, particularly when mounted in quinoline and viewed under polarised light. Polarised light examination (Fig. 3.14) also shows that the pore volume is 5% at the periphery but increases to at least 25% in the centre.

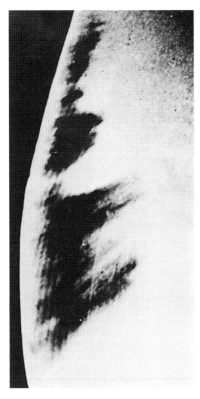

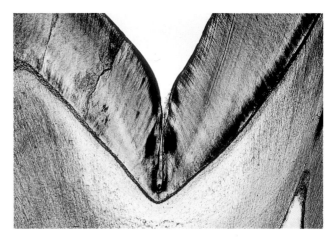

Fig. 3.16 Undecalcified section showing early enamel lesions in the enamel surrounding and deep to an occlusal pit.

Fig. 3.15 Early interproximal caries. A microradiograph of the same section as in Figures 3.12–14, showing radiolucency following the same pattern, the intact surface zone and accentuation of the striae of Retzius. (Kindly lent by the late Professor A I Darling.)

Microradiography, which will detect demineralisation in excess of 5%, shows that the area of radiolucency corresponds closely with the size and shape of the body of the lesion, in contrast to the surface zone which appears relatively radiopaque (Fig. 3.15). Alternating radiopaque and radiolucent lines, about 30 μm apart, can also be seen passing obliquely through the subsurface region. The radiolucent lines show an apparently preferential demineralisation and probably represent the striae of Retzius. At higher magnifications, still finer lines running at right angles to the enamel surface, and others parallel to the surface, may be discerned. These lines may represent preferential demineralisation along the junctional sites mentioned earlier, and represent the prism boundaries and the cross striations, respectively.

The *surface zone* represents one of the most important changes in enamel caries in terms of prevention and management of the disease. It shows the paradoxical feature that it has not merely remained intact during this stage of the attack but remains more heavily mineralised and radiopaque than the deeper zones. It has a pore volume of only 1%.

When the surface zone is removed and the enamel is exposed to an acid buffer, the more highly mineralised surface zone reappears over the deeper changes described earlier. The surface zone therefore appears to form partly by remineralisation. The remineralising salts may come either from those concen-

trated in the plaque or from precipitation of calcium and phosphate ions diffusing outwards as the deeper zones are demineralised.

In pit and fissure caries the same changes take place but as acid diffuses out from the pit the lesion forms a ring round it. However, in a two-dimensional view, the same zones as in smooth surface caries are seen on either side of the fissure (Fig. 3.16).

As noted earlier, the initial attack on enamel appears to be by highly mobile hydrogen ions permeating the organic matrix enabling them to attack the surface of the apatite crystals. The apatite crystals become progressively smaller. Microdissection of the translucent zone has shown that the apatite crystals have declined in diameter from the normal of 35–40 nm to 25–30 nm and in the body of the lesion to 10–30 nm. In the dark zone, by contrast, enamel crystals appeared to have grown to 50–100 nm and in the surface zone to 35–40 nm. These findings also suggest that demineralisation and remineralisation are alternating processes. However, as the lesion progresses and cavitation develops, demineralisation comes to dominate the process.

In broad general terms therefore, enamel crystallites are progressively dissolved until disintegration becomes visible microscopically. Defects eventually become large enough to allow bacteria to enter.

There is evidence of preferential destruction of the prism cores, and experimentally a similar effect is seen when enamel is exposed to dilute acid (Figs 3.17 and 3.18). Whatever the precise nature of these changes, bacteria do not physically penetrate enamel until acid destruction of the tissue has provided pathways large enough for them to enter (Fig. 3.20).

Cavity formation

Once bacteria have penetrated the enamel they reach the amelodentinal junction and spread laterally to undermine the enamel. This has three major effects. First, the enamel loses the support of the dentine and is therefore greatly weakened. Second, it is attacked from beneath (Fig. 3.21). Third, spread of bacteria along the amelodentinal junction allows them to attack the dentine

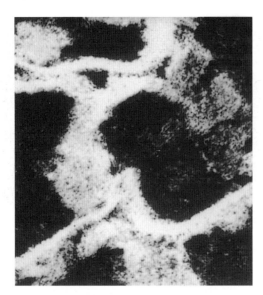

Fig. 3.17 Chalky enamel. An electronphotomicrograph of chalky enamel produced by the action of very dilute acid. The crystallites of calcium salts remain intact in the prism sheaths, while the prism cores and some of the interprismatic substance have been destroyed. The same appearance is seen in chalky enamel caused by early caries. (From a picture kindly lent by Dr K Little.)

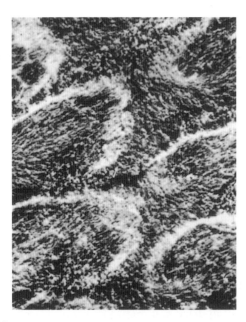

Fig. 3.18 The organic matrix of developing enamel. An electronphotomicrograph of a section across the lines of the prisms before calcification showing the matrix to be more dense in the region of the prism sheaths than in the prism cores or interprismatic substance. (From a photograph kindly lent by Dr K Little.)

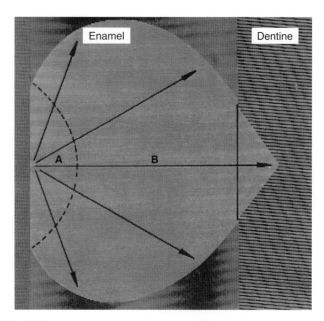

Fig. 3.19 Diagram summarising the main features of the precavitation phase of enamel caries as indicated here in this final stage of acid attack on enamel before bacterial invasion, decalcification of dentine has begun. The area (A) would be radiolucent in a bite-wing film but the area (B) could be visualised only in a section by polarised light microscopy or microradiography. Clinically the enamel would appear solid and intact but the surface would be marked by an opaque white spot over the area (A) as seen in Figure 3.11 (From McCracken A W, Cawson R A 1983 Clinical and oral microbiology. McGraw-Hill.)

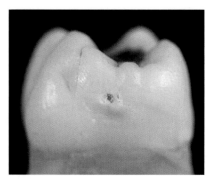

Fig. 3.20 Early cavitation in enamel caries. The surface layer of the white spot lesion has broken down, allowing plaque bacteria into the enamel.

As undermining of the enamel continues, it starts to collapse under the stress of mastication and to fragment around the edge of the (clinically obvious) cavity. By this stage, bacterial damage to the dentine is extensive.

The process of enamel caries is summarised in Table 3.15.

PATHOLOGY OF DENTINE CARIES

The *initial (non-bacterial) lesion* forms deep to carious enamel before a cavity has formed. Diffusion of acid into the dentine leaves its collagenous matrix intact at this stage. However, once

over a wide area (Fig. 3.21). Thus the primary lesion provides the bridgehead for the attack on enamel, but undermining of the enamel determines the area of a cavity. Clinically this is frequently evident when there is no more than a pinhole lesion in an occlusal pit, but cutting away the surrounding enamel shows it to be widely undermined.

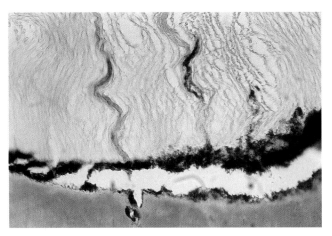

Fig. 3.21 Enamel caries. Infection has spread along the amelodentinal junction undermining and invading the deep surface of the enamel. The terminations of the dentinal tubules are also infected but destruction, at this stage, is mainly at the expense of the enamel.

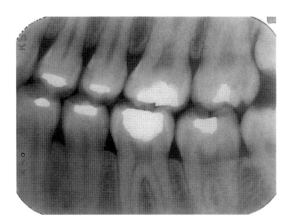

Fig. 3.22 Bite-wing radiograph showing interproximal caries below many of the contact points.

bacteria have penetrated the enamel, they spread along the amelodentinal junction to attack the dentine over a wide area. The lesion is therefore conical with its apex towards the pulp (Fig. 3.23).

The *infected lesion* is facilitated by the dentinal tubules which form a pathway open to bacteria. After demineralisation, the dentine matrix is progressively destroyed by proteolysis.

Streptococci play the major role in the attack on enamel, but lactobacilli may be as important in dentine caries. As the lesion progresses, the bacterial population becomes increasingly mixed

---

Table 3.15 Stages of enamel caries

- Permeation of the organic matrix by hydrogen ions causes submicroscopic changes
- The early damage is submicroscopic and seen as a series of zones of differing translucency
- Microradiography confirms that these changes represent areas of increasing demineralisation
- The surface zone is largely formed by remineralisation
- There is alternating demineralisation and remineralisation but demineralisation is predominant as cavity formation progresses
- Bacteria cannot invade enamel until demineralisation provides pathways large enough for them to enter

---

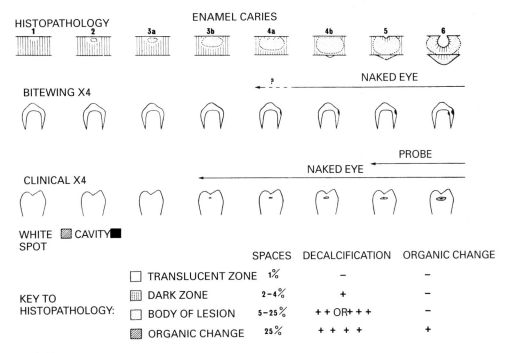

Fig. 3.23 This diagram summarises the sequential changes in enamel from the stage of the initial lesion to early cavity formation and relates the different stages in the development of the lesion with the radiographic appearances and clinical findings. (Diagram kindly lent by the late Professor I A Darling and reproduced by courtesy of the Editor of the British Dental Journal 1959; 107:27–30.)

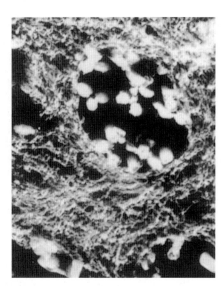

Fig. 3.24 Infection of the dentinal tubules. This electronphotomicrograph shows bacteria in the lumen of the tubules. Between the tubules is the collagenous matrix of the dentine. (From a picture kindly lent by Dr K Little.)

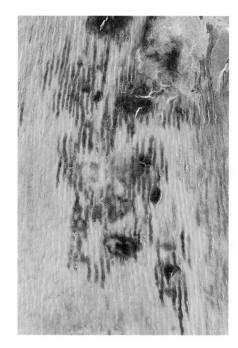

Fig. 3.25 Caries of dentine. Infected tubules and fusiform masses of bacteria have expanded into the softened tissue. Adjacent tubules in the demineralised dentine have been bent and pushed aside by these masses.

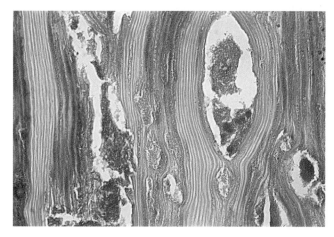

Fig. 3.26 Advanced dentine caries. The dentine is disintegrating (left). To the right is a large liquefaction focus and tubules packed with bacteria.

and their relative contributions to dentine destruction become more difficult to disentangle.

At first, the decalcified dentine retains its normal morphology, and no bacteria can be seen. Once bacteria have reached the amelodentinal junction they extend down the tubules, soon fill them and spread along any lateral branches. The tubules become distended into spindle shapes by the expanding masses of bacteria and their products, which the softened matrix cannot confine. As a result, adjacent less heavily infected tubules become bent. Later still, the intervening tubule walls are destroyed and collections of bacteria in adjacent tubules coalesce to form irregular *liquefaction foci*. These in turn coalesce to form progressively more widespread tissue destruction (Figs 3.25 and 3.26).

In some areas bacteria also spread laterally, and, occasionally, large bacteria-filled clefts form at right angles to the general direction of the tubules. Clinically, these clefts may allow carious dentine sometimes to be excavated in flakes in a plane parallel to the surface (Fig. 3.27).

The main events in dentine caries are summarised in Table 3.16.

Protective reactions of dentine and pulp under caries

The reactions in dentine are mainly due to odontoblast activity, so that dentine and pulp should be considered as one tissue. These reactions are not specific and may be provoked by other irritants such as attrition, erosion, abrasion and restorative procedures. Reactionary changes in dentine start even before cavity formation in enamel but are more likely to develop significantly under slowly progressing caries.

Reactionary changes in dentine are summarised in Table 3.17.

These reactionary changes start to develop early but at best can only slow the advance of dental caries. Even sclerotic dentine is vulnerable to bacterial acid and proteolysis and once bacteria have penetrated the normal dentine they can invade any reactionary dentine to reach the pulp (Figs 3.28–3.31).

Root surface caries

When the neck of the tooth becomes exposed by recession of the gingival margin in later life a stagnation area may be formed and the cementum attacked. Cementum is readily decalcified

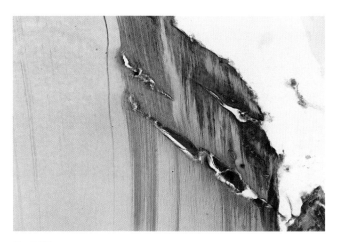

Fig. 3.27 Clefts in carious dentine. Infection is tracking along the tubules but has also spread across the tubules, forming heavily infected clefts. The appearances suggest that there are lines of weakness in the dentine, along which infection spreads easily.

Table 3.16   Key events in the development of dentine caries

- Non-bacterial, precavitation, acid softening of matrix
- Migration of pioneer bacteria along tubules
- Distortion of tubules by expanding masses of bacteria
- Breakdown of intervening matrix forming liquefaction foci
- Progressive disintegration of remaining matrix tissue

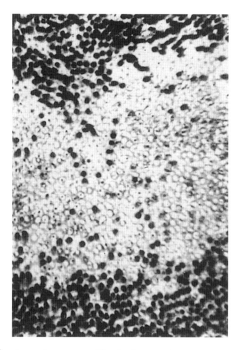

Fig. 3.28 A translucent zone. The dentinal tubules are seen in cross-section. Those in the centre of the picture have become obliterated by calcification of their contents; only the original outline of the tubules remains visible and the zone appears translucent to transmitted light. On either side are patent tubules filled with stain. (Kindly lent by Dr G C Blake, and reproduced by courtesy of the Honorary Editors, Proceedings of the Royal Society of Medicine 1958; 51:678.)

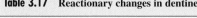

Table 3.17   Reactionary changes in dentine

Response	Key facts
Tubular sclerosis	Peritubular dentine reduces the size of the dentinal tubules, preventing bacterial penetration and generating a more heavily mineralised dentine. Tubular sclerosis usually forms in a band about halfway between the pulp and amelodentinal junction. It forms a translucent zone which may be visible radiographically and is detectable with hand instruments when excavating caries
Regular reactionary dentine	Forms at the pulp dentine interface and retains the tubular structure of dentine. Forms in response to mild stimuli and may obliterate pulp horns, increasing the dentine thickness between caries and pulp. Unfortunately it often forms most on the floor and sides of the pulp chamber where it is of little value in defence against caries
Irregular reactionary dentine	Forms in response to moderate or severe insult by caries and correspondingly ranges from dentine with irregular tubules to a disorganised bone-like mineralised tissue ('eburnoid')
Dead tracts	Formed when odontoblasts die and their tubules become sealed off. If peritubular dentine formation was extensive before odontoblast death the dead tract may be sclerotic and inhibit advance of caries. If not it may allow more rapid progress

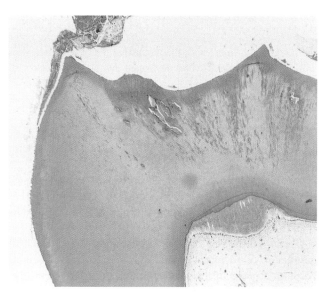

Fig. 3.29 Regular reactionary dentine below occlusal caries. Bacteria extend more than half the distance from the amelodentinal junction to the pulp and the underlying pulp horn has been obliterated by reactionary dentine. The reactionary dentine bulges into the pulp. Note the lack of inflammation in the pulp.

and presents little barrier to infection. The cementum therefore softens beneath the plaque over a wide area, producing a saucer-shaped cavity, and the underlying dentine is soon involved. Cementum is invaded along the direction of Sharpey's fibres. Infection spreads between the lamellae along

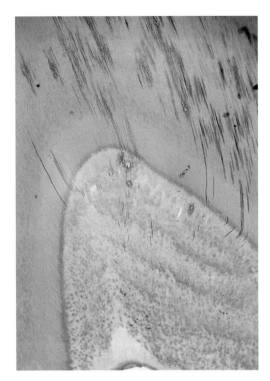

Fig. 3.30 Secondary (reactionary) dentine and caries. Regular, tubular, secondary dentine has formed under a carious cavity. A line marks the junction of the primary and secondary dentine where the tubules change direction. Bacteria spreading down the tubules of the primary tissue have extended along the junction and into the tubules of the reactionary dentine.

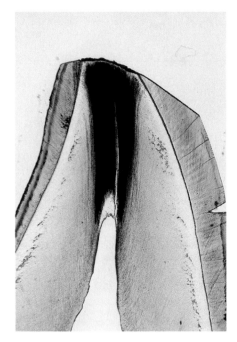

Fig. 3.31 A dead tract. The empty tubules below the worn incisal edge have been filled with a stain to which they are permeable from the surface, so that the whole zone appears black. At the proximal end of the tubules the dead tract has been sealed off by impermeable reactionary dentine through which the stain cannot penetrate. The pulp is thus protected from irritants penetrating along the dentinal tubules.

the incremental lines, with the result that the dentine becomes split up and progressively destroyed by a combination of demineralisation and proteolysis. The further progress of caries in the underlying dentine is essentially similar to that in other parts of the tooth.

Arrested caries and remineralisation

Precavity (white spot) interstitial caries may become arrested when the adjacent tooth is lost so that the stagnation area is removed. The lesion may become remineralised by minerals from the saliva.

Dentine caries may occasionally be arrested as a result of destruction of so much enamel that a wide area of dentine becomes exposed. If this surface is then subjected to attrition, plaque deposition may be prevented. More frequently, but still uncommonly, dentine is exposed by attrition and remains caries-free for the same reason. It becomes smooth, polished and stained (see Fig. 4.31).

Under favourable conditions carious demineralisation can be reversed and early lesions can remineralise. Use of fluorides and consumption of a less cariogenic diet may cause a surface

lesion in enamel to heal entirely. Even under natural conditions, approximately 50% of interproximal enamel lesions may show no radiographic evidence of progression for 3 years. Similarly, in some patients, secondary caries may not necessarily develop at the margins of restorations overhanging the enamel.

Adult and childhood caries

In adults, caries usually progresses slowly and a small cavity may take several months to develop. By contrast, childhood caries, particularly of deciduous teeth, may be so rapid that the pulp becomes exposed long before the tooth is due to be shed.

Pulpitis

Pulpitis follows penetration of dentine by bacteria or their metabolites and represents the breakdown of the protective hard dental tissues and opening of the soft tissues to infection.

Clinical aspects of reactions to caries

The reactive changes described above render the dentine immediately under a carious cavity more or less impermeable, unless caries is advancing very rapidly.

SUGGESTED FURTHER READING

Bowen W H 1999 Wither or whither caries research? Caries Res 33:1–3

Brathall D 1992 Caries, views and perspectives. Scand J Dent Res 100:47–51

Carlsson J 1989 Microbial aspects of frequent intake of products with high sugar concentrations. Scand J Dent Res 97:110–114

Costerton J W et al 1987 Bacterial biofilms in nature and disease. Ann Rev Microbiol 41:435–464

Frank M J 1990 Structural events in the caries process in enamel, cementum and dentine. J Dent Res 69(Spec Iss):559–566

Gibbons R J 1989 Bacterial adhesion to oral tissues: a model for infectious diseases. J Dent Res 68:750–760

Hardie J M, Whiley R A 1999 Plaque microbiology of crown caries. In *Dental Plaque revisited*. Ed Newman H N, Wilson M. Bioline, Cardiff

Kishimoto D, Hay D I, Gibbons R J 1989 A human salivary protein which promotes adhesion of *Streptococcus mutans* serotype c strains to hydroxyapatite. Infect Immun 57:3702–3707

Levine R S 1989 Saliva: 2. Saliva and dental caries. Dental Update 14:158–165

Liang L, Drake D, Doyle R J 1989 Stability of the glucan-binding lectin of oral streptococci. J Dent Res 68(Spec Iss):1677

McHugh W D 1999 Dental plaque: thirty years on. In *Dental plaque revisited*. Ed Newman H N, Wilson M. Bioline, Cardiff

Mergenhagen S E et al 1987 Molecular basis of bacterial adhesion in the oral cavity. Rev Infect Dis 9(Suppl 5):S467–475

Moller H, Scroder U 1986 Early natural subsurface caries. A SEM study of the enamel surface before and after remineralisation. Caries Res 20:97–102

Newbrun E 1989 Frequent sugar intake — then and now: interpretation of the main results. Scand J Dent Res 97:103–109

Roberts M W, Li S-H 1987 Oral findings in anorexia nervosa and bulimia nervosa: a study of 47 cases. JADA 115:407–410

Rugg-Gunn A J, Hackett A F, Appleton D R 1987 Relative cariogenicity of starch and sugars in a 2-year longitudinal study of 405 English schoolchildren. Caries Res 21:464–473

Russell M W, Hajishengallis G, Childers N K et al 1999 Secretory immunity in defense against cariogenic Mutans streptococci. Caries Res 33:4–15

Shaw J H 1987 Causes and control of dental caries. N Engl J Med 317:996–1003

Shellis R P, Dibdin G H 1988 Analysis of the buffer systems in dental plaque. J Dent Res 67:438–446

Tabak L A, Bowen W H 1989 Role of saliva (pellicle), diet and nutrition on plaque formation. J Dent Res 68(Spec Iss):1560–1566

Van Houte J 1994 Role of micro-organisms in caries etiology. J Dent Res 73:672–681

Woodward M, Walker A R P 1994 Sugar consumption and dental caries: evidence from 90 countries. Br Dent J 176:297–302

Pulpitis, apical periodontitis, resorption and hypercementosis

PULPITIS

Pulpitis is the most common cause of dental pain and loss of teeth in younger persons. The usual cause is caries penetrating the dentine but there are other possibilities (Table 4.1). Pulpitis, if untreated, is followed by death of the pulp and spread of infection through the apical foramina into the periapical tissues. This in turn causes periapical periodontitis.

Table 4.1 Causes of pulpitis

- Dental caries
- Traumatic exposure of the pulp
- Fracture of a crown or cusp
- Cracked tooth syndrome
- Thermal or chemical irritation

Dental caries is by far the most common cause and is usually obvious unless it has extended under the edge of a restoration.

Exposure during cavity preparation allows bacteria to enter the pulp and also damages it mechanically (Fig. 4.1).

Fracture may either open the pulp chamber or leave so thin a covering of dentine that bacteria can enter.

A tooth, particularly a restored premolar, may split, usually under masticatory stress (Fig. 4.2). These minute cracks are often invisible, but allow bacteria into the pulp chamber. The affected tooth may sometimes be identified by applying pressure to the occlusal fissure with a ball-ended burnisher to open up the crack. Pulp pain usually then results. Alternatively the crack may be made visible with oblique transillumination or, possibly more easily, by wetting the crown of the tooth with a dye such as fluorescein and visualising it with ultraviolet light.

Over-rapid cavity cutting, especially of deep cavities, can cause immediate damage to the pulp. Large unlined metal restorations may also allow continuous low-grade thermal stimuli to damage the pulp over a longer period. Some restorations without a protective lining, particularly, in the past were sufficiently irritant to kill the pulp.

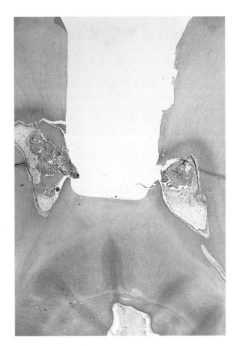

Fig. 4.1 Traumatic exposure. The pulp has been exposed during cavity preparation and dentine chippings and larger fragments have been driven into the pulp. The tooth was extracted before a strong inflammatory reaction has had time to develop but it is clear that some inflammatory cells have already localised around the debris which will have introduced many bacteria to the pulp.

Clinical features

Acute pulpitis

In the early stages the tooth is hypersensitive. Very cold or hot food causes a stab of pain which stops as soon as the irritant is removed. As inflammation progresses, pain becomes more persistent and there may be prolonged attacks of toothache. The pain may start spontaneously, often when the patient is trying to get to sleep.

The pain is partly due to the pressure on the irritated nerve endings by inflammatory infiltrate within the rigid pulp chamber and partly due to release of pain-producing substances from the damaged tissue. The pain at its worst is excruciatingly severe, sharp and stabbing in character. It is little affected by simple analgesics.

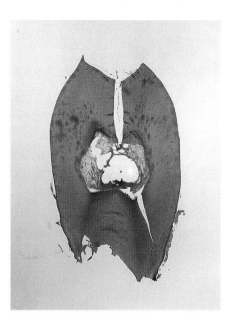

Fig. 4.2 Cracked tooth. The pulp died beneath this crack which was undetected clinically but which has opened up after decalcification of the tooth.

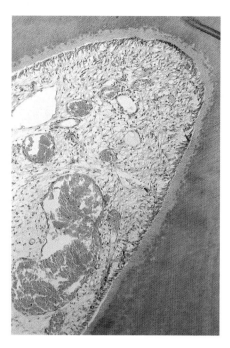

Fig. 4.3 Pulpal hyperaemia. While bacteria are still some distance from the pulp, acid permeating along the dentinal tubules gives rise to hyperaemia, oedema and a light cellular inflammatory infiltrate in the pulp.

Chronic pulpitis

The pulps of individual teeth are not precisely represented on the sensory cortex. The pulp pain is therefore poorly localised and may be felt in any of the teeth of the upper or lower jaw of the affected side. Rarely, pain may be referred to a more distant site such as the ear. Pulp pain is not provoked by pressure on the tooth. The patient can chew in comfort unless there is a large open cavity allowing fragments of food to press on the pulp through the softened dentine. Many pulps under large carious cavities die painlessly. The first indication is then development of periapical periodontitis, either with pain or seen by chance in a radiograph. In other cases there are bouts of dull pain, brought on by hot or cold stimuli or coming on spontaneously. There are often prolonged remissions.

Pathology

Pulpitis is caused by a mixed infection which usually enters from the mouth via a carious cavity.

Acute closed pulpitis

Histologically, there is initial hyperaemia limited to the area immediately beneth the irritant (Fig. 4.3). Infiltration by inflammatory cells and destruction of odontoblasts and adjacent mesenchyme follow. A limited areas of necrosis may result in formation of a minute abscess, localised by granulation tissue (Figs 4.4–4.6). Later, inflammation spreads until the pulp is obliterated by dilated blood vessels and acute inflammatory cells (Fig. 4.7). Necrosis follows.

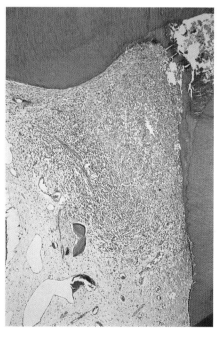

Fig. 4.4 Acute pulpitis. Beneath the carious exposure (top right) a dense inflammatory infiltrate is accumulating. More deeply, the pulp is intensely hyperaemic.

Chronic closed pulpitis

The main features are a predominantly mononuclear cell infiltrate and a more vigorous connective tissue reaction. A small area of pulpal necrosis and pus formation may be localised by a well-defined wall of granulation tissue, and a minute abscess

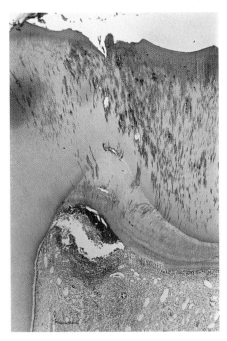

Fig. 4.5 Acute pulpitis. Infection has penetrated the reactionary dentine causing inflammation to spread down the pulp and pus to form in the corner.

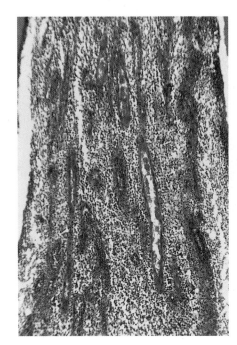

Fig. 4.7 Acute pulpitis – terminal stage. The entire pulp has been destroyed and replaced by inflammatory cells and dilated vessels.

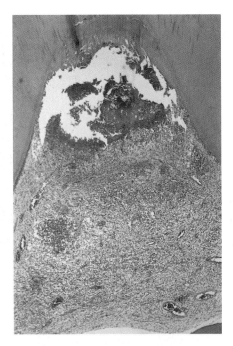

Fig. 4.6 Acute caries and pulpitis. Infection has penetrated to the pulp. Part of the pulp has been destroyed, and an abscess has formed, containing a bead of pus.

may thus form. The remainder of the pulp may then appear normal.

Rarely, inflammation may be well localised beneath an exposure so that a partial calcific barrier forms beneath the lesion, or considerable amounts of reactionary dentine continue

to form round the opening. Such changes are particularly likely to follow pulp capping. Calcific barriers (seen radiographically as 'dentine bridges') are frequently poorly formed, and inflammation progresses beneath them (Figs 4.8 and 4.9). However, in successful cases, formation of a complete barrier of tubular reactionary dentine may allow preservation of the remainder of the pulp.

The chief factor hampering pulpal survival is its enclosure within the rigid walls of the pulp chamber and, in fully formed teeth, the limited aperture for the apical vessels. In acute inflammation, these vessels can readily be compressed by inflammatory oedema and thrombose. The blood supply of the pulp is thus cut off and dies. This may be rapid in the case of acute pulpitis, or delayed in chronic lesions. The relatively prolonged survival of chronically inflamed pulps is shown by the persistence of symptoms over a long period. However, pulp death is the end result.

Open pulpitis

Occasionally the pulp survives but is chronically inflamed, beneath a wide exposure, despite the heavy infection (Fig. 4.10). This is traditionally believed to be associated with open apices which allow an adequate blood supply.

Chronic hyperplastic pulpitis (pulp polyp). Rarely, despite wide exposure and heavy infection, the pulp not merely survives but proliferates through the opening. This may even happen in fully formed teeth.

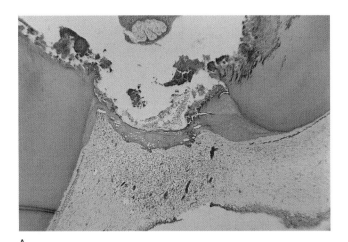

A

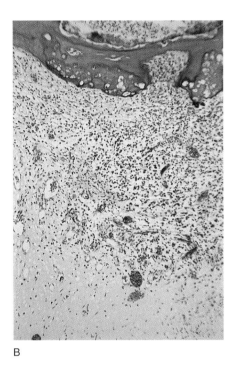

B

Fig. 4.8 Chronic pulpitis. **A.** Another pulpitis and formation of a calcific barrier. **B.** This higher power view shows the calcific barrier in more detail, in particular its irregular structure and failure to hold back the infection.

Clinically, a pulp polyp appears as a dusky red or pinkish soft nodule protruding into the cavity. It is painless but may be tender and bleed on probing. It should be distinguished from proliferating gingival tissue extending over the edge of the cavity by tracing its attachment (Fig. 4.11).

Histologically, few odontoblasts survive and the pulp becomes replaced by granulation tissue (Fig. 4.12). As this mass grows out into the cavity in the tooth it can become epithelialised and covered by a layer of well-formed stratified squamous epithelium. This protects the mass and allows inflammation under it to subside the fibrous tissue to replace the granulation tissue. This degree of pulpal proliferation can be seen in teeth with fully formed roots (Fig. 4.13).

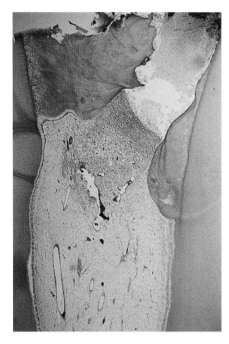

Fig. 4.9 Pulp capping. The procedure has allowed the pulp to survive until reactionary dentine has proliferated greatly beside the exposure. Failure of the procedure is indicated by the inflammatory cells concentrated below the opening.

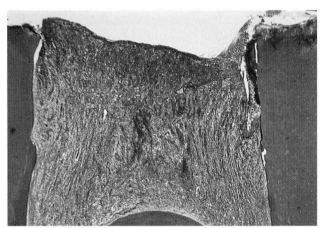

Fig. 4.10 Open pulpitis. Beneath the wide exposure the pulp has survived in the form of granulation tissue with the most dense inflammatory infiltrate beneath the open surface.

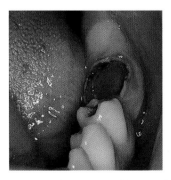

Fig. 4.11 Pulp polyp. An inflamed nodule of granulation tissue can be seen growing from the pulp chamber of this broken down first permanent molar.

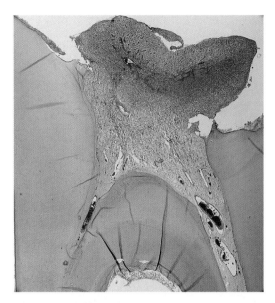

Fig. 4.12 Pulp polyp. A hyperplastic nodule of tissue is growing out through a wide exposure of the pulp. The masses of inflammatory cells and the many new vessels are characteristic of granulation tissue.

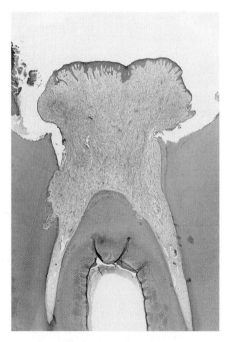

Fig. 4.13 Pulp polyp. In this broken down molar, granulation tissue is proliferating from the pulp cavity and has acquired an epithelial covering over much of its surface. Note also the internal resorption (left) as a result of pulpal inflammation.

Management

The chances of survival of an inflamed pulp are poor and treatment options are limited (Table 4.2).

Open pulpitis is usually associated with gross cavity formation and it is rarely possible to save the tooth, despite the vitality of the pulp. Key features of pulpitis are summarised in Table 4.3.

Table 4.2 Treatment options for pulpitis
● Extraction
● Endodontic treatment
● Pulp capping

Table 4.3 Key features of pulpitis
● Pulpitis is caused by infection or irritation of the pulp, usually by caries
● Severe stabbing pain in a tooth, triggered by hot or cold food or starting spontaneously, indicates acute irreversible pulpitis
● Pulp pain is poorly localised
● Chronic pulpitis is often symptomless
● Untreated pulpitis usually leads to death of the pulp and spread of infection to the periapical tissues

---

PULP CALCIFICATIONS

Pulp stones

Rounded masses of dentine may form within the pulp and can be seen in radiographs as small opacities. In the past they were thought to cause symptoms but are developmental anomalies. For unknown reasons, they are common in the teeth of patients with Ehlers–Danlos (floppy joint) syndrome, a genetic defect of collagen formation.

Histologically, pulp stones consist of dentine which may show complete or incomplete tubule formation (Fig. 4.14). A distinction used to be drawn between free and attached pulp stones. However, this is frequently an illusion caused by a plane of section which fails to pass through the connection between the pulp stone and the pulp wall.

DIFFUSE CALCIFICATION

Amorphous dystrophic calcifications may sometimes be seen histologically in the pulp and are thought to be an age-related degenerative change.

Pulp stones and diffuse calcification are of no clinical significance except insofar as they may obstruct endodontic treatment. Otherwise they can be ignored.

PERIAPICAL PERIODONTITIS

Periapical inflammation is usually due to spread of infection following death of the pulp (Table 4.4). It characteristically causes tenderness of the tooth in its socket. Local (periapical) periodontitis must be distinguished from chronic (marginal) periodontitis, in which infection and destruction of the

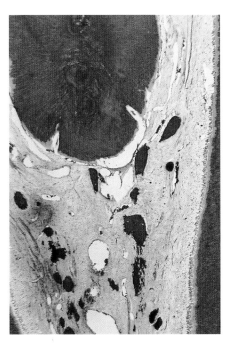

Fig. 4.14 Pulp stones. A rounded nodule of calcified tissue in which some irregular tubules may be seen is present in the pulp. Smaller stones and amorphous calcifications surround the main mass (trichrome stain).

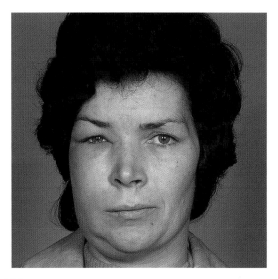

Fig. 4.15 Oedema due to acute apical periodontitis. An acute periapical infection of a canine has perforated the buccal plate of bone causing oedema of the face; this quickly subsided when the infection was treated.

Table 4.4 Causes of apical periodontitis

- Infection
- Trauma
- Chemical irritation

supporting tissues spread from chronic infection of the gingival margins (Ch. 5).

Infection is far the most common cause. The usual sequence of events is caries, pulpitis, death of the pulp and periodontitis.

The pulp sometimes dies from a blow which damages the apical vessels. The necrotic pulp probably becomes infected by bacteria from the gingival margins, leading to apical periodontitis. A high filling, or biting suddenly on a hard object, sometimes cause an acute but usually transient periodontitis.

During endodontic treatment, instruments may be pushed through the apex or side of the root, damaging the periodontal membrane and carrying infected debris from the pulp chamber into the wound.

Irritant antiseptics used to sterilise a root canal can escape through the apex and damage the surrounding tissues. A root-canal filling may also extend beyond the apex with similar effect.

ACUTE APICAL PERIODONTITIS

Clinical features

The patient may give a history of pain due to previous pulpitis. When periodontitis develops, escape of exudate into the periodontal ligament causes the tooth to be extruded by a minute amount and the bite to fall more heavily on it. The tooth is at first uncomfortable, then increasingly tender, even to mere touch. Hot or cold substances do not cause pain in the tooth. As inflammation becomes more severe and pus starts to form, pain becomes intense and throbbing in character. There is often a large carious cavity or filling in the affected tooth, or it may be discoloured due to death of the pulp earlier. At this stage the gingiva over the root is red and tender, but there is no swelling while inflammation is confined within the bone.

Radiographs give little information because bony changes have had too short a time to develop. Immediately round the apex the lamina dura may appear slightly hazy and the periodontal space may be slightly widened. When acute periodontitis is due to exacerbation of a chronic infection, the original lesion can be seen as an area of radiolucency at the apex.

Exudate may penetrate overlying bone and periosteum a day or so after the onset of pain, allowing relief of the pressure. Pain quickly abates but exudate, if it cannot escape, distends the soft tissues to form a swelling. When an upper canine is affected, the swelling quickly spreads to the face and eyelid and may close the eye on that side (Fig. 4.15). In spite of the alarming appearance, the swelling is due only to oedema. It subsides when the tooth is extracted or the infection is drained.

The regional lymph nodes may be enlarged and tender, but general symptoms are usually slight or absent.

Inflammation typically remains localised. Further spread of infection can cause inflammation of the surrounding bone (osteomyelitis) or cellulitis (Ch. 6) but only exceedingly rarely.

Pathology

Acute apical periodontitis is a typical acute inflammatory reaction with engorged blood vessels and packing of the tissue

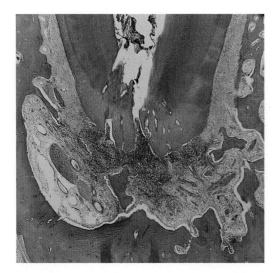

Fig. 4.16 Acute apical periodontitis. In this early acute lesion inflammatory cells, mainly neutrophil polymorphonuclear leukocytes, are seen clustered around the apex of a non-vital tooth. The inflammatory cells are spreading around and into bone and there has not yet been time for significant bone resorption to develop.

with neutrophils (Fig. 4.16). These changes are initially localised to the immediate vicinity of the apex as a consequence of the rich blood supply to this area. The immediately adjacent lamina dura becomes resorbed and an abscess cavity may form if not aborted by treatment (Table 4.5).

Table 4.5 Possible complications of acute apical periodontitis
● Suppuration ● Regional lymphadenopathy ● Spreading infection

Treatment

Extraction of the diseased tooth removes the source of infection and drains the exudate. This is the simplest and most effective treatment. Antibiotics should not be given for simple acute periodontitis if immediate dental treatment is available. Alternative treatment is to retain the tooth by endodontic treatment, which should also serve to drain the infection.

CHRONIC APICAL PERIODONTITIS

Clinical features

Chronic periodontitis is a low-grade infection. It may follow an acute infection that has been inadequately drained and incompletely resolved. The tooth is non-vital and may be slightly tender to percussion but otherwise symptoms may be minimal. Frequently, chronic periodontitis is first recognised as a rounded area of radiolucency at the apex of a tooth (an 'apical

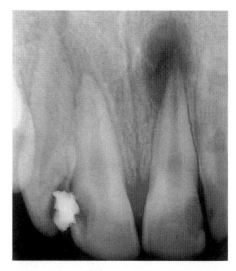

Fig. 4.17 Chronic apical abscess. Periapical bone resorption has developed as a result of inflammation. The area of radiolucency corresponds with the histological changes seen in the next figure.

granuloma') in a routine radiograph (Fig. 4.17). The area is usually about 5 mm in diameter and has well-defined margins. A distinct cortex is sometimes interpreted as early cyst formation, but this cannot be confirmed without a biopsy.

Table 4.6 Possible complications of chronic apical periodontitis
● Periapical granuloma formation ● Radicular cyst formation ● Suppuration and sinus formation ● Acute exacerbations

Pathology

Chronic periodontitis is a typical chronic inflammatory reaction characterised by lymphocytes, macrophages and plasma cells. Infection is confined by inflammatory cells, and granulation tissue surrounds the area. The granulation tissue grows into a rounded mass (a 'granuloma'), and osteoclasts resorb the bone to accommodate it (Figs 4.18 and 4.19).

Despite absence of symptoms, there is no spontaneous healing because of the persistent reservoir of infection in the root canal. Instead, granulation tissue proliferates round the focus of irritation at the tooth apex and surrounding bone is resorbed to leave a round area of radiolucency. Healing only follows extraction, effective endodontic treatment or apicectomy (Fig. 4.20).

Variable degrees of proliferation of the epithelial rests of Malassez in a periapical granuloma at the apex of a dead tooth are common (Fig. 4.21). Epithelial proliferation may be sufficient to lead ultimately to cyst formation and is the most common cause of jaw cysts.

This epithelium forms irregular strands or loops. Sometimes a microscopic cyst cavity, with a lining of hyperplastic

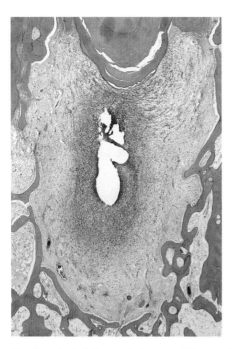

Fig. 4.18 Chronic periapical abscess. At the apex of the non-vital tooth is an abscess cavity surrounded by a thick fibrous wall densely infiltrated by inflammatory cells, predominantly neutrophils. Periapical bone has been resorbed and the trabeculae reorientated around the mass.

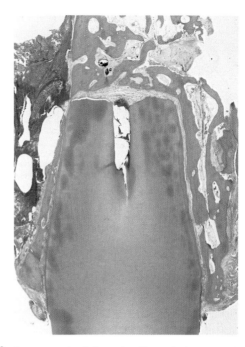

Fig. 4.20 Low power detail shows the effects of apicectomy. The chronic inflammatory reaction has entirely cleared. New bone has formed to replace the excised apex and there is a condensation of connective tissue across the deep end of the root canal filling.

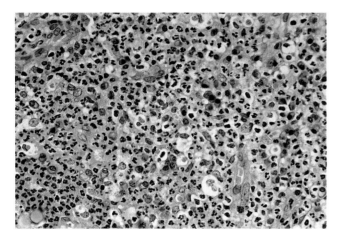

Fig. 4.19 High power of an apical granuloma showing neutrophils, lymphocytes and plasma cells in loose oedematous fibrous tissue.

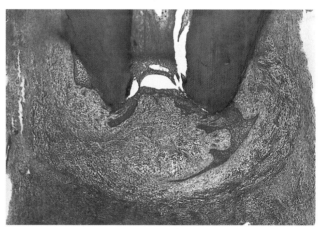

Fig. 4.21 Epithelial proliferation in an apical granuloma. Inflammation induces proliferation of odontogenic epithelium in rests of Malassez. This change may lead to cyst formation (Ch. 7).

epithelium, forms and represents the earliest stage of radicular cyst. In other cases the epithelium is scanty or destroyed by the inflammation.

Periapical granulomas usually remain localised within the bone. Occasionally, there is abscess formation and pus may reach the surface by resorption of the bone (usually on the buccal surface of the gingiva) immediately over the apex of the tooth. A nodule of granulation tissue forms in response to the irritation by pus and marks the opening of the sinus.

An uncommon complication, but sometimes the first sign of periapical periodontitis, is the tracking of a sinus onto the skin surface. This most frequently happens on or near the chin as a result of a long-forgotten blow and death of a lower incisor

(Fig. 4.22). In such cases the crown of the damaged tooth is usually discoloured (Fig. 4.23) and may be chipped. A radiograph shows the periapical area of bone destruction. Many patients fail to associate the sinus with dental infection but competent endodontic treatment causes the sinus to heal remarkably quickly.

Treatment

According to the state of the rest of the dentition, extraction or endodontic treatment are the main options. Competent endo-

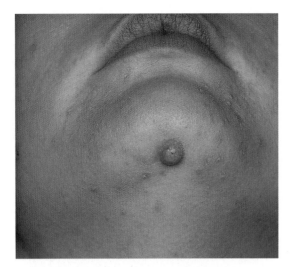

Fig. 4.22 A persistent skin sinus from a lower incisor rendered non-vital by a blow some time previously. This young woman was seen and treated unsuccessfully for 2 years by her doctor, surgeons and dermatologists before anyone looked at her teeth.

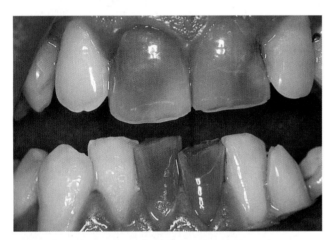

Fig. 4.23 Non-vital incisor teeth, in this case as a result of trauma. Haemorrhage and products of autolysis of the pulp discolour the dentine and darken the teeth.

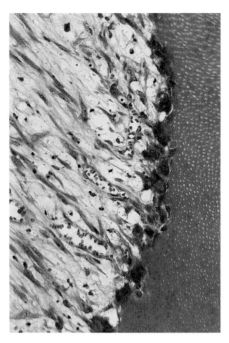

Fig. 4.24 Resorption during periapical periodontitis. Active osteoclastic resorption of dentine is continuing in the presence of inflammatory exudate. This is a common change but usually minor in extent.

dontic treatment leads to healing even if cystic change has started. Persistence of chronic periodontitis after root canal treatment is usually due to technical faults, and apicectomy may be required (see Fig. 4.20).

RESORPTION OF TEETH

The deciduous teeth are progressively loosened and ultimately shed as a result of progressive resorption of the roots as a physiological process arising from the pressure of the underlying successors. Resorption of permanent teeth is always pathological.

Whenever resorption takes place, there is usually some attempt at repair by apposition of cementum or bone. During resorption of deciduous teeth a period of resorption is followed by one of repair, so that clinically the looseness of these teeth varies before they are shed.

Resorption is rarely important but very occasionally results from some destructive disease such as a tumour. Hypercementosis is also rarely important but may occasionally be a cause of difficult extractions.

Pathology

Pressure is probably the main factor. However, in some cases no cause is apparent. Resorption is mainly carried out by osteoclasts which, during active phases, may be seen in lacunae in the hard tissue with which their cytoplasm appears to merge (Fig. 4.24). When resorption is very slow, osteoclasts may not be seen and, being intermittent in their action, disappear during inactive periods. Humoral mediators such as prostaglandins may also contribute to bone resorption.

Resorption of deciduous teeth

Resorption of deciduous teeth occasionally leads to a few minor complications.

Ankylosis. In the resting stages of resorption excessive repair tissue may be deposited until the root becomes fused to the adjacent bone. This may prevent the tooth from being shed and the permanent successor from erupting. If not removed, the ankylosed tooth becomes partially submerged by the continued growth of the surrounding alveolar ridge. The tooth should be removed, surgically if necessary, to allow the successor to erupt.

Separation of an apex. Resorption may be irregular so that part of the tooth is cut off. The fragment remains buried or eventually appears on the surface.

Failure of resorption. Absence or misplacement of a permanent successor is the usual cause. The deciduous tooth may then remain in the arch for many years.

Resorption of permanent teeth

Resorption of permanent teeth is usually limited in extent, but may rarely destroy a large part of them. There are various causes (Table 4.7).

Table 4.7 **Important causes of resorption of permanent teeth**

- Periapical periodontitis. The most common cause but is usually slight
- Impacted teeth pressing on the root of an adjacent tooth
- Unerupted teeth. Over the course of years these may undergo resorption or hypercementosis, or both
- Replanted teeth. These are sometimes rapidly and grossly resorbed
- Neoplasms. Resorption of related teeth is a typical sign of an intraosseous neoplasm such as an ameloblastoma
- Idiopathic resorption, peripheral and internal

Cementum is most readily resorbed while enamel is the most resistant. When an impacted tooth presses on the roots of another, these are resorbed, but sometimes the crown of the impacted tooth may be destroyed.

Idiopathic resorption

Internal resorption ('pink spot') is a curious and uncommon condition in which dentine is resorbed from within the pulp. Resorption tends to be localised, producing the characteristic sign of a well-defined rounded area of radiolucency in the crown (Fig. 4.25). This may affect an incisor tooth, and a rounded pink area appears where the vascular pulp has become visible through the attenuated hard tissue. The cause is unknown but it may possibly be a late result of damage to the blood supply of the pulp by a blow.

Idiopathic internal resorption can also affect any part of other teeth but causes no signs until the pulp is opened and allows access to infection. Alternatively resorption may be detected by chance in a routine radiograph.

External resorption may be localised or generalised. Very rarely resorption may start, for unknown reasons, on the surface of the root near the apex, and affect many teeth. Over the course of years, more than half the root may be destroyed. The lost tissue is partially repaired by bone-like tissue.

Localised root resorption is also uncommon and of unknown cause. A limited area of the root is attacked from its external surface and resorption goes on until the pulp is reached. Treatment is ineffective.

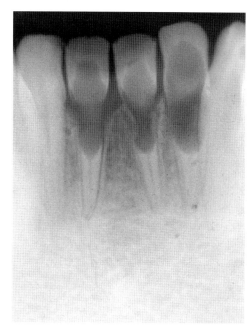

Fig. 4.25 Idiopathic internal resorption ('pink spot'). In this unusually severe example, resorption has progressed into the roots of three lower incisors.

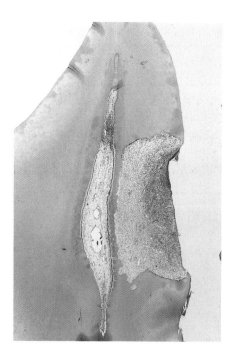

Fig. 4.26 Idiopathic external resorption. A localised area of destruction of dentine produced by osteoclastic activity. The cavity is filled with proliferating connective tissue. The pulp shows no reaction and the sparing of the circumpulpal dentine until a late stage is a characteristic feature of external resorption.

Pathology

Vascular granulation tissue replaces the part of the periodontal ligament or pulp. Osteoclasts border the affected dentine or enamel. Inflammatory changes may be superimposed if the

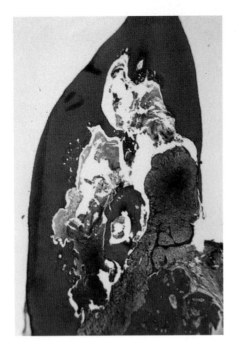

Fig. 4.27 Idiopathic resorption. A grossly resorbed central incisor with a widely perforated pulp wall. The pulp has been replaced by granulation tissue and bony repair tissue has been laid down more deeply.

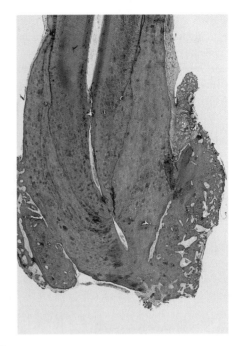

Fig. 4.28 Hypercementosis in Paget's disease. An irregular craggy mass of bone-like cementum has been formed over thickened regular and acellular cementum.

pulp chamber has been opened by destruction of its walls. Irregular repair with bone or cementum may take place (Figs 4.26 and 4.27).

Treatment

Idiopathic resorption is usually untreatable. However, if a pink spot in an incisor tooth is noticed at an early stage endodontic treatment should be carried out before the pulp chamber becomes exposed.

HYPERCEMENTOSIS

Apposition of excessive amounts of cementum is not uncommon and due to several possible causes (Table 4.8).

Increased thickness of cementum is not itself a disease, and no treatment is necessary. If hypercementosis is gross, as in Paget's disease, extractions become difficult (Fig. 4.28).

Table 4.8 Causes of hypercementosis

● Ageing
● Periapical periodontitis. A common cause but minor in amount. Close to the apex there is usually a little resorption, but coronally, cementum is laid down, forming a shoulder
● Functionless and unerupted teeth. Hypercementosis and resorption may alternate
● Paget's disease. Alternating, irregular apposition and resorption, with apposition predominating, produce an irregular mass of cementum on the root with a histological 'mosaic' pattern
● Cementoblastoma (Ch. 8)

Concrescence

Rarely hypercementosis causes fusion of the roots of adjacent teeth (Figs 4.29 and 4.30). It is rarely noticed until an attempt is made to extract one of the teeth. The two teeth are then found to move in unison, and surgical intervention becomes necessary.

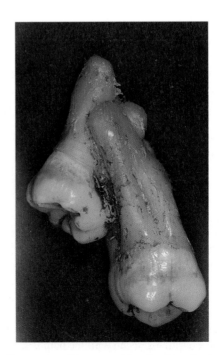

Fig. 4.29 Concrescence. Two upper molars fused together by cementum.

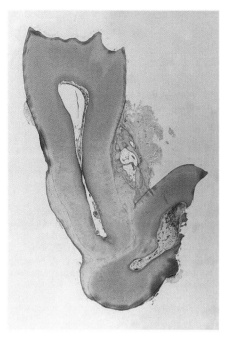

Fig. 4.30 Concrescence. Histological section of fused teeth reveals that the teeth are joined by cementum and not dentine.

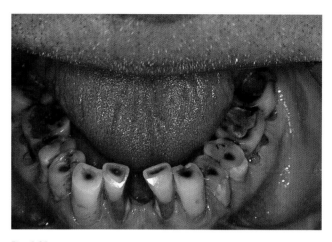

Fig. 4.31 Attrition. Excessive wear of the occlusal surfaces of the teeth, as a result of an abrasive diet. The site of the pulp of several teeth is marked by reactionary dentine which is porous and stained. Teeth remain vital.

CHRONIC (NON-CARIOUS) INJURIES TO TEETH

Non-carious chronic damage to the teeth may be referred to as *tooth-wear*. The latter may be caused by attrition, abrasion or erosion, or combinations of these influences.

Attrition

Attrition is tooth-to-tooth wear, and results more rapidly from a gritty diet and may be seen in immigrants from developing countries or in ancient skulls. Attrition may also be seen in the elderly and can result from a subconscious tooth grinding habit which may be nocturnal and is termed *bruxism*.

Attrition can eventually flatten the masticatory surfaces and expose the dentine. Reactionary dentine formation in response to this slow process protects the pulp (Fig. 4.31).

Bruxism

Bruxism is the term given to periodic repetitive clenching or rhythmic forceful grinding of the teeth. Some 10–20% of the population report the habit but the incidence rises to 90% when mild subconcious grinding is included. It has an equal sex incidence, is commoner in children and young adults and uncommon after middle age. The aetiology is unknown but probably multifactorial. Bruxism is performed during light sleep and some consider it primarily a sleep disorder. Bruxism is also common in those with disability (Ch. 33). Grinding the teeth is often also a subconscious response to frustration and

though usually then brief, may be acquired as a more prolonged habit and damage the teeth.

Bruxism is divided into nocturnal and daytime types. In nocturnal bruxism the teeth are clenched or ground many times each night but for only a few seconds at a time. Even so, the forces exerted and the total time of occlusal contact is much longer than normal. Bruxism is often performed in a protrusive or lateral excursion so that the forces are borne on few teeth and in an unfavourable direction. The resulting attrition can be deeply destructive, particularly in a Class II division 2 occlusion. The signs of bruxism are shown in Table 4.9.

Table 4.9 Features and effects of bruxism

- Noise during grinding
- Attrition, wear facets and occasionally sensitivity
- Fracture of cusps and restorations
- Mobility of teeth
- Hypertrophy of masseter and anterior temporalis muscles
- Myalgia and limitation of jaw movement
- Tenderness on palpation of masticatory muscles

Only the grinding itself is diagnostic. Attrition may also be seen in the elderly particularly as a result of physiological wear (see above). The muscle pain of bruxism is felt in the morning, and is the same as muscle pain after exercise. However, most 'bruxists' experience no pain and pain does not correlate with the severity of the grinding or clenching.

Bruxism is often considered to be linked to pain dysfunction syndrome, but the association is not strong (Ch. 11). It has also been suggested that bruxism may result from occlusal interference but bruxism may even be carried out with complete dentures.

Management

Bruxism should be treated conservatively and any intervention should be reversible. Reassurance and explanation are often all that are required and stress management such as relaxation, hypnosis or sleep advice may be tried.

Appliances are widely prescribed but there is no firm evidence to support their use. Claims that appliances act by changing the vertical dimension, relieving occlusal interference, repositioning the condyles, changing mandibular posture or preventing periodontal ligament proprioception are unproven and their mechanisms of action are unknown. Nevertheless, appliances frequently appear to be effective and they are useful to protect against severe attrition. Appliances may be attached to upper and lower arches, including flat bite planes and various types of occlusal splints. All should be worn at night only and initially for one month. If there is no improvement, treatment should be discontinued to prevent adverse effects on the soft tissues and occlusion. If effective, the appliances may be worn intermittently during exacerbations. Soft vacuum-formed appliances are cheap and readily fitted as a short-term diagnostic aid but are quickly worn out by determined bruxism. Any type of appliance occasionally worsens bruxism. If bruxism appears related to anxiety, a short course of an anxiolytic such as diazepam may help break the habit. Occlusal adjustment has been shown to be ineffective and should be avoided.

Those who indulge in bruxism during the day may grind, clench, or perform other parafunctional habits such as cheek, tongue or nail biting or tongue thrusting. Appliances probably do not help daytime bruxism.

Abrasion

Abrasion of the necks of the teeth is seen mainly in the elderly as a consequence of overvigorous tooth brushing or use of an abrasive dentifrice. The exposed dentine is shiny and smooth. Eventually, grooves worn into the necks of the teeth can be so deep as to extend into the pulp chamber but reactionary dentine protects the pulp (Figs 4.32 and 4.33). The crown of the tooth may even break off without exposing the pulp.

Erosion

Erosion is progressive dissolution of tooth substance by exposure to acids. It appears to be a growing problem as a result of overconsumption of soft drinks or fruit juices, or both (Fig. 4.34, see also Fig. 30.2).

Chronic regurgitation of gastric secretions, typically as a consequence of chronic pyloric stenosis, can cause a characteristic erosion particularly of the palatal surfaces of the upper teeth (see Fig. 29.1). Similar damage can result from self-induced vomiting. The latter is characteristic of bulimia, a psychological disorder in which there are episodes of binge gorging followed by self-induced vomiting to maintain a thin figure.

In the past, industrial exposure to corrosive chemicals was a significant cause of dental erosion.

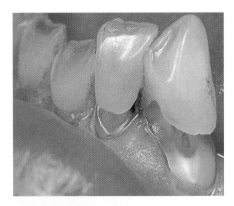

Fig. 4.32 Attrition and abrasion. Chronic physical trauma to the teeth produced by chewing and over-vigorous use of a toothbrush respectively. The incisal edges of the teeth have worn into polished facets, in the centres of which the yellowish dentine is visible. The necks of the two nearest teeth have been deeply incised by tooth brushing, also exposing dentine. The pulp has been obliterated by secondary dentine formation but its original site can be seen in the centre of the exposed dentine.

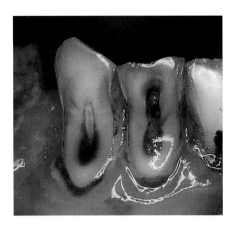

Fig. 4.33 Mixed pattern tooth loss. In this case, an element of erosion may be present. Note the shiny polished surface produced by abrasion.

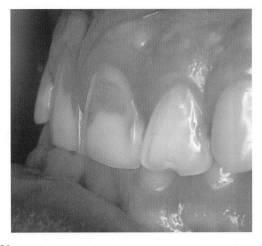

Fig. 4.34 Erosion. Saucer-shaped defects on the labial enamel resulting from acid drinks being trapped between the upper lip and teeth.

SUGGESTED FURTHER READING

Bergenholtz G 1981 Inflammatory response of the dental pulp to bacterial irritation. J Endod 7:100–104

Brook I, Frazier E H, Gher M E 1996 Microbiology of periapical abscesses and associated maxillary sinusitis. J Periodontol 67:608–610

Currie W J R, Ho V 1993 An unexpected death associated with an acute dentoalveolar abscess. Br J Oral Maxillofac Surg 31:296–298

Kuc I, Peters E, Pan J 2000 Comparison of clinical and histologic diagnoses in periapical lesions. Oral Surg Oral Med Oral Pathol Radiol Endod 89:333–337

Lewis M A O, MacFarlane T W, McGowan D A 1986 Quantitative bacteriology of acute dentoalveolar abscesses. J Med Microbiol 21:101–104

Morse D R, Furst M L, Belot R M et al 1987 Infectious flare-ups and serious sequelae following endodontic treatment: a prospective randomised trial on antibiotic prophylaxis in cases of asymptomatic pulpal-periapical lesions. Oral Surg Oral Med Oral Pathol 64:96–109

Trowbridge H O 1981 Pathogenesis of pulpitis resulting from dental caries. J Endod 7:52–60

Wright E F, Gullickson D C 1996 Identifying acute pulpalgia as a factor in TMD pain. JADA 127:773–780

Gingivitis and periodontitis

THE NORMAL PERIODONTAL TISSUES

The gingival tissues comprise a series of anatomical regions (Table 5.1).

Table 5.1 Anatomical regions of normal healthy gingival tissue

- *Junctional epithelium.* Extends from the amelocemental junction to the floor of the gingival sulcus and forms the epithelial attachment to the tooth surface
- *Sulcular epithelium.* Lines the gingival sulcus and joins the epithelial attachment to the free gingiva
- *Free gingiva.* Coronal to the amelocemental junction and attached gingiva, and includes the tips of the interdental papillae
- *Attached gingiva.* Extends apically from the free gingiva to the mucogingival junction and is bound down to the superficial periodontal fibres and periosteum.

Histologically, gingival epithelium is stratified squamous: the free and attached gingiva are parakeratinised. The epithelial attachment consists of flattened stratified squamous epithelium adhering to enamel (Fig. 5.1). The attachment apparatus consists of a basal lamina and hemidesmosomes. The attachment to the enamel appears histologically as a clear cuticle (Fig. 5.2). It forms an effective seal, protecting the underlying connective tissues. The epithelial attachment is so firmly adherent to the tooth surface that mechanical damage, which would otherwise pull the epithelium from the tooth, tears apart the epithelial cells (Fig. 5.2). This epithelium has a relatively high turnover rate and the epithelial attachment is probably actively maintained and reformed. This enables the attachment to migrate apically until it becomes attached to cementum when periodontitis develops.

The attached gingiva is firmly bound down to the underlying bone to form a tough mucoperiosteum. Its stippled appearance is due to the intersections of its underlying epithelial ridges at the junction with the connective tissue.

The alveolar mucosa is continuous with the attached gingiva but is sharply demarcated by its smooth surface, darker colour and increasing separation from the bone.

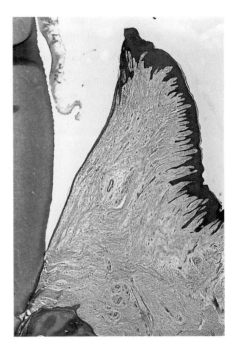

Fig. 5.1 Gingival sulcus and epithelial attachment. This sagittal section of a specimen from a woman of 27 shows the normal appearances. Enamel removed by decalcification of the specimen has left the triangular space. The epithelial attachment forms a line from the top of the papilla to the amelocemental junction; its enamel surface, the actual line of attachment, is sharply defined. The gingival sulcus, minute in extent, is formed where the papilla curves away from the line of the enamel surface. There is hardly any inflammatory infiltrate.

Gingival and periodontal fibres

The principal fibres of the periodontal ligament form fibrous bundles interspersed by loose connective tissue containing blood vessels and nerves. These components provide a viscoelastic supportive mechanism resisting both compressive and tensile forces on the teeth. The normal thickness of the periodontal ligament is about 0.1–0.3 mm.

The principal fibres are arranged in a series of fairly well-defined groups (Table 5.2).

The periodontal ligament fibres are embedded in cementum at their inner ends and in the lamina dura at their outer ends. New fibres replacing those which have aged, or forming in

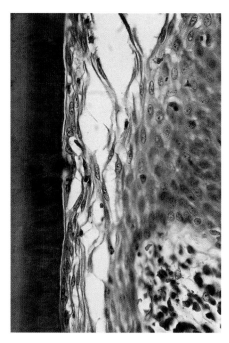

Fig. 5.2 The strength of the epithelial attachment. On this tooth the epithelial attachment has migrated on to the surface of the cementum as a result of periodontal disease. The epithelium has been torn away from the tooth but the tear is within the junctional epithelium, leaving some of its cells still adherent to the cementum and attached by a clear cuticle. A similar strength is seen when the junctional epithelium is attached to enamel.

Table 5.2 Principal fibres of the periodontal ligament

- *Oblique fibres* form a suspensory ligament from socket to root in coronal to apical directions
- *Horizontal fibres* form a dense group attaching neck of tooth to rim of socket
- *Transeptal fibres* of the horizontal group are not attached to alveolar bone but pass superficially to it and join adjacent teeth together. They protect the interdental gingiva by resisting forces that would otherwise separate the teeth and open the contact points
- *Gingival fibres* form a cuff round the neck of the tooth supporting the soft tissues. They resist separation of the gingivae from the tooth and help to prevent formation of pockets

---

response to new functional stresses, are attached by apposition of further layers of cementum which becomes thicker with age. The lamina dura is a layer of compact bone continuous, at the mouths of the sockets, with the cortical bone of the jaw. The radiographic appearance of the lamina dura has limited diagnostic value in periodontics as its presence largely depends on the alignment of the beam.

Gingival fluid (exudate)

In health, a minute amount of fluid can be collected from the gingival margins. It differs in composition from saliva which contains IgA while gingival fluid has a variable but significant

content of IgG, IgM and leucocytes. Unlike saliva, gingival fluid is not a secretion (there are no glands in this region) but is inflammatory exudate. It therefore increases greatly with the degree of inflammation.

Nomenclature and classification of periodontal disease

The term *periodontal disease* usually refers only to plaque-related inflammatory disease of the dental supporting tissues. A wide variety of diseases of the oral mucosa can also affect the gingivae occasionally, so that conditions as diverse as tuberculosis or lichen planus can produce lesions in this area. Such conditions do not play any significant part in the development of periodontal disease in its commonly accepted sense.

Chronic gingivitis is, with few exceptions, the preliminary stage to the development of chronic periodontitis, but clinically no sharp dividing line can be drawn between chronic gingivitis and the onset of periodontitis. Nevertheless, the distinction is important in that chronic gingivitis can generally be cured by plaque control. By contrast, loss of bone and tooth support due to chronic periodontitis are largely irreversible.

The main *clinical* types of periodontal disease are grouped together on the basis of what seems to be the predominant pathological process (Table 5.3).

Table 5.3 Types of periodontal disease

I.   Gingivitis and periodontitis
- Chronic gingivitis (common plaque-related type)
- Chronic adult periodontitis (common, plaque-related type)

II. Less common types of gingivitis
- Acute necrotising ulcerative gingivitis
- HIV-associated gingivitis
- Herpetic gingivostomatitis (Ch. 12)
- Wegener's granulomatosis (Ch. 28)

III. Uncommon types of periodontitis
- Prepubertal periodontitis
- Juvenile periodontitis
- Rapidly progressive periodontitis
- HIV-associated periodontitis
- Acute leukaemic periodontal destruction

IV. Miscellaneous periodontal disorders
- Gingival hyperplasia
    Familial
    Drug-related
- Periodontal atrophy
- Periodontal (lateral) abscess
- Pericoronitis

CHRONIC GINGIVITIS

Clinical features

Chronic gingivitis is asymptomatic, low grade inflammation of the gingivae. The latter become red and slightly swollen with oedema (Fig. 5.3). Plaque, deposited along the gingival margins, is readily detectable. In most patients, chronic gingivitis is

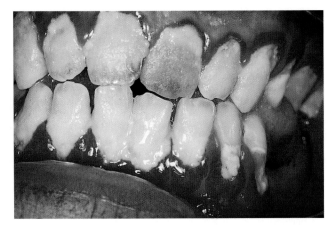

Fig. 5.3   Gingivitis. A florid, bright-red band of gingival inflammation results from very poor oral hygiene. Thick accumulations of plaque are visible on all tooth surfaces.

Table 5.4   Factors contributing to or exacerbating chronic gingivitis

Local
  ● Poor toothbrushing technique
  ● Dental irregularities providing stagnation areas
  ● Restorations or appliances causing stagnation areas
Systemic
  ● Pregnancy
  ● Down's syndrome
  ● Poorly-controlled diabetes mellitus

due to local factors and in particular, ineffective toothbrushing. It should be curable by effective oral hygiene.

Chronic hyperplastic gingivitis is a term sometimes given to chronic gingivitis in which inflammtory oedema is prominent. However there is no soft tissue hyperplasia. Maintenance of strict oral hygiene brings resolution.

Systemic disorders can exacerbate chronic gingivitis but rarely play a significant role (Table 5.4).

Pathology

Gingivitis is an inflammatory response to plaque bacteria. By definition, inflammation is restricted to the gingival margins and does not affect the periodontal ligament or bone (Fig. 5.4).

The development of gingivitis has been arbitrarily divided into three histological stages (Tables 5.5 and 5.6) while the fourth stage refers to chronic periodontitis. It must be appreciated that these stages are artificially distinguished, being largely based on animal studies.

Variations in plaque bacteria with stage of disease

Healthy (uninflamed) gingivae.   The plaque is supragingival and thin (10 to 20 cells thick). Gram-positive bacteria predominate and include *Actinomyces* species, *Rothia*, viridans streptococci and *S. epidermidis*. In elderly patients in perio-

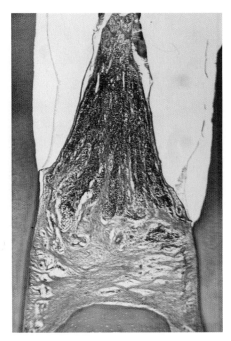

Fig. 5.4   Chronic gingivitis. The epithelial attachment remains at the level of the amelocemental junction and inflammatory cells are concentrated in the gingiva.

Table 5.5   'Initial stage' chronic gingivitis
● Develops within 24–48 hours of exposure to plaque ● Plaque related to gingival sulcus ● Vasodilatation ● Infiltration predominantly of neutrophils ● Leakage of exudate into gingival sulcus

Table 5.6   Established chronic gingivitis
● Dense, predominantly plasmacytic infiltrate ● Infiltrate fills but limited to interdental papillae ● Destruction of superficial connective tissue fibres ● Deepened gingival crevice ● Epithelial attachment remains at or near amelocemental junction ● Alveolar bone and periodontal ligament remain intact

dontal health, Gram-positive bacteria, particularly streptococci, form the largest single group (50% of the predominant cultivable flora), while gram-negative bacteria only account for 30%. The latter include porphyromonas and fusobacterium species.

Early (and experimental) gingivitis.   If toothbrushing is neglected for several days, plaque grows in thickness and is typically 100 to 300 cells thick. In the earliest stages bacteria proliferate but the plaque remains Gram-positive in character and *Actinomyces* species become predominant.

Chronic gingivitis.   With the passage of time, persistence of plaque leads to chronic inflammation, and Gram-negative

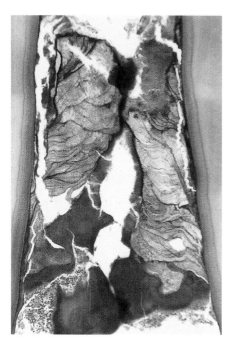

Fig. 5.5 Subgingival calculus showing the layered structure resulting from incremental deposition. The calculus has a brown colour as a result of blood and bacterial pigment within it. A thick layer of plaque adheres to the deep surface.

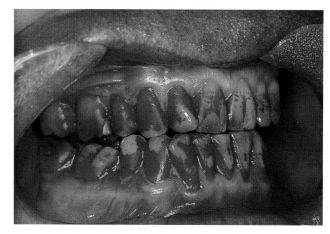

Fig. 5.6 Accumulation of plaque stained after 24 hours by disclosing solution.

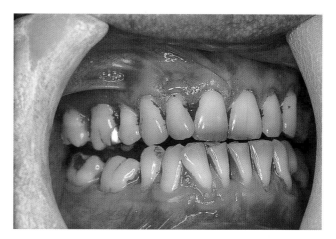

Fig. 5.7 The effects of tooth brushing in the same patient. Plaque remains interdentally in most areas, explaining why gingivitis is often localised here.

organisms become increasingly prominent. *Veillonella*, *Fusobacterium* and *Campylobacter* species become conspicuous.

Calculus

Calculus is calcified plaque. The calcification is less significant than the bacterial content which induces inflammation and, later, tissue destruction. However, calculus distorts the gingival crevice and by extending the stagnation area probably promotes even greater bacterial proliferation (Fig. 5.5). Supragingival calculus mainly forms opposite the orifices of the major salivary glands in the lower incisor and upper first molar areas. It cannot be removed by the patient and provides a rough, plaque-retentive surface.

Several compounds, such as pyrophosphates, added to dentifrices have been shown to reduce calculus formation to variable degrees. However, any clinical benefit has not been unequivocally established.

Management

Chronic gingivitis is readily recognisable from the clinical features already described. Gentle probing shows absence of pocketing and radiographs show intact crestal alveolar bone. The diagnosis is confirmed by resolution of gingivitis when effective oral hygiene measures (including calculus removal and effective toothbrushing habits) become established (Figs 5.6 and 5.7). Any exacerbating factors must be dealt with if possible.

Pregnancy gingivitis

Pre-existing gingivitis may become more severe in the first two months of pregnancy (see Fig. 31.9). Inflammatory erythema and oedema typically become more severe and a localised vascular lesion (a *pregnancy tumour*) may develop. The latter has the same structure as a pyogenic granuloma (Ch. 19).

Pregnancy gingivitis can be much ameliorated or abolished by a strict oral hygiene regime, and improves after parturition. However, if a pregnancy tumour persists, it should be excised.

Down's syndrome

In Down's syndrome, gingivitis is exacerbated by excessive plaque formation and difficulties in establishing effective tooth-brushing habits. The multiple immunodeficiencies typical of this disorder contribute. Progress to periodontitis and early tooth loss are frequent consequences (see Figs 33.3 and 33.4).

Diabetes mellitus

In poorly-controlled diabetes, periodontal health may deteriorate sharply. In well-controlled diabetes, acceleration of gingivitis may not be noticeable. However, it appears that, overall, diabetics suffer somewhat more severe periodontal disease and slightly earlier tooth loss than healthy, control populations. The neutrophil defect typical of this disease is probably the main factor involved.

CHRONIC ADULT PERIODONTITIS

Clinical features

Chronic periodontitis (the 'advanced lesion') is the chief cause of tooth loss in later adult life, but symptoms are typically minimal. Many patients remain unaware of the disease until teeth become loose.

Gingivitis persists and patients may complain of gingival bleeding or an unpleasant taste. Later, gingival recession or loosening of the teeth may become conspicuous. Periodontitis is a potent and common cause of foul-smelling breath (halitosis). The congested gingival margins become purplish-red, flabby and swollen. The interdental papillae 'split' and can be separated from the teeth. Later the papillae are destroyed and the gingival margin tends to become straight with a swollen, rounded edge.

Pressure on the gingival margins causes bleeding, and sometimes pus can be expressed from round the necks of the teeth. Bacterial plaque and calculus are widespread.

Loss of attachment leads to pocketing which allows a probe to be passed down between teeth and gingiva. In pockets the rough surface of subgingival calculus can be felt. Eventually, teeth become increasingly loose and dull to percussion.

Radiography

The earliest change is loss of definition and blunting of the tips of the alveolar crests. Bone resorption usually progresses in a regular manner and its level remains the same along a row of teeth. A straight line can be drawn along the crest of the alveolar bone (horizontal bone loss — Fig. 5.8). Complex patterns of bone loss may also be seen, probably due to the effects of variable degrees of loss of attachment superimposed upon the underlying anatomical features. Thus in areas where bone is thin, destruction results in horizontal bone loss, but where alveolar bone is thicker, partial destruction gives rise to vertical or angular bone defects.

Aetiology and pathology

Conditions promoting stagnation and maintenance of infection at the gingival margins have been discussed earlier. Persistence of infection at the gingival margins leads to progressive in-

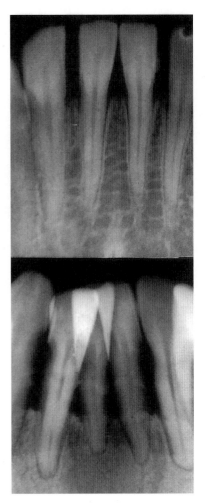

Fig. 5.8 Early and severe horizontal bone loss in advanced chronic adult periodontitis.

flammation and destruction of the supporting tissues. Usually, local factors are most important in the progres of chronic periodontitis, but for reasons which are unclear, there is wide individual response.

The main features of the pathology of chronic periodontitis are summarised in Table 5.7.

Plaque

Bacterial plaque, a dense mat of bacteria (Table 5.8), extends from the gingival margins into pockets.

Subgingival calculus

Extension and calcification of plaque leads to formation of subgingival calculus within periodontal pockets. The deposits are thin, more widely distributed, harder, darker and more firmly attached than supragingival calculus. Calculus appears laminated histologically, with altered staining, probably due to breakdown products from blood cells oozing into the pockets (Fig. 5.9). Subgingival calculus helps to perpetuate chronic

Table 5.7 Pathological processes in chronic periodontitis

- Chronic inflammation
- Destruction of periodontal ligament fibres
- Resorption of alveolar bone
- Migration of the epithelial attachment towards the apex
- Formation of pockets around the teeth
- Formation of subgingival plaque and calculus

Table 5.8 Important bacteria associated with periodontal disease

Actinobacillus actinomycetemcomitans
Actinomyces viscosus
Capnocytophaga species*
Eikenella corrodens
*Fusobacterium nucleatum**
*Porphyromonas gingivalis**
*Prevotella intermedia**
Treponemas and other spirochaetes*
Wolinella recta

(* = anaerobes)

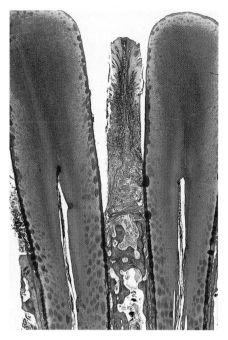

Fig. 5.10 Established chronic periodontitis. In this woman of 33, periodontal pockets have extended well beyond the amelocemental junction and inflammatory cells fill the interdental gingiva.

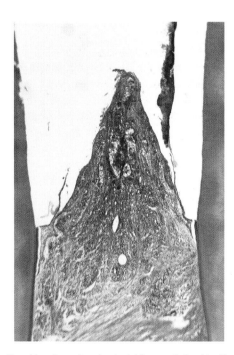

Fig. 5.9 Transition from chronic gingivitis to periodontitis. No pocket has yet formed but the epithelial attachment has extended on to the cementum and inflammation has spread deeper still.

periodontitis. It forms a reservoir of bacteria, helping to sustain inflammation, and acts as a barrier to healing.

Chronic inflammation

Plasma cells typically predominate but are accompanied by lymphocytes and neutrophils which migrate into pockets.

Inflammatory cells infiltrate the connective tissue and spread between the principal fibres (Fig. 5.10). Dense masses of these cells accumulate, especially under the epithelium in the connective tissue apposed to plaque and calculus.

Pocketing

Pocketing, a characteristic feature of chronic periodontitis, is due to the slower destruction of gingival soft tissues than of periodontal ligament and bone (Fig. 5.11). Less frequently, where gingival tissue is thin, it may be lost at the same rate as the supporting tissues, and gingival recession results. Pockets round the teeth provide a protected environment in which bacteria grow more freely. There is no effective drainage and the wall of the pocket presents a large area where bacteria or their products can irritate the tissues. Pockets also favour the growth of anaerobes which probably contribute greatly to tissue destruction.

Pockets surround the teeth. One wall is formed by cementum, the other soft tissue replacing the destroyed bone and periodontal fibres. The outer wall consists of connective tissue infiltrated by chronic inflammatory cells and lined by epithelium continuous with the gingival epithelium at the pocket mouth. The epithelial attachment forms the deep boundary. The epithelium is often hyperplastic but blood vessels may extend through it almost to its surface.

'Ulceration' of the lining is often described but rarely seen histologically.

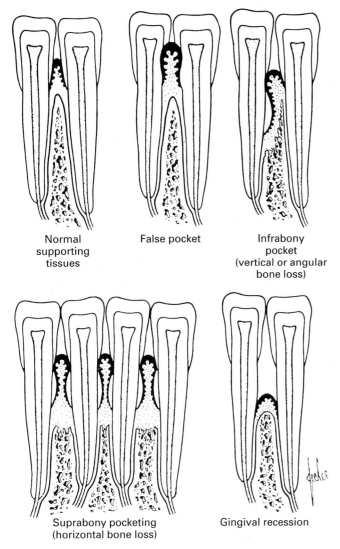

Normal
supporting
tissues

False pocket

Infrabony
pocket
(vertical or angular
bone loss)

Suprabony pocketing
(horizontal bone loss)

Gingival recession

Fig. 5.11 Pocket formation in periodontal disease. A simplified diagram to show the relationship between periodontal soft tissues and alveolar bone in the different presentations of periodontal disease.

Epithelial migration

The epithelial attachment migrates from enamel on to cementum, forming the floor of the pocket (Fig. 5.12). The attachment to cementum is strong, and a clear refractile cuticle (see Fig. 5.2) can sometimes be seen joining the epithelium to the root surface. The length of the epithelial attachment is variable but may extend several millimetres.

Destruction of periodontal fibres

Periodontal fibres are destroyed progressively from the gingival margin down to the level of the floor of the pocket. More deeply, the fibres retain their normal appearance.

Destruction of alveolar bone

Bone destruction starts at the alveolar crest. The usual level of

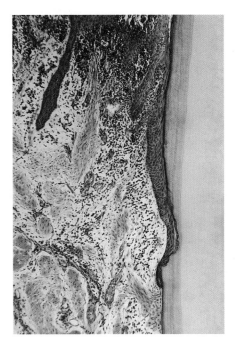

Fig. 5.12 Chronic periodontitis. The epithelial attachment has extended well down on to the cementum, but the inflammatory cells are concentrated superficially in the gingiva.

the remaining bone is just deep to the floor of the pocket where the superficial fibres of the periodontal ligament are attached. The zone of inflammation is separated from the underlying bone by a zone of fibrous tissue. This so-called fibrous walling-off is typical of chronic periodontitis and invariably present (Fig. 5.10). It has been suggested that the inflammatory lesion may extend beyond this to affect the alveolar bone and remaining periodontal ligament during periods of active disease, but histological evidence of this is lacking. Osteoclasts are rarely seen, probably because their action is intermittent and the rate of bone destruction extremely slow.

Osteoporosis and premature alveolar bone loss

Confirmation that osteoporosis may be related to premature alveolar bone loss has been handicapped by the difficulties in measuring bone mineral density (BMD) accurately. However, it has been confirmed that diminished bone mineral density measured by dual X-ray absorptiometry in several parts of the skeleton, showed a highly significant correlation with the thickness of the mandibular alveolar process in the first premolar region.

Other studies have also shown that age-related bone loss is greater in women than men after the age of 50 years. There is also a significant increase in mandibular cortical porosity and concomittant decline in bone mass, with an estimated loss of bone mineral content of 1.5% per year in women, but only 0.9% in men.

These findings may possibly explain the apparently anomalous finding in British national surveys of dental health

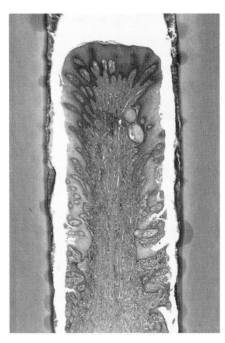

Fig. 5.13 Advanced chronic periodontitis. The cementum on the pocket walls is covered with a thin layer of plaque. The epithelium of the pocket lining is hyperplastic and the pocket extends beyond the lower edge of the picture.

that women tend to lose their teeth earlier despite more regular attendance for treatment.

Role of specific bacteria in destructive periodontitis

With formation of pockets and subgingival plaque there is enormous proliferation of bacteria of all kinds. Subgingival plaque appears to have a dense zone attached to the tooth surface where the bacteria are mainly Gram-positive. By contrast plaque related to the pocket wall is less densely packed but involves many Gram-negative bacteria, including anaerobes and spirochaetes. Bacteria particularly associated with destructive disease include *Porphyromonas gingivalis, Actinobacillus actinomycetemcomitans, B. intermedius, Wolinella recta*, spirochaetes with axial filaments, or in other cases *Eikenella corrodens*, and other corroding bacteria. The latter's colonies cause pitting ('corrosion') of the surface of culture media.

Also present are *Fusobacterium nucleatum* and as yet unidentified anaerobic vibrios and spirochaetes. Where there is severe and relatively acute bone loss associated with severe inflammation, in young adults, for example, *Actinobacillus actinomycetemcomitans* and *Porphyromonas gingivalis* appear to be particularly important. Where inflammation is minimal in spite of extensive bone loss there may be greater numbers of *Prevotella melaninogenica* and *Eikenella corrodens*. Many of the bacteria implicated in destructive periodontitis are dangerous pathogens and in other body sites can cause severe

or lethal systemic infections. For example, *Capnocytophaga ochraceus, Selenomonas sputigena* and *Eikenella corrodens* have been implicated in life-threatening infections, particularly in patients with granulocytopenia.

In human periodontal disease, it remains unclear which particular types of bacteria are responsible for tissue destruction. However, inoculation of specific bacteria into the mouths of germ-free animals has yielded somewhat unexpected results. Thus, various Gram-positive bacteria typically produced large amounts of plaque but Gram-negative bacteria did not. Certain bacteria of either group could induce or accelerate periodontal tissue damage but there was typically little inflammation or lymphocytic infiltration of the tissues. In Gram-positive infections also, few osteoclasts were seen. However, *A. viscosus* in particular, produces a bone-resorbing factor. Gram-negative bacteria also stimulated osteoclastic activity, and numerous osteoclasts were seen at the sites of tissue destruction.

That individual species of bacteria may be responsible for periodontal tissue destruction is also suggested by the finding in monkeys that the severity of periodontal damage correlates well with the numbers of *Porphyromonas gingivalis* which can be isolated. Further, antimicrobial treatment that suppressed *P. gingivalis*, led to healing and bone regeneration. Greater numbers of *P. gingivalis* also appear to be associated with enhanced periodontal disease activity in humans.

Bacterial mediators of tissue damage

Periodontal destruction may result from the actions of bacterial products or indirectly from immunologically mediated processes or both in varying degree. Bacterial products (virulence factors) that may contribute to tissue damage include enzymes, toxins and bone-resorbing factors.

Enzymes. Destruction of periodontal fibres may be due to collagenases. Prevotella species, for example, produce collagenase, trypsin, fibrinolysin, hyaluronidase, chondroitin sulphatase, heparinase, aribonuclease and deoxyribonuclease. Cytotoxic metabolic products such as indole, ammonia and hydrogen sulphide may also contribute. Porphyromonas species, especially *P. gingivalis*, are regularly associated with human destructive periodontitis.

Toxins. Certain strains of *A. actinomycetemcomitans* produce a powerful leukotoxin, while *P. gingivalis* and *P. intermedius* produce an epitheliotoxin.

Endotoxin, a lipopolysaccharide (LPS) component of Gram-negative bacteria cell walls, is released after cell lysis. It can liberate lysosomal enzymes from phagocytes and activate complement via the alternative pathway. Endotoxins can therefore mediate an inflammatory response. Endotoxins from some bacteria can enhance osteoclastic resorption to variable degrees and in this respect, endotoxin from *P. gingivalis* is ten times more potent than that from *A. actinomycetemcomitans*. The Gram-positive cell wall component, lipoteichoic acid (LTA) is also a potent mediator of inflammation and enhances bone resorption.

Bone resorbing factors. *A. viscosus* produces factors which induce decalcification of bone in vitro. Lipopolysaccharide can also induce bone resorption under experimental conditions, as can crude soluble extracts of human supragingival plaque and some other bacterial products. Bacterial factors can also cause bone resorption by stimulating release of, or acting synergistically with lymphokines, osteoclast activating factors and prostaglandin E_2.

Interference with host defence mechanisms

Other virulence factors act by interfering with host defences. Substances (leukotoxins) cytotoxic for human leucocytes are produced by *A. actinomycetemcomitans* in particular. This bacterium is involved in juvenile periodontitis and can also cause osteomyelitis and infective endocarditis in humans. Other bacterial factors potentially capable of damaging host defences are immunoglobulin proteases. *N. gonorrhoea* can produce IgA proteases which help it overcome mucosal defences and contributes to the inability of infected persons to develop protective immunity. Several of the oral viridans streptococci have also been shown to produce IgA proteases. Lipopolysaccharides, dextran and levan may also be immunosuppressive, but under different circumstances may be immunopotentiating.

Smoking

Smokers have greater susceptibility to periodontitis but paradoxically less gingivitis. The reasons for this are not understood but smoking is known to interfere with inflammatory and immune reactions probably by activating endothelial and inflammatory cells inappropriately in the lungs and circulation, and by inducing them to secrete cytokines and other compounds. Also, nicotine is a vasoconstrictor, though its effects on the gingiva have proved difficult to measure. Overall, smokers have greater loss of attachment, early tooth loss and respond less well to treatment.

Immunological processes in periodontal disease

Immunological mechanisms are involved in periodontal disease, as they are in every microbial disease. Antibodies are produced against plaque bacterial antigens. These may for example mediate opsonisation and killing of bacteria by neutrophils and macrophages. Complement is also activated by antigen/antibody complexes and contributes to the inflammatory reaction. In the process of inflammation, microbes are killed but there may also be some damage to host tissues in so-called innocent bystander damage.

Many T lymphocytes are also present and may be involved in cell-mediated reactions to plaque pathogens. Other hypersensitivity reactions may also participate.

However, it must be appreciated that the immunological reactions in chronic periodontitis are essentially protective. With loss of normal immune competence, as in conditions of neutropenia for example, periodontal destruction may be greatly accelerated. Severely destructive periodontitis may also be seen in AIDS.

The remarkable feature of periodontal disease is that, despite the presence of innumerable major pathogens in periodontal pockets, tissue destruction is so slow. In an otherwise healthy person it is not uncommon for half a century to pass before 1 cm of alveolar bone is lost. This represents a loss of an average of 0.2 mm of bone loss a year.

Progress of chronic periodontitis

Chronic periodontitis, once established, is self-perpetuating. Pockets cannot drain effectively and favour proliferation of bacteria. The epithelial lining, plaque and subgingival calculus effectively obstruct healing. Further destruction of periodontal fibres and alveolar bone causes the pockets to deepen. The natural termination of the process is loosening and exfoliation of the teeth.

General principles of management of chronic periodontitis

The main components of the management of periodontal disease are summarised in Table 5.9.

Table 5.9 General principles of management of periodontal disease

- Control of bacterial plaque
- Establishment of healthy gingiva accessible to plaque control
- Minimisation of periodontal tissue loss
- Use of antibiotics in selected cases
- Mucogingival surgery in selected cases

It may be depressing for readers who have steeped themselves in the complexities of the immunology of periodontal disease to find that its management largely depends on time-honoured, manual methods of plaque control.

Effective daily plaque removal by the patient is imperative for success. Conscientious toothbrushing and interdental cleaning with aids such as floss, wooden sticks, or small brushes, as necessary, are required. These simple measures will bring about complete resolution of simple gingivitis as mentioned earlier.

Anything hampering plaque control, particularly calculus and faulty restorations, should be dealt with. Other conditions promoting stagnation (Table 5.10) may be more difficult to eliminate.

Table 5.10 Factors promoting stagnation and persistence of plaque

- Calculus
- Overhanging restorations
- Food packing due to faulty contact points
- Irregularities of the teeth
- Mouthbreathing
- Pocketing

Treatment of periodontal pockets

Successful treatment depends upon thorough supragingival and subgingival plaque removal. The latter may achieved by *subgingival scaling* or *root planing* which also removes some cementum to ensure plaque elimination from surface irregularities. The aim is to produce a root surface to which the detached gingival tissue may adhere. Such methods should result in resolution of inflammation in the pocket wall. The junctional epithelial attachment to the root surface may extend in length coronally, and there is usually shrinkage of the gingival margin, thus exposing more root surface. The clinical result is greater recession, shallower probing depth and less bleeding on probing. Failure to achieve clinical improvement is due to either a lapse in plaque control by the patient or failure to remove subgingival plaque (Table 5.11).

Table 5.11 Factors compromising subgingival plaque removal

- Excessive pocket depth
- Distorted root morphology and furcations
- Inaccessible root surfaces (e.g. distal surfaces of posterior teeth)
- Operator competence

Failure of benefit from root planing is shown by:

- Bleeding or exudation of pus on probing the depth of pocket
- Increasing probing depths
- Radiographic deterioration of bone levels.

Subgingival scaling or root planing will not remove subgingival plaque entirely and may force pocket bacteria into the tissues. However, competent performance of these procedures reduces bacterial bulk, changes the composition of the flora and frequently produces clinical improvement.

When root planing fails, mucogingival surgery may be used to excise pockets to enable the patient to keep the root surfaces clean. The earliest form of resective surgery was gingivectomy*. This is still a useful procedure, particularly in patients with false pockets due to fibrous gingival hyperplasia and unresponsive to non-surgical treatment. However gingivectomy is unsuitable for (1) pockets extending beyond the mucogingival junction such that excision would remove all the keratinised gingiva and (2) the base of the pocket is apical to the bone crest. Gingivectomy for deep pocketing also exposes the necks of the teeth and produces a 'horse-tooth' appearance unacceptable to most patients.

Flap operations

Surgical approaches usually depend on elevation of flaps and are designed to remove the inner lining of the pocket whilst preserving the outer keratinised gingiva. Inflamed tissue is

---

*Gingivectomy dates back at least 800 years. Crusaders' gums were so swollen by scurvy they had to have them cut away to enable them to eat.

curetted away and the root surfaces are cleaned. The flaps are then sutured back around the necks of the teeth. The flap can be replaced at or near the preoperative level or it can be repositioned apically so that it just covers the alveolar crest. The former approach requires that the flap must reattach to the denuded root surface, whereas the latter aims to eliminate the pocket. Apical placement of the flap may produce an aesthetically undesirable result, and exposure of complex root forms may not facilitate plaque control by the patient.

Reattachment surgery

The ultimate goal of this technique is the promotion of new cementum apposition to anchor periodontal fibres to a healthier root surface. This ideal result ('new attachment') would obviously be the most satisfactory method of treatment. Unfortunately it has been largely unsuccessful, mainly as a consequence of rapid re-epithelialisation of the root surface and production of a long junctional epithelium. Until recently, methods designed to retard or redirect epithelial migration at the healing dentogingival junction have not been successful. A new connective tissue attachment will probably only form if cells from the remaining healthy periodontal ligament repopulate the root surface. Insertion of a barrier membrane between the flap and root surface may prevent epithelial and gingival connective tissue ingrowth ('guided tissue regeneration'). Histological evidence suggests that new attachment that forms after this procedure is only in relatively small amounts.

Limitations of periodontal surgery

Periodontal surgery may be of little benefit when multirooted teeth have furcation involvement. When one root is more severely affected than another, resection of the affected root or half the tooth (hemisection) may be succesful.

Overall, however, clinical trials comparing gingivectomy and various flap procedures have shown minimal differences in results under conditions where the standard of plaque control is high. If plaque control is poor they are equally ineffective and may lead to greater loss of periodontal support. Most patients with periodontal disease can be successfully treated by a non-surgical approach, and when surgical and non-surgical treatment have been compared, similar results have been obtained. Surgery may have advantages when treating deep pockets, while the non-surgical approach is better for shallower pockets.

Antibiotics for control of plaque bacteria

Antibiotics reaching periodontal plaque cause considerable disturbance of the bacterial flora and have the potential for destroying important pathogens. It might be suspected that this effect would be transient, but it must be borne in mind that the complex interdependent ecosystem of plaque bacteria associated with periodontal disease is built up over a period of years. Although plaque bacteria can undoubtedly develop resistance, anaerobes generally do not lose antibiotic sensitivity as readily as many aerobes.

In the USA especially, antibiotics have been used particularly for the management of periodontal disease responding poorly to conventional treatment. Overall, tetracyclines seem to be the most effective. They have the widest spectrum of activity of all antibiotics, and the side-effects, particularly of topical applications, are minimal. Even when given systemically, tetracyclines may reach concentrations in the gingival sulcus several times greater than serum levels. They also bind to calcified tissues such as cementum. In various studies, tetracyclines appear to have produced significant changes in the composition of plaque. They have brought clinical improvement, particularly when combined with conventional treatment such as root planing.

Tetracycline-containing plastic fibres have also been placed in the gingival sulcus for direct delivery of a high local concentration. Putative plaque pathogens such as porphyromonas species and other anaerobes were not found to have repopulated the plaque within the period of follow-up. Though the use of antibiotics in the management of periodontal disease is not universally accepted, it seems likely that they can produce long-term reduction in plaque pathogenicity. By interfering with complex bacterial ecosystems, less harmful species may proliferate. With the small doses used in topical applications, significant adverse effects seem unlikely to be troublesome.

However, some long-term studies have shown little or no benefit from the use of tetracyclines over scaling and root-planing alone.

Treatment of advanced periodontal disease

Once pocketing has extended beyond the point where treatment can be beneficial, the teeth should be extracted. Deep pockets are a source of sepsis which may have remote effects such as infective endocarditis. Deep pockets are most frequent in elderly patients, who have the highest susceptibility to and mortality from infective endocarditis. At the local level, if infection is allowed to persist, excessive resorption of the alveolar bone may cause difficulties in retaining dentures.

Prognosis in periodontal disease

Reliable predictions about the results of treatment cannot always be made but some factors obviously affect the outcome (Table 5.12).

Table 5.12 Factors affecting prognosis of periodontal disease
● Oral hygiene status and motivation
● Degree of bone loss
● Age
● Tooth factors
● Host resistance

Much depends on the level of oral hygiene maintained by patients and whether they are sufficiently strongly motivated to co-operate in a long regime of treatment. The degree of attachment loss, as shown by pocket depth and radiographic assessment, clearly determine whether teeth can be saved. However, in patients with the same amount of destruction of supporting tissues, the older the patient the better the prognosis, as the disease is of slower progress. Dental factors such as tooth type, root length, root anatomy and degree of furcation involvement can significantly affect the response to periodontal surgery. If also the teeth are heavily restored or have had faulty endodontic treatment or have already been lost, extensive periodontal treatment may be inappropriate (Figs 5.14, 5.15 and 5.32).

Despite intensive investigation, there remains, for no clear reasons, a 'high-risk' group for periodontitis who suffer more extensive bone loss than others of similar age.

COMPLICATIONS OF CHRONIC PERIODONTITIS

Complications can be local or systemic (Table 5.13).

Of the systemic complications, infective endocarditis is discussed in Chapter 27. It only needs to be emphasised here that bacteraemias resulting from movement of teeth in their sockets are most severe and most likely to lead to infective endocarditis in the elderly with advanced chronic periodontitis.

More controversial is the role of chronic periodontitis in contributing to atherosclerosis and its consequences, myocardial infarction or stroke.

It is widely believed now that chronic infection contributes to the development of atherosclerosis and several large surveys have shown an association between the latter and chronic

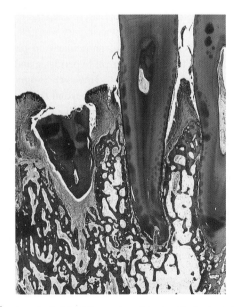

Fig. 5.14 A neglected dentition such as this, despite the buried root and advanced bone loss round the other tooth, might nevertheless be suitable for expert periodontal care.

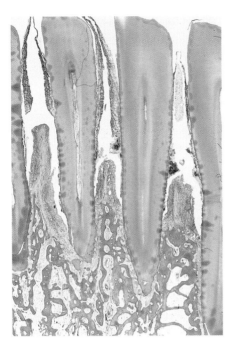

Fig. 5.15 Attempts at periodontal surgery to preserve teeth such as these are hopeless. With so little supporting bone it is surprising that they have remained in place at all.

Table 5.13 Complications of chronic periodontitis

Local
● Periodontal abscess
Systemic
● Infective endocarditis
● Atherosclerosis and cardiovascular disease (?)

periodontitis. However, the importance of chronic periodontitis in this effect remains unproven and many other candidate infections have been proposed.

PERIODONTAL (LATERAL) ABSCESS

Periodontal abscess results from acute infection of a periodontal pocket. It sometimes follows treatment such as root planing when trauma to the pocket lining implants bacteria into the tissues. Otherwise the causes are uncertain but an abscess may result from some change in the pocket flora or damage by a foreign body such as a fish bone driven through the floor of a pocket. Food packing down between the teeth with poor contact points may also contribute. Drainage through the pocket mouth is poor, and made worse by inflammatory oedema and soft tissue swelling.

Clinical features

The onset is rapid. Gingival tenderness progresses to throbbing

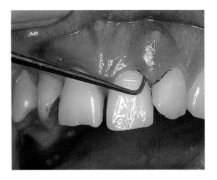

Fig. 5.16 Periodontal abscess. The abscess is pointing on the alveolar mucosa well above the attached gingiva. The probe is inserted deeply in the pocket communicating with the abscess.

pain. The tooth affected is vital and tender to percussion. The overlying gingiva is red and swollen. Pus may exude from the pocket, but a deep periodontal abscess may point on the alveolar mucosa, forming a sinus. More generalised chronic periodontitis is usually associated. The vitality of the tooth and its less severe tenderness usually distinguished a lateral abscess from acute apical periodontitis. The great depth of the pocket from which pus may exude helps to make the diagnosis clear (Fig. 5.16).

Radiographic changes are not visible until after about a week. A radiolucent area may then be seen beside the tooth.

Pathology

The bony wall of the pocket is actively resorbed by many osteoclasts. There is dense infiltration by neutrophils and pus formation (Figs 5.17 and 5.18). The pocket deepens rapidly by destruction of periodontal fibres, sometimes to the apex of the tooth. Alveolar bone in the floor of the original pocket is destroyed, and the pocket extends between the tooth and alveolar bone. An intrabony pocket may thus form.

Treatment

A periodontal abscess should be drained. Infected tissue can removed by subgingival curettage, and the root surfaces thoroughly debrided. Occasionally incision through the overlying gingiva is needed. However, if periodontal disease is severe and widespread, it may be appropriate to extract the affected tooth.

JUVENILE PERIODONTITIS

Juvenile periodontitis is uncommon, having a prevalence of about 1:1000, with males and females equally affected. Its onset may be around puberty or earlier. It appears to comprise a spectrum of disorders and only generalisations can be made about it here.

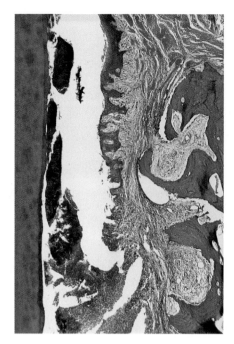

Fig. 5.17 Acute periodontal abscess. There is well-advanced chronic periodontitis, but acute inflammatory changes have developed in this pocket with destruction of periodontal ligament and alveolar bone with formation of an abscess and a deep intrabony pocket from a man of 55.

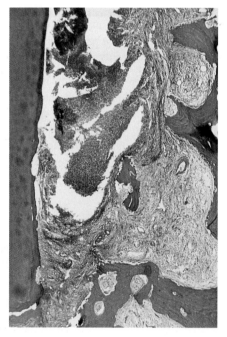

Fig. 5.18 Periodontal abscess. Higher power view of the floor of the pocket shows the purulent inflammation and gross resorption of alveolar bone extending to the apex.

The main features are rapid breakdown of the periodontal tissues of permanent first molars and incisors. There is also a rare, more generalised form which appears to be a less clearly definable disease entity. Several systemic diseases can cause premature periodontal destruction but the term 'juvenile

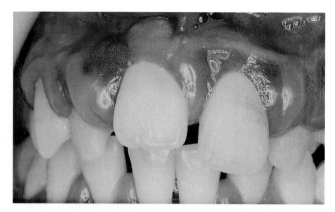

Fig. 5.19 Localised juvenile periodontitis. Drifting of upper central incisors due to gross loss of attachment. There is some marginal inflammation but oral hygiene is good and the clinical appearance belies the periodontal destruction.

periodontitis' is usually reserved for cases in which clinically significant organic disease is absent.

Aetiology

There is a familial predisposition but the immediate cause may be a specific bacterial infection and an associated neutrophil defect. The bacterium commonly found in the diseased sites is *Actinobacillus actinomycetemcomitans*, strains of which produce a potent leukotoxin. Antibodies to this bacterium and the leukotoxin are found in the serum and gingival fluid. Neutrophils from many patients have a defect in chemotaxis and reduced surface receptor binding capacity. The defect may be genetically determined, while acquisition of the organism is probably from other family members.

Clinical features

The incisor and first molar teeth are usually the most severely affected. Gingivitis is minimal or absent and the main feature is drifting and loosening of teeth, most noticeably in the front of the mouth. The teeth may also tilt or become extruded (Fig. 5.19).

Radiography

Deep, angular bone loss and displacement of the anterior teeth are typical findings (Fig. 5.20). The remarkable symmetry seen in this condition is often such as to make the sides of the mouth appear almost as mirror images of each other.

Pathology

Little material has become available for histological examination, but there is degeneration of principal periodontal fibres, which become replaced by a loose oedematous network of connective tissue, without significant inflammatory infiltration. Alveolar bone is resorbed.

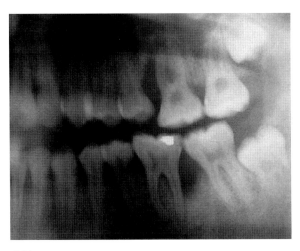

Fig. 5.20 Juvenile periodontitis. Patient aged 17 years showing severe bone destruction around first permanent molars. Probing depths exceeded 10 mm. One first permanent molar was affected on the contralateral side but in this case the central incisors were spared.

Treatment

Severely affected teeth may require extraction. Currently, early surgical treatment and tetracycline administration are advised. Surgical excision of the pocket lining may help to eradicate bacteria colonising the epithelial lining and possibly, bacteria within the diseased tissue. Tetracycline is effective against *A. actinomycetemcomitans* and given for 2–3 weeks. This treatment may be dramatically successful in the early stages of the disease.

There is a tendency for the condition to slow down or burn out in some individuals in their twenties. The residual disease is referred to as *post-juvenile periodontitis*.

Other causes of early-onset periodontal destruction

Very rarely, severe periodontal destruction may affect the deciduous and permanent dentition in a condition termed *prepubertal periodontitis*. These children have profound neutrophil or monocyte dysfunction, or both, and suffer from other infections such as otitis media. Another form of generalised severe periodontitis which affects young individuals in their twenties and early thirties may also be associated with a phagocyte defect and is referred to as 'rapidly progressive periodontitis' or 'aggressive periodontitis'. Recognised causes of premature periodontal destruction are summarised in Table 5.14.

It should be noted that the pathological mechanisms of these different types of premature periodontal tissue destruction are diverse. In the immunodeficiencies, there is acceleration of the usual bacterial processes of tissue destruction. By contrast, in the genetic syndromes mentioned above there are structural defects in the periodontal tissues, while in Langerhans cell histiocytosis there is tumour-like destruction of the periodontal tissues.

Table 5.14 Systemic causes of premature periodontal tissue destruction

- Immunodeficiencies
    Down's syndrome (Ch. 34)
    Leucopenia (Ch. 25)
    Severe, uncontrolled diabetes mellitus
    HIV infection
    Papillon–Lefèvre syndrome
- Genetic syndromes
    Hypophosphatasia
    Ehlers–Danlos syndrome (type VIII)
- Others
    Eosinophilic granuloma (Langerhans' cell histiocytosis — Ch. 9)

All (except Down's syndrome) are uncommon or rare, but are important to distinguish from early onset periodontitis in that the underlying disorder may threaten the patient's health or life.

Immunodeficiencies

Some types of immunodeficiency disease are associated with premature destructive periodontitis. Down's syndrome, in which there are multiple immunodeficiencies, is the most common example. Agranulocytosis and acute leukaemia may also be associated with necrotising gingivitis and periodontal tissue destruction. Agranulocytosis is mainly a disease of adults, while the common childhood type of acute leukaemia (acute lymphocytic leukaemia) typically does not show periodontal destruction. The importance of cyclic neutropenia has been greatly exaggerated. It is little more than a pathological curiosity and early-onset periodontitis is by no means always associated. It should be emphasised that early-onset periodontitis in patients with immunodeficiency disorders (unlike 'idiopathic' juvenile periodontitis) is typically associated with abnormal susceptibility to non-oral infections.

Papillon–Lefèvre syndrome

Papillon–Lefèvre syndrome is an exceedingly rare autosomal recessive disorder. The main features are, typically, hyperkeratosis of palms and soles starting in infancy, and early onset periodontal destruction. As a cause of the latter, *A. actinomycetemcomitans* has frequently been implicated. However, it has been shown that there is loss-of-function mutation in the cathepsin C gene. Those with the disease are homozygous for the mutation and completely lack cathepsin C activity. Carriers are heterozygous, have low cathepsin C activity but suffer no ill-effects. Parents of children with Papillon–Lefèvre syndrome have low cathepsin C activity, but do not seem to have premature periodontal destruction.

Cathepsin C, a lysosomal protease, plays an essential role in activating granule serine proteases in bone marrow-derived effector cells, particularly neutrophils. Lack of activation of these enzymes impairs host responses to bacteria in periodontal pockets. The possibility that depressed cathepsin C activity may be responsible for common types of periodontitis seems unlikely.

There is also speculation that cathepsin C might also have a role in the abnormal kertosis in Papillon–Lefèvre syndrome.

Ehlers–Danlos syndrome (Type VIII)

Ehlers–Danlos syndrome is an important cause of floppy joint syndromes and its main oral effects are on the temporomandibular joint, where it can be responsible for recurrent dislocations. However, in the Type VIII variant which is inherited as an autosomal dominant, there is bruising, soft and hyperextensible skin, and hypermobile joints. Early onset periodontal disease is related to a defect in collagen formation but the molecular defect is unknown. Teeth are commonly lost by the age of 30 years.

Langerhans' cell histiocytosis (eosinophilic granuloma)

Eosinophilic granuloma is a tumour or tumour-like disease (Ch. 9). A typical effect is destruction of the bone of the jaw with formation of a tumour-like mass. It can also cause a distinctive type of periodontal tissue destruction which exposes the roots of the teeth. Radiographically, this gives an appearance described as 'teeth floating on air'.

Hypophosphatasia

Hypophosphatasia is a rare genetic disorder which can have severe skeletal effects as a result of failure of development of mature bone. There may also be failure of cementum formation causing loosening or exfoliation of the teeth without signs of gingivitis or periodontitis. Premature loss of the deciduous teeth, especially the incisors, is characteristic and occasionally the only overt manifestation of the disease.

ACUTE PERICORONITIS

Incomplete eruption of a wisdom tooth produces a large stagnation area under the gum flap. It can easily become infected, causing pericoronitis. Several factors (Table 5.15) may contribute.

Pericoronitis is caused by a mixed infection and various pathogens of dental plaque, particularly anaerobes, can be causative.

Table 5.15 Factors contributing to pericoronitis

- Impaction of food and plaque accumulation under the gum flap
- An upper tooth biting on the gum flap
- Acute ulcerative gingivitis (rarely)

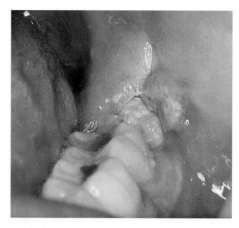

Fig. 5.21 Pericoronitis. A pocket has formed between the gingiva and the crown of a partially erupted third molar, which is overlaid by the operculum.

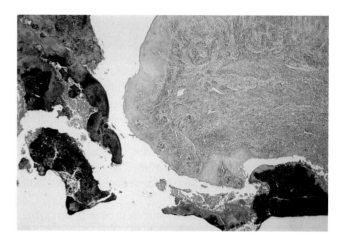

Fig. 5.22 Pericoronitis. Section through the operculum shows the heavy deposits of microbial plaque beneath it and along its anterior edge (left) (Gram stain).

Clinical features

Young adults are affected. The main symptoms are soreness and tenderness around the partially erupted tooth (Figs 5.21 and 5.22). There is pain, swelling, difficulty in opening the mouth, lymphadenopathy, sometimes slight fever and, in severe cases, suppuration and abscess formation. Swelling and difficulty in opening the mouth may be severe enough to prevent examination of the area.

Management

Food debris should be removed from under the gum flap by irrigation. The position of the affected tooth, its relationship to the second molar, and any complicating factors should be determined by radiography.

In mild cases it may be enough for patients to keep the mouth clean and to use hot mouth rinses whenever symptoms develop, until the inflammation subsides. This may happen naturally by further eruption or by extraction of the tooth after the infection has been overcome.

If radiographs show that the third molar is badly misplaced, impacted or carious, it should be extracted after inflammation has subsided.

When an upper tooth is biting on the flap it is often preferable to extract it, especially if the lower tooth is ultimately to be removed. If there are strong reasons for retaining the upper tooth, the cusps should be ground away sufficiently to prevent it from traumatising the flap. Trichloracetic acid used very sparingly on cotton wool pledget, followed by glycerine, is often useful to reduce the operculum.

In severe cases, particularly when there is fever and lymphadenopathy, metronidazole or penicillin or both should be given.

Spread of infection (cellulitis or osteomyelitis) may follow extraction of the tooth while infection is still acute, but is rare.

ACUTE NECROTISING ULCERATIVE GINGIVITIS

Acute ulcerative gingivitis is a distinct and specific disease which can cause significant periodontal tissue damage but does not often contribute to chronic periodontal disease. The following account describes the disease in HIV-negative persons.

Clinical features

The incidence of ulcerative gingivitis has declined sharply in the Western world since the second world war. It typically affects apparently healthy young adults, usually those with neglected mouths.

Typical features are summarised in Table 5.16.

Crater-shaped or punched-out ulcers form initially at the tips of the interdental papillae. Ulcers are sharply defined by erythema and oedema; their surface is covered by a greyish or yellowish tenacious slough. Removal of the slough causes free bleeding.

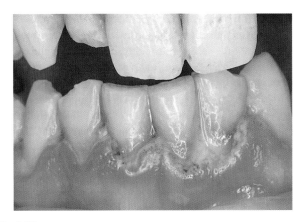

Fig. 5.23 Acute necrotising ulcerative gingivitis. The characteristic features of the lesion, the crater-shaped ulcers starting at the tips of the interdental papillae, are covered by a slough, as shown here.

Lesions remain restricted to the gingivae and supporting tissues. They mainly spread along the gingival margins and deeply, destroying interdental soft and hard tissues, but rarely across the attached gingiva. Deep spread can cause rapid destruction of both soft tissues and bone, producing triangular spaces between the teeth (Fig. 5.23).

If treatment is delayed the end result can be considered distortion of the normal gingival contours, promoting stagnation and possibly recurrences or chronic periodontal disease.

In the past particularly, localised spread to immediately adjacent oral mucosa was occasionally seen but acute ulcerative gingivitis is not an oral mucosal infection.

Aetiology

The bacteria responsible are a complex of spirochaetes and fusiforms (Fig. 5.24). These organisms may be present in small numbers in the healthy gingival flora. With the onset of ulcer-

Table 5.16 Typical features of acute necrotizing ulcerative gingivitis

- Young adult males mainly affected
- Often cigarette smokers and/or with minor respiratory infection
- Cratered ulcers starting at the tips of the interdental papillae
- Ulcers spread along gingival margins
- Gingival soreness and bleeding
- Foul breath
- No significant lymphadenopathy
- No fever or systemic upset
- Smears from ulcers dominated by Gram-negative spirochaetes and fusiform bacteria
- Responds to oral hygiene and metronidazole in immunocompetent patients

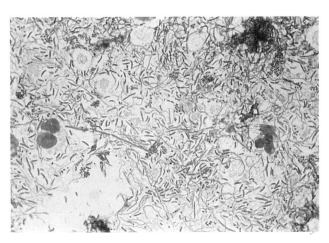

Fig. 5.24 A smear from an ulcer of acute necrotising ulcerative gingivitis shows the dense proliferation of *Treponema vincentii* and *Fusobacterium nucleatum*.

ative gingivitis, both bacteria proliferate until they dominate the bacterial picture in smears from the lesions. This overwhelming proliferation of the spirochaete and fusobacterium at the site of tissue destruction, invasion of the tissues by spirochaetes seen by electron microscopy, and the sharp fall in their numbers with effective treatment indicate that they are the responsible agents. Nevertheless, it is still uncertain whether this spirochaetal complex is the sole cause of ulcerative gingivitis and other bacteria have been implicated (Table 5.17).

Table 5.17 Bacteria implicated in acute ulcerative gingivitis

- *Treponema vincentii*
- *Fusobacterium fusiformis*
- *Prevotella intermedia*
- *Porphyromonas gingivalis*
- *Selenomonas sputigena*
- *Leptotrichia buccalis*

Despite doubts about the precise identity of the bacterial cause of acute ulcerative gingivitis, it is clearly an anaerobic infection and responds rapidly to metronidazole.

Host factors

Ulcerative gingivitis is a disease of otherwise healthy young adults usually with neglected, dirty mouths. However, ulcerative gingivitis may also develop in children having immunosuppressive treatment and in patients with HIV infection (see below).

Local factors appear to be important and ulcerative gingivitis does not appear to be transmissible. Ulcerative gingivitis ('trench mouth') was almost epidemic among soldiers in the 1914–1918 war and civilians subjected to bombing in the 1939–1945 war. Malnutrition has been excluded as a factor during these periods but being shelled or bombed can (reasonably enough) be regarded as stressful. Other evidence also suggests that chronic anxiety may be a predisposing factor in this infection. Smoking and upper respiratory infections have also been implicated. However, ulcerative gingivitis is relatively rarely seen in the UK now (Table 5.18) and the etiology remains uncertain.

Table 5.18 Differential diagnosis of acute necrotising ulcerative gingivitis

- Primary herpetic gingivostomatitis
- HIV-associated acute ulcerative gingivitis (see below)
- Gingival ulceration in acute leukaemia or aplastic anaemia

Treatment

Oral hygiene (debridement) is essential. Metronidazole (200 mg by mouth, taken after food three times a day for three days)

greatly accelerates resolution. Side-effects are few, apart from interaction with alcohol, and rarely significant.

Follow-up treatment — rehabilitation of the mouth. Once the acute phase has subsided the state of oral hygiene should be brought to as high a standard as possible to lessen the risk of recurrence.

HIV-ASSOCIATED GINGIVITIS

HIV-positive persons can suffer severe necrotising ulcerative gingivitis as their immune function declines. Clinically, it resembles ulcerative gingivitis in HIV-negative persons but rapidly progresses to HIV-associated periodontitis.

A distinctive HIV-associated gingivitis can be an early sign and precede other opportunistic infections. It appears as a distinct erythematous band extending along the free and attached gingiva. Clinically, it resembles so-called desquamative gingivitis (Ch. 13) rather than common chronic gingivitis, but profuse bleeding is characteristic (Table 5.19).

Table 5.19 Typical features of HIV-associated gingivitis

- Well demarcated band of erythema along free and attached gingiva
- Resembles 'desquamative gingivitis' clinically
- Profuse bleeding
- Bacteria similar to those from periodontal pockets

The etiology of HIV-associated gingivitis is unclear, especially as the bacteria isolated from it are similar to those from advanced chronic periodontitis.

HIV-ASSOCIATED PERIODONTITIS

HIV-associated ulcerative gingivitis as described earlier is associated with soft-tissue necrosis and rapid destruction of the periodontal tissues. It is typically intensely painful. There is little deep pocketing because soft tissue and bone are lost virtually simultaneously. More than 90% of the attachment can be lost within 3–6 months, and the soft-tissue necrosis can lead to exposure of bone and sequestration.

The pain of HIV-associated periodontitis is usually aching in character and felt within the jaw rather than in the gingivae. It may be felt before tissue destruction becomes obvious. HIV-associated gingivitis and periodontitis are usually generalised but are sometimes localised to one or more discrete areas.

Bacteriologically, HIV-associated periodontitis resembles that of classical periodontitis in HIV-negative persons. It is typically associated with a low CD4 count and a poor prognosis for the patient.

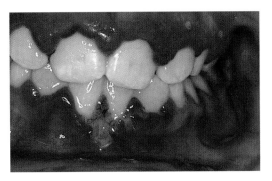

Fig. 5.25 Acute herpetic gingivostomatitis. There is diffuse reddening of the attached gingiva with ulceration in the lower incisor region extending beyond the attached gingiva (see also Ch. 12).

Table 5.20 Causes of gingival enlargement

- Fibrous gingival hyperplasia
  Genetic
  Drug-associated
  Phenytoin
  Calcium channel blockers
  Cyclosporin
- Inflammatory gingival swelling
  Chronic 'hyperplastic' gingivitis
  Pregnancy gingivitis
  Leukaemia infiltration
  Wegener's granulomatosis
  Sarcoidosis
  Orofacial granulomatosis
  Scurvy

Management

Debridement and removal of any sequestra under local anaesthesia, chlorhexidine mouth rinses, systemic metronidazole and analgesics may be effective. Additional broad-spectrum antibiotics have been recommended by some but increase the risk of thrush, to which these patients are particularly susceptible. If thrush is present or develops, antifungal drugs are required.

HERPETIC GINGIVOSTOMATITIS

In children particularly, primary herpetic stomatitis is associated with acute gingivitis. The gingivae are conspicuously erythematous and oedematous (Fig. 5.25). Herpetic ulcers may form on the tips of the interdental papillae or on any other anatomical regions of the gingivae, but are not an essential feature. Unlike ulcerative gingivitis, herpetic vesicles and ulcers extend widely over the oral mucosa. Lymphadenopathy is associated and systemic upset may be severe.

Smears from the lesions show typical viral damaged cells and the gingivitis resolves with control of the virus. This may be hastened by use of aciclovir (Ch. 12).

MISCELLANEOUS PERIODONTAL DISORDERS

Gingival swelling

Gingival swelling may be due to fibrous hyperplasia or to non-fibrous inflammatory or other infiltrations (Table 5.20).

Hereditary gingival fibromatosis

Gingival fibromatosis is a feature of several heritable disorders. All are rare but the most common type is an autosomal dominant syndrome in which gingival fibromatosis may be associated with hypertrichosis and mental retardation.

Gingival enlargement may precede eruption of the teeth or

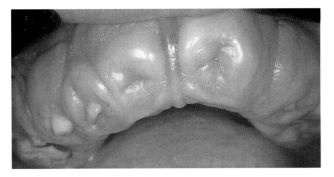

Fig. 5.26 Hereditary gingival fibromatosis. Fibrous overgrowth of the gingiva has covered the crowns of the teeth and almost buried them (pseudo-anodontia).

may not develop until later in childhood. The gingivae may be so grossly enlarged as completely to bury the teeth and are pale, firm and smooth or stippled in texture (Fig. 5.26). The facial features may also be coarse and thickened, simulating acromegaly, and there may be excessive hairiness (hypertrichosis). Epilepsy or mental retardation are rare features.

Histologically, the gingival tissue consists of thick bundles of collagenous connective tissue with little or no inflammatory exudate (Fig. 5.27).

The excess gingival tissue can only be removed surgically but is likely to re-form. Gingivectomy should be delayed as long as possible, preferably until after puberty, when the rate of growth of the tissues is slower. Maintenance of oral hygiene is important to prevent infection becoming established in the deep false pockets. However, inflammation is frequently insignificant.

Drug-induced hyperplasia

Long-term use of the anti-epileptic drug phenytoin (Epanutin*) can cause gingival hyperplasia. The overgrowth principally

*Phenytoin is sometimes referred to as Dilantin by a generation that has not caught up with current drug names. Dilantin is an American proprietary name for phenytoin and does not exist in Britain.

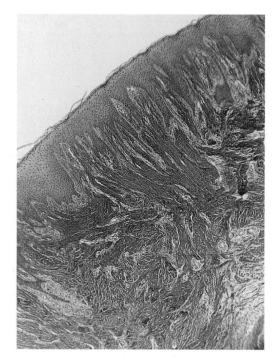

Fig. 5.27 Gingival fibromatosis. Both the genetic and drug-induced types share this histological picture of gross fibrous proliferation (red) and (frequently, as here) absence of inflammation.

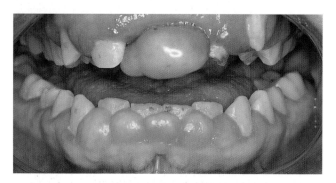

Fig. 5.28 Gingival hyperplasia due to phenytoin. Characteristically (unlike Fig. 5.26), the fibrous overgrowth has originated in the interdental papillae, which become bulbous but remain firm and pale. Localised gross enlargement such as that around the upper central incisor may result and can form a plaque trap.

involves the interdental papillae, which become bulbous and overlap the teeth (Fig. 5.28). Typically the gingivae are firm and pale, and the stippled texture is exaggerated, producing an orange-peel appearance.

Infection appears to contribute and overgrowth of the gingivae can sometimes be kept under control by rigorous oral hygiene. Frequently, however, gingivectomy becomes necessary or is demanded by patients who are embarrassed by what they regard as a stigma of their disease.

Clinically similar changes are seen with use of calcium-channel blockers such as nifedipine and diltiazem (for hypertension or angina), and with immunosuppressive drug cyclosporin. Clinically they all cause preferential enlargement

of the interdental papillae and histologically they all resemble the genetic type of gingival hyperplasia.

INFLAMMATORY GINGIVAL SWELLINGS

Chronic 'hyperplastic' and pregnancy gingivitis have been discussed earlier.

Wegener's granulomatosis

Wegener's granulomatosis (Ch. 28) is an uncommon, frequently lethal disease of which the typical features are granulomatous ulceration of the nasopharynx, pulmonary cavitation and renal damage. Occasionally, the first sign is a characteristic form of proliferative gingivitis, bright or dusky red in colour and with a granular surface, to which the term 'strawberry gums' has been applied. Recognition of this type of gingivitis and confirmation of the diagnosis by biopsy which shows the characteristic giant cells, may be life-saving by enabling treatment to start exceptionally early.

Sarcoidosis and orofacial granulomatosis

As discussed in Chapters 28 and 29, these diseases can give rise to gingival swelling in which granuloma formation is seen histologically. They cannot be distinguished by gingival biopsy alone.

Acute leukaemia

Gingival swelling is most frequently seen in acute myelo-monocytic leukaemia. The abnormal white cells are unable to perform their normal defensive function and cannot control infection at the gingival margins. The abnormal leucocytes pack the area until the gingivae become swollen with leukaemic cells (Fig. 5.29). These cells are so defective that infection progresses, leading to ulceration and breakdown of the tissues.

Clinically the gingivae are swollen, shiny, pale or purplish in colour and frequently ulcerated (Fig. 5.30). Other signs of leukaemia (pallor, purpura or lassitude) may also be seen.

Topical antibiotics or chlorhexidine and improved oral hygiene may lead to regression of the swelling (Fig. 5.31), but the patient's general prognosis is poor.

Scurvy

Grossly swollen and congested gingivae are a classical sign of scurvy, but though the disease is largely of historical interest, occasional cases are reported even now.

The gingival swelling is due to a combination of chronic inflammation and an exaggeration of the inflammatory congestion due to scorbutic purpura. The diagnosis should only be made on clear evidence of dietary deficiency and of purpura. In these cases treatment with vitamin C and adequate oral hygiene relieves the gingival condition.

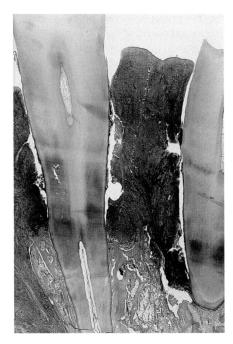

Fig. 5.29 Acute myelomonocytic leukaemia. The gingival swelling can be seen to be due to packing of the gingivae with leukaemic cells. The periodontal tissues have broken down as a result of the poor resistance to infection.

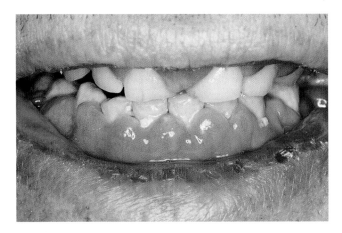

Fig. 5.30 Acute myelomonocytic leukaemia. The gingival margins are swollen and soft due to the leukaemic infiltrate.

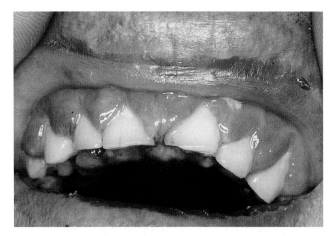

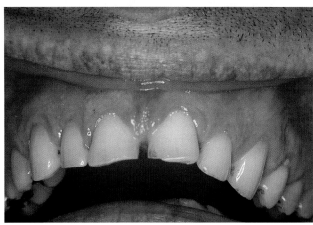

Fig. 5.31 Acute leukaemia. Gross leukaemic infiltration has caused the gingival margins to reach the incisal edges of the teeth (upper picture). The benefits of plaque control with an antibiotic mouth rinse and oral hygiene, have restored the normal appearance (lower picture).

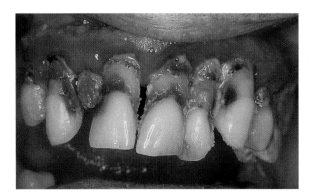

Fig. 5.32 Advanced periodontitis with recession. In this neglected mouth, deposits of plaque and supragingival calculus adhere to the exposed roots, which are vulnerable to caries.

GINGIVAL RECESSION

Recession of the gingivae and eventual exposure of the roots is common (Figs 5.32 and 5.33). It is usually but not invariably associated with ageing, as susceptibility to it varies. The major predisposing factor is thinness of the gingival tissue. This is readily damaged by trauma from forceful toothbrushing and plaque-induced inflammation. One hypothesis suggests that epithelial proliferation of the junctional epithelium in inflam-

mation results in an epithelial 'bridge' extending to the external gingival epithelium across the narrow band of inflamed connective tissue. This is followed by remodelling of the gingival margin. It seems likely that plaque-induced loss of attachment in areas of thick tissue can lead to pocket formation, whereas

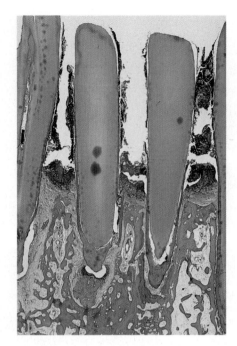

Fig. 5.33 Periodontitis with recession. In this case, gingival destruction is almost as great as the degree of bone resorption so that excessively long clinical crowns have been produced. Supragingival calculus and a dense inflammatory infiltrate in the gingiva can be seen.

thin tissue is destroyed entirely. The resulting receded gingival margins often appear relatively uninflamed.

Gingival abrasion

Abrasion causes recession of the gingivae and damage to the teeth. Early changes may be seen in some young adults and severe examples in later life. Forceful toothbrushing with a stiff brush used with a sawing motion across the teeth and use of an abrasive dentifrice is the usual cause. Grooves are worn into the necks of the teeth, and reactionary dentine forms beneath. Eventually the necks of teeth may be cut so deeply that the crowns break off, but the pulp remains covered by reactionary dentine (see Fig. 4.32). The gingival margins recede but they remain conspicuously firm, pale and healthy where they are worn away. Nearby, there may be chronic gingivitis interstitially where the toothbrush fails to reach.

Treatment of gingival recession

Recession of the gingivae sometimes causes patients to fear that they will soon lose their teeth. In older patients, where enough alveolar bone remains, the teeth can remain in useful function for many years and patients can be reassured. The main requirement is to keep the gingival margins plaque-free, especially in the enlarged interstitial spaces. In the case of abrasive gingival recession, the patient must also be shown how to keep the teeth clean without causing further damage. Various surgical procedures have been devised to correct localised areas of gingival recession or to produce thicker zones of gingiva which, it is hoped, are more resistant to recession.

An early result of abrasion is exposure of the dentine, which may be hypersensitive. Many treatments for it have been introduced, but their number betrays their limitations. Traditional remedies are topical applications of strong astringents such as zinc chloride or silver nitrate. Proprietary preparations such as Tresiolan and Durophat may be more effective.

SUGGESTED FURTHER READING

Armitage G C 1999 Development of a classification system for periodontal diseases and conditions. Ann Periodontol 4:1–6

Bozzo L, Almeida O P, Scully C, Aldred M J 1994 Hereditary gingival fibromatosis. Report of an extensive four-generation pedigree. Oral Surg Oral Med Oral Pathol 78:452–454

Corbet E F, Davies W I R 1993 The role of supragingival plaque in the control of progressive periodontal disease. J Clin Periodontol 20:307–313

De Vree H, Steenackers K, De Boever J A 2000 Periodontal treatment of rapid progressive periodontitis in 2 siblings with Papillon–Lefèvre syndrome: 15-year follow-up. J Clin Periodontol 27:354–360

Fairbrother K J, Heasman P F 2000 Anticalculus agents. J Clin Periodontol 27:285–301

Feres M, Haffajee A D, Goncalves C et al 1999 Systemic doxycycline administration in the treatment of periodontal infections (1). Effect on the subgingival microflora. J Clin Periodontol 26:775–783

Fine D H 1994 Microbial identification and antibiotic sensitivity testing, an aid for patients refractory to periodontal therapy. J Clin Periodontol 21:98–106

Grossi S G, Zambon J J, Ho A W et al 1994 Assessment of risk for periodontal disease. I. Risk indicators for attachment loss. J Periodontol 65:260–267

Grossi S G, Genco R J, Machtei E E et al 1995 Assessment of risk for periodontal disease. II. Risk factors for alveolar bone loss. J Periodontol 66:23–29

Hildebolt C F 1997 Osteoporosis and oral bone loss. Dentomaxillofacial Radiol 26:3–15

Holmstrup P, Westergaard J 1994 Periodontal disease in HIV-infected patients. J Clin Periodontol 21:270–280

Hornung G M, Cohen M E 1995 Necrotizing ulcerative gingivitis, periodontitis, and stomatitis: clinical staging and predisposing factors. J Periodontol 66:990–998

Ishikawa I, Umeda M, Laosrisin N 1994 Clinical, bacteriological and immunological examinations and the treatment process of two Papillon–Lefèvre patients. J Clin Periodontol 65:364–271

Jeffcoat M K, Chestnut C H 1993 Systemic osteoporosis and oral bone loss. Evidence shows increased risk. J Am Dent Assoc 124:49–56

Johnson B D, Engel D 1986 Acute necrotising ulcerative gingivitis: a review of diagnosis, etiology and treatment. J Periodontol 57: 141–150

Johnson N W, Bain C A Tobacco and oral disease. EU-Working Group on Tobacco and Oral Health. 2000 Br Dent J 189:200–206

Jonasson G, Kiliaridis S, Gunnarsson R 1999 Cervical thickness of the mandibular alveolar process and skeletal bone mineral density. Acta Odontol Scand 57:155–161

Liljenberg B, Lindhe J, Berglundh T et al 1994 Some microbiological, histopathological and immunohistochemical characteristics of progressive periodontal disease. J Clin Periodontol 21:720–727

Liede K E, Haukka J K, Hietanen J H P et al 1999 The association between smoking cessation and periodontal status and salivary proteinase levels. J Periodontol 70:1361–1368

Linden G J, Mullaly B H 1994 Cigarette smoking and periodontal destruction in young adults. J Periodontol 65:718–723

Löe H, Brown J 1991 Early onset periodontitis in the United States of America. J Periodontol 62:608–616

Luke D A 1992 The structure and function of the dentogingival junction and periodontal ligament. Br Dent J 172:187–190

Margiotta V, Pizza I, Pizza G, Barbaro A 1996 Cyclosporin- and nifedepine-induced gingival overgrowth in renal transplant patients: correlations with periodontal and pharmacological parameters, and HLA-antigens. Oral Pathol Med 25:128–134

Nery E B, Eson R G, Lee K K et al 1995 Prevalence of nifedipine-induced gingival hyperplasia. J Periodontol 66:572–578

Palmer R M, Scott D A, Meeking T N et al 1999 Potential mechanisms of susceptibility to periodontitis in tobacco smokers. J Periodont Res 34:363–369

Plagmann H-C, Kocher T, Kuhrau N, Caliebe A 1994 Periodontal manifestation of hypophosphatasia. A family case report. J Clin Periodontol 21:710–716

Praytino S W, Addy M, Wade W G 1993 Does gingivitis lead to periodontitis in young adults? Lancet 342:471–472

Renvert S, Dahlén G, Wikström M 1996 Treatment of periodontal disease based on microbiological diagnosis. Relation between microbiological and clinical parameters during 5 years. J Periodontol 67:562–571

Robinson P G, Winkler J R, Palmer G et al 1994 The diagnosis of periodontal conditions associated with HIV infection. J Periodontol 65:236–243

Ronderos M, Jacobs D R, Himes J H et al 2000 Associations of periodontal disease with femoral bone mineral density and estrogen therapy: cross-sectional evaluation of US adults from NANES III. J Clin Periodontol 27:778–786

Smith G L F 1994 Diagnosis of periodontal disease activity by detection of key microbial antigens. J Clin Periodontol 21:615–620

Socransky S S, Haffajee A D 1992 The bacteriology of destructive periodontal disease: current concepts. J Periodontol 63:322–331

Socransky S S, Haffajee A D 1991 Microbial mechanisms in the pathogenesis of destructive periodontal disease: a critical assessment. J Periodontol 26:322–331

Thakker N 2000 Genetic analysis of Papillon–Lefèvre syndrome. Oral Diseases 6:263

Timmerman M F, van der Weijden G A, van Steenbergen T J M et al 1996 Evaluation of the long-term efficacy and safety of locally applied minocycline in adult periontitis patients. J Clin Periodontol 23:707–716

Williams D M, Hughes F J, Odell E W, Farthing P M 1992 *Pathology of periodontal disease*. Oxford, Oxford University Press

6 Major infections of the mouth, jaws and perioral tissues

Severe oral and perioral infections are uncommon. It is hardly surprising, however, in view of the vast number of bacteria in the mouth, that oral and perioral infections are of local origin. Periodontal pockets in particular contain great concentrations of bacteria, many of which are potent pathogens. Moreover these bacteria can give rise to serious systemic infections, such as infective endocarditis. Also, in the past particularly, but occasionally today, they can be life-threatening or fatal by direct spread.

ACUTE OSTEOMYELITIS OF THE JAWS

Osteomyelitis of the jaws is mainly a disease of adults with several potential sources of infection (Table 6.1).

Table 6.1 Acute osteomyelitis of the jaws: potential sources of infection

- Periapical infection
- A periodontal pocket involved in a fracture
- Acute necrotising gingivitis or pericoronitis (even more rarely)
- Penetrating, contaminated injuries (open fractures or gunshot wounds)

Important predisposing causes are summarised in Table 6.2.

The effect of immunodeficiency is variable and acute osteomyelitis of the jaw is uncommon in HIV infection.

Table 6.2 Important predisposing conditions for osteomyelitis

Local damage to or disease of the jaws
- Fractures including gunshot wounds
- Radiation damage
- Paget's disease or osteopetrosis (Ch. 5)

Impaired immune defences
- Acute leukaemia
- Poorly controlled diabetes mellitus
- Sickle cell anaemia
- Chronic alcoholism or malnutrition

Clinical features

Most patients with osteomyelitis are adult males with infection of the mandible. Osteomyelitis of the maxilla is a rare disease of neonates or infants after either birth injuries or uncontrolled middle ear infection.

Early complaints are severe, throbbing, deep-seated pain, and swelling with external swelling due to inflammatory oedema. Later, distension of the periosteum with pus, and finally subperiosteal bone formation cause the swelling to become firm. The overlying gingiva is red, swollen and tender.

Associated teeth are tender. They may become loose and pus may exude from an open socket or gingival margins. Muscle oedema causes difficulty in opening the mouth and swallowing. Regional lymph nodes are enlarged and tender, and anaesthesia or paraesthesia of the lower lip is characteristic.

Frequently the patient remains well but in the acute phase there may be fever and leucocytosis. A severely ill, or very pale patient suggests underlying disease which requires investigation.

Radiographic changes do not appear until after at least 10 days. Loss of trabecular pattern and areas of radiolucency indicate bone destruction. These areas have ill-defined margins and have a fluffy or moth-eaten appearance (Fig. 6.1). Areas of dead bone appear as relatively dense areas which become more sharply defined as they are progressively separated as sequestra. Later, in young persons particularly, subperiosteal new bone formation causes a buccal swelling and appears as a thin, curved strip of new bone below the lower border of the jaw in lateral radiographs.

Pathology

Oral bacteria, particularly anaerobes such as *Bacteroides*, *Porphyromonas* or *Prevotella* species are important causes but the infection is often mixed. Staphylococci may be responsible when they enter from the skin via an open fracture.

The mandible has a relatively limited blood supply and dense bone with thick cortical plates. Infection causes acute inflammation in the medullary soft tissues and inflammatory exudate spreads infection through the marrow spaces. It also compresses blood vessels confined in the rigid boundaries of the vascular canals. Thrombosis and obstruction then lead to further bone

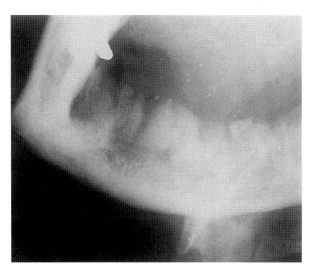

Fig. 6.1 Osteomyelitis of the mandible following dental extractions. The outlines of the extraction sockets can be seen, together with dense sequestra of bone lying in a poorly circumscribed radiolucency.

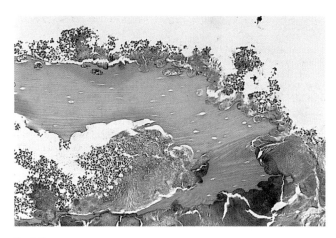

Fig. 6.2 High power view of a sequestrum showing non-vital bone (the osteocyte lacunae are empty), and eroded outline with superficial lacunae produced by osteoclastic resorption, and a dense surface growth of bacteria.

necrosis. Dead bone is recognisable microscopically by lacunae empty of osteocytes but filled with neutrophils and colonies of bacteria which proliferate in the dead tissue (Fig. 6.2).

Pus, formed by liquefaction of necrotic soft tissue and inflammatory cells, is forced along the medulla and eventually reaches the subperiosteal region by resorption of bone. Distension of the periosteum by pus stimulates subperiosteal bone formation but perforation of the periosteum by pus and formation of sinuses on the skin or oral mucosa are rarely seen now.

At the boundaries between infected and healthy tissue, osteoclasts resorb the periphery of the dead bone which eventually becomes separated as a sequestrum (Fig. 6.3). Once infection starts to localise, new bone forms around it, particularly subperiosteally.

Where bone has died and been removed, healing is by granulation with formation of coarse fibrous bone in the

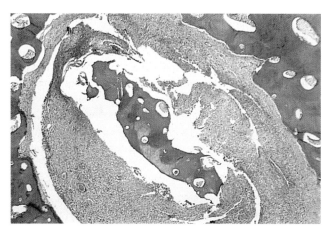

Fig. 6.3 Late-stage chronic osteomyelitis. A sequestrum trapped in a cavity within the bone. It is surrounded by fibrous tissue containing an infiltrate of inflammatory cells. Surgical intervention is needed to remove an infected sequestrum such as this.

proliferating connective tissue. After resolution, fibrous bone is gradually replaced by compact bone and remodelled to restore normal morphology.

Management

The main requirements are summarised in Table 6.3.

Table 6.3 Summary of management of osteomyelitis

Essential measures
- Bacterial sampling and culture
- Vigorous (empirical) antibiotic treatment
- Drainage
- Give specific antibiotics based on culture and sensitivities
- Give analgesics
- Debridement
- Remove source of infection, if possible.

Adjunctive treatment
- Sequestrectomy
- Decortication if necessary
- Hyperbaric oxygen*
- Resection and reconstruction for extensive bone destruction

*Mainly of value for osteoradionecrosis and possibly, anaerobic infections

Bacteriological diagnosis. A specimen of pus or a swab from the depths of the lesion must first be taken for culture and sensitivity testing.

Antimicrobial treatment. Immediately a specimen has been obtained, vigorous antibiotic treatment should be started. Initially, penicillin, 600–1200 mg daily can be given by injection (if the patient is not allergic), with metronidazole 200–400 mg 8-hourly. Clindamycin penetrates avascular tissue better and is frequently effective. The regimen is adjusted later in the light of the bacteriological findings.

Debridement. Removal of foreign or necrotic material and immobilisation of any fracture are necessary if there has been a gunshot wound or other contaminating injury.

Drainage. Pressure should be relieved by tooth extraction, bur holes or decortication, as necessary, and exudate drained into the mouth or externally.

Removal of sequestra. Dead bone should not be forcibly separated and vigorous curetting is inadvisable, but in the late stages a loosened sequestrum may have to be removed. Teeth should be extracted only if loosened by tissue destruction.

Adjunctive treatment. Decortication or hyperbaric oxygen therapy, or both, may be required, particularly in radiation-associated osteomyelitis.

Table 6.4 Acute osteomyelitis of the jaws: key features
● Mandible mainly affected, usually in adult males ● Infection of dental origin – anaerobes are important ● Pain and swelling of jaw ● Teeth in the area are tender: gingivae are red and swollen ● Sometimes paraesthesia of the lip ● Minimal systemic upset ● After about 10 days, radiographs show moth-eaten pattern of bone destruction ● Good response to prompt antibiotic treatment and debridement

Complications

Anaesthesia of the lower lip usually recovers with elimination of the infection. Rare complications include pathological fracture caused by extensive bone destruction, chronic osteomyelitis after inadequate treatment, cellulitis due to spread of exceptionally virulent bacteria or septicaemia in an immunodeficient patient.

Key features of osteomyelitis of the jaws are summarised in Table 6.4.

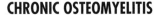

CHRONIC OSTEOMYELITIS

Rarely, inadequately treated acute osteomyelitis may lead to *chronic suppurative osteomyelitis*, which may also be a complication of irradiation (Fig. 6.4). Persistent low-grade infection is associated with bone destruction and granulation tissue formation, but little suppuration.

Chronic osteomyelitis can also arise de novo as a result of infection by weakly virulent bacteria or in avascular bone. Radiographic appearances are variable but sometimes distinctive.

CHRONIC NON-SUPPURATIVE OSTEOMYELITIS

The following types of so-called chronic osteomyelitis are mostly localised bone reactions to a source of inflammation or infection. Suppuration and infiltration of marrow spaces by inflammatory cells are absent and bacteria are not readily cultivable. Their key features are summarised in Tables 6.5, 6.6 and 6.7.

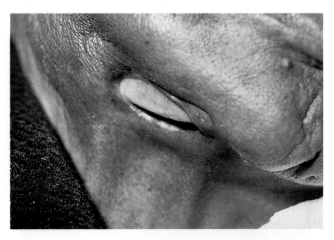

Fig. 6.4 Chronic osteomyelitis secondary to radiotherapy. Part of the necrotic portion of the mandible is visible, having ulcerated through the skin.

Table 6.5 Diffuse sclerosing osteomyelitis: key features
● Adults ● No sex predeliction ● Sclerosis round site of periapical or periodontal chronic inflammation ● No pain or swelling ● Radiographically resembles but is distinct from florid cemento-osseous dysplasia *Pathology* ● Bone sclerosis and remodelling ● Scanty marrow spaces and little or no inflammatory infiltrate, though adjacent to area of inflammation *Treatment* ● Elimination of originating source of inflammation, but sclerotic areas remain radiographically

Table 6.6 Focal sclerosing osteomyelitis: key features
● Rare bony reaction to low-grade periapical infection or unusually strong host defensive response ● Children and young adults affected ● Premolar or molar region of mandible affected ● Bone sclerosis associated with a nonvital or pulpitic tooth ● Localised but uniform radiodensity related to tooth with widened periodontal ligament space or periapical area ● No expansion of the jaw Pathology ● Dense sclerotic bone with scanty connective tissue or inflammatory cells Treatment ● Elimination of the source of inflammation by extraction or endodontic treatment

Chronic specific osteomyelitis

Syphilitic, actinomycotic and tuberculous osteomyelitis of the jaws are recognised entities but largely of historical interest.

Table 6.7 Proliferative periostitis ('Garré's osteomyelitis'*): key features

- Adolescents mainly affected
- Usually associated with periapical but sometimes other inflammatory foci
- Periosteal reaction affecting lower border of mandible causing 'onion skin' thickening and swelling of bone
Pathology
- Parallel layers of highly cellular woven bone interspersed with scantily inflamed connective tissue
- Small sequestra if present
Treatment
- Eliminate focus of infection
- Bone gradually remodels after 6 to 12 months

*Garré's osteomyelitis is a misnomer. In his original description he made no mention of proliferative changes in the lesion, X-rays had not then been invented and he provided no histological back-up.

SCLEROTIC BONE ISLANDS (IDIOPATHIC OSTEOSCLEROSIS)

Areas of sclerosis in the jaw are sometimes seen by chance in routine, particularly panoramic, radiographs. They should not be mistaken for a low-grade bone infection (particularly if first noticed after a surgical procedure) as they have sometimes been. Operative interference should be avoided as it may lead to complications and medicolegal claims, without being beneficial.

ALVEOLAR OSTEITIS

Alveolar osteitis (dry socket) can hardly be termed a major infection but can be mistaken clinically for osteomyelitis, which can rarely follow. It is by far the most frequent painful complication of extractions. Nevertheless, it is uncommon overall.

Aetiology

Alveolar osteitis is frequently unpredictable and without any obvious predisposing cause but numerous possible aetiological factors exist (Table 6.8).

Difficult disimpactions of third molars frequently lead to painful alveolar osteitis. However, the blood supply to the area

Table 6.8 Possible aetiological factors for alveolar osteitis

- Excessive extraction trauma
- Limited local blood supply
- Local anaesthesia
- Oral contraceptives
- Osteosclerotic disease
- Radiotherapy

often appears to be critical. In healthy persons alveolar osteitis virtually only affects the lower molar region where the bone is more dense and less vascular than elsewhere. Alveolar osteitis is also an expected complication of extractions in Paget's disease and particularly after radiotherapy where endarteritis causes ischaemia of the bone. Alveolar osteitis is also more frequent in susceptible patients, when local anaesthesia is used.

Loss of clot from the extraction socket was traditionally ascribed to bacterial proteolytic enzymes. However, it appears frequently to be due to excessive local fibrinolytic activity. The alveolar bone and other oral tissues have a high content of fibrinolysin activators (plasmin) which are released when the bone is traumatised. Nevertheless, once the clot has been destroyed, infection from the mouth is inevitable and anaerobes are likely to play a major role.

The oestrogen component of oral contraceptives apparently enhances serum fibrinolytic activity and, reportedly, is also associated with a higher incidence of alveolar osteitis.

Clinical features

Women are more frequently affected. Pain usually starts a few days after the extraction, but sometimes may be delayed for a week or more. It is deep-seated, severe and aching or throbbing. The mucosa around the socket is red and tender. There is no clot in the socket, which contains, instead, saliva and often decomposing food debris (Fig. 6.5). When debris is washed away, whitish, dead bone may be seen or may be felt as a rough area with a probe. Sometimes the socket becomes concealed by granulations growing in from the gingival margins. Pain often

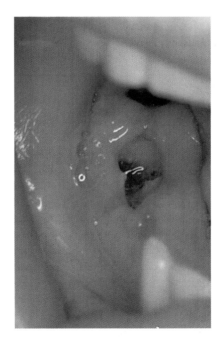

Fig. 6.5 Dry socket. Typical appearances of chronic alveolar osteitis; the socket is empty and the bony lamina dura is visible.

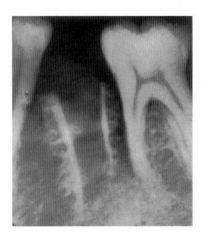

Fig. 6.6 Sequestration in a severe dry socket. Almost the whole of the lamina dura and attached trabeculae have become necrotic, forming a sequestrum. Healing is delayed while the sequestrum remains in place. Most dry sockets are not associated with sequestration, or with only small sequestra.

continues for a week or two, or occasionally longer. Sequestration of the socket may sometimes be seen radiographically (Fig. 6.6).

Pathology

The initial event is destruction of the clot which normally fills the socket. This leaves an open socket in which infected food and other debris accumulates in direct contact with the bone. Bone damaged during the extraction, particularly the dense bone of the lamina dura, dies. The necrotic bone lodges bacteria which proliferate freely, protected from leucocytes unable to reach them through this avascular material. In the surrounding tissue, inflammation usually localises infection to the socket walls. Dead bone is gradually separated by osteoclasts, and sequestra are usually shed in tiny fragments. Healing is by granulation from the base and walls of the socket.

Prevention

Since damage to bone appears to be an important predisposing factor, extractions should obviously be carried out with minimal trauma. Immediately after the extraction the socket edges should be squeezed firmly together and held for a few minutes until the clot has formed. In the case of disimpactions of third molars, where alveolar osteitis is more common, prophylactic antibiotics are often given. Their value is unproven and there is no indication for using antibiotics for routine dental extractions. However, in patients who have had irradiation for oral cancer or osteosclerotic Paget's disease where there is extensive infection, antibiotic cover should be given and the tooth removed surgically, with as little damage as possible to surrounding bone.

There remain a few patients who otherwise appear to be well but are especially prone to alveolar osteitis which follows every extraction under local anaesthesia including regional blocks. In

such patients, dry socket may be preventable if general anaesthesia is used.

Treatment

Local conditions strongly favour persistence of infection, and it is more surprising that the infection is well localised than that it responds poorly to treatment. It is important to explain this to patients and to warn them that they may have a week or more of discomfort. It is also important to explain that the pain is not due, as patients usually think, to a broken root.

Treatment should aim to keep the open socket clean and to protect exposed bone. The socket should be irrigated with mild warm antiseptic, then filled with an obtundant dressing containing some non-irritant antiseptic to prevent food and debris from accumulating. This should be followed by frequent use of hot mouth-rinses. Many socket dressings has been formulated but a convenient proprietary preparation is Alvogel. It is easy to manipulate, and patients report that it gives a sensation of warmth in place of the pain. Apart from being obtundant and antiseptic, the socket dressing should preferably be soft, adhere to the socket wall and be absorbable. Non-absorbable dressings must be removed as soon as possible to allow the socket to heal. Most cases become free from pain after one or two dressings.

Key features of alveolar osteitis are summarised in Table 6.9.

Table 6.9 Alveolar osteitis: key features

- The most common painful complication of dental extractions
- Loss of clot normally filling extraction socket
- Loss of clot may be due to excessive local fibrinolytic action or bacterial enzymes or both
- Bare, whitish lamina dura exposed in socket
- Pain relieved by irrigation and repeated dressing of socket
- Dead bone usually shed as crumb-like fragments
- Eventual healing of socket from its base by granulation

FASCIAL SPACE INFECTIONS (CERVICOFACIAL CELLULITIS)

Usually, acute periapical infections result in abscess formation. In an abscess, bacteria cause localised tissue necrosis and pus forms by the action of neutrophil proteolytic enzymes. The process is localised by granulation tissue forming the abscess wall. However, the surrounding soft tissues may become swollen by diffusion of fluid (inflammatory exudate) into them.

Fascial space infections are a form of *cellulitis* in which, unlike an abscess, bacteria spread in the soft tissues. Fasciae covering muscle bundles are normally in close apposition. If these fasciae are forced apart, avascular spaces are created. If localisation of an infection by virulent bacteria fails, inflammatory exudate opens up the fascial spaces carrying bacteria with it

MAJOR INFECTIONS OF THE MOUTH, JAWS AND PERIORAL TISSUES

CHAPTER 6

into the tissue planes. The latter extend from the base of the skull to the mediastinum. Unlike simple inflammatory oedema therefore, the exudate in cellulitis forms the vehicle for the spread of the infection.

Deep fascial space infections cause gross inflammatory exudate and tissue oedema, associated with fever and toxaemia. Before the advent of antibiotics the mortality was high and the disease is still life-threatening if treatment is delayed. The main types are sublingual, submandibular (Fig. 6.7) and parapharyngeal. *Ludwig's angina* involves several of these regions.

The characteristic features are diffuse swelling, pain, fever and malaise. The swelling is tense and tender, with a characteristic board-like firmness. The overlying skin is taut and shiny. Pain and oedema limit opening the mouth and often cause dysphagia. Systemic upset is severe with worsening fever, toxaemia and leucocytosis. The regional lymph nodes are swollen and tender.

In Ludwig's angina particularly, airway obstruction can quickly result in asphyxia.

Pathology

Anaerobic bacteria are mainly responsible and infection mainly spreads from mandibular third molars whose apices are closely related to several fascial spaces (Figs 6.7 and 6.8). Fasciae covering muscles and other structures are normally adherent but

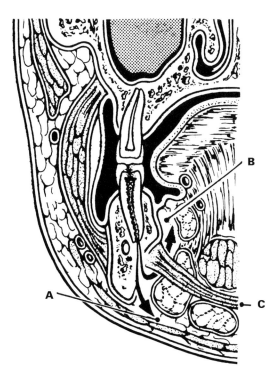

Fig. 6.7 Paths of infection spread from lower molars. By penetrating the lingual plate of the jaw below the attachment of myelohyoid (C) infection immediately enters the submandibular space (A). Below the mylohyoid is the main body of the submandibular salivary gland with its deep process curving around the posterior border of the muscle; infection from the third molar can follow the same route to enter the sublingual space (B).

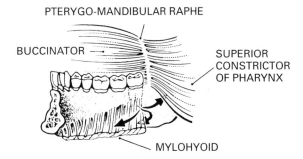

Fig. 6.8 Paths of infection from the third molar. The diagram shows the lingual aspect of the jaw and indicates how infection penetrating from the lingual plate of bone can enter the sublingual space above, or the submandibular space below, the mylohyoid muscle which forms the major structure of the floor of the mouth. Moreover, since this point is at the junction of the oral cavity and pharynx, infection can also spread backwards to reach the lateral surface of superior constrictor, i.e. the lateral pharyngeal space.

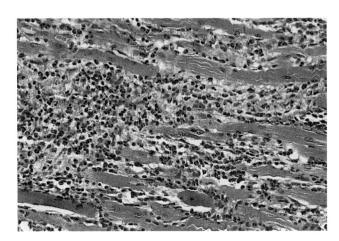

Fig. 6.9 Cellulitis. Infection spreading through the tissues is accompanied by a dense infiltrate of neutrophils, here separating muscle bundles in a facial muscle.

can be spread apart by inflammatory exudate. Spaces created in this way are almost avascular and inflammatory exudate carries bacteria widely through them (Fig. 6.9).

Ludwig's angina is a severe form of cellulitis which usually arises from the lower second or third molars. It involves the sublingual and submandibular spaces bilaterally almost simultaneously and readily spreads into the lateral pharyngeal and pterygoid spaces and can extend into the mediastinum.

The main features are rapidly spreading sublingual and submandibular cellulitis with painful, brawny swelling of the upper part of the neck and the floor of the mouth on both sides (Fig. 6.10). With involvement of the parapharyngeal space, the swelling tracks down the neck (Figs 6.11 and 6.12), and oedema can quickly spread to the glottis.

Swallowing and opening the mouth become difficult, and the tongue may be pushed up against the soft palate. The latter or oedema of the glottis causes worsening respiratory obstruction. The patient soon becomes desperately ill, with fever, respiratory distress, headache and malaise.

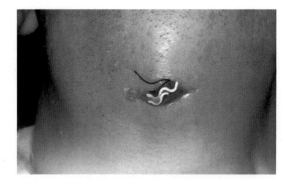

Fig. 6.10 Ludwig's angina. Incision and drainage of the front of the neck to relieve the pressure of exudate which compromises the airway. The neck is grossly swollen, shiny and dusky in hue; the edges of the wound have pulled apart, indicating the distension of these normally lax tissues.

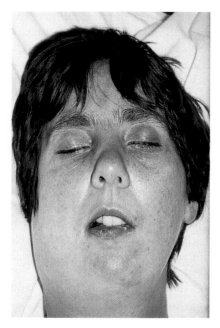

Fig. 6.12 Ludwig's angina. There is cellulitis and gross oedema of the right submandibular and sublingual spaces extending on to the left side and into the neck and parapharyngeal space. (By kind permission of Professor J D Langdon.)

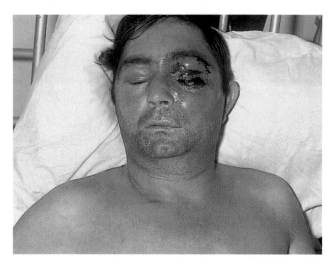

Fig. 6.11 Facial cellulitis arising from an infected upper tooth. The tissues are red, tense and shiny and the patient is incapacitated by the systemic effects of infection. (By kind permission of Professor J D Langdon.)

Table 6.10   Fascial space infections: key features

- Potentially life-threatening infections due to spread of bacteria into perioral fascial spaces
- Infection usually arises from lower second or third molars
- Ludwig's angina comprises bilateral involvement of sublingual and submandibular spaces and readily spreads into lateral pharyngeal and pterygoid spaces
- Affected tissues swollen and of board-like hardness
- Severe systemic upset associated
- Glottic oedema or spread into the mediastinum may be fatal

Management

The main requirements are (1) immediate admission to hospital, (2) procurement of a sample for culture and sensitivity testing, (3) aggressive antibiotic treatment, (4) securing the airway by tracheostomy if necessary, and (5) drainage of the swelling to reduce pressure.

Key features of fascial space infections are summarised in Table 6.10.

CAVERNOUS SINUS THROMBOSIS

Cavernous sinus thrombosis is an uncommon life-threatening complication of infection that can sometimes originate from an upper anterior tooth. Blindness or death can result.

Clinically, gross oedema of the eyelid is associated with pulsatile exophthalmos due to venous obstruction. Cyanosis,

proptosis, a fixed dilated pupil and limited eye movement rapidly develop. The patient is seriously ill with rigors, a high swinging fever and deteriorating sight.

Early recognition and treatment of cavernous sinus thrombosis is essential. The main measures are use of antibiotics, drainage of pus and possibly anticoagulant treatment. There is a 50% mortality and 50% of survivors may lose the sight of one or both eyes.

MAXILLOFACIAL GANGRENE (NOMA, CANCRUM ORIS)

Noma is an overwelmingly severe oral infection, extending on to and destroying part of the face, and fatal if inadequately treated. It has been described as a 'severe scourge to mankind' as children are mainly affected.

Noma was common among starving prisoners in Nazi concentration camps, particularly children, in the 1940s and

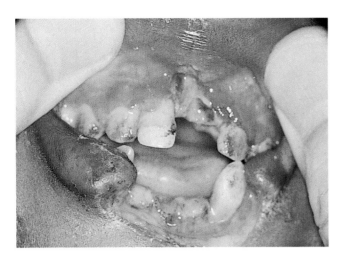

Fig. 6.13 Cancrum oris. In the maxilla there is extension of necrotising gingivitis into the alveolar process and in the lower arch anteriorly, resulting in destruction of much of the lower lip.

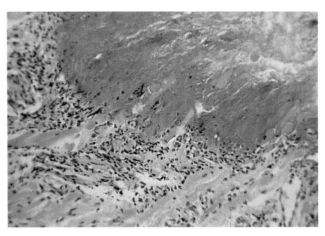

Fig. 6.14 Cancrum oris. Muscle has been invaded by spirochaetes and fusiforms. There is rapid necrosis and only a light inflammatory response of neutrophils.

invariably fatal. Later, attention was drawn to the disease in Africa in the 1960s. Otherwise, noma has virtually disappeared from developed countries, and for decades the disease has been largely ignored. However, it is so widespread in sub-Saharan Africa as to have become a subject for international concern and a World Health Organization project to assess prevalence and preventive measures has been instituted. In Niger alone, where severe malnutrition, poor oral hygiene and debilitating diseases are contributory, there are estimated to be over 100 000 cases. Political unrest has in many cases contributed to the poverty which is a major factor in the aetiology. Noma has also been seen in HIV-positive patients, but only rarely, despite the severity of the immune deficiency.

Apart from occasional adults with AIDS, children under 10 years are affected. Aetiological factors include severe malnutrition, poor oral and general hygiene, and contributory infections such as measles which impair immunity. The main bacteria isolated are anaerobes including *Fusobacterium necrophorum*, *Prevotella intermedia* and spirochaetes. *F. necrophorum* is a commensal in the gut of herbivores and also a cause of necrotising infections in animals. It has been suggested that *F. necrophorum* plays an important role in noma in Africa as a result of patients living in close proximity and often sharing drinking water with cattle.

Noma starts within the oral cavity from an acute necrotising ulcerative gingivitis associated with extensive oedema, but extends outwards, rapidly destroying soft tissues and bone (Fig. 6.13). The gangrenous process starts as a painful, small, reddish-purple spot or indurated papule which ulcerates. The ulcer spreads to involve the labiogingival fold, adjacent mucosa and underlying bone. Diffuse oedema of the face, foetor and profuse salivation are associated. As the overlying tissues become ischaemic the skin turns blue-black.

The gangrenous area becomes increasingly sharply demarcated and ultimately sloughs away. Muscle, invaded by spirochaetes and fusiform bacteria, undergoes rapid necrosis associated with only a weak inflammatory response (Fig. 6.14). The slough is

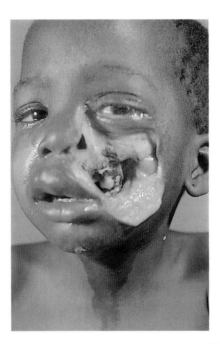

Fig. 6.15 Cancrum oris. Gross destruction and sloughing of facial tissues as a result of spread of infection from the maxillary gingivae. A molar tooth is visible centrally in the defect. (By kind permission of Professor R D Emslie.)

cone-shaped, with its apex superficially so that the underlying destruction of hard and soft tissues is more extensive than external appearances suggest. As the slough separates, the bone dies: sequestration and exfoliation of teeth follow. A gaping facial defect is left (Fig. 6.15).

Management

Malnutrition and underlying infections must be treated. A combination of penicillin or an aminoglycoside and metronidazole will usually control the local infection, but debridement of necrotic soft tissue is also needed. After control of the infection and recovery of health, reconstructive surgery is usually required to prevent permanent mutilation.

Remarkably, at the end of World War II, some children with noma, who survived until release from Nazi concentration camps, responded rapidly to a high calorie diet, nicotinic acid and injections of a sulphonamide.

ACTINOMYCOSIS

Actinomycosis is a chronic, suppurative infection caused by a filamentous bacterium, usually *Actinomyces israelii*. Though common in the past, it has become rare.

Bacteria causing actinomycosis are common in the normal mouth. Injuries, especially dental extractions or fractures of the jaw, can provide a pathway and sometimes precede infection but in fact, rarely do so. Most patients were previously healthy and it is uncommon even in patients with AIDS. The pathogenesis is therefore unclear.

Clinically, men are predominantly affected, typically between the ages of 30 and 60 years. A chronic soft tissue swelling near the angle of the jaw in the upper neck is the usual complaint. The swelling is dusky-red or purplish, firm and slightly tender. The skin eventually breaks down as discharging sinuses form. There is often difficulty in opening the mouth but pain is minimal. Healing leads to scarring and puckering of the skin and in the absence of treatment, a large fibrotic mass can form, covered by scarred and pigmented skin, on which several sinuses open. However, such a picture is rarely now seen. Currently, the usual clinical features are a persistent subcutaneous collection of pus or a sinus, unresponsive to conventional, short courses of antibiotics.

Pathology

A. israelii spreads by direct extension through the tissues and causes chronic suppurative inflammation. In the tissues, colonies of actinomyces form rounded masses of filaments with peripheral, radially-arranged club-shaped thickenings. Neutrophils mass round the colonies; pus forms centrally, chronic inflammatory cells surround the focus and an abscess wall of connective tissues forms (Fig. 6.16).

The abscess eventually points on the skin, discharging pus in which so-called sulphur granules (colonies of actinomyces) may be visible. The abscess continues to discharge and surrounding tissues become fibrotic. Nevertheless, infection spreads to cause further abscesses. Untreated, the area can become honey-combed with abscesses and sinuses, and widespread fibrosis.

Management

Actinomycosis should be suspected if a skin sinus fails to heal after a possible focus has been found and eliminated. A fresh specimen of pus is needed. A positive diagnosis can rarely be

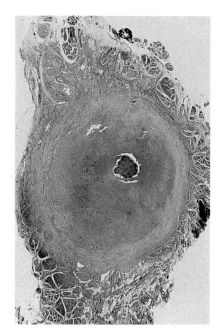

Fig. 6.16 Actinomycosis. This single, complete loculus was from an early case of actinomycosis that followed dental extraction. The colony of actinomyces with its paler staining periphery (a 'sulphur' granule) is in the centre; around it is a dense collection of inflammatory cells, surrounded in turn by proliferating fibrous tissue. It will be apparent that an antibiotic cannot readily penetrate such a fibrous mass and must be given in large doses to be effective.

made without 'sulphur granules' which may be found by rinsing the pus with sterile saline. The laboratory should be warned that actinomycosis is suspected, to enable appropriate media to be used and the culture maintained long enough for these slow-growing organisms to develop.

Frequently, small amounts of penicillin have been given earlier. These are insufficient to control the infection but make bacteriological diagnosis difficult.

The mainstay of treatment is penicillin, which should be continued for 4–6 weeks or occasionally longer, as pockets of surviving organisms may persist in the depths of the lesion to cause relapse. Abscesses should be drained surgically as they form. For patients allergic to penicillin, erythromycin can be given.

The key features of actinomycosis are given in Table 6.11.

Table 6.11 Actinomycosis: key features

- Chronic infection by filamentous bacterium, usually *A. israelii*
- Infection spreads through the tissues to produce multiple abscesses and sinuses, in severe cases
- More usually now, there is only a localised subcutaneous collection of pus
- Microscopy shows colonies of actinomyces with peripheral, radially-arranged club-shaped thickenings
- Pus forms centrally and connective tissue forms an abscess wall
- Sulphur granules (colonies of actinomyces) from the pus, required for culture
- Responds to prolonged treatment with penicillin or tetracycline
- Surgical drainage of locules of pus may be needed

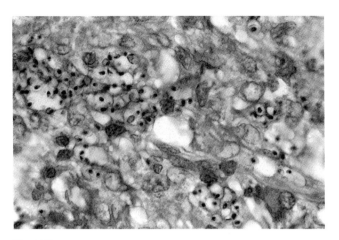

Fig. 6.17 Histoplasmosis. Part of an oral biopsy under high power, showing typical round yeast forms with their clear haloes (PAS stain).

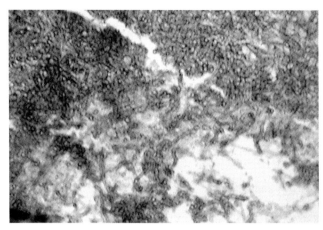

Fig. 6.18 Aspergillosis. Tissue densely infiltrated by aspergillus hyphae. In this section stained with PAS stain the septate hyphae appear as tubes with a red PAS-positive wall.

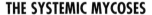

Table 6.12 **Some systemic mycoses than can affect the mouth**

- Histoplasmosis
- Rhinocerebral mucormycosis
- Rhinocerebral aspergillosis
- Cryptococcosis
- Paracoccidioidomycosis (South American blastomycosis)

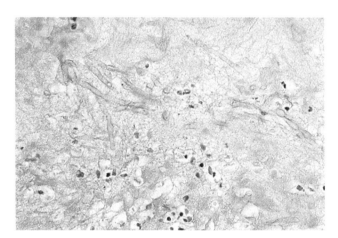

Fig. 6.19 Mucormycosis. Necrotic tissue infiltrated by the broad, knobbly branching hyphae of *Mucor* sp.

THE SYSTEMIC MYCOSES

The systemic mycoses are rare in Britain but may be seen in immunocompromised patients or in those from endemic areas such as South America. Though superficial candidosis is common, there are surprisingly few reports of oral lesions due to systemic mycoses in AIDS patients. Cryptococcosis is the most common mycosis in AIDS and is sometimes the presenting disease. Clinically, most of the systemic mycoses can cause oral lesions at some stage, and often then give rise to a nodular and ulcerated mass, which can be tumour-like in appearance. (Fig. 6.20). Mulberry-like gingival ulcerations with bleeding and purulent foci have been described in paracoccidiomycosis in a patient with AIDS.

Microscopically, most systemic mycoses give rise to granulomas similar to those of tuberculosis but there may also be abscess formation. Characteristic yeast forms or hyphae may sometimes be seen with special stains such as PAS (Figs 6.17–6.19). However, microscopy may not be diagnostic and culture of unfixed material may be necessary.

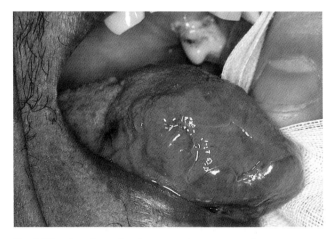

Fig. 6.20 Histoplasmosis. The gross nodular swelling of the tongue and ulceration are typical of many of the systemic mycoses.

Treatment

Amphotericin remains the most generally effective drug for most systemic mycoses but given intravenously can cause renal damage and severe hypersensitivity reactions. Liposomal amphotericin is less toxic and as effective. Ketoconazole and its analogues have mainly been used for maintenance.

SYSTEMIC INFECTIONS BY ORAL BACTERIA

The mouth harbours a great variety of microbes and virulent pathogens, particularly in periodontal pockets, but high levels of immunity keep the infection localised. Oral bacteria, even some such as *Leptotrichia buccalis* which were long thought to be harmless, once they reach the blood stream of immunocompromised patients, can cause septicaemias, which can be fatal.

Infective endocarditis

A special example of a systemic infection of dental origin is infective endocarditis, which can occasionally follow dental operations, particularly extractions, and cause irreparable damage to heart valves (Ch. 27).

Lung and brain abscesses

Some of these abscesses are due to oral anaerobic bacteria which are probably aspirated during sleep to cause a lung abscess and a secondary brain abscess. Isolated brain abscesses caused by oral bacteria are recognised but difficult to explain.

Immunodeficiency states

In severe immunodeficiency states, such as immunosuppression for organ transplants, lymphoreticular diseases, or neutropenia due to cytotoxic chemotherapy, bacteraemias of oral origin can sometimes cause septicaemias. Viridans streptococcal bacteriaemia is a recognised complication of neutropenia, but is not due to dental manipulations. Mucosal ulceration due to cytotoxic drugs is believed to be the portal of entry.

If antibiotic cover is thought necessary for dental operations, particularly extractions or periodontal treatment a combination of amoxycillin 3 g plus metronidazole 400 mg by mouth, one hour before operations may possibly offer some protection and can be repeated six hours later, if thought desirable. However, there is no definitive prophylactic regimen, as the causes are varied and unpredictable.

Prosthetic joint replacements

There is no evidence of a significant risk of infection of prosthetic joints from dental operations.

SUGGESTED FURTHER READING

Akula S K, Creticos C M, Weldon-Linne C M 1989 Gangrenous stomatitis in AIDS. Lancet 1:955

Aldesberger L 1946 Medical observations in Auschwitz concentration camp. Lancet 1:317

Barrios T J, Aria A A, Brahay C 1995 Cancrum oris in an HIV-positive patient. J Oral Maxillofac Surg 53:851–855

Bochud P-Y, Clandra T, Francioli P 1994 Bacteremia due to viridans streptococci in neutropenic patients: a review. Am J Med 97:256

Cawson R A, Binnie W H, Barrett A W, Wright J 2001 *Color atlas of oral disease*, 3rd Edn. Mosby-Wolfe, London

Cawson R A, Langdon J D, Eveson J W 1996 *Surgical pathology of the mouth and jaws*. Wright, Oxford

Chow A W 1992 Life-threatening infections of the head and neck. Clin Infect Dis 14:991–1004

Cohen M E, Simecek J W 1995 Effects of gender-related factors on the incidence of localized alveolar osteitis. Oral Surg Oral Med Oral Pathol Oral Radiol Endod 79:416–422

Denning D W 2000 Early diagnosis of invasive aspergillosis. Lancet 355:423

Diamond R D 1991 The growing problem of mycoses in patients infected with the human immunodeficiency virus. Rev Infect Dis 13:480–486

Emslie R D 1963 Cancrum oris. Dent Pract Dent Rec 13:481–494

Enwonu C O, Falker W A, Idigbe E O 2000 Oro-facial gangrene (noma/cancrum oris): pathogenetic mechanisms. Crit Rev Oral Biol Med 11:159–171

Enwonwu C O, Falker W A, Idigbe E O, Savage K O 1999 Noma (cancrum oris): questions and answers. Oral Diseases 5:144–149

Geist J R, Katz J O 1990 The frequency and distribution of idiopathic osteosclerosis. Oral Surg Oral Med Oral Pathol 69:388–393

Giovani E M, Mantesso A, Locucca S V L et al 2000 Paracoccidioidomycosis in an HIV-positive patient: a case report with gingival aspects. Oral Diseases 6:327–329

Glueck C J, McMahon R E, Bouquot J et al 1996 Thrombophilia, hypofibrinolysis, and alveolar osteonecrosis of the jaws. Oral Surg Oral Med Oral Pathol Radiol Endod 81:557–566

Griffin J M, Bach D E, Nespeca J A, Marshall K J 1983 Noma. Report of two cases. Oral Surg 56:605–607

Har-El G, Aroesty J H, Shaha A, Lucente F E 1992 Changing trends in deep neck abscess. A retrospective study of 110 patients. Oral Surg Oral Med Oral Pathol 77:446–450

Indresano A T, Haug R H, Hoffman M J 1992 The third molar as cause of deep space infections. J Oral Maxillofac Surg 50:33–35

Jansma J, Vissink A, Spijkervet F K L, Roodenburg J L N, Panders A K, Vermey A et al 1992 Protocol for the prevention and treatment of oral sequelae resulting from head and neck radiation therapy. Cancer 70:2171

Koorbusch G F, Fotos P, Goll T K 1992 Retrospective study of osteomyelitis. Etiology, demographics, risk factors and management in 35 cases. Oral Surg Oral Med Oral Pathol 74:149–154

Kuriyama T, Karasawa T, Nakagawa K et al 2000 Bacteriologic features and antimicrobial susceptibility in isolates from orofacial odontogenic infections. Oral Surg Oral Med Oral Pathol Oral Radiol Endod 90:600–608

Larsen P E 1992 Alveolar osteitis after removal of impacted mandibular third molars. Identification of the patient at risk. Oral Surg Oral Med Oral Pathol 72:393–397

Lortholary O, Denning D W, Dupont B 1999 Endemic mycosis: a treatment update. J Antimicrob Chemother 43:321–331

Marple B F 1999 Ludwig angina. A review of current airway management. Arch Otolaryngol Head Neck Surg. 125:596–600

Martinez D, Burgueno M, Forteza G et al 1992 Invasive maxillary aspergillosis after dental extraction. Oral Surg Oral Med Oral Pathol 74:466–468

Maximew W G, Wood R E, Liu F-F 1991 Postradiation dental extractions without hyperbaric oxygen. Oral Surg Oral Med Oral Pathol 72:270–274

McDonnell D 1993 Dense bone islands. A review of 107 patients. Oral Surg Oral Med Oral Pathol 76:124–128

Notani K-I, Sato O, Hashimoto I et al 2000 Intracranial *Aspergillus* infection from the paranasal sinus. Oral Surg Oral Med Oral Pathol Radiol Endod 89:9–11

Ogundiya D A, Keith D A, Mirowski J 1989 Cavernous sinus thrombosis and blindness as a complication of an odontogenic infection. Report of a case and review of the literature. J Oral Maxillofac Surg 47:1317

Pascale R, Del Valle G A, Moreau P et al 1995 Viridans streptococcal bacteraemia in patients with neutropenia. Lancet 345:1607–1609

Peterson L J 1993 Contemporary management of deep neck infections. J Oral Maxillofac Surg 51:226–231

Richard P, Del Valle G A, Moreau P et al 1995 Viridans streptococcal bacteraemia in patients with neutropenia. Lancet 345:1607–1609

Sakamoto H, Aoki T, Kise Y et al 2000 Descending necrotizing mediastinitis due to odontogenic infections. Oral Surg Oral Med Oral Pathol Radiol Endod 89:412–419

Schneider L C, Mesa M L 1990 Differences between florid osseous dysplasia and chronic diffuse sclerosing osteomyelitis. Oral Surg Oral Med Oral Pathol 70:308–312

Scully C, de Almeida O 1992 Orofacial manifestations of the systemic mycoses. J Oral Pathol Med 21:289–294

Shroyer J V, Lew D, Abreo F, Unhold G P 1991 Osteomyelitis of the mandible as a result of sickle cell disease. Report and literature review. Oral Surg Oral Med Oral Pathol 72:25–28

Smithe O P, Prentice H G, Madden G M, Nazareth B 1990 Lingual cellulitis causing upper airways obstruction in neutropenic patients. BMJ 300:24

Sposto M R, Mendes-Giannini, Moraes M J et al 1994 Paracoccidioidomycosis manifesting as oral lesions: clinical, cytological and serological investigation. J Oral Pathol Med 23:85–87

Sposto M R, Scully C, de Almeida O P et al 1993 Oral paracoccidioidomycosis. A study of 36 South American patients. Oral Surg Oral Med Oral Pathol 75:461–465

Tempest M N 1966 Cancrum oris. Br J Surg 53:949–969

Thorn J J, Hansen H S, Specht L et al 2000 Osteoradionecrosis of the jaws: clinical characteristics and relation to the field of irradiation. J Oral Maxillofac Surg 58:1088–1093

Tibbles P M, Edelsberg J S 1996 Hyperbaric oxygen therapy. N Engl J Med 334:1642–1648

Tsumoda R, Suda S, Fukaya T et al 2000 Descending necrotizing mediastinitis caused by odontogenic infection: a case report. J Oral Maxillofac Surg 58:240–242

Van Merkensteyn J P R, Balm A J M, Bakker A J M, Borgmeyer-Hoelen A M M J 1994 Hyperbaric oxygen treatment of osteoradionecrosis of the mandible with repeated pathological fracture. Report of a case. Oral Surg Oral Med Oral Pathol 77:461–464

Cysts of the jaws

Cysts are the most common cause of chronic swellings of the jaws. They are more common in the jaws than in any other bone because of the many rests of odontogenic epithelium remaining in the tissues. Cysts formed from this epithelium (odontogenic cysts) account for most cysts of the jaws. By far the most common is the radicular (periodontal or 'dental') cyst.

> Cysts are pathological fluid-filled cavities lined by epithelium

Typical features of jaw cysts

Most jaw cysts behave similarly and usually grow slowly and expansively. They differ mainly in their relationship to a tooth, and the radiographic features are usually a good guide as to their nature (Table 7.1). Even when it is not possible to decide the nature of a cyst, this affects treatment only with less common types. However, it is particularly important to distinguish keratocysts and unicystic ameloblastomas from common types. These occasionally have identical radiographic appearances, and diagnosis ultimately depends on histopathology.

Table 7.1 Key features of jaw cysts

- Form sharply-defined radiolucencies with smooth borders
- Fluid may be aspirated and thin-walled cysts may be transilluminated
- Grow slowly, displacing rather than resorbing teeth
- Symptomless unless infected and are frequently chance radiographic findings
- Rarely large enough to cause pathological fracture
- Form compressible and fluctuant swellings if extending into soft tissues
- Appear bluish when close to the mucosal surface

The classification of cysts is summarised in Table 7.2.

This classification, though widely accepted, has to a slight extent been superseded by more recent findings. Moreover for practical reasons, this order of entities will not be adhered to here.

Other cystic or cyst-like lesions

Cystic odontogenic tumours are not included in the above classification, but cystic ameloblastomas and calcifying

Table 7.2 Classification of cysts of the jaws (WHO — modified)

Developmental cysts
Odontogenic
   'Gingival cysts' of infants (Epstein pearls)
   Odontogenic keratocyst ('primordial' cyst)
   Dentigerous (follicular) cyst
   Eruption cyst
   Lateral periodontal cyst
   Gingival cyst of adults
   Glandular odontogenic; sialo-odontogenic cyst
Non-odontogenic cysts
   Nasopalatine duct cyst
   Nasolabial cyst
Inflammatory odontogenic cysts
Radicular
   Residual
   Lateral
Paradental

odontogenic (ghost cell) cysts can be mistaken radiographically for radicular or other non-neoplastic cysts as discussed later.

Also excluded from the above classification are cysts without epithelial lining (pseudocysts), namely solitary (simple) bone cysts and aneurysmal bone cysts. These also are cystic only in their radiographic appearances. They are skeletal diseases and affect the jaws only occasionally, as discussed in Chapter 9.

Odontogenic cysts (not surprisingly) affect the tooth-bearing region of the jaws. Most non-odontogenic, true cysts are developmental, and form in the region of the anterior maxilla. Their relative frequency is shown in Table 7.3, though figures in the different surveys vary as a result of differences in categorisation, what kinds of cysts are included, and other factors.

Table 7.3 Relative frequency of different types of jaw cysts

Radicular (periodontal)	65–70%
Dentigerous	15–18%
Odontogenic keratocysts	3–5%
Nasopalatine	5–10%
Lateral periodontal	< 1%
Paradental	< 1%

Radicular cysts are discussed first as being the most common type, whose treatment forms the basis for that of most other jaw cysts.

RADICULAR CYSTS

Clinical features

Radicular cysts are the most common cause of major, chronic swellings and the most common type of cyst of the jaws. They are rarely seen before the age of 10 and are most frequent between the ages of 20 and 60 years. They are more common in males than females, roughly in the proportion of 3 to 2. The maxilla is affected more than three times as frequently as the mandible.

Radicular cysts, like other cysts of the jaws, cause slowly progressive painless swellings, with no symptoms until they become large enough to be conspicuous (Fig. 7.1). If infection enters, the swelling becomes painful and may rapidly expand, partly due to inflammatory oedema. The swelling is rounded and at first hard. Later, when the bone has been reduced to eggshell thickness, a crackling sensation may be felt on pressure. Finally, part of the wall is resorbed entirely away, leaving a soft fluctuant swelling, bluish in colour, beneath the mucous membrane. The dead tooth from which the cyst has originated is (by definition) present, and its relationship to the cyst will be apparent in a radiograph (Fig. 7.2).

Practical point   Always determine the vitality of teeth associated with a jaw cyst

---

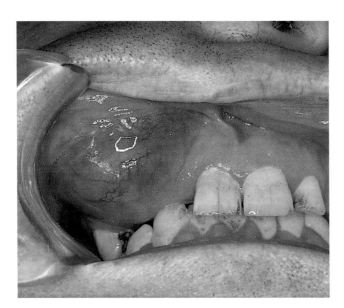

Fig. 7.1   Typical clinical appearance of a large cyst. This radicular cyst in the right maxillary alveolar process forms a rounded swelling with a bluish colour.

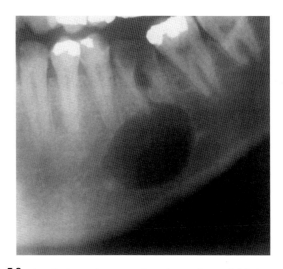

Fig. 7.2   A radicular cyst on a grossly carious and non-vital first permanent molar. A rounded and sharply defined area of radiolucency is associated with the apices of the roots.

Pathogenesis and pathology

The main factors responsible for cyst development are summarised in Table 7.4.

Table 7.4   **Major factors in the pathogenesis of cyst formation**

- Proliferation of epithelial lining and fibrous capsule
- Hydrostatic pressure of cyst fluid
- Resorption of surrounding bone

Epithelial proliferation

Infection from the pulp chamber induces inflammation and proliferation of the epithelial rests of Malassez. If infection can be eliminated from the root canal, small radicular cysts (up to 1 or 2 cm diameter) may regress without surgery.

Hydrostatic effects of cyst fluids

That radicular and many other cysts expand in balloon-like fashion, wherever the local anatomy permits, indicates that internal pressure is a factor in their growth. The hydrostatic pressure within cysts is about 70 cm of water and therefore higher than the capillary blood pressure.

Cyst fluid is largely inflammatory exudate and contains high concentrations of proteins, some of high molecular weight which can exert osmotic pressure. Consistent with the inflammation usually present in cyst walls, cyst fluid may contain cholesterol, breakdown products of blood cells, exfoliated epithelial cells, and fibrin.

The cyst wall does not seem to act entirely as a simple semi-permeable membrane. Low-molecular-weight proteins are present in similar concentrations to those in the plasma but there are smaller amounts of high-molecular-weight proteins. The capillaries in the cyst wall are more permeable as a result of inflammation and contribute varying amounts of immuno-globulins and other proteins. The net effect is that pressure is created by osmotic tension within the cyst cavity.

Bone-resorbing factors

Experimentally, cyst tissues in culture release bone-resorbing factors. These are predominantly prostaglandins E2 and E3. Different types of cysts and tumours may produce different quantities of prostaglandins but if so, it is unclear whether this affects the mode of growth of the cyst. Collagenases are present in the walls of keratocysts, but their contribution to cyst growth is also unclear.

Pathology

All stages can be seen from a periapical granuloma containing a few strands of proliferating epithelium derived from the epithelial rests of Malassez (Figs 7.3 and 7.4), to an enlarging cyst with a hyperplastic epithelial lining and dense inflammatory infiltrate. Epithelial proliferation results from irritant products leaking from an infected root canal to cause chronic periapical inflammation.

The epithelial lining consists of stratified squamous epithelium of variable thickness. It lacks a well-defined basal cell layer and is sometimes incomplete. Early, active epithelial proliferation is associated with obvious chronic inflammation and may then be thick, irregular and hyperplastic or appear net-like (Fig. 7.5),

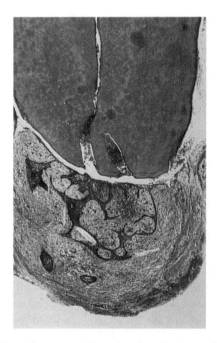

Fig. 7.3 The earliest stages of formation of a radicular cyst. Some periapical granulomas, such as this, contain proliferating strands of odontogenic epithelium. In places the epithelium has broken down centrally to form small epithelium-lined spaces.

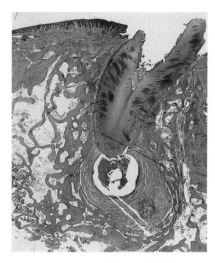

Fig. 7.4 A developing radicular cyst. An epithelium-lined cavity has formed in this large periapical granuloma. There is a thick fibrous capsule infiltrated by chronic inflammatory cells. The alveolar bone has been resorbed and remodelled to accommodate the slowly expanding swelling.

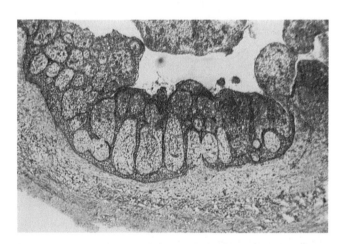

Fig. 7.5 Radicular cyst. The epithelial lining often assumes this arcaded pattern with numerous inflammatory cells beneath its surface.

forming rings and arcades (Fig. 7.6). Hyaline bodies may be seen in the epithelium (Fig. 7.7) and mucous cells are often present as a result of metaplasia (Fig. 7.8). Long-standing cysts typically have a thin flattened epithelial lining, a thick fibrous wall and minimal inflammatory infiltrate.

The cyst capsule and wall. The capsule consists of collagenous fibrous connective tissue. During active growth the capsule is vascular and infiltrated by chronic inflammatory cells adjacent to the proliferating epithelium. Plasma cells are often prominent or predominant, and are a response to antigens leaking through the tooth apex.

In the bony wall there is osteoclastic activity and resorption. Beyond the zone of resorption there is usually active bone formation. The net effect is that a cyst expands but retains a bony wall, even after it has extended beyond the normal bony contours. This bony wall nevertheless becomes progressively thinner since repair is slower than resorption, until it forms a

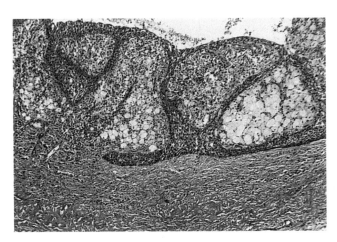

Fig. 7.6 Higher power of the lining of a radicular cyst. The arcaded epithelium contains numerous neutrophils emigrating into the lumen and there are pale staining areas of foamy macrophages in the inner wall.

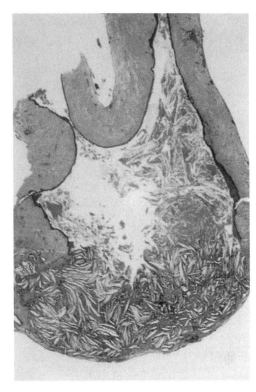

Fig. 7.9 Cholesterol clefts in a cyst wall. This low power view shows the relationship of cholesterol clefts to the cyst. Cholesterol crystals are formed in the fibrous wall. The epithelium overlying this focus has broken down and the cholesterol leaks into the cyst contents. Elsewhere the lumen is lined by a flattened layer of squamous epithelium.

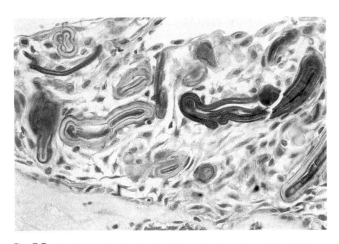

Fig. 7.7 Hyaline or Rushton bodies. These translucent or pink staining lamellar bodies are formed by the cyst lining epithelium and indicate the odontogenic origin of a cyst.

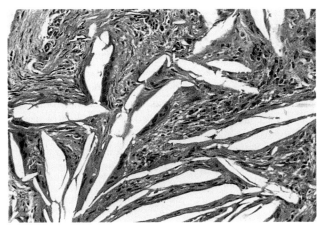

Fig. 7.10 Cholesterol clefts. Cholesterol has been dissolved out during preparation of the section, leaving clefts. The crystals are treated as foreign bodies and flattened multinucleate foreign body giant cells are seen along the edges of several clefts.

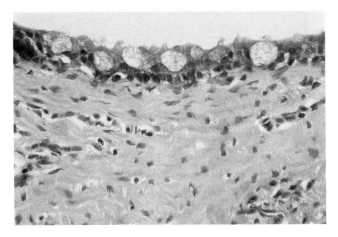

Fig. 7.8 Mucous metaplasia in a radicular cyst. The numerous goblet cells can be seen but are more typical of dentigerous cysts.

mere eggshell, then ultimately disappears altogether. The cyst then starts to distend the soft tissues and appears as a soft bluish swelling (Fig. 7.1).

Clefts. Within the cyst capsule there are often areas split up by fine needle-shaped clefts (Figs 7.9 and 7.10). These are left by cholesterol dissolved-out during preparation for sectioning. The cholesterol is derived from breakdown of blood cells. Small clefts are enclosed by foreign body giant cells, and

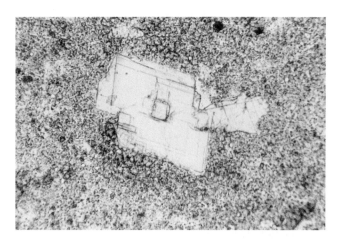

Fig. 7.11 Cholesterol crystals from a cyst aspirate indicating the presence of inflammation. The rectangular shape with a notched corner is characteristic.

Table 7.5 Radicular cyst: key features

- Form in bone in relation to the root of a non-vital tooth
- Arise by epithelial proliferation in an apical granuloma
- Are usually asymptomatic unless infected
- Diagnosis is by the combination of radiographic appearances, a non-vital tooth and appropriate histological appearances
- Clinical and radiographic features are usually adequate for planning treatment
- Do not recur after competent enucleation
- Residual cysts can remain after the causative tooth has been extracted and diagnosis is then less obvious
- Cholesterol crystals often seen in the cyst fluid but not specific to radicular cysts

extravasated red cells and blood pigment are associated. Clefts may also be seen extending into the cyst contents but are formed in the cyst wall.

Cyst fluid. The fluid is usually watery and opalescent but sometimes more viscid and yellowish, and sometimes shimmers with cholesterol crystals. A smear of this fluid may show typical notched cholesterol crystals microscopically (Fig. 7.11). Histologically, the protein content of the fluid is usually seen as amorphous eosinophilic material, often containing broken-down leucocytes and cells distended with fat globules.

Radiography

A radicular cyst appears as a rounded, radiolucent area with a sharply defined outline. A condensed radiopaque periphery is present only if growth is unusually slow and is usually more prominent in long-standing cysts. The dead tooth from which the cyst has arisen can be seen and often has a large carious cavity. Adjacent teeth may be tilted or displaced a little or occasionally become slightly mobile. Very large cysts in the maxilla may extend in any available direction and become irregular. Infection of a cyst causes the outline to become hazy as a result of greater vascularity and resorption of the surrounding bone.

Key features of radicular cysts are summarised in Table 7.5.

Residual and lateral radicular cysts

A radicular cyst may persist after extraction of the causative tooth. Residual cysts are a common cause of swelling of the edentulous jaw in older persons (Figs 7.12 and 7.13). Residual cysts may interfere with the fit of dentures, but may slowly regress spontaneously. This is suggested by the progressive thinning of the lining (Fig. 7.14).

Lateral radicular cysts can occasionally form at the side of a nonvital tooth as a result of the opening of a lateral branch of the root canal. They are rare and must be distinguished from

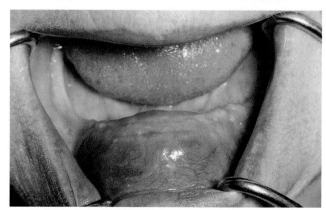

Fig. 7.12 Residual cyst. The causative tooth has been extracted leaving the cyst in situ. See also Figure 7.13.

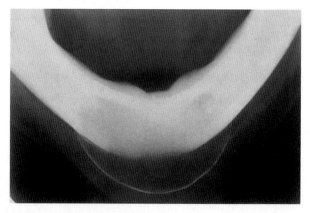

Fig. 7.13 Radiographic appearance of the residual cyst shown in Figure 7.12. Note the thin bulging periosteal new bone layer which can give rise to the clinical sign of eggshell crackling. (Figures 7.12 and 7.13 kindly lent by Mr P Robinson.)

lateral periodontal cysts which are another entity as discussed later.

Differential diagnosis

There are many causes of circumscribed areas of radiolucency in the jaws (Table 7.6).

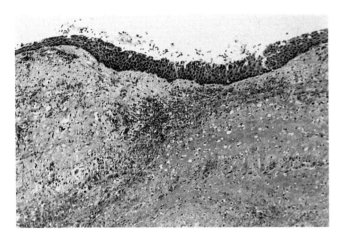

Fig. 7.14 Lining of a residual cyst. There is only a minor degree of inflammation and the epithelium forms a thin regular layer.

Table 7.6 Differential diagnosis of cyst-like areas of radiolucency

- Anatomical structures (maxillary antrum and foramina)
- Pseudocysts (Ch. 10)
- Neoplasms, particularly ameloblastoma (Ch. 8)
- Giant cell granuloma of the jaws (Ch. 9)
- Hyperparathyroidism (Ch. 10)
- Cherubism (Ch. 10)

Radicular cysts are usually readily recognised by their clinical and radiographic features. The cystic nature of a lesion can be confirmed by aspirating its contents through a needle inserted through the wall under aseptic conditions. The detection of fluid does not distinguish one cyst from another or a cystic neoplasm from a true cyst. The presence of cholesterol crystals is not of diagnostic significance.

Histologically, the lining of simple stratified squamous epithelium with an inflammatory infiltrate confirms the diagnosis. Distinguishing features of other types of cysts are discussed below.

Neoplasms. Benign (odontogenic) tumours or occasionally an ameloblastoma may resemble a simple cyst radiographically. Resorption of adjacent teeth suggests a neoplasm rather than a cyst but is not diagnostic in itself. It is essential that the whole of a cyst lining be available for examination, since part of the lining, even though neoplastic, may appear as a thin layer of flattened stratified squamous epithelium like that of a simple cyst.

Rarely a metastasis in the jaw may cause a sharply defined area of radiolucency. More often it causes a lesion with a hazy outline and irregular shape. Tumours also tend to be painful and to grow more rapidly than cysts. Nevertheless, it may be difficult or impossible to distinguish them from infected cysts radiographically, but at operation the solid nature of a tumour will be obvious and histological examination will confirm the diagnosis.

Treatment

Enucleation and primary closure

Enucleation is the usual method and usually entirely effective (Table 7.7). The affected (dead) tooth may be extracted or root-filled and preserved. A mucoperiosteal flap over the cyst is raised and a window is opened in the bone to give adequate access. The cyst is then carefully separated from its bony wall. The entire cyst is removed intact and should be sent in fixative for histological examination. The edges of the bone cavity are smoothed off, free bleeding is controlled and the cavity is irrigated to remove debris. The mucoperiosteal flap is replaced and sutured in place. The sutures should be left for at least 10 days.

Table 7.7 Advantages and limitations of enucleation of cysts

Advantages	Possible disadvantages
The cavity usually heals without complications	Infection of the clot filling the cavity
Little aftercare is necessary	Recurrence due to incomplete removal of the lining
The complete lining is available for histological examination	Serious haemorrhage (primary or secondary)
	Damage to apices of vital teeth projecting into the cyst cavity
	Damage to the inferior dental nerve
	Opening the antrum when enucleating a large maxillary cyst
	Fracture of the jaw if an exceptionally large mandibular cyst is enucleated

Any disadvantages are largely theoretical and in competent hands even very large cysts can be enucleated safely. Recurrence is remarkably rare. There are few contraindications: they are relative rather than absolute.

Marsupialisation

Marsupialisation is a largely outmoded treatment for radicular cysts. The cyst is opened essentially as for enucleation but the lining is sutured to the mucous membrane at the margins of the opening. The aim is to produce a self-cleansing cavity which becomes in effect, an invagination of the oral tissues. However, considerable aftercare is needed to keep the cavity clean. The cavity is initially packed with ribbon gauze and after the margins have healed a plug or extension to a denture is made to close the opening. Food debris has to be regularly washed out, but once the cavity has filled up from the base and sides sufficiently to become self-cleansing the plug can be removed. The cavity usually becomes closed by regrowth of the surrounding tissue and restoration of the normal contour of the part. However, the orifice may close and the cyst re-form.

Also, the complete lining is not available for histological examination.

The main application of marsupialisation is for temporary decompression of exceptionally large cysts where fracture of the jaw is a risk. When enough new bone has formed, the cyst can be enucleated. Occasionally retention of the tooth in a dentigerous cyst is needed and marsupialisation may allow it to erupt.

PARADENTAL CYSTS

Paradental cysts occasionally result from inflammation round partially erupted teeth, particularly mandibular third molars. They affect males predominantly, usually between the ages of 20–25 years. The affected tooth is vital but typically shows pericoronitis. Histologically the cyst resembles a radicular cyst but for a more intense inflammatory infiltrate in the wall.

Enucleation is effective.

DENTIGEROUS CYSTS

A dentigerous cyst surrounds the crown of a tooth and is a dilatation of the follicle (Figs 7.15 and 7.16). The cyst is attached to the neck of the tooth, prevents its eruption and may displace it for a considerable distance.

Clinical features

Dentigerous cysts are more than twice as common in males as females. They are uncommon in children and most often found between the ages of 20 and 50.

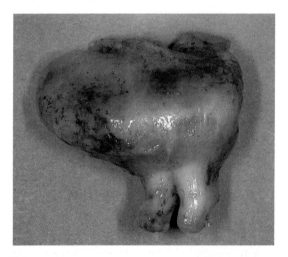

Fig. 7.15   Dentigerous cyst. This cyst has been removed together with its associated tooth. The cyst surrounds the crown and is attached at the cementoenamel junction.

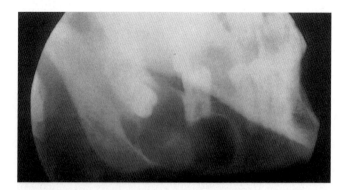

Fig. 7.16   Dentigerous cyst. The cyst has developed around the crown of the buried third molar (left), but has extended forward to involve the root of a vital second molar. It should not, however, be confused with a radicular cyst arising from the latter.

Like other cysts, uncomplicated dentigerous cysts cause no symptoms until the swelling becomes noticeable. Alternatively a dentigerous cyst may be a chance radiographic finding or found when the cause is sought for a missing tooth. Infection of a dentigerous cyst causes the usual symptoms of pain and accelerated swelling.

Radiography

The cavity is well circumscribed, rounded and unilocular and contains the crown of a tooth displaced from its normal position (Fig. 7.16). Occasionally there may be pseudoloculation as a result of trabeculation or ridging of the bony wall. The slow growth of dentigerous cysts usually results in a sclerotic bony outline and a well-defined cortex. The affected tooth is often displaced a considerable distance, and a third molar, for instance, may be pushed to the lower border of the mandible. Rarely, if the cyst remains unrecognised for a long period the enclosed tooth may become resorbed (Fig. 7.17).

These features readily distinguish a dentigerous cyst from a radicular cyst. However, a keratocyst or ameloblastoma may occasionally envelop the crown of the tooth, and either of these may create the radiographic appearance of a dentigerous cyst. The diagnosis ultimately therefore depends on histological examination.

Pathogenesis and pathology

Attachment of the cyst lining at or near the amelocemental junction suggests that dentigerous cysts arise as a result of cystic change in the remains of the enamel organ after enamel formation is complete. Division between the remnants of the internal enamel epithelium covering the enamel and the external enamel epithelium, forming the greater part of the cyst

> Dentigerous cysts contain the crown of an unerupted tooth and have an epithelial lining derived from enamel epithelium, attached to the tooth at the amelodentinal junction

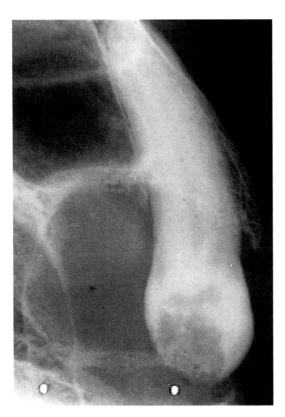

Fig. 7.17 Resorption of tooth associated with a dentigerous cyst. The crown of this buried canine within the cyst shows resorption. This is unusual and is seen only in long-neglected cysts, as in this otherwise edentulous patient.

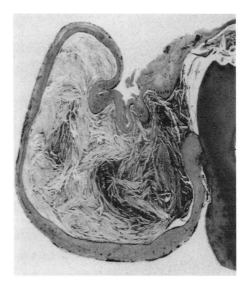

Fig. 7.18 Dentigerous cyst. The cyst surrounds the crown of this molar and the wall is attached to its cementoenamel junction. There is a uniform, thin epithelial lining with minimal inflammatory infiltrate. Cholesterol clefts are numerous in the lumen, a result of the formation of cholesterol crystals in the wall.

lining, can occasionally be seen at the attachment of the cyst to the neck of tooth (Figs 7.18 and 7.19).

Progressive growth of the cyst leads to dilatation of the dental follicle. Factors triggering these changes are not known. However, there is a strong association between failure of eruption of teeth and formation of dentigerous cysts which predominantly affect teeth which are particularly prone to failure of eruption, namely, maxillary canines and mandibular third molars in particular.

The lining of dentigerous cysts typically consists of thin, sometimes bilaminar, stratified epithelium (Fig. 7.20), frequently with numerous mucous cells. This epithelium may occasionally keratinise by metaplasia. The fibrous wall is similar to that of radicular cysts, but inflammatory changes are typically absent (Fig. 7.21).

Management principles

If the tooth is in a favourable position and space is available, it may occasionally be possible to marsupialise a dentigerous cyst to allow the tooth to erupt. Alternatively, the tooth can be transplanted to the alveolar ridge or extracted, as appropriate, and the cyst enucleated.

Key features of dentigerous cysts are summarised in Table 7.8.

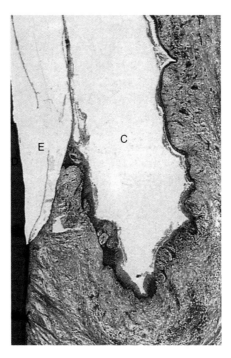

Fig. 7.19 Dentigerous cyst. To the left is the dentine (D). (E) is the enamel space left after decalcification and is separated from the cyst cavity (C) by a thin layer left by the inner enamel epithelium. The cyst itself appears to have formed as a result of accumulation of fluid between the inner and outer enamel epithelium and by continued proliferation of the latter to form the cyst lining, which joins the tooth at the epithelial attachment.

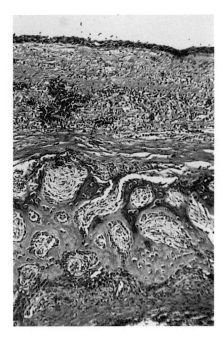

Fig. 7.20 Section through the full thickness of the wall of a dentigerous cyst. There is minimal inflammation and the epithelium is only two or three cells thick. Beyond the fibrous tissue the outermost layer of the wall is formed by woven bone, a feature common to most types of intraosseous cyst.

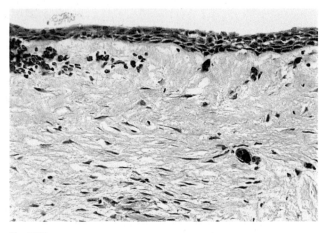

Fig. 7.21 Dentigerous cyst. In this uncomplicated cyst there is no inflammation and the wall comprises a layer of fibrous tissue lined by a thin layer of stratified squamous epithelium.

Table 7.8 Dentigerous cysts: key features

- Arise in bone and contain the crown of an unerupted tooth which is usually displaced
- Are most frequently associated with unerupted third molars and canines
- Clinical and radiographic features usually provide an accurate preoperative diagnosis but confirmation is histological
- May be mistaken radiographically for an odontogenic keratocyst or ameloblastoma
- Respond to enucleation or marsupialisation and do not recur after treatment

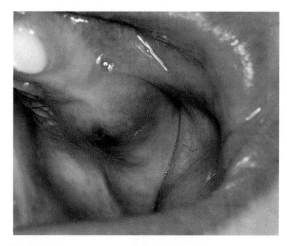

Fig. 7.22 An eruption cyst over an erupting upper molar. There has been bleeding into the cyst cavity as a result of trauma.

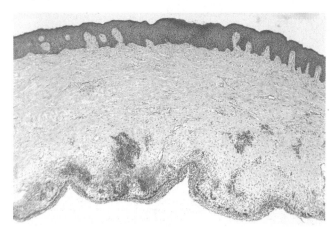

Fig. 7.23 Roof of an eruption cyst. At the upper surface is the keratinised epithelium of the alveolar ridge and, below, separated by a thin layer of relatively uninflamed fibrous tissue, the lining of an eruption cyst.

ERUPTION CYST

An eruption cyst occasionally forms over a tooth about to erupt. Strictly speaking an eruption cyst is a soft-tissue cyst but probably arises from enamel organ epithelium after enamel formation is complete and is, in effect, a superficial dentigerous cyst.

Clinical features

Eruption cysts affect children and involve teeth having no predecessors (deciduous teeth or permanent molars). The cyst lies superficially in the gingiva overlying the unerupted tooth and appears as a soft, rounded, bluish swelling (Fig. 7.22). The epithelial lining is separated from the alveolar mucosa by a thin layer of fibrous tissue (Fig. 7.23).

Management

The cyst roof may be removed to allow the tooth to erupt, but most eruption cysts probably burst spontaneously and never come to surgery.

ODONTOGENIC KERATOCYSTS

Keratocysts are uncommon but important because of their strong tendency — unlike most other cysts — to recur after removal.

Clinical features

Most series have recorded a peak incidence between ages 20 to 30 years but other large series have shown peaks between 50 and 70 years. The mandible is usually affected. At least 50% of keratocysts form in the angle of the mandible, extending forwards into the body and upwards into the ramus. Keratocysts, like other jaw cysts, are symptomless until the bone is expanded or they become infected. The main difference is that expansion of the jaw is much less than the radiographic extent of the cyst. Hence clinical signs often fail to appear until the cyst is well advanced, and relatively extensive cysts are occasionally found by chance in radiographs.

Radiography

Keratocysts appear as well-defined radiolucent areas, either more or less rounded with a scalloped margin, or multiloculated and simulating an ameloblastoma (Fig. 7.24). The bony wall

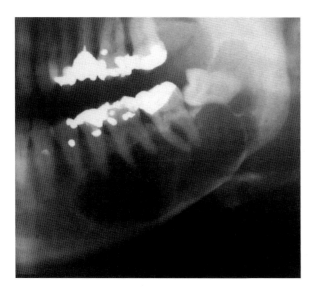

Fig. 7.24 Odontogenic keratocyst. Part of a panoramic tomogram showing typical appearances. The cyst is multilocular and has extended a considerable distance along the medullary cavity without appreciable expansion or displacement of the teeth.

appears sharply demarcated. Occasionally, a keratocyst may envelop an unerupted tooth and be indistinguishable radiographically from a dentigerous cyst. Roots of adjacent teeth may become displaced.

Key features of dentigerous cysts are summarised in Table 7.9.

Table 7.9 Odontogenic keratocyst: key features

- Form intraosseously, most frequently in the posterior alveolar ridge or angle of mandible
- May grow round a tooth
- Sometimes multilocular radiographically
- Spread extensively along marrow spaces before expanding the jaw
- Frequently recur after enucleation
- Do not respond to marsupialisation
- Definitive diagnosis only by histopathology although clinical and radiographic features may allow fairly accurate preoperative diagnosis
- May be confused with ameloblastoma or with dentigerous cysts radiographically
- May be part of the jaw cyst/basal cell naevus syndrome

Pathogenesis and pathology

Keratocysts probably arise from any of the primordial epithelia (the dental lamina or its remains) or, as originally believed, from the enamel organ before tooth formation. However, it is difficult to reconcile such origins with the appearance of keratocysts in middle age and their relatively rapid epithelial turnover. The aetiology of keratocysts is therefore speculative.

Radioactive labelling used to estimate mitotic activity suggests that keratocyst lining may be proliferating more actively than mucosal epithelium. Mural growth therefore appears to be more important in the enlargement of keratocysts than osmotic pressure exerted by the cyst's contents. This active mural growth and epithelial proliferation is probably a factor determining the frequency with which keratocysts recur.

Two types of keratocyst are recognised. They have slightly different demographic characteristics (Table 7.10), but the

Table 7.10 Important features of keratocysts

Feature	Parakeratotic	Orthokeratotic
Relative frequency (%)	88	12
Sex %		
Male = 61.5% overall	62	57
Female = 38.5% overall	38	43
Age at presentation (years)	34	40
Association with impacted tooth (%)	48	76
Midline location (%)	6	16
Pain (%)	15	9
Radiographic appearance	Usually multilocular	Frequently monolocular
Recurrence rate (%)	43	4

Table 7.11 Typical histological features of keratocysts

- Epithelial lining of uniform thickness
- Flat lower border of epithelium
- Clearly defined basal layer of tall cells in parakeratinised cysts (Fig. 7.25)
- Thin eosinophilic layer of pre-keratin in parakeratinised cysts
- Cyst lining typically much folded (Fig. 7.26)
- Epithelial lining weakly attached to the fibrous wall
- Abundant orthokeratin formation and well-defined granular cell layer in orthokeratinised cysts (Fig. 7.27)
- Thin fibrous wall
- Inflammatory cells typically absent or scanty

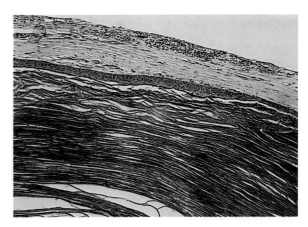

Fig. 7.27 Odontogenic keratocyst (orthokeratinised variant). There is a thick layer of keratin at the epithelial surface and filling the lumen.

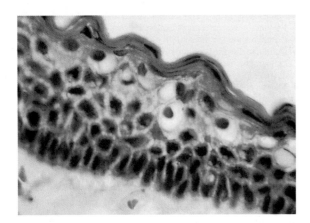

Fig. 7.25 Parakeratinised odontogenic keratocyst. High power showing the typical features of the epithelial lining: a flat basement membrane; elongated palisaded basal cells; 10–20 cells in thickness and with a corrugated parakeratotic surface.

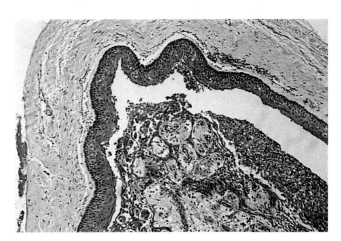

Fig. 7.28 Inflamed odontogenic keratocyst. Around the periphery the cyst shows the typical features of a thin, uninflamed fibrous wall and regular epithelium with a flat basement membrane but, centrally, inflammation in a mural nodule has resulted in loss of typical features and hyperplastic strands of non-keratinised epithelium have formed.

Growth of keratocysts is by extension of finger-like processes into marrow spaces rather than by expansion. Growth of the wall being greater than expansion of the cyst cavity, causes the lining to become much folded (Fig. 7.26).

Management

The diagnosis should preferably be confirmed before operation, both to exclude an ameloblastoma and also because of the problem of removing keratocysts entirely.

Aspiration is unlikely to be helpful. Squames in the cyst fluid are not in themselves diagnostic as other cysts can form keratin and, very rarely, a carcinoma with cystic change may shed squames into its interior.

Keratocyst fluid has a low soluble protein content but, in practice, biopsy confirms the diagnosis more reliably and quickly.

On confirmation of the diagnosis, treatment should be by complete enucleation. This is usually difficult as the lining is

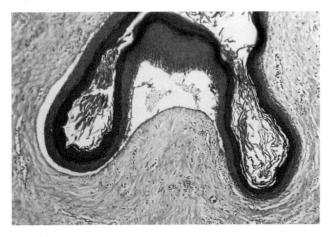

Fig. 7.26 Odontogenic keratocyst. Folding of the wall and separation of the epithelium from the connective tissue wall are characteristic features.

important difference is that parakeratotic cysts are far more likely to recur than orthokeratotic cysts.

The histological appearances of the lining of keratocysts are characteristic (Table 7.11).

If inflammation becomes superimposed the epithelial lining can lose its characteristic features and come to resemble that of a radicular cyst (Fig. 7.28).

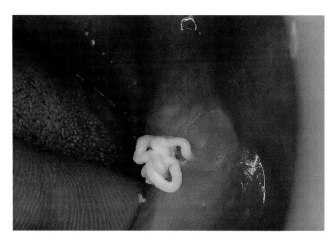

Fig. 7.29 Orthokeratinised keratocyst. Perforation of and pressure on the cyst roof has caused keratin to extrude and has helped to confirm the diagnosis.

friable (particularly if inflamed) but treatment should be thorough, to try to be certain that every fragment of lining has been removed.

Resection provides the lowest recurrence rate but at the cost of considerable morbidity. Enucleation alone is likely to lead to a recurrence rate of up to 60%. However, treating the cyst lining with Carnoy's fluid improves the results of enucleation. The purpose is to fix the lining and make it easier to remove intact. Preliminary decompression also improves the prognosis.

Recurrence

Recurrence rates are affected by various factors (Table 7.12).

A major factor leading to recurrence is the difficulty in removing every trace of the epithelial lining. Its more vigorous proliferative activity than that of other cyst linings may allow a few remaining epithelial cells to readily form another cyst. Formation of another cyst from other dental lamina remnants is not strictly a recurrence but the fact that recurrences can appear up to 40 years after enucleation suggests this may happen. Otherwise recurrence is often within the first 5 years after treatment. Vigorous treatment is likely to reduce the risk of recurrence, but there is no absolute certainty of a cure, and patients should be followed up with regular radiographic examinations.

The basal cell carcinoma/jaw cyst (Gorlin–Goltz) syndrome

This syndrome, often called the Gorlin–Goltz syndrome, is heritable as an autosomal dominant trait. It consists essentially of the triad of multiple basal cell naevi, keratocysts of the jaws and skeletal anomalies. However, many other defects may be associated. It is caused by mutations in the *patched* (PTCH) tumour suppressor gene. This gene is important in developmental patterning and also controls the cell cycle via the *hedgehog* (HH) signalling pathway. The anomaly maps to chromosome 9q, and is also found in sporadic, non-syndromal tumours such as basal cell carcinomas, trichoepitheliomas and medulloblastomas, but which can also be part of the syndrome.

Mutations within PTCH may also be found in sporadic keratocysts.

The main features of the syndrome are listed in Table 7.13, though a great many other abnormalities may be present as the phenotype varies between families. Unusually, inheritance of the mutation in only one allele is sufficient to cause many of the syndromic features. When the second allele is inactivated, basal cell carcinomas and odontogenic keratocysts develop.

A great variety of other abnormalities may be present, and effects on the patient depend on the predominant manifestation. Thus in some cases there are innumerable basal cell carcinomas. Though termed 'naevoid' these tumours differ from typical basal carcinomas only in their early onset and slower growth. Other patients have many jaw cysts, necessitating repeated operations. Cleft lip or palate or both is seen in a small proportion of these patients. Otherwise, the importance of this syndrome, from the dental viewpoint, is treatment of the keratocysts and to warn the patient of the likelihood of development of further cysts which must be dealt with by orthodox means as they arise. If neglected, these cysts can cause complications like other jaw cysts. Structurally the cysts, like other keratocysts, are more common in the body or ramus of the mandible. Otherwise they are rarely distinguishable histologically from the more common type of keratocysts, but may have many daughter cysts in the walls (Fig. 7.33). The great majority are parakeratinised and have a strong tendency to recur after treatment.

Table 7.12   Possible reasons for recurrence of keratocysts

- Thin, fragile linings, difficult to enucleate intact
- Fingerlike cyst extensions into cancellous bone
- Daughter cysts sometimes present in the wall
- More rapid proliferation of keratocyst epithelium
- Other dental lamina remnants may produce another keratocyst (pseudo-recurrence)
- Inferior standard of surgical treatment

Table 7.13   Key features of Gorlin–Goltz syndrome

- Characteristic facies with frontal and parietal bossing and broad nasal root (Fig. 7.30)
- Multiple keratocysts of the jaws (Figs 7.31 and 7.32)
- Multiple, naevoid basal cell carcinomas of the skin
- Skeletal anomalies (usually of a minor nature) such as bifid ribs and abnormalities of the vertebrae
- Intracranial anomalies may include calcification of the falx cerebri and abnormally shaped sella turcica
- Cleft lip and palate in approximately 5%

GINGIVAL CYSTS

Dental lamina cysts of the newborn (Bohn's nodules)

Up to 80% of newborn infants have small nodules or cysts in the gingivae, due to proliferation of the epithelial rests of Serres (Fig. 7.34). Most resolve spontaneously.

Cysts (Epstein's pearls) may also arise from nonodontogenic epithelium along the midpalatine raphe. These may enlarge sufficiently to appear as creamy-coloured swellings a few millimetres in diameter, but also resolve spontaneously in a matter of months.

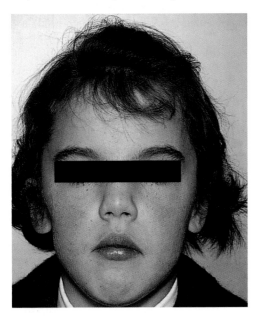

Fig. 7.30 Basal cell naevus (Gorlin's syndrome). The typical facies with a broad nasal root and mild frontal bossing.

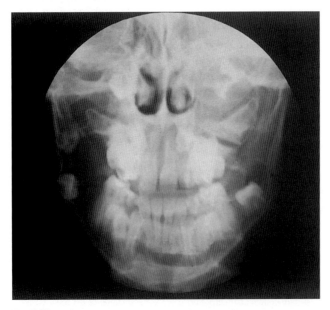

Fig. 7.31 PA jaws of the same patient with the basal cell naevus (Gorlin's) syndrome shown in Figure 7.30. Odontogenic keratocysts are present in the ramus and angle of the mandible on both sides, that on the right causing significant expansion.

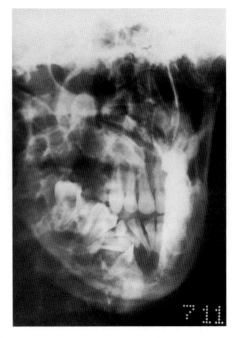

Fig. 7.32 Oblique lateral radiograph of a patient with the basal cell naevus (Gorlin's) syndrome. A very large odontogenic keratocyst involves the whole ramus and body, causing considerable expansion, especially at the lower border

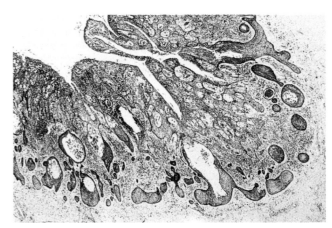

Fig. 7.33 Odontogenic keratocyst in the basal cell naevus syndrome. Although the cysts in syndrome patients are often indistinguishable from typical odontogenic keratocysts, there may be extensive islands of epithelium in the cyst wall and many daughter cysts.

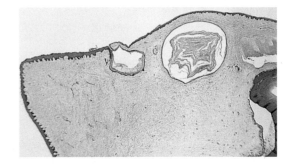

Fig. 7.34 Gingival cyst of the new born (Bohn's nodules). This section from an embryo shows cyst formation in the rests of Serres superficial to the developing teeth. The cysts are lined by keratinising epithelium.

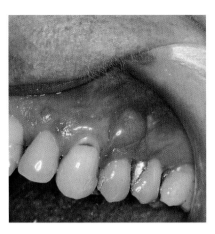

Fig. 7.35 Gingival cyst of adult. Typical presentation as a superficial cyst in the attached gingiva of a premolar tooth.

Gingival cysts of adults

Gingival cysts are exceedingly rare. They usually form after the age of approximately 40. Clinically, they form dome-shaped swellings less than 1 cm in diameter and sometimes erode the underlying bone (Fig. 7.35). They are lined by very thin, flat, stratified squamous epithelium and my contain fluid or layers of keratin. They are unlikely to recur after enucleation.

LATERAL PERIODONTAL CYSTS

These uncommon intraosseous cysts are developmental and form beside a vital tooth. They are usually seen by chance in routine radiographs and resemble other odontogenic cysts radiographically, apart from their position beside a tooth (Fig. 7.36), near the crest of the ridge. They cause no symptoms unless they erode through the bone to extend into the gingiva.

Microscopically, the lining is squamous or cuboidal epithelium, frequently only one or two cells thick, but

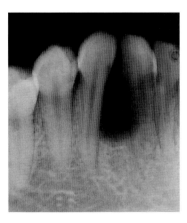

Fig. 7.36 Lateral periodontal cyst. Typical radiographic appearance showing a well-demarcated rounded radiolucency between the roots of the lateral incisor and canine, the roots of which have been displaced.

sometimes with focal thickenings. Some of the cells may have clear cytoplasm and resemble those seen in the dental lamina.

The cyst should be enucleated and the related tooth can be retained if healthy.

Botryoid odontogenic cysts

The botryoid odontogenic cyst is probably a variant of, and even more rare than, the lateral periodontal cyst. It typically affects the mandibular premolar to canine region in adults over 50.

Microscopically, it is typically multilocular with fine fibrous septa. The lining consists of flattened non-keratinised epithelium interspersed with clear, glycogen-containing cells and sporadic budlike proliferations protruding into the cyst. It should be enucleated or conservatively excised as it has a strong tendency to recur.

Glandular odontogenic cyst

The glandular odontogenic cyst is another rare entity with many features in common with botryoid odontogenic cysts but there are pools of mucin and mucous cells in variable numbers within the epithelium. It is frequently also multilocular and has a strong tendency to recur.

Table 7.14 Key features of lateral periodontal cyst and variants

Lateral periodontal cysts
- Developmental cysts that form beside a vital tooth
- Usually seen by chance in routine radiographs
- Resemble other odontogenic cysts radiographically, apart from position near the crest of the ridge
- Cause no symptoms but can erode through the bone to extend into the gingiva
- Microscopically, the lining is squamous or cuboidal epithelium, frequently only one or two cells thick, sometimes with focal thickenings
- Some cells may have clear cytoplasm
- Respond to enucleation
- The related tooth can be retained if healthy

Botryoid odontogenic cysts
- Probably a variant of lateral periodontal cyst, but more rare.
- Typically affect the mandibular premolar to canine region in adults over 50.
- Microscopically, typically multilocular* with fine fibrous septa.
- Lined by flattened non-keratinised epithelium interspersed with clear, glycogen-containing cells
- Also sporadic budlike proliferations protrude into the lumen
- Has a strong tendency to recur after enucleation
- Should be conservatively excised

Glandular odontogenic cyst
- Also rare and with many features in common with botryoid odontogenic cysts
- Frequently multilocular*
- Microscopically, pools of mucin and mucous cells present in the epithelium
- Has a strong tendency to recur
- Should be conservatively excised

*Multilocularity not necessarily visible in radiographs

NASOPALATINE DUCT CYSTS

The nasopalatine duct connects the organ of Jacobson in the nasal septum to the palate in many animals. Jacobson's organ is joined centrally to an accessory olfactory bulb. Cats, for instance, may sometimes be noticed to sense an interesting odour by inhaling through the mouth, and in most species Jacobson's organ is used to assess the state of sexual readiness of potential mates. Disappointingly therefore, Jacobson's organ has disappeared in man, and only a few epithelial cells lying along the line of the nasopalatine duct, persist. These cells can give rise to nasopalatine duct cysts.

Nasopalatine cysts, which form in the midline of the anterior maxilla, are uncommon. The nasopalatine, incisive canal, median palatine, palatine papilla and median alveolar cysts are variants of the same lesion, varying slightly in position in relation to the postulated line of the incisive canal.

Clinical features

Nasopalatine duct cysts are slow-growing and resemble other cysts of the jaws clinically, apart from their site. Occasionally they cause intermittent discharge with a salty taste. If allowed to grow sufficiently large, nasopalatine cysts may cause a swelling in the midline of the anterior part of the palate (Fig. 7.37), particularly when superficial (so-called palatine papilla cyst).

Radiography shows a rounded radiolucent area with a well-defined often sclerotic margin in the anterior part of the midline of the maxilla (Fig. 7.38). They occasionally appear heart-shaped because of radiographic superimposition of the nasal spine. They are usually symmetrical but may be slightly larger to one side. The anterior palatine fossa must be distinguished from a small nasopalatine cyst. The maximum size of a normal fossa is up to 6 or 7 mm.

Key features of nasopalatine duct cysts are summarised in Table 7.15.

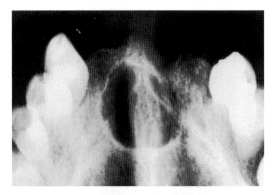
Fig. 7.38 Nasopalatine cyst. The usual appearance is a rounded or pear-shaped area of radiolucency, mainly in the midline.

Table 7.15   Nasopalatine duct cyst: key features

- Often asymptomatic, chance radiographic findings
- Form in the incisive canal region
- Arise from vestiges of the nasopalatine duct and may be lined by columnar respiratory epithelium
- The long spheno-palatine nerve and vessels may be present in the wall
- Can usually be recognised radiographically
- Histological examination necessary to exclude other cyst types arising at this site
- Do not recur after enucleation

Pathogenesis and pathology

Nasopalatine cysts arise from the epithelium of the nasopalatine duct in the incisive canal. In man, vestiges of a primitive organ of smell in the incisive canal can be found in the form of incomplete epithelium-lined ducts, cords of epithelial cells, or merely epithelial rests.

The epithelial lining is usually either stratified squamous epithelium or ciliated columnar (respiratory) epithelium or both together (Fig. 7.39). Mucous glands are often and neurovascular bundles are sometimes present in the wall (Fig. 7.40). These are

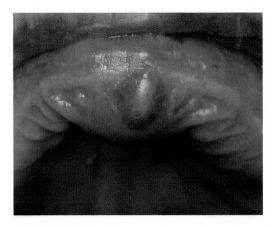
Fig. 7.37 Nasopalatine cyst. Typical presentation with a dome-shaped bluish enlargement overlying the incisive canal.

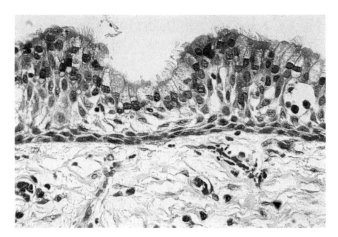
Fig. 7.39 Nasopalatine cyst. The lining, in part at least, may consist of respiratory (ciliated columnar) epithelium, as here.

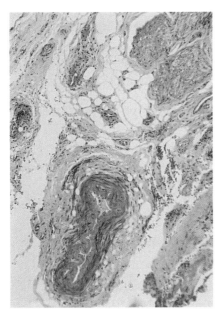

Fig. 7.40 Nasopalatine cyst. Nerves and blood vessels of the incisive canal in the cyst wall.

the long sphenopalatine nerve and vessels which pass through the incisive canal and are often removed with the cyst.

Treatment

Nasopalatine duct cysts should be enucleated. Recurrence is unlikely.

NASOLABIAL CYST

This very uncommon cyst forms outside the bone in the soft tissues, deep to the nasolabial fold. It probably arises from remnants of the nasolabial duct and is occasionally bilateral.

The lining is pseudo-stratified columnar epithelium with or without some stratified columnar epithelium. If allowed to grow sufficiently large, the cyst produces a swelling of the upper lip and distorts the nostril. Treatment is usually by simple excision but occasionally may be complicated if the cyst has perforated the nasal mucosa and discharged into the nose.

CYSTIC NEOPLASMS

Unicystic ameloblastoma

Most ameloblastomas contain microcysts but the unicystic variant has a lining of flattened tumour cells which resemble those of non-neoplastic cysts and a nodule of tumour in the wall or bulging into the lumen. Unicystic ameloblastomas frequently mimic dentigerous cysts radiographically (Ch. 8).

Calcifying odontogenic cyst

This uncommon lesion may be a cystic neoplasm: solid variants are rare (Ch. 8). The cyst lining consists of epithelium, often with palisading of the basal cells which may resemble ameloblasts. The most striking feature is areas of abnormal keratinisation producing swollen cells whose outlines and nuclei become progressively paler (ghost cells).

NEOPLASTIC CHANGE WITHIN CYSTS

Neoplasms, either ameloblastomas or carcinomas, could conceivably arise from the epithelial lining of cysts. There is scant evidence that ameloblastomas arise in this way, and the idea almost certainly results from incorrect radiographic interpretation or faulty histological diagnosis.

There are a few well-authenticated cases of carcinomas arising from cyst linings but they are exceedingly rare. It is essential to exclude other possibilities before such a diagnosis is made. Since cysts of the jaws are common, a neoplasm might develop coincidentally nearby and grow until it involves and fuses with the cyst wall.

SO-CALLED GLOBULOMAXILLARY CYSTS

These exceedingly rare cysts have been traditionally ascribed to proliferation of sequestered epithelium along the line of fusion of embryonic processes. It is now accepted that this view of embryological development is incorrect and there is no evidence that epithelium becomes buried in this fashion. Most so-called globulomaxillary cysts are usually found to be odontogenic cysts of various types.

CYSTS OF THE SOFT TISSUES

Some cysts described earlier form in or extend into the soft tissues overlying the jaws. However, most soft tissue cysts are nonodontogenic. The most common soft tissue cysts are mucoceles (extravasation or retention cysts) and the ranula which originate in minor salivary glands (Ch. 18) but the sublingual dermoid is a developmental anomaly.

Sublingual dermoid

These cysts probably form as a result of some abnormality of development of the branchial arches or pharyngeal pouches.

Clinical features

Dermoid cysts develop between the hyoid and jaw or may form immediately beneath the tongue (Fig. 7.41). They are sometimes filled with desquamated keratin giving them a semi-

117

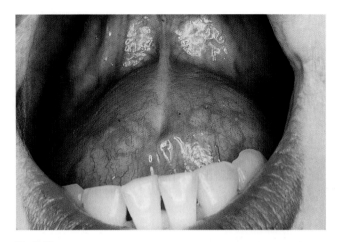

Fig. 7.41 Sublingual dermoid cyst. This is an unusually large specimen but appears even larger because the patient is raising and protruding her tongue. This cyst, unlike a ranula, can be seen to have a thick wall because it has arisen in the deeper tissues of the floor of the mouth.

solid, putty-like consistency. A sublingual dermoid is more deeply placed than a ranula; the latter is obviously superficial, having a thin wall and a bluish appearance. A dermoid causes no symptoms until large enough to interfere with speech or eating. Nevertheless, a large swelling can be accommodated in the floor of the mouth without disability and can be completely concealed by the tongue in its normal resting position.

Pathology

The lining of *epidermoid* cysts is keratinising stratified squamous epithelium alone. Less often, cysts also have dermal appendages in the wall and are then referred to as *dermoid* cysts. Still others are lined partly by keratinising stratified squamous epithelium and partly by respiratory (ciliated columnar stratified) epithelium.

These cysts should be dissected out.

SUGGESTED FURTHER READING

Ackerman G L, Cohen M, Altini M 1987 The paradental cyst: a clinicopathological study of 57 cases. Oral Surg Oral Med Oral Pathol 64:308–312

Altini M, Shear M 1992 The lateral periodontal cyst: an update. J Oral Pathol Med 21:245–250

Blanas N, Freund B, Schwartz M et al 2000 Systematic review of the treatment and prognosis of the odontogenic keratocyst. Oral Surg Oral Med Oral Pathol Radiol Endod 90:553–558

Browne R M (Ed) 1991 *Investigative pathology of odontogenic cysts*. CRC Press, Boca Raton

Cawson R A, Binnie W H, Barrett A W, Wright J M 2001 *Oral disease*, 3rd Edn. Mosby-Wolfe, London

Cawson R A, Binnie W H, Barrett A W, Wright J M 1988 *Lucas's Pathology of tumors of the oral tissues*. Churchill Livingstone, Edinburgh

Cawson R A, Langdon J D, Eveson J W 1996 *Surgical pathology of the mouth and jaws*. Wright, Oxford

Craigh G T 1976 The paradental cyst. A specific inflammatory odontogenic cyst. Br Dent J 141:9–14

Crowley T E, Kaugars G E, Gunsolley J C 1992 Odontogenic keratocysts: a clinical and histologic comparison of the parakeratin and orthokeratin variants. J Oral Maxillofac Surg 50:22–26

Friedrichsen S W 1993 Long-term progression of a traumatic bone cyst. A case report. Oral Surg Oral Med Oral Pathol 76:421–424

Gurol M, Burkes J, Jacoway J 1995 Botryoid odontogenic cyst: analysis of 33 cases. J Periodontol 66:1069–1073

Hernandez G A, Castro A, Castro G, Amador E 1993 Aneurysmal bone cyst versus hemangioma of the mandible. Report of a long-term follow-up of a self-limiting case. Oral Surg Oral Med Oral Pathol 76:790–796

Hussain K, Edmondson H D, Browne R M 1995 Glandular odontogenic cysts. Diagnosis and treatment. Oral Surg Oral Med Oral Pathol 79:593–603

Kuroi M 1980 Simple bone cyst of the jaw: review of the literature and report of a case. J Oral Surg 38:456–459

Li T-J, Browne R M, Matthews J B 1994 Quantification of PCNA$^+$ cells within odontogenic jaw cyst epithelium. J Oral Pathol Med 23:184–189

Lombardi T, Odell E W, Morgan P R 1995 p53 immunohistochemistry of odontogenic keratocysts in relation to recurrence, basal cell budding and basal-cell naevus syndrome. Arch Oral Biol 40:1081–1084

Meiselman F 1994 Surgical management of the odontogenic keratocyst: conservative approach. J Oral Maxillofac Surg 520:960–963

Philipsen H P, Reichart P A 1998 Unicystic ameloblastoma. A review of 193 cases from the literature. Oral Oncol 34:317–325

Semba I, Kitano M, Mimura T, Sonoda S, Miyawaki A 1994 Glandular odontogenic cyst: analysis of cytokeratin expression and clinicopathological features. J Oral Pathol Med 23:377–382

Shear M 1994 Developmental odontogenic cysts. An update. J Oral Pathol Med 23:1–11

Shear M 1992 *Cysts of the oral regions*, 3rd Edn. Wright PSG; Bristol

Swanson K S, Kaugars G E, Gunsolley J C 1991 Nasopalatine duct cyst: an analysis of 334 cases. J Oral Maxillofac Surg 49:268–271

Weathers D R, Waldron C A 1973 Unusual multilocular cysts of the jaws (botryoid odontogenic cysts) Oral Surg Oral Med Oral Pathol 36:235–241

William T P, Connor F A 1994 Surgical management of the odontogenic keratocyst: aggressive approach. J Oral Maxillofac Surg 520:964–966

Woolgar J A, Rippin J W, Browne R M 1987 A comparative histological study of odontogenic keratocysts in basal cell naevus syndrome and control patients. J Oral Pathol 16:75–80

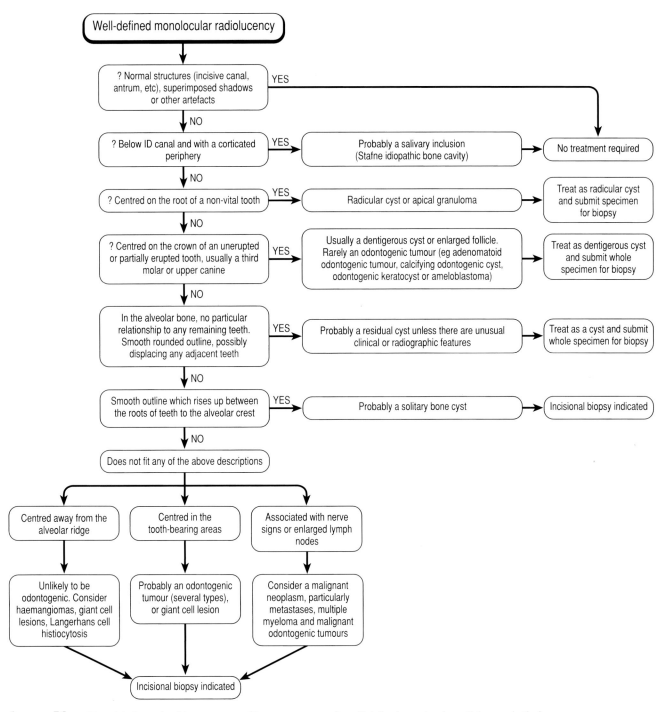

Summary 7.1 Differential diagnosis of the common and important causes of a well-defined monolocular radiolucency in the jaws.

CHAPTER
7

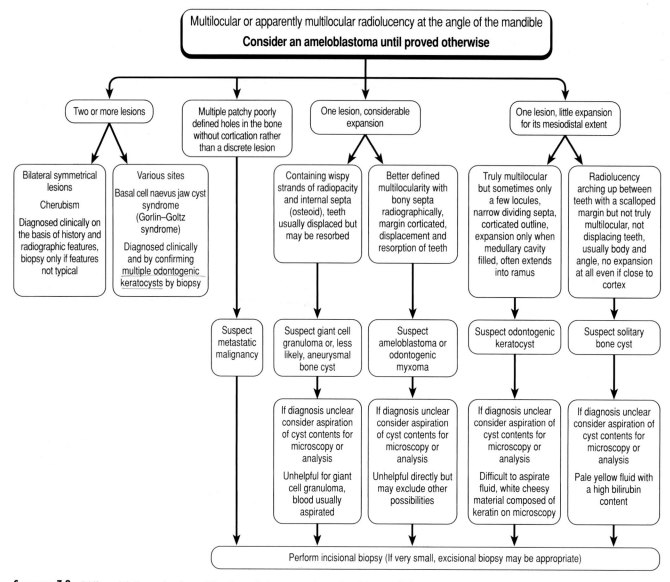

Summary 7.2   Differential diagnosis of a multilocular radiolucency at the angle of the mandible.

Odontogenic tumours and tumour-like lesions of the jaws

Tumours or tumour-like swellings of the jaws can be odontogenic or non-odontogenic (Table 8.1).

Table 8.1   **Important causes of tumours (swellings) of the jaws**

- Cysts, predominantly odontogenic cysts
- Odontogenic tumours
- Giant cell lesions
- Fibro-osseous lesions
- Primary (nonodontogenic) neoplasms of bone
- Metastatic neoplasms

Odontogenic tumours are the most common neoplasms of the jaws and have been classified by the WHO as shown in Table 8.2. However, some tumours are not recognised in this classification, and it will not be followed exactly in the subsequent text.

Table 8.2   **Important types of odontogenic tumours**

- Benign epithelial neoplasms
  Ameloblastoma
  Adenomatoid odontogenic tumour
  Calcifying odontogenic tumour
  Calcifying epithelial odontogenic tumour
  Clear cell odontogenic carcinoma
  Calcifying (ghost cell) odontogenic cyst
  Squamous odontogenic tumour
- Benign mixed epithelial and connective tissue neoplasms
  Ameloblastic fibroma
- Benign connective tissue
  Odontogenic fibroma
  Odontogenic myxoma
  Cementoblastoma
- Hamartomas
  Odontomas
- Malignant epithelial neoplasms
  Odontogenic carcinomas
- Malignant connective tissue
  Odontogenic sarcomas

AMELOBLASTOMA

Ameloblastomas are the most common neoplasms of the jaws. They are usually first recognised between the ages of 30 and 50,

and rare in children and old people. Eighty per cent form in the mandible; of these, 70% develop in the posterior molar region, and often involve the ramus. They are symptomless until the swelling becomes obtrusive (Fig. 8.1).

Radiographically, ameloblastomas typically form rounded, cyst-like, radiolucent areas with moderately well-defined margins and typically appear multilocular (Fig. 8.2). Lingual

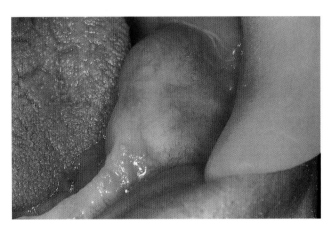

Fig. 8.1   Ameloblastoma. Typical presentation. There is a rounded, bony swelling of the posterior alveolar bone, body and angle of the mandible. There is no ulceration, a feature only seen in very large tumours which have perforated the cortex.

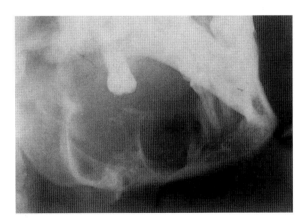

Fig. 8.2   Ameloblastoma. The typical radiological appearance of ameloblastoma is a multilocular cyst or multiple cyst cavities of different sizes, as shown here.

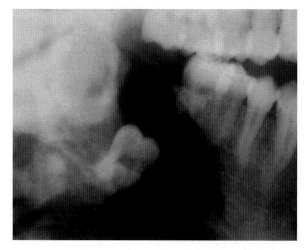

Fig. 8.3 Ameloblastoma. This ameloblastoma forms a monolocular radiolucency enveloping the crown of an unerupted tooth. The radiological appearance mimics a dentigerous cyst, reinforcing the maxim that ameloblastoma should be considered in the differential diagnosis of every radiolucency at the angle of the mandible.

expansion may sometimes be seen, but is not pathognomonic of ameloblastoma. Other variants are a honeycomb pattern, a single well-defined cavity indistinguishable from a radicular or, rarely, a dentigerous cyst (Fig. 8.3). However, differentiation from non-neoplastic cysts and other tumours or tumour-like lesions of the jaws is not possible by radiography alone.

Pathology

Follicular ameloblastomas are the most common and most readily recognisable type, with islands and trabeculae of epithelial cells in a connective tissue stroma (Fig. 8.4). These epithelial processes consist of a well-organised single layer of tall, columnar, ameloblast-like cells which have nuclei at the opposite pole to the basement membrane (reversed polarity), and surround a core of loosely arranged polyhedral or angular cells, resembling stellate reticulum (Fig. 8.5).

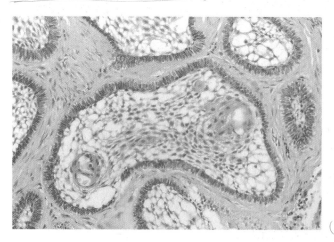

Fig. 8.4 Ameloblastoma. Islands of follicular ameloblastoma comprising stellate reticulum and a peripheral layer of elongated ameloblast-like cells.

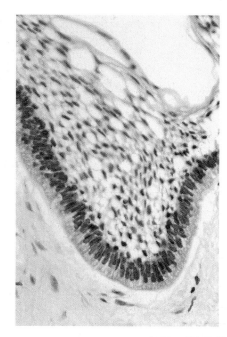

Fig. 8.5 Ameloblastoma. At high power in this follicular ameloblastoma the palisaded, elongated peripheral cells with reversed polarity are seen to be very similar in appearance to ameloblasts.

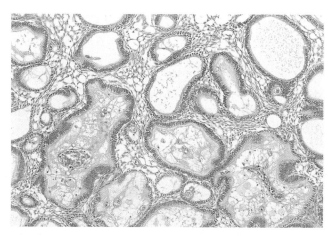

Fig. 8.6 Ameloblastoma. Plexiform ameloblastoma composed of interconnecting strands of epithelium surrounding islands of connective tissue. Several of the stromal islands have degenerated to form small cystic cavities.

Cyst formation is common, particularly as microcysts within a predominantly solid tumour. Such cysts may develop either within the epithelial islands or result from cystic degeneration of the connective tissue stroma (Fig. 8.6). Less frequently the whole tumour may be cystic, as discussed later.

Plexiform ameloblastomas consist mainly of thin trabeculae of small, darkly staining epithelial cells in a sparsely cellular connective tissue stroma (Fig. 8.7).

Acanthomatous ameloblastomas show squamous metaplasia of the central cores of neoplastic epithelium (Fig. 8.8).

Basal cell ameloblastomas are rare but consist of more darkly staining cells predominantly in a trabecular pattern with little

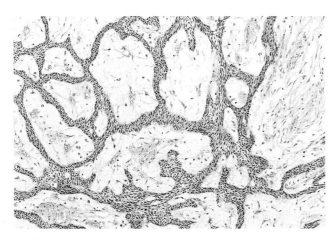

Fig. 8.7 Ameloblastoma, plexiform type. There are thin, interlacing strands of epithelium but typical ameloblasts are not seen.

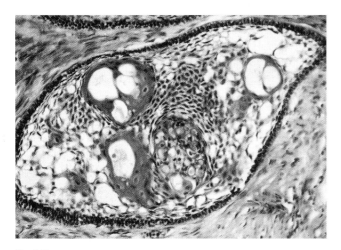

Fig. 8.8 Squamous metaplasia in an ameloblastoma. Stellate reticulum-like cells have undergone squamous metaplasia to form keratin.

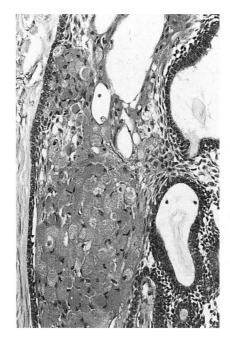

Fig. 8.9 Ameloblastoma. Granular cell change in an ameloblastoma. Ameloblast and stellate reticulum-like cells have undergone degenerative change to form large pink granular cells. In some tumours this change is extensive and the term 'granular cell ameloblastoma' is applied.

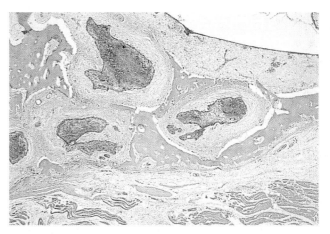

Fig. 8.10 Ameloblastoma. Islands of ameloblastoma penetrating surrounding bone at the periphery of the lesion. Such bony infiltration demands that ameloblastoma is excised with a margin rather than curetted.

evidence of palisading at the periphery. They have been mistaken for basal cell carcinomas.

Granular cell ameloblastomas are also rare. They usually resemble the follicular type, but the epithelium, particularly in the central areas of the tumour islands, forms sheets of large eosinophilic granular cells (Fig. 8.9).

These varied histological appearances have not been convincingly shown to affect the tumour's behaviour.

Management

The diagnosis must be confirmed by biopsy. Treatment is by wide excision, preferably taking up to 2 cm of apparently normal bone around the margin. Complete excision is curative but enucleation is followed by recurrence (Fig. 8.10).

Complete excision of a large ameloblastoma may mean total resection of the jaw and bone grafting. However, ameloblastomas only gradually erode compact bone and the lower border may be spared. An extensive operation can therefore be avoided by leaving the lower border of the jaw intact and

extending the resection subperiosteally. Bony repair causes much of the jaw to re-form. Regular radiographic follow-up is essential as any recurrence may not appear for several years. Limited re-operation can be performed if necessary. The patient must be warned of the necessity of regular follow-up and, possibly, of a further operation. Spread of ameloblastomas into the soft tissues is difficult to manage (Fig. 8.11).

Unicystic ameloblastoma

This is a distinct entity. Persons between the ages of 10 and 19 years are predominantly affected. Over 80% of these cystic

123

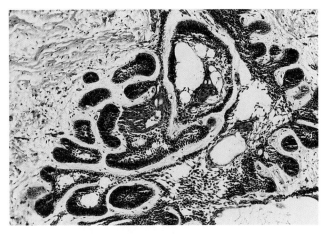

Fig. 8.11   Ameloblastoma. Soft tissue spread after repeated inadequate excisions.

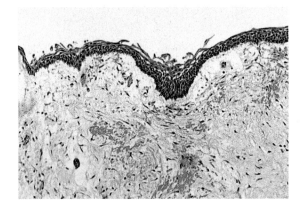

Fig. 8.12   Cystic ameloblastoma. Part of the lining of a large cyst within an ameloblastoma showing how the epithelium has become flattened and lost its typical features. Histological diagnosis may not be possible unless solid tumour is included in the specimen.

tumours enclose the crown of a tooth and mimic dentigerous cysts radiographically.

Histologically, the tumour forms the cyst wall and may proliferate into the lumen. Tumour cells forming the cyst wall are flattened and easily mistaken for those of a non-neoplastic cyst (Fig. 8.12).

Unicystic ameloblastomas, as described above, differ from the solid types in that they can be enucleated with a low risk of recurrence. A 10% recurrence rate 10 years after enucleation can be expected. However, in some unicystic ameloblastomas tumour tissue extends from the cyst wall into the surrounding tissues. These have a high risk of recurrence after enucleation. The diagnosis of unicystic ameloblastoma therefore cannot be made on a unilocular radiographic appearance or a single

> The possibility that any radiolucency at the angle of the mandible might be an ameloblastoma should not be dismissed until the diagnosis is confirmed by biopsy

incisional biopsy. Multiple areas need to be evaluated to confirm that the tumor does not extend beyond the cyst wall.

Maxillary ameloblastomas are particularly dangerous partly because the bones are considerably thinner than those of the mandible and present weak barriers to spread. Maxillary ameloblastomas tend to form in the posterior segment and to grow upwards to invade the sinonasal passages, pterygomaxillary fossa, orbit, cranium and brain. They are thus frequently lethal.

Key features of ameloblastomas are summarised in Table 8.3.

Malignant ameloblastoma and ameloblastic carcinoma

Both of these exceptionally rare tumours are little more than pathological curiosities — though not to the patient of course.

Malignant ameloblastoma is a histologically typical ameloblastoma, which nevertheless gives rise to pulmonary metastases which retain the microscopic appearances of the primary. Some cases appear to have resulted from aspiration implantation. If so, local excision of the secondary deposit should be curative. Other cases are histologically typical ameloblastomas which have metastasised to various sites. Neither the primary tumour nor metastases significantly differ histologically, from conventional, non-metastasising ameloblastomas. It is therefore not possible to predict on the basis of morphology alone, whether an ameloblastoma will metastasise. However, the chances of it so doing are remote.

Ameloblastic carcinoma is a tumour which initially resembles an ameloblastoma histologically, but loses differentiation and behaves malignantly. It spreads to lymph nodes or beyond. Later, the microscopic appearances become similar to a squamous cell carcinoma. Rarely, the progressive loss of differentiation can be seen in successive specimens from the same patient and confirms the diagnosis (Fig. 8.13). The treatment is that of an intraosseous carcinoma but the prognosis is poor if metastases are present.

ADENOMATOID ODONTOGENIC TUMOUR

Adenomatoid odontogenic tumour is uncommon, completely benign, and probably a hamartoma.

Table 8.3   Ameloblastoma: key features

- Neoplasm of odontogenic epithelium
- The most common odontogenic neoplasm
- Usually presents between ages 30 and 50
- Locally invasive but does not metastasise
- Typically asymptomatic and appears as a multilocular cyst radiographically
- Most commonly forms in posterior mandible
- Treated by excision with a margin of normal tissue
- Maxillary ameloblastomas can invade the cranial base and be lethal

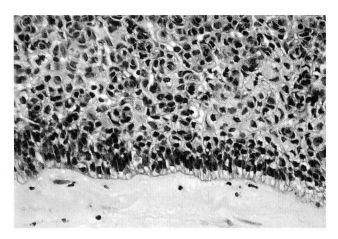

Fig. 8.13 Ameloblastic carcinoma. Very rarely a malignant variant of the ameloblastoma is encountered. Histologically they may be indistinguishable from other carcinomas, but in some cases, as here, a peripheral layer of palisaded ameloblast-like cells remains, indicating the tumour's nature.

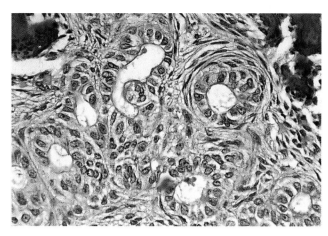

Fig. 8.15 Adenomatoid odontogenic tumour. At higher power the duct-like spaces which give the tumour its name are seen.

Clinically, adenomatoid odontogenic tumours are found either in late adolescence or young adults. Females are twice as frequently affected as males. The tumour is most frequently sited in the anterior maxilla and forms a very slow-growing swelling. Alternatively it may be noticed by chance on a radiograph where it frequently simulates a radicular or dentigerous cyst. Most specimens are only a few centimetres in diameter.

Pathology

A well-defined capsule encloses whorls and strands of epithelium, among which are microcysts, resembling ducts cut in cross-section and lined by columnar cells similar to ameloblasts (Figs 8.14 and 8.15). These microcysts may contain homogeneous eosinophilic material. Microcysts have led to the tumours being called adenomatoid, but they are not ducts and are never seen cut longitudinally. Fragments of amorphous or crystalline calcification may also be seen among the sheets of epithelial cells.

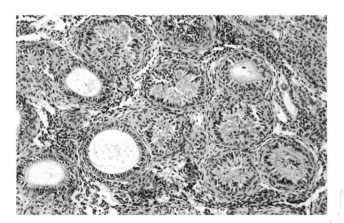

Fig. 8.14 Adenomatoid odontogenic tumour. Low magnification shows duct-like microcysts and convoluted structures. The stroma is scanty.

These lesions shell out readily, enucleation is curative and recurrence is almost unknown.

Key features of adenomatoid odontogenic tumour are summarised in Table 8.4.

Table 8.4 Adenomatoid odontogenic tumour: key features

- Rare
- Hamartoma of odontogenic epithelium
- Usually presents between ages 15 and 20
- Most common in the anterior maxilla
- Often appears radiographically as a unilocular dentigerous cyst
- Responds to enucleation

CALCIFYING EPITHELIAL ODONTOGENIC TUMOUR

This tumour, with bizarre microscopic features, is often termed a Pindborg tumour, after its discoverer. Though rare, it is important, because it could be mistaken for a poorly differentiated carcinoma microscopically.

Clinically, adults are mainly affected at an average age of about 40. The typical site is the posterior body of the mandible, which is twice as frequently involved as the maxilla. Symptoms are usually lacking until a swelling appears. Radiographs show a translucent area with poorly defined margins and, usually, increasing radiopacities within the tumour as it matures.

Pathology

Calcifying epithelial odontogenic tumours consist of sheets or strands of epithelial cells in a connective tissue stroma (Fig. 8.16). The epithelial cells are polyhedral and typically have distinct outlines and intercellular bridges. Gross variation in nuclear size, including giant nuclei, is frequently striking (Fig. 8.17). These nuclei are usually hyperchromatic and, though mitoses are rare, produce an alarming resemblance to a poorly-

125

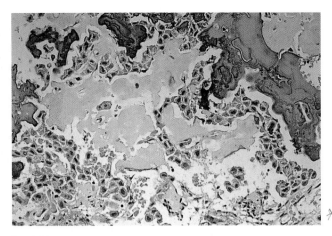

Fig. 8.16 Calcifying epithelial odontogenic tumour (Pindborg tumour). The tumour is composed of strands and sheets of polyhedral epithelial cells lying in pale pink staining amyloid-like material. Some of this material has mineralised, stains a darker blue colour and gives rise to radiopacities within the lesion.

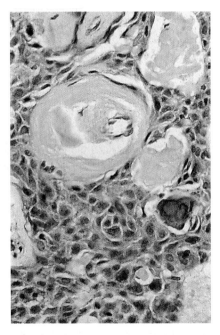

Fig. 8.17 Calcifying epithelial odontogenic tumour. At higher power the epithelial cells are seen to have sharply defined cell membranes resembling squamous epithelium and pleomorphic hyperchromatic nuclei. The pale pink material is amyloid-like.

differentiated carcinoma. However, unlike most carcinomas, a stromal inflammatory reaction is typically absent. Within the tumour, there are typically homogeneous hyaline areas, with the staining characteristics of amyloid. These may calcify and form concentric rings in and around degenerating epithelial cells and may form large masses. Clear cells may also be present.

Calcifying epithelial odontogenic tumours are not encapsulated, are locally invasive and behave similarly to ameloblastomas. Diagnosis depends on histological examination. It is particularly important to distinguish this pleomorphic tumour

Table 8.5 Calcifying epithelial odontogenic tumour: key features
● Rare neoplasm of odontogenic epithelium ● Usually presents between ages 30 and 50 ● Many bizarre pleomorphic and hyperchromatic nuclei and formation of amyloid-like material ● Solid tumour, mixed radiolucency ● Most commonly forms in posterior mandible ● Locally invasive but does not metastasise ● Treated by excision with a small margin

from a poorly differentiated carcinoma to avoid overtreatment. Complete excision of the tumour with a border of normal bone should be curative, but recurrence follows incomplete excision.

Key features of calcifying epithelial odontogenic tumour are summarised in Table 8.5.

CLEAR CELL ODONTOGENIC CARCINOMA

This very rare neoplasm affects elderly patients (60 to 74 years). Symptoms include mild pain or tenderness, or loosening of teeth of either jaw associated with expansion of the jaw and a ragged area of radiolucency.

Pathology

Clear cell odontogenic carcinoma is poorly circumscribed and consists mainly of clear cells with a central nucleus and a well-defined cell membrane. They form large sheets, separated by thin fibrous septa (Fig. 8.18). Inflammatory cells are scanty but areas of haemorrhage may be seen. Nervous tissue may be enveloped and the tumour invades surrounding tissues. Important differences from calcifying epithelial odontogenic tumour are the lesser degree of nuclear pleomorphism and the lack of calcifications or amyloid-like material.

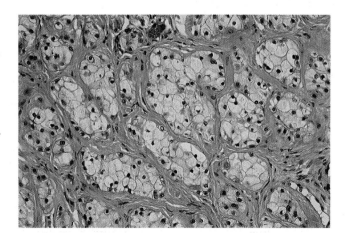

Fig. 8.18 Clear cell odontogenic carcinoma. This rare epithelial odontogenic tumour is composed of pale-staining clear cells.

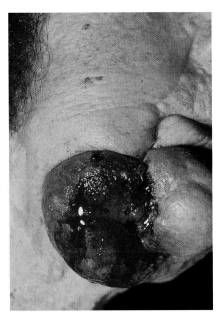

Fig. 8.19 Clear cell odontogenic carcinomas. This neglected tumour has fungated through the cheek.

Treatment. This tumour is capable of metastasising to regional nodes and distant organs and has occasionally been fatal. Wide excision followed by radiotherapy is required (Fig. 8.19).

CALCIFYING (GHOST CELL) ODONTOGENIC CYST

The calcifying odontogenic cyst is rare and the solid form is even less common. It is a benign neoplasm but has a malignant variant.

Clinically, almost any age and either jaw can be affected. The site is most often anterior to the first molar but occasionally it is the gingival mucosa and the underlying bone is merely indented. On radiographs, the appearance is usually cystic but it may be multilocular or contain flecks of calcification. Occasionally roots of adjacent teeth are eroded.

Pathology

The lining of cystic areas consists of squamous epithelium with cuboidal or ameloblast-like basal cells (Figs 8.20 and 8.21). This epithelium is sometimes thick and can contain areas resembling stellate reticulum. Solid variants of this tumour may therefore resemble an ameloblastoma.

The most conspicuous feature is abnormal keratinisation producing areas of swollen, eosinophilic cells which become progressively paler, leaving only their outlines (ghost cells) or hyaline masses (Fig. 8.22). The ghost cells typically calcify in patchy fashion, and where this keratin-like material comes into contact with connective tissue it excites a foreign body reaction. Approximately 10% of calcifying odontogenic cysts are associated with odontomas or other odontogenic tumours.

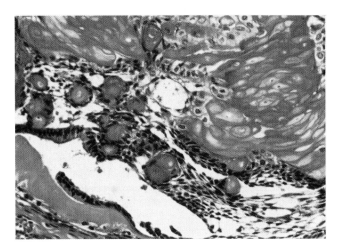

Fig. 8.20 Calcyfing odontogenic cyst. There are some amelobast-like cells (left), a layer of cells resembling stellate reticulum, and a mass of epithelial ghost cells.

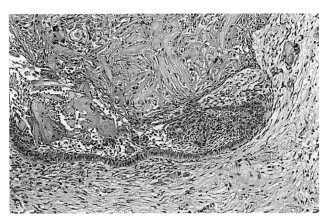

Fig. 8.21 Calcifying odontogenic cyst. There is a thin lining of epithelium with a basal layer of columnar cells and the lumen is filled by ghost cells shed into the cyst cavity.

The behaviour of a calcifying odontogenic cyst is similar to that of a non-neoplastic cyst, overlying bone is only occasionally eroded and enucleation is usually effective. Key features are summarised in Table 8.6.

Table 8.6 Calcifying odontogenic cyst: key features

- Rare
- Probably a neoplasm of odontogenic epithelium
- Wide age range
- Radiographically unilocular often undistinguishable from non-neoplastic jaw cysts
- Calcifications in the cyst wall may suggest the diagnosis
- Forms at any site in alveolar ridge, usually posteriorly
- Occasionally forms in soft tissue of the gingiva
- Diagnosis by finding ghost and ameloblast-like cells histologically
- Usually responds to enucleation like a nonneoplastic cyst
- Solid lesions may be more aggressive

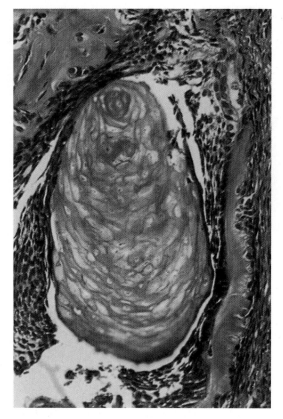

Fig. 8.22 Calcifying odontogenic cyst with ghost cells.

SQUAMOUS ODONTOGENIC TUMOUR

This rare tumour mainly affects young adults and involves the alveolar process of either jaw, close to the roots of erupted teeth.

Radiographically, the squamous odontogenic tumour can mimic severe bone loss from periodontitis or produce a cyst-like area.

Pathology

Circumscribed, rounded, or more irregular islands of squamous epithelium with flattened peripheral cells are set in a fibrous stroma (Fig. 8.23). Foci of keratin or parakeratin may form in the epithelium, which may also contain laminated calcifications or globular eosinophilic structures.

This tumour is benign, though there may occasionally be invasion of adjacent structures by maxillary lesions. However, curettage and extraction of any teeth involved appears usually to be effective.

AMELOBLASTIC FIBROMA

This tumour, though rare, is important in the differential diagnosis of ameloblastoma.

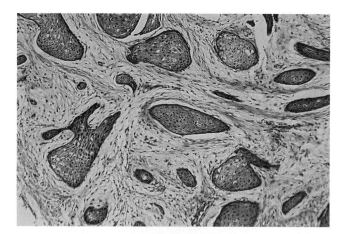

Fig. 8.23 Squamous odontogenic tumour. The lesion is composed of islands of squamous epithelium without peripheral palisaded cells.

Clinically, ameloblastic fibromas usually affect young persons (of average age 15 years). They are slow-growing and usually asymptomatic, but eventually expand the jaw. Radiographically, they can appear as a multi- or unilocular cysts in the posterior body of the mandible.

Pathology

Both the epithelium and connective tissue are neoplastic. The epithelium consists of ameloblast-like or more cuboidal cells surrounding others resembling stellate reticulum or more compact epithelium. The epithelium is sharply circumscribed by a basal membrane and forms islands, strands or mushroom-like proliferations in a loose but cellular, fibromyxoid connective tissue, which resembles the immature dentine papilla (Figs 8.24 and 8.25).

An ameloblastic fibroma may rarely be combined with mixed calcifying dental tissues (ameloblastic fibro-odontoma), and radiographs typically show the densely opaque dental tissues in the otherwise radiolucent area.

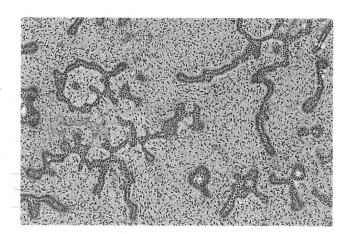

Fig. 8.24 Ameloblastic fibroma. The appearance is somewhat similar to that of ameloblastoma but the pattern of budding strands is distinctive and the connective tissue resembles the undifferentiated mesenchyme of the dental papilla.

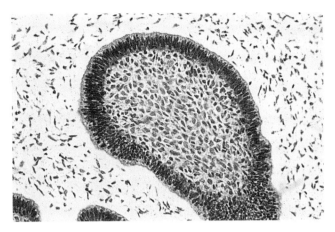

Fig. 8.25 Ameloblastic fibroma. At higher power the resemblance to dental papilla, ameloblasts and stellate reticulum is seen more clearly.

Ameloblastic fibroma and fibro-odontoma are benign. They do not infiltrate bone and separate readily from their bony walls. Conservative resection is effective, but, if incomplete, recurrence follows. However, there is a potential for malignant change. Key features are summarised in Table 8.7.

Table 8.7 Ameloblastic fibroma: key features
● Rare
● Neoplasm of both odontogenic epithelium and mesenchyme
● Usually seen in children or young adults
● Solid lesion but appears as unilocular or multilocular radiolucency
● Treated by excision with a small margin
● Can undergo malignant change

Ameloblastic sarcoma (ameloblastic fibrosarcoma)

This is the rare malignant counterpart of ameloblastic fibroma. It is invasive and destructive but has little tendency to metastasise. Reports suggest that approximately 50% arise from ameloblastic fibromas.

ODONTOGENIC MYXOMA

The odontogenic myxoma is peculiar to the jaws and consists of dental mesenchyme.

Clinically, young people are predominantly affected. The tumour gives rise to a fusiform swelling and a radiolucent area with scalloped margins or a soap-bubble appearance (Fig. 8.26).

Pathology

Myxomas consist of scanty spindle-shaped or angular cells with long, fine, anastomosing processes, distributed in loose mucoid material (Figs 8.27 and 8.28). A few collagen fibres may also form, and there may be small, scattered epithelial rests. The margins of the tumour are ill-defined and peripheral bone is progressively resorbed.

Myxomas are benign, but can infiltrate widely. Wide excision is required but, in spite of vigorous treatment, some tumours persist, and have been seen over 30 years after the original operations. By this time they appear inactive and are symptomless.

Rare variants with a more cellular and pleomorphic microscopic picture may be categorised as myxosarcomas but appear

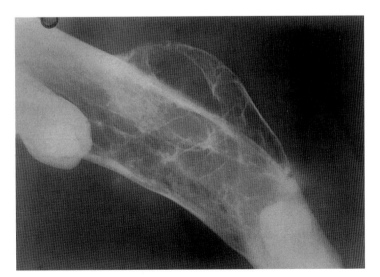

Fig. 8.26 Odontogenic myxoma of the mandible. An occlusal view showing the finely trabeculated, soap-bubble appearance and gross expansion of the mandible. Evidence of residual tumour was still present after 35 years in spite of vigorous treatment, both surgery and radiotherapy, in its earlier stages.

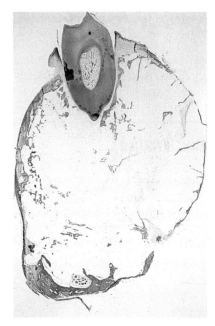

Fig. 8.27 Odontogenic myxoma. This cross-section of the mandible through a myxoma shows extensive bony resorption and gross expansion. The pale staining myxoid lesion gives the tumour an empty appearance.

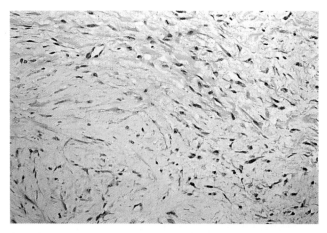

Fig. 8.28 Odontogenic myxoma. High power view showing the typical appearance of sparse fibroblasts lying in a myxoid or ground substance-rich matrix.

to have little or no potential for metastasis. Key features are summarised in Table 8.8.

Table 8.8 Odontogenic myxoma: key features
• Rare
• Neoplasm of odontogenic mesenchyme
• Usually seen in young adults
• Benign but prone to recurrence
• Forms a multilocular, sometimes soap-bubble radiolucency
• Most common site is posterior mandible
• Treated by excision

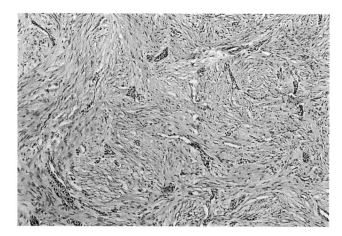

Fig. 8.29 Odontogenic fibroma. This rare mesenchymal odontogenic tumour consists of fibrous tissue containing rests and strands of odontogenic epithelium resembling those found in the periodontal ligament.

ODONTOGENIC FIBROMA

The odontogenic origin of this rare tumour is suggested by its endosteal site and the presence of epithelial rests.

Clinically, odontogenic fibroma more frequently affects the mandible. It forms a slow-growing asymptomatic mass which may eventually expand the jaw. If found by chance in a radiograph, it appears as a sharply defined, rounded lucent area in a tooth-bearing region.

Pathology

Odontogenic fibromas consist of spindle-shaped fibroblasts and bundles of whorled collagen fibres (Fig. 8.29), and may contain strands of odontogenic epithelium.

Odontogenic fibromas are benign and shell out from their surroundings.

TUMOURS AND DYSPLASIAS OF CEMENTUM

CEMENTOBLASTOMA

Cementoblastoma is a neoplasm of cementum. Lesions formerly categorised as cementomas or cemental dysplasias are now categorised as fibro-osseous lesions as discussed below, as is cemento-ossifying fibroma.

Cementoblastoma is a benign neoplasm and forms a mass of cementum-like tissue as an irregular or rounded mass attached to the root of a tooth, usually a mandibular first molar.

Clinically, cementoblastomas mainly affect young adults, particularly males, typically below the age of 25. They are slow-growing and the jaw is not usually expanded. A cemento-blastoma only rarely causes gross bony swelling and pain.

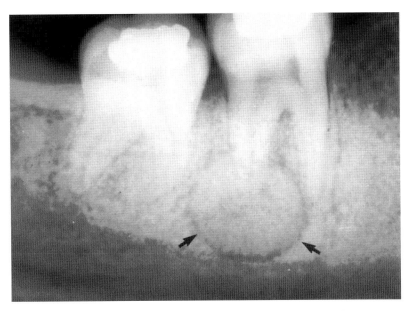

Fig. 8.30 Periapical radiograph showing the typical appearances of a cementoblastoma, a radiopaque mass with a radiolucent rim attached to the root apex. (By kind permission of Mr E Whaites.)

Radiographically, there is typically a radiopaque mass with a thin radiolucent margin, attached to the roots of a tooth (Fig. 8.30). The mass may be rounded or irregular in shape and mottled in texture. Resorption of related roots is common, but the tooth remains vital.

Pathology

The mass consists of cementum which often contains many reversal lines, resembling Paget's disease. Cells are enclosed within the cementum, and in the irregular spaces are many osteoclasts and osteoblast-like cells (Figs 8.31 and 8.32). The cellular appearance may sometimes appear so active as to be mistaken for an osteosarcoma.

Peripherally, there is a broad zone of unmineralised tissue and a connective tissue capsule. These appearances are essentially the same as those of an osteoblastoma, a rare bone tumour. They are only distinguishable by the cementoblastoma's relationship to a tooth (Fig. 8.33).

Cementoblastomas are benign, and, if completely excised and the tooth extracted, there should be no recurrence. Incomplete removal leads to continued growth. Key features are summarised in Table 8.9.

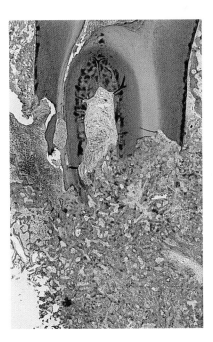

Fig. 8.31 Cementoblastoma. A dense mass of interconnected trabeculae of osteoid is fused to the resorbed roots of the first permanent molar.

CEMENTO-OSSIFYING FIBROMA

So-called cementifying and ossifying fibromas are not regarded as separate entities.

Cemento-ossifying fibroma is uncommon. It is well circumscribed and undergoes slow expansile growth, usually in the mandibular premolar or molar region, and typically causes a painless swelling. Patients are usually between 20 and 40 years, but the age range is wide. Females are affected several times more frequently than males.

Cemento-ossifying fibroma is radiolucent with varying degrees of calcification and has well defined margins radiographically (Fig. 8.34). Calcifications tend to be concentrated centrally and some specimens appear largely radiopaque with a thin radiolucent rim. Roots of related teeth can be displaced.

131

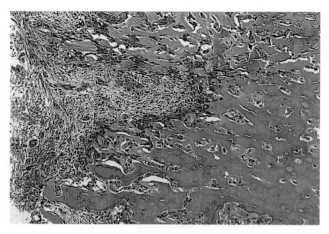

Fig. 8.32 Cementoblastoma. At high power at the periphery of the lesion there are radiating seams of osteoid with a thick layer of atypical cementoblasts on their surface.

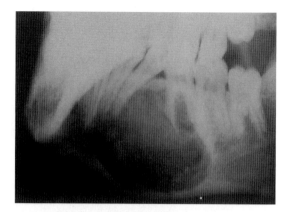

Fig. 8.34 Cemento-ossifying fibroma. The tumour forms a characteristic rounded well-circumscribed lesion radiographically, cloudily radiolucent in its earlier and radiopaque in its later stages. It is slow-growing, as can be seen by the displacement of the teeth.

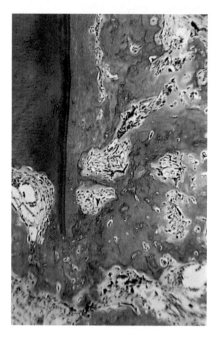

Fig. 8.33 Resorbed root at the centre of a cementoblastoma showing continuity of cementum with the mineralised tissue of the lesion.

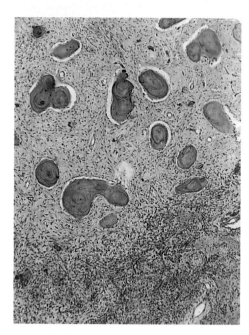

Fig. 8.35 Cemento-ossifying fibroma. This example contains densely mineralised and darkly staining islands of cementum-like tissue lying in cellular fibrous tissue. Towards the actively growing margin of the lesion (lower part) the fibrous tissue is more cellular and is forming woven bone.

Table 8.9 Cementoblastoma: key features

- Neoplasm of cementoblasts (odontogenic mesenchyme)
- Usually seen in young adults
- Benign
- Radiopaque with a narrow lucent rim
- Most commonly is at the apex of a vital lower first molar
- Treated by enucleation

Microscopy

Cemento-ossifying fibromas are well demarcated from the surrounding bone. The appearances are widely variable and range from predominantly fibrous tumors with variable degress

of cellularity and scanty calcifications to densely calcified nodules with little stroma.

The types of calcifications include trabeculae of woven bone with osteoblastic rimming, which frequently form a reticular pattern. Other patterns are dystrophic calcifications or predominantly acellular, rounded calcifications resembling cementicles (Fig. 8.35). These calcifications gradually grow, fuse, and ultimately form a dense mass (Fig. 8.36). Most so-called cementifying fibromas show mixed spherical calcifications and bone trabeculae.

Cemento-ossifying fibroma may be also classified with the fibro-osseous lesions as discussed in Chapter 10.

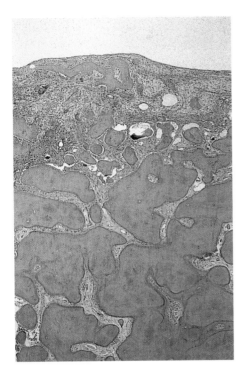

Fig. 8.36 Cemento-ossifying fibroma. In this mature lesion there are large coalescing islands of dense bone and little fibrous tissue. Note the well-demarcated periphery of fibrous tissue which has shelled away from the adjacent bone during removal.

Histologically, cemento-ossifying fibroma may be indistinguishable from limited areas of fibrous dysplasia or cemento-osseous dysplasias. However, the clinical and radiographic findings should allow the distinctions to be made.

Management

The patterns of calcifications have no effect on the tumour's behaviour. Cemento-ossifying fibromas may have a definable capsule and can be readily enucleated. Occasionally, large tumours which have distorted the jaw require local resection and bone grafting, but recurrence is rare. However, if an associated tooth is extracted, a densely calcified cemento-ossifying fibroma can become a focus for chronic osteomyelitis. If this happens, wide excision becomes necessary.

Juvenile active ('aggressive') ossifying fibroma

The term *juvenile ossifying fibroma* is sometimes restricted to tumours which particularly affect patients of 15 years or younger. They are mostly found in extragnathic bones. However, some affect the maxilla or, rarely, the mandible. Jaw lesions tend to be asymptomatic but expansion is common.

Two distinctive microscopic patterns have been reported. The 'trabecular' type is characteristic of the so-called juvenile ossifying fibroma and shows a loose, fibroblastic stroma containing very fine, lace-like trabeculae of immature osteoid

entrapping plump osteoblasts. Mitoses may be seen and focal collections of giant cells are common.

The 'psammomatoid' variant consists of an exceedingly cellular fibroblastic stroma containing compact, rounded calcifications.

Some of these lesions have been locally aggressive and shown a tendency to recur. However, there are no definitive histologic criteria for distinguishing these tumours from more typical cemento-ossifying fibromas. Despite the cellular ('active') appearance of the juvenile type, conservative surgery is typically effective.

NON-NEOPLASTIC ODONTOGENIC LESIONS

CEMENTO-OSSEOUS DYPLASIAS

These are non-neoplastic proliferations. They are of periodontal ligament origin and all the variants involve the same pathological processes and differ mainly in their extent and radiographic appearances.

Periapical cemental dysplasia

Periapical cemental dysplasia affects women (particularly the middle-aged) more than 10 times as frequently as men, and is also more common in blacks. It typically involves the mandibular incisor region, but can affect several sites or be generalised.

They are asymptomatic but can be seen early in radiographs, as rounded radiolucent areas related to the apices of the teeth. These simulate periapical granulomas but related teeth are vital. Later, increasing calcification, starting centrally, causes the masses to become densely radiopaque, but all stages of development may be seen in multiple lesions.

Pathology

The lesions resemble cemento-ossifying fibromas histologically and consist, in their early stages, of cellular fibrous tissue containing foci of cementum-like tissue. Progressive calcification leads to the formation of a solid, bone-like mass. Early lesions need to be distinguished from periapical granulomas by dental investigation. Further treatment is unnecessary, as the disorder is self-limiting.

Florid cemento-osseous dysplasia and gigantiform cementoma

This is probably a florid form of periapical cemental dysplasia and affects a similar group of persons. The sclerotic masses are frequently symmetrical and may involve all four quadrants. They are asymptomatic unless they become infected, but can expand the jaw.

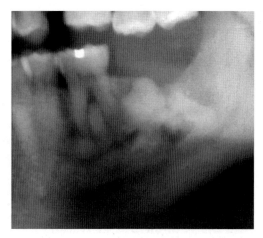

Fig. 8.37 Florid cemento-osseous dysplasia. Section of a panoramic tomogram showing the typical appearances of multiple irregular radiopaque masses centred on the roots of the teeth. The periphery of each is radiolucent. Similar lesions were present on the contralateral side of the mandible.

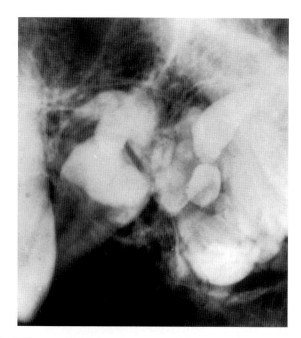

Fig. 8.38 Compound odontoma. The mass consists of many denticles which overlap each other in the radiograph but are nevertheless just visible as individual tooth-like structures.

Radiographically, florid cemento-osseous dysplasia appears as radiopaque, somewhat irregular masses without a radiolucent border and in the past has been mistaken for chronic osteomyelitis (Fig. 8.37).

Microscopically, the appearances are generally similar to periapical cemental dysplasia.

Gigantiform cementoma is a rare familial variant of florid cemento-osseous dysplasia.

Focal cemento-osseous dysplasia

This term is given to changes similar to florid osseous dysplasia but forming a single lesion.

Management of cemento-osseous dysplasias

Infection of these lesions by unwise extractions or other means must be avoided. Osteomyelitis resulting from such causes is difficult to treat because of the widespread sclerosis in the late stages. Wide excision may then be required to allow resolution. Treatment is otherwise not indicated except rarely for cosmetic reasons.

ODONTOMAS (ODONTOMES)

Odontomas are developmental malformations (hamartomas) of dental tissues, not neoplasms. Like teeth, once fully calcified they do not develop further. Even when the morphology is grossly distorted (as in complex odontomas), the pulp, dentine, enamel and cementum are in normal anatomical relationships with one another, and, also like teeth, odontomas may erupt.

Odontomas affect the maxilla slightly more frequently than the mandible and are often recognised in early adolescence by the dense opacity of the enamel component in routine radiographs. When odontomas have erupted, infection develops in one of the many stagnation areas, and abscess formation commonly follows. In other cases, odontomas displace teeth or block their eruption or become involved in cyst formation.

Compound odontomas

These consist of many separate, small, tooth-like structures (denticles), probably produced by localised, multiple budding-off from the dental lamina and formation of many tooth germs.

Clinically, a compound odontoma usually forms in the anterior part of the jaws and gives rise to a painless swelling. The denticles may be seen radiographically as separate densely-calcified bodies (Fig. 8.38).

Histologically, the denticles are embedded in fibrous connective tissue, and have a fibrous capsule (Figs 8.39 and 8.40).

The mass should be enucleated as a potential obstruction to tooth eruption or cyst formation.

Complex odontoma

Complex odontomas consist of an irregular mass of hard and soft dental tissues, having no morphological resemblance to a tooth and frequently forming a cauliflower-like mass.

Clinically, complex odontomas are usually seen in young

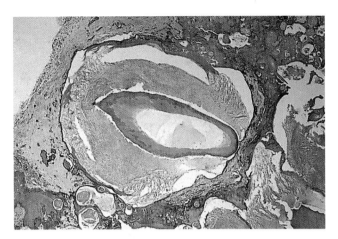

Fig. 8.39 Compound odontoma. A denticle of dentine surrounded by enamel matrix is lying within more irregular calcified tissues.

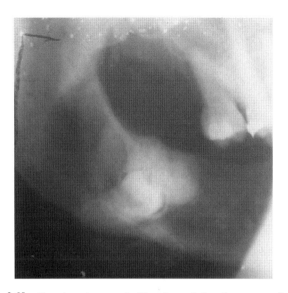

Fig. 8.41 Complex odontoma. In this radiograph the odontoma overlies the crown of a buried molar and shows the typical dense amorphous area of radiopacity.

persons, but may escape diagnosis until late in life. Typically, a hard painless swelling is present, but the mass may start to erupt and infection follows. The mass may also undergo cystic change or resorption. Radiographically, when calcification is complete, an irregular radiopaque mass is seen containing areas of densely radiopaque enamel (Fig. 8.41).

Histologically, the mass consists of all the dental tissues in a disordered arrangement, but frequently with a radial pattern. The pulp is usually finely branched so that the mass is perforated, like a sponge, by small branches of pulp (Fig. 8.42). Key features are summarised in Table 8.10.

The mass should be removed by conservative surgery.

Table 8.10 Odontomas: key features

- Hamartomas of odontogenic epithelium and mesenchyme
- Usually found between ages 10 and 20 years
- Benign
- Develop like surrounding teeth with initial (crypt-like) radiolucent phase, intermediate stage of mixed radiolucency, finally densely radiopaque
- May be compound (many small teeth) or complex (disordered mass of dental hard tissue)
- Most common sites are anterior maxilla and posterior mandible
- Respond to enucleation

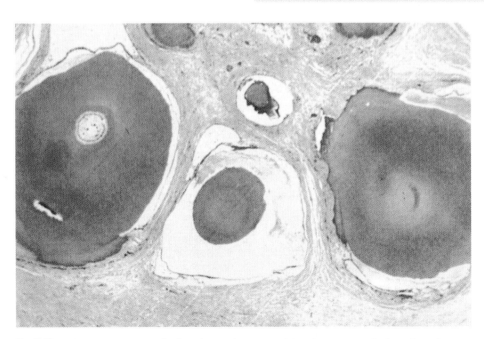

Fig. 8.40 Compound odontoma. Sections from various areas of the odontoma, seen in the radiograph shown in Figure 8.38, show denticles of dentine and enamel cut in various planes, and more irregular calcified tissues, within a connective tissue capsule.

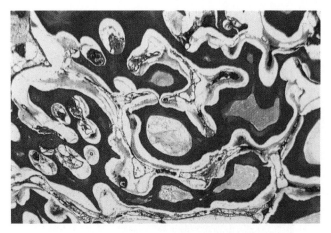

Fig. 8.42 Complex odontoma. A disorganised mass of dentine, enamel and cementum penetrated by fine divisions of pulp.

Other types of odontomas

In the past, complex classifications have been devised to include such developmental anomalies as *dilated, invaginated* and *geminated* odontomas. These abnormalities are, in part, obviously tooth-like. Dilated and gestant odontomas arise by invagination of cells of the enamel organ or of the epithelial sheath of Hertwig, which actively proliferate until they expand the developing tooth. Gestant odontomas range in severity from a cingular pit in an otherwise normal upper lateral incisor to the so-called *dens in dente*. Minor morphological anomalies such as these have been discussed in Chapter 2.

'Dentinoma'. Calcified masses called 'dentinomas' have rarely been described. However, dentine forms only under the inductive effect of ameloblasts and the existence of dentinomas is no longer accepted.

Mixed odontogenic tumours. Very occasionally odontomas and odontogenic tumours are combined.

SUGGESTED FURTHER READING

Baden E, Doyle J, Mesa M, Fabie M, Lederman D, Eichen M 1993 Squamous odontogenic tumour. Report of three cases including the first extraosseous case. Oral Surg Oral Med Oral Pathol 75:733–738

Bang G, Koppang H S, Hansen L S, Gilhuus-Moe, Aksdal E et al 1989 Clear cell odontogenic carcinoma: report of three cases with pulmonary and lymph node metastases. J Oral Pathol Med 18:113–118

Bredenkamp J K, Zimmerman M C, Mickel R A 1989 Maxillary ameloblastoma. A potentially lethal neoplasm. Arch Otolaryngol Head Neck Surg 115:99–104

Bruce R A, Jackson I T 1991 Ameloblastic carcinoma. Report of an aggressive case and review of the literature. J Cranio Max Fac Surg 19:267–271

Buchner A 1991 The central (intraosseous) calcifying odontogenic cyst: an analysis of 215 cases. J Oral Maxillofac Surg 49:330–339

Buchner A, Merrell P W, Hansen L S, Leider A S 1991 Peripheral (extraosseous) calcifying odontogenic cyst. A review of forty-five cases. Oral Surg Oral Med Oral Pathol 72:65–70

Cawson R A 1972 Myxoma of the mandible with a 35 year follow-up. Br Oral Surg 10:59–63

Cawson R A, Binnie W H, Barrett A W, Wright J M 2001 *Oral disease*, 3rd Edn. Mosby-Wolfe, London

Cawson R A, Binnie W H, Barrett A W, Wright J M 1998 *Lucas's Pathology of tumors of the oral tissues*. Churchill Livingstone, Edinburgh

Daley T D, Wysocki G P 1994 Peripheral odontogenic fibroma. Oral Surg Oral Med Oral Pathol 78:329–336

Franklin C D, Pindborg J J 1976 The calcifying epithelial odontogenic tumor. A review and analysis of 113 cases. Oral Surg 42:753–765

Gardner D G, Corio R L 1984 Plexiform unicystic ameloblastoma. A variant of ameloblastoma with low-recurrence rate after enucleation. Cancer 53:1730–1735

Gerol M, Burkes E J 1995 Peripheral ameloblastoma. J Periodontol 66:1065–1068

Gorlin R J, Pindborg J J, Redman R S, Williamson J J, Hansen L S 1964 The calcifying odontogenic cyst — A new entity and possible analogue of the cutaneous epithelioma of Malherbe. Cancer 17:723–729

Handlers J P, Abrams A M, Melrose R J, Danforth R 1991 Central odontogenic fibroma: clinicopathologic features of 19 cases and review of the literature. J Oral Maxillofac Surg 49:46–54

Holmlund A, Anneroth G, Lundquist G, Nordenram A 1991 Ameloblastomas originating from odontogenic cysts. J Oral Pathol Med 20:318–321

Hong S P, Ellis G L, Hartman K S 1991 Calcifying odontogenic cyst: a review of ninety-two cases with reevaluation of their nature as neoplasms, the nature of ghost cells, and subclassification. Oral Surg Oral Med Oral Pathol 72:56–64

Kaugars G E, Miller M E, Abbey L M 1989 Odontomas. Oral Surg Oral Med Oral Pathol 67:172–176

Keszler A, Dominguez F V, Giannunzio G 1995 Myxoma in childhood: an analysis of 10 cases. J Oral Maxillofac Surg 53:518–521

McCoy B P, Carroll M K O, Hall J M 1992 Carcinoma arising in a dentinogenic ghost cell tumor. Oral Surg Oral Med Oral Pathol 74:371–378

Muller S, Parker D C, Kapadia S B, Budnick S D, Barnes E L 1995 Ameloblastic fibrosarcoma of the jaw. A clinicopathologic and DNA analysis of five cases and review of the literature. Oral Surg Oral Med Oral Pathol 79:469–477

Peltola J, Magnusson B, Hopponen R-P, Borrman H 1994 Odontogenic myxoma — a radiographic study of 21 tumours. Br J Oral Maxillofac Surg 32:298–301

Philipsen H P, Reichart P A 1998 Unicystic ameloblastoma. A review of 193 cases from the literature. Oral Oncol 34:317–325

Philipsen H P, Reichert P A, Zhang K J, Nikai H, Yu Q X 1991 Adenomatoid odontogenic tumor: biologic profile base on 499 cases. J Oral Pathol Med 20:149–158

Pindborg J J, Kramer I R H, Shear M 1992 *Histological typing of odontogenic tumours*, 2nd Edn. World Health Organization. Springer Verlag, Berlin

Reichart P A, Philipsen H P, Sonner S 1995 Ameloblastoma: biological profile of 3677 cases. Oral Oncol Eur J Cancer 31B:86–99

Ulmansky M, Hjorting-Hansen E, Praetorius F, Haque M F 1994 Benign cementoblastoma. A review and five new cases. Oral Surg Oral Med Oral Pathol 77:48–55

Williams H K, Mangham C, Speight P M 1999 Juvenile ossifying fibroma. An analysis of eight cases and a comparison with other fibro-osseous lesions. J Oral Pathol Med 29:13–18

Williams T P 1993 Management of ameloblastoma: a changing perspective. J Oral Maxillofac Surg 51:1064–1070

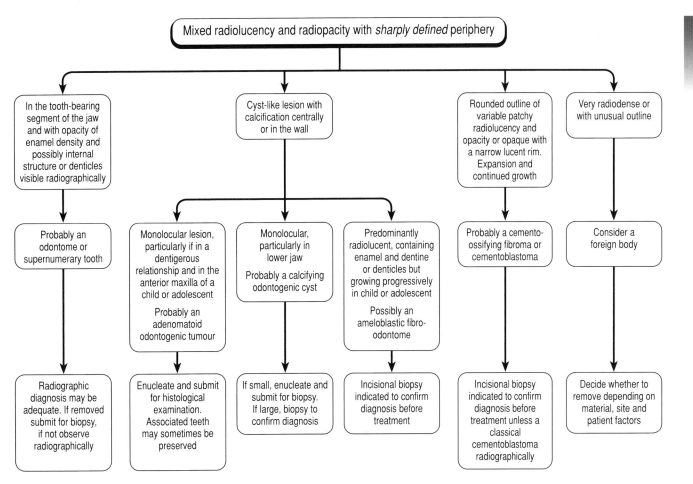

Summary 8.1 Differential diagnosis and management of sharply defined mixed radiolucencies in the jaws.

Non-odontogenic tumours of the jaws

Almost any type of tumour can arise in the jaws but most of them are considerably more common in other parts of the skeleton. Only the more important examples (Table 9.1) are considered here.

OSTEOMA AND OTHER BONY OVERGROWTHS

True tumours consisting of bone (either compact or cancellous) are occasionally seen, but localised overgrowths of bone (exostoses) are more common. They consist of lamellae of compact bone, but large specimens may have a core of cancellous bone. Small exostoses may form irregularly on the surface of the alveolar processes (Fig. 9.1) and specific variants are *torus palatinus* and *torus mandibularis*. They differ from other exostoses only in that they develop in characteristic sites and are symmetrical.

Torus palatinus commonly forms towards the posterior of the midline of the hard palate (Fig. 9.2). The swelling is rounded and symmetrical, sometimes with a midline groove. It is not usually noticed until middle age and, if it interferes with the fitting of a denture, should be removed.

Tori mandibularis form on the lingual aspect of the mandible opposite the mental foramen. They are typically bilateral,

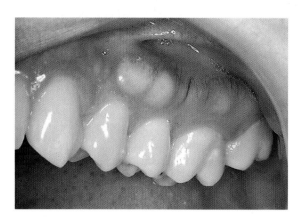

Fig. 9.1 Exostoses. Bony exostoses, aside from tori, are found most frequently buccally on the alveolar bone and are often symmetrically arranged.

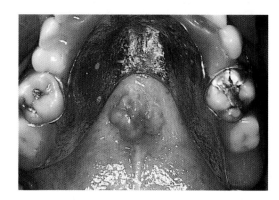

Fig. 9.2 Torus palatinus. Palatal tori range from small smooth elevations to lobular swellings such as this. The bone is covered by only a thin mucosa which is prone to trauma.

forming hard, rounded swellings (Fig. 9.3). The management is the same as that of torus palatinus.

Compact and cancellous osteoma

Compact osteomas consist of lamellae of bone, sometimes in layers like an onion but not in haversian systems (Fig. 9.4). This dense bone contains occasional vascular spaces, and grows very slowly. Cancellous osteomas consist of slender trabeculae of

Table 9.1 Non-odontogenic tumours of bone

- Primary — benign
    Osteoma
    Osteochondroma
    Cemento-ossifying fibroma
    Central giant-cell granuloma
    Haemangioma
    Melanotic neuroectodermal tumour
- Primary — malignant
    Osteosarcoma
    Chondrosarcoma
    Ewing's sarcoma
    Multifocal or potentially multifocal:
        Myeloma
        Langerhans cell histiocytosis
- Metastatic
    Carcinoma

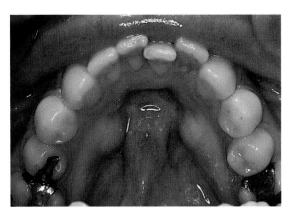

Fig. 9.3 Mandibular tori. The typical appearance of bilateral tori lingual to the lower premolars.

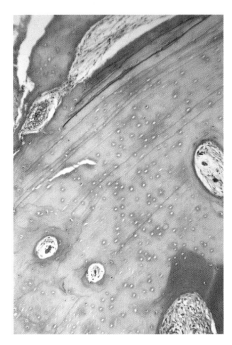

Fig. 9.4 Compact osteoma. Dense bone is laid down in lamellae with occasional vascular spaces, but there is no attempt to form Haversian systems.

bone, with interstitial marrow spaces and a lamellated cortex (Fig. 9.5).

Osteomas should be excised only if they become large enough to cause symptoms or interfere with the fitting of a denture.

Gardner's syndrome

Gardner's syndrome comprises multiple osteomas of the jaw, polyposis coli with a high malignant potential, and often other abnormalities such as dental defects and epidermal cysts or fibromas. It is inherited as an autosomal dominant trait but penetrance is weak.

Early recognition of these oral features should prompt bowel radiography or endoscopy and possibly prophylactic colectomy.

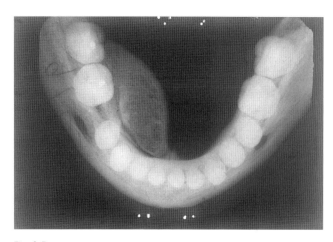

Fig. 9.5 Cancellous osteoma of the mandible. The tumour has arisen from a relatively narrow base lingually to the molars but has been moulded forward during growth by pressure of the tongue. The trabecular pattern of cancellous bone can be seen. A torus mandibularis arises further forward on the jaw, arises from a broad base and is usually bilateral.

OSTEOCHONDROMA (CARTILAGE-CAPPED OSTEOMA)

These bony overgrowths grow by ossification beneath a cartilaginous cap. Most arise from the region of the coronoid or condylar process and form a hard bony protuberance which can interfere with joint function. The cartilaginous cap may not be visible in radiographs. Almost any age can be affected.

Pathology

The lesion is subperiosteal and has a cap of hyaline cartilage where the cartilage cells are sometimes regularly aligned or irregular and contain minute foci of ossification (Fig. 9.6). As age advances, the mass progressively ossifies.

These tumours are benign and usually cease to grow after skeletal maturation. Removal is therefore curative.

CEMENTO-OSSIFYING FIBROMA

Cemento-ossifying fibroma has been discussed in Chapter 9, as its presence in the jaw and cemental content suggest an odontogenic origin.

GIANT-CELL ('REPARATIVE') GRANULOMA

Giant-cell granulomas are hyperplastic rather than neoplastic. The giant-cell tumour (osteoclastoma), by contrast, is an aggressive neoplasm which chiefly affects the limbs but virtually never the jaws.

Pathogenesis. The earlier name 'giant-cell reparative granuloma' derives from the unconvincing idea (also applied to

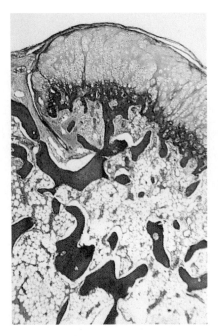

Fig. 9.6 Osteochondroma. There is a superficial cap of hyaline cartilage which undergoes endochondral ossification to form normal trabeculae of lamellar bone. The marrow spaces contain normal marrow continuous with those in the underlying bone.

solitary bone cysts) that it was a reaction to trauma which caused intramedullary haemorrhage. They are probably developmental.

Giant-cell granuloma is usually seen in young people under 20, and in females twice as frequently as males. The mandible, anterior to the first molars, where the teeth have had deciduous predecessors, is the usual site. There is frequently only a painless swelling, but growth is sometimes rapid and the mass can, rarely, erode through the bone, particularly of the alveolar ridge, to produce a purplish soft-tissue swelling (Fig. 9.7).

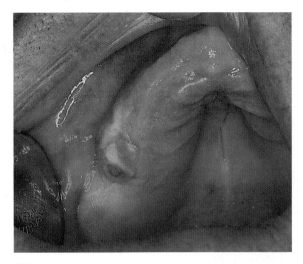

Fig. 9.7 Giant cell granuloma. This maxillary lesion has perforated the cortex and formed an ulcerated bluish soft-tissue mass on the alveolar ridge. The underlying alveolar bone is considerably expanded.

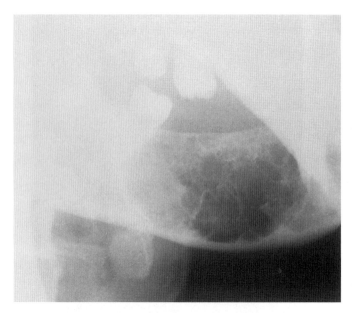

Fig. 9.8 Giant cell granuloma. Characteristic radiographic appearance of an expansile radiolucency with scalloped margins containing numerous thin internal septa of wispy bone and osteoid.

Radiographs show a rounded cyst-like radiolucent area, often faintly loculated or with a soap-bubble appearance (Fig. 9.8). Roots of teeth can be displaced or occasionally, resorbed.

Pathology and management

Giant-cell granuloma forms a lobulated mass of proliferating vascular connective tissue packed with giant cells (osteoclasts) (Figs 9.9 and 9.10). Signs of bleeding into the mass and deposits of haemosiderin are frequently seen. Fibroblastic proliferation or prominent osteoid and bone formation are common. There are no changes in blood chemistry.

Curettage of giant-cell granulomas is usually adequate and wide excision unnecessary; small fragments that may be left behind may cause little trouble, rarely require further treatment and may resolve spontaneously. Recurrence follows incomplete

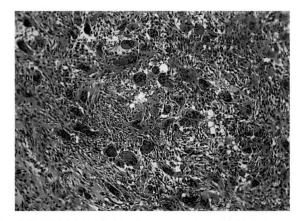

Fig. 9.9 Giant cell granuloma. The tissue is vascular and contains much extravasated blood, around which giant cells are clustered.

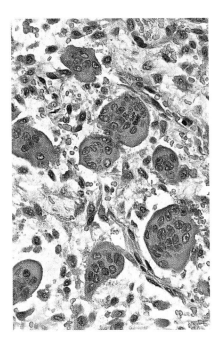

Fig. 9.10 Giant cell granuloma. High power showing the osteoclast-like giant cells with numerous, evenly dispersed nuclei.

Table 9.2 Central giant cell granuloma: key features

- Benign hyperplastic lesion of unknown aetiology
- More common in young females but seen over a wide age range
- Very expansile and may be destructive. May penetrate cortical bone and periosteum
- Solid but appears as unilocular or multilocular cyst-like radiolucency
- Forms in alveolar ridge, anterior to 6s, more frequently in the mandible but often in the maxilla
- No changes in blood chemistry
- Treated by curettage but second operation sometimes required

removal and a further limited operation may become necessary. Key features are summarised in Table 9.2.

Other giant cell lesions of the jaws

Several other jaw lesions (Table 9.3) can resemble a giant cell granuloma microscopically, and must be considered in the differential diagnosis.

HAEMANGIOMA OF BONE

Haemangiomas are rare tumours of bone, but a relatively high proportion are in the mandible, particularly in women.

Clinically, haemangiomas cause progressive painless swellings which, when the overlying bone is resorbed, may become pulsatile. Teeth may be loosened and there may be bleeding, particularly from the gingival margins involved by the tumour.

Table 9.3 Differential diagnosis of giant cell lesions of the jaws

- *Hyperparathyroidism.* Histologically indistinguishable from giant cell granuloma but serum calcium levels are raised (Ch. 10)
- *Cherubism.* May be indistinguishable from giant-cell granuloma histologically, but lesions are symmetrical, near the angles of the mandible (Ch. 10)
- *Giant-cell tumour (osteoclastoma).* Aggressive tumour of long bones. Broadly similar histologically to giant-cell granuloma but a distinct entity in terms of behaviour
- *Aneurysmal bone cysts* may contain many giant cells but consist predominantly of multiple blood-filled spaces (Ch. 10)
- *Fibrous dysplasia.* Only limited foci of giant cells. No defined margins radiographically. Growth ceases with skeletal maturity (Ch. 10)

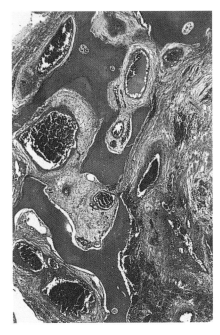

Fig. 9.11 Haemangioma of bone. The marrow spaces contain very large blood-filled sinuses with thin walls and the lesion is poorly localised and permeates between the bony trabeculae.

Radiographically there is a rounded or pseudoloculated radiolucent area with ill-defined margins or a soap-bubble appearance.

Pathology

Haemangiomas of bone are essentially similar to those in soft tissues. They are usually cavernous (Fig. 9.11), but there is also an arteriovenous type (fast-flow angioma) which has large feeder arteries, tends to expand rapidly and is likely to bleed severely if opened.

Management

A haemangioma may not be suspected if its vascularity is not obvious. Opening it or extracting a related tooth may therefore release torrents of blood, occasionally with fatal results. However, once the diagnosis has been made, wide en bloc resection is the only practical treatment. If there are identifiable feeder vessels selective arterial embolisation makes surgery considerably safer.

MELANOTIC NEUROECTODERMAL TUMOUR OF INFANCY (PROGONOMA)

This rare tumour, which arises from the neural crest, may appear in the anterior maxilla in the first few months of life. It is usually painless, and slowly expansive, but occasionally grows rapidly.

Radiograpically, there is an area of bone destruction, frequently with ragged margins, and displacement of the developing teeth (Fig. 9.12). However, the tumour is benign, though it can recur.

Pathology

There are pigmented and non-pigmented cells in a fibrous stroma. The pigmented cells have large pale nuclei and are filled with coarse melanin-containing cytoplasmic granules (Fig. 9.13). They form solid groups or line small spaces. The non-pigmented cells have large, densely hyperchromatic nuclei and form small groups, either in the stroma or in the spaces lined by the pigmented cells (Fig. 9.14).

Management

The tumour is non-encapsulated but usually separates easily from the bone at operation. Conservative treatment is usually curative but, even when excision is incomplete, recurrence is rare. Irradiation is contraindicated. Key features are summarised in Table 9.4.

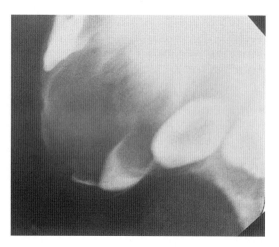

Fig. 9.12 Melanotic neuroectodermal tumour of infancy. The anterior maxilla of this neonate contains an expansile radiolucency which has displaced tooth germs and eroded the alveolar bone.

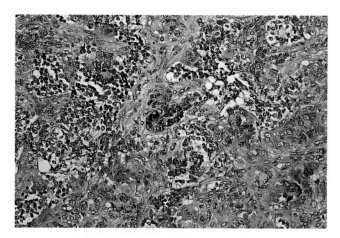

Fig. 9.13 Melanotic neuroectodermal tumour of infancy. Pale pink staining epithelial cells, some of which are pigmented (centrally), arranged in clusters and surrounded by small, round, darkly staining tumour cells.

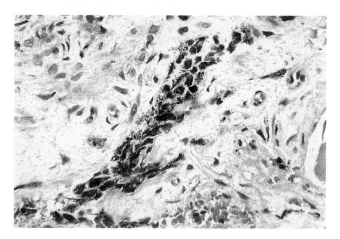

Fig. 9.14 Melanotic neuroectodermal tumour of infancy. Higher power showing the melanin pigment granules within a strand of epithelium.

Table 9.4 Melanotic neuroectodermal tumour of infancy: key features

- Very rare
- Congenital or appears in first few months
- Presents as expansion of anterior maxilla, typically bluish in colour
- Benign but destroys bone
- Responds to conservative excision or curettage

MALIGNANT NEOPLASMS OF BONE

Osteosarcoma

Osteosarcoma is highly malignant and the most common *primary* (non-odontogenic) neoplasm of bone, but overall is rare, especially in the jaws.

Osteosarcomas rarely have identifiable causes but a few develop late in life after irradiation or Paget's disease of bone, but the latter type virtually never affects jaws.

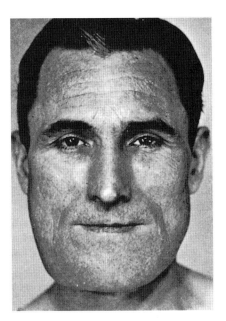
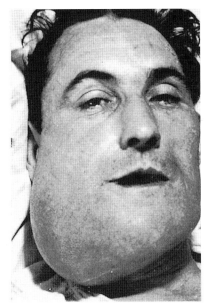

Fig. 9.15 Osteosarcoma. The pictures show the progress of the tumour over a period of 3 months. The patient died with metastases in the lungs, about a month after the second picture was taken. (Taken before the advent of colour photography.)

Osteosarcoma of the jaws is typically seen between the ages of 30 and 40. Males are slightly more frequently affected, and the body of the mandible is a common site. There is typically a firm swelling which grows noticeably in a few months and becomes painful (Fig. 9.15). Teeth may be loosened and there may be paraesthesia or loss of sensation in the mental nerve area. Metastases to the lungs may develop early.

Radiographically, appearances are variable but irregular bone destruction usually predominates over bone formation. Bone formation in a soft-tissue mass is highly characteristic (Fig. 9.16). A sun-ray appearance or Codman's triangles at the margins, due to lifting of the periosteum and new bone formation, are rarely seen and not specific to osteosarcoma. Radiographs of the chest should also be taken, as secondary deposits may be present.

Pathology

The neoplastic osteoblasts vary in size and shape, they may be small and angular or large and hyperchromatic (Fig. 9.17).

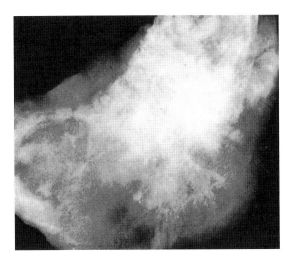

Fig. 9.16 Osteosarcoma. Radiograph of the jaw removed from the patient seen in Figure 9.15 shows the irregular bone destruction and pattern of new bone formation which replaces the normal structure.

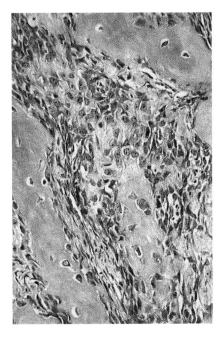

Fig. 9.17 Osteosarcoma. Trabeculae of abnormal woven bone surrounded by atypical cells in which mitoses are frequent and pleomorphism is conspicuous.

CHAPTER
9

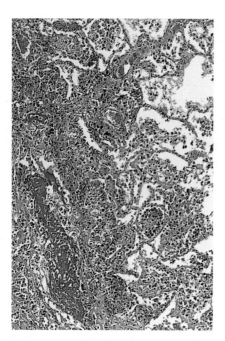

Fig. 9.18 Osteosarcoma. A post-mortem specimen of lung from the same patient shown in Figure 9.15. Malignant cells infiltrate the alveoli and are forming woven bone (left).

Mitoses may be seen, particularly in the more highly cellular areas. Giant cells may be conspicuous, but many cells are nondescript. Bone formation does not necessarily predominate and osteoid formation is the main diagnostic criterion and is seen in metastases (Fig. 9.18). Cartilage and fibrous tissue are usually also present and sometimes predominate but usually only in part of the tumour. A small biopsy may, therefore, show only a single tissue, such as cartilage, and be mistaken for a chondrosarcoma.

Key features are summarised in Table 9.5.

Table 9.5 Osteosarcoma of the jaws: key features

● Rare
● Patients' mean age is about 35
● Occasionally follows irradiation
● Usually affects the mandible
● Radiographically, bone formation is seen in a soft tissue mass
● Treated by radical surgery, sometimes with additional chemotherapy
● Slightly better prognosis than osteosarcoma of the long bones

Management

Osteosarcoma is rapidly invasive and can metastasise early. Treatment is by early mandibulectomy or maxillectomy together with wide excision of any soft-tissue extensions of the tumour. This may be combined with radiotherapy and/or chemotherapy. The prognosis depends mainly on the extent of the tumour at operation and deteriorates with spread to the soft tissues, to lymph nodes (in about 10% of cases), or to the base of the skull.

In approximately 50%, there is local recurrence within a year of treatment and a sharp deterioration in prognosis. The 5-year survival rate may range from 40% for tumours less than 5 cm in diameter to zero for tumours over 15 cm.

CHONDROMA AND CHONDROSARCOMA

The diagnosis of chondroma of the jaws should generally be avoided as most prove to be chondrosarcomas. They are rare tumours of the maxillary bones.

Histologically, chondromas consist of hyaline cartilage, but the cells are irregular in size and distribution. Calcification or ossification may develop. However, about 20% of chondrosarcomas in the maxillofacial area were originally thought to have been chondromas.

Management. Excision should include a wide margin of normal tissue, because of the difficulty in distinguishing benign from malignant tumours.

Chondrosarcoma

Chondrosarcomas of the jaws affect adults at an average age of about 45. The anterior maxilla is the site in 60% of cases.

Pain, swelling or loosening of teeth associated with a radiolucent area are typical. The radiolucency can be well or poorly circumscribed, or may appear multilocular. Calcifications are frequently present and may be widespread and dense.

Pathology

The cartilage in jaw tumours is usually comparatively well-formed or, less often, poorly differentiated or myxoid (Fig. 9.19). The chondrocytes are pleomorphic, often binucleate and may show mitotic activity (Fig. 9.20).

Maxillofacial chondrosarcomas are aggressive, and local recurrence or persistent tumour is the main cause of death. Lungs or other bones are the usual sites of distant spread but fewer than 10% of these tumours metastasise.

Chondrosarcomas must be widely excised as early as possible, but this can be difficult in the maxillofacial region. Inadequate excision usually leads to recurrences beyond the original site and deterioration of the prognosis. The response to radiotherapy is usually poor.

Mesenchymal chondrosarcoma is an uncommon but highly malignant variant. It is a highly cellular tumour in which there are only small foci of tissue recognisable as poorly-formed cartilage. It is sometimes very vascular.

EWING'S SARCOMA

Ewing's sarcoma is rare but, when it affects the head and neck region, has a predilection for the body of the mandible.

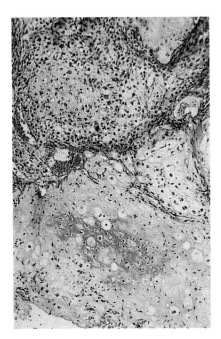

Fig. 9.19 Chondrosarcoma. Lobules of abnormal hyaline cartilage are formed in a disorganised fashion by sheets of malignant cells.

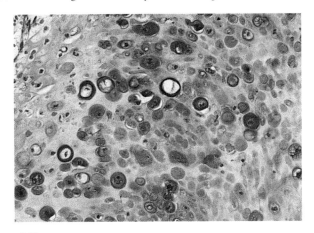

Fig. 9.20 Chondrosarcoma. Higher power of cartilage within a chondrosarcoma showing the abnormal chondrocytes and disorganised mineralisation.

Clinically, patients are usually children or young adults. Typical symptoms are bone swelling and often pain, progressing over a period of months. Teeth may loosen and the overlying mucosa ulcerate. Fever, leukocytosis, a raised ESR and anaemia may be associated and indicate a poor prognosis.

Pathology

Ewing's sarcoma cells resemble lymphocytes but are about twice their size and are of neuroectodermal origin. They have a darkly staining nucleus and a rim of cytoplasm, which is typically vacuolated and stains for glycogen. The cells form diffuse sheets or loose lobules, separated by septa. Distant spread is usually to the lungs and other bones. Lymph nodes are occasionally involved.

The initial treatment is wide excision or, if not possible, megavoltage irradiation. Combination chemotherapy should also be given and appears to have improved the survival rate but increases the risk of lymphoid tumours later.

MULTIPLE MYELOMA

Multiple myeloma is a neoplasm of plasma cells which produce a monoclonal immunoglobulin. It causes multiple foci of bone destruction, bone pain and tenderness. Rarely a jaw lesion or a complication such as oral amyloidosis may be the first symptom. Proliferation of myeloma cells in the marrow frequently causes anaemia and sometimes thrombocytopenia. Infections may result from depressed production of normal immunoglobulins. Occasionally myeloma is detected before symptoms appear, by the chance finding, in a routine examination, of a greatly raised ESR as a result of overproduction of immunoglobulin (usually IgG).

Skeletal radiographs typically show multiple punched-out areas of radiolucency, particularly in the vault of the skull.

Pathology

Myeloma appears as sheets of neoplastic plasma cells which may be well or poorly differentiated (Figs 9.21 and 9.22). Diagnosis depends on marrow biopsy and confirmation by serum electrophoresis showing a monoclonal band (Fig. 9.23). Light chain overproduction is common and leads to Bence-Jones proteinuria and often amyloidosis.

There is frequently an initial response to combination chemotherapy, but fewer than 20% of patients survive for 5 or more years. Dental treatment may be complicated by anaemia, haemorrhagic tendencies, or increased susceptibility to infection.

Intravenous bisphonates have been shown to delay the onset of lytic lesions or severe osteoporosis, and help symptom control. Thalidomide is also being investigated for its therapeutic value.

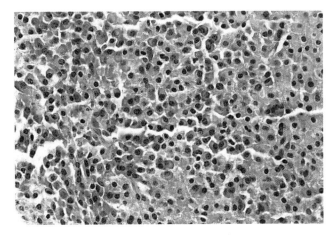

Fig. 9.21 Multiple myeloma. The lesion is composed of a uniform and dense infiltrate of neoplastic plasma cells with darker than normal staining nuclei.

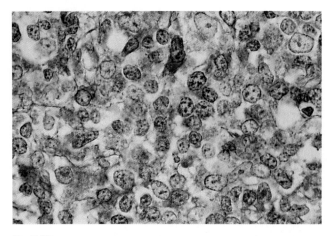

Fig. 9.22 Multiple myeloma. Immunocytochemistry for λ light chain results in a brown positive stain in all cells, indicating a monoclonal and therefore neoplastic proliferation of plasma cells.

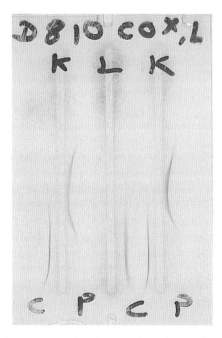

Fig. 9.23 Immunoelectrophoresis comparing patient's and control serum for their content of κ and λ light chains. The patient has a raised level of κ light chain.

SOLITARY (EXTRAMEDULLARY) PLASMACYTOMA

Approximately 80% of these rare tumours form in the soft tissues of the head and neck region. Multiple myeloma develops in up to 50% of patients within 2 years.

Solitary plasmacytoma of bone occasionally affects the jaw. Bone pain, tenderness, or a swelling and a sharply defined area of radiolucency are typical. Treatment is by radiotherapy. The prognosis is significantly better than for soft-tissue plasmacytoma. Over 65% of patients survive for 10 or more years, but the majority eventually develop multiple myeloma.

Histologically the appearances of solitary and multiple myeloma are the same. Key features are summarised in Table 9.6.

Table 9.6   Multiple myeloma: key features
• Myeloma is a malignant bone-seeking neoplasm of plasma cells
• Radiographically, punched-out lesions appear particularly in the skull
• Similar lesions may appear in the jaws
• Malignant plasma cells show varying degrees of dedifferentiation
• Monoclonal immunoglobulin (usually IgG) produced
• Anaemia, purpura or immunodeficiency may be associated
• Light chain production can lead to amyloidosis causing macroglossia in 20%
• Short-term benefit only from combination chemotherapy
• Solitary (soft tissue or intraosseous) myelomas rare but may affect maxillofacial region. They progress to multiple myeloma

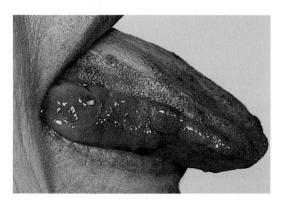

Fig. 9.24 Amyloidosis. These slightly yellow nodules on the lateral border of an enlarged tongue are characteristic of amyloidosis.

AMYLOIDOSIS

Amyloidosis is a typical product of myeloma and is the deposition in the tissues of an abnormal protein with characteristic staining properties. In over 20% of cases of overproduction of immunoglobulin light chains, amyloid is deposited in the mouth, particularly the tongue, to cause macroglossia or localised swellings or both (Figs 9.24 and 9.25) (see Ch. 14).

LANGERHANS' CELL HISTIOCYTOSIS (HISTIOCYTOSIS X)

Langerhans' cells resemble histiocytes but are dendritic, antigen-presenting cells within epithelia. They occasionally give rise to bone tumours. Three forms are recognised;

1. Solitary eosinophilic granuloma
2. Multifocal eosinophilic granuloma (including Hand–Schuller–Christian disease)
3. Letterer–Siwe syndrome.

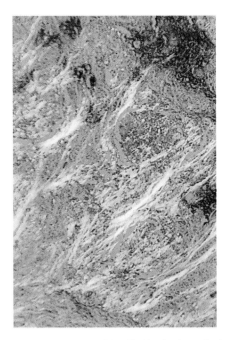

Fig. 9.25 Amyloidosis. Amyloid identified in the tissues by its green birefringence under polarised light when stained with Congo red.

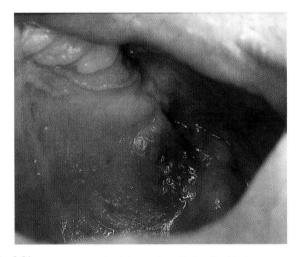

Fig. 9.26 Langerhans' cell histiocytosis. This localised lesion (eosinophilic granuloma) has produced an ulcerated mass on the maxillary alveolar ridge. The clinical appearances are non-specific.

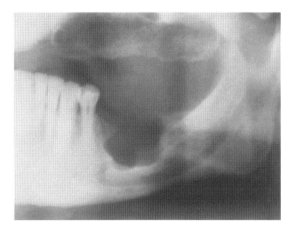

Fig. 9.27 Langerhans' cell histiocytosis. This localised lesion (eosinophilic granuloma) shows the characteristic appearance of a well-defined radiolucency scooped out of the alveolar bone. The margin is corticated in places, but less well-defined elsewhere.

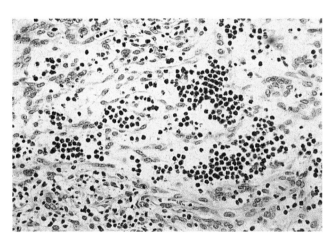

Fig. 9.28 Langerhans' cell histiocytosis. Clusters of eosinophils in a background of paler staining Langerhans' cells.

In these tumours, both the surface markers of Langerhans' cells and, by electron microscopy, characteristic Birbeck granules may be recognisable.

Solitary eosinophilic granuloma

Solitary eosinophilic granuloma of the jaw causes localised bone destruction with swelling and often pain (Fig. 9.26). Occasionally, gross periodontal destruction exposes the roots of the teeth. A rounded area of radiolucency with indistinct margins (Fig. 9.27) and an appearance of teeth 'floating in air' are typical.

Pathology. There are varying proportions of histiocyte-like Langerhans' cells and eosinophils, sometimes with other types of granulocytes (Fig. 9.28). The Langerhans' cells have pale, vesiculated and often lobulated nuclei, and weakly eosinophilic cytoplasm (Fig. 9.29). For diagnosis, positive staining of Langerhans' cells for S-100 protein and CD1a antigen electron microscopy are confirmatory.

The response to curettage is usually good and spontaneous regression is also possible.

Hand–Schuller–Christian disease

This term was given to histiocytosis causing exophthalmos, diabetes insipidus and lytic skull lesions, but this triad is present in only a minority. Usually the skull, axial skeleton and femora, and also sometimes the viscera (hepatosplenomegaly) or the skin may be involved.

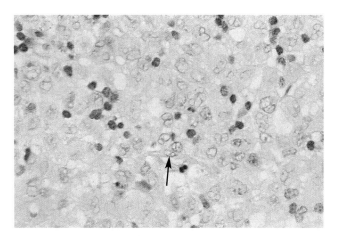

Fig. 9.29 Langerhans' cell histiocytosis. Higher power showing the pale staining Langerhans' cells with their characteristic folded, bilobed (coffee bean) nuclei.

Letterer–Siwe syndrome

This aggressive form of histiocytosis affects infants or young children. Progression to widespread disease, with involvement of skin, viscera and bones, can be rapidly fatal, despite treatment by irradiation and/or chemotherapy.

Overall, the behaviour of Langerhans' cell histiocytosis is unpredictable, but the younger the patient and the greater the number of organ systems affected, the worse the prognosis. Key features are summarised in Table 9.7.

Table 9.7   **Langerhans' cell histiocytosis: key features**
● Isolated or multifocal tumours of Langerhans' (histiocyte-like) cells
● In adults can give rise to benign chronic mass (eosinophilic granuloma)
● Eosinophilic granulomas form sharply-demarcated radiolucencies
● Alveolar bone around teeth may be destroyed (teeth floating in air appearance)
● May mimic juvenile periodontitis radiographically
● In childhood is frequently a disseminated malignant disease
● Diagnosis is by biopsy
● Solitary lesions respond to curettage or resection
● Children may require chemotherapy. Significant mortality in infants

METASTATIC TUMOURS

Carcinoma of various organs (Table 9.8) are common and the most frequent metastases reaching the jaw by the bloodstream.

Rarely a malignant deposit in the jaw causes the first symptoms and can lead to diagnosis of the primary. More often the neoplasm has been treated earlier. In either case a metastasis in the jaw is indicative of life-threatening disease. Patients are usually middle-aged or elderly.

Table 9.8   Important sites of primary tumours metastasising to the jaws
● Breast
● Bronchus
● Prostate
● Thyroid
● Kidney

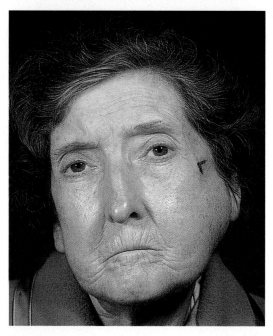

Fig. 9.30 Metastatic carcinoma of the mandible. Swelling developed in the ramus quite suddenly in this apparently fit patient. Investigations showed a deposit of poorly differentiated carcinoma in the jaw and signs of a bronchial carcinoma.

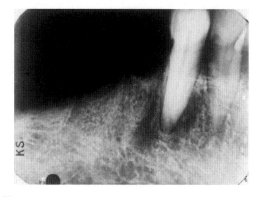

Fig. 9.31 Metastatic bronchogenic carcinoma. This small metastasis in the alveolar bone has produced a poorly-demarcated, patchy radiolucency and destroyed the lamina dura around the root apex. Such small lesions have been mistaken for periapical granulomas radiographically.

Common symptoms are pain or swelling of the jaw (Fig. 9.30), and there may be paraesthesia or anaesthesia of the lip. There is typically an area of radiolucency with a hazy outline (Figs 9.31 and 9.32). It sometimes simulates an infected cyst or

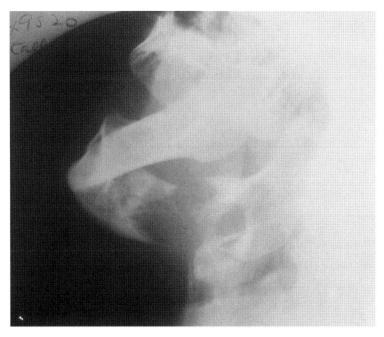

Fig. 9.32 Metastatic carcinoma in the mandible. A large and poorly defined radiolucent metastasis has destroyed most of the posterior body of the mandible, resulting in a pathological fracture.

may be quite irregular and simulate osteomyelitis. Sometimes the entire mandible may have a moth-eaten appearance. Bone sclerosis is a typical result of prostatic carcinoma.

Pathology

Secondary deposits are usually adenocarcinomas but depend on the nature of the primary growth. Osteoclastic bone destruction at the periphery of the deposit is the most common effect (Fig. 9.33). After histological confirmation of the diagnosis, a careful history, especially of previous operations, may be required.

General and blood examinations, and a skeletal survey will show the extent of the disease. The primary growth should be treated if still feasible. In most cases bony metastases imply that palliative treatment is the best that can be achieved. Irradiation may sometimes make the lesion in the jaw regress for a time and lessen pain.

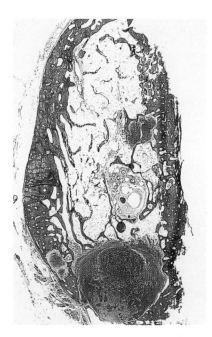

Fig. 9.33 Metastatic carcinoma in the jaw. Section across a mandible shows a deposit of carcinoma which has destroyed the cortex of the bone and is extending into the medulla.

SUGGESTED FURTHER READING

CHAPTER 9

Auclair P L, Cuenin P, Kratochvil F J, Slater L J, Ellis G L 1988 A clinical and histomorphologic comparison of the central giant cell granuloma and the giant cell tumor. Oral Surg Oral Med Oral Pathol 66:197–208

Barrera-Franco J L, Flores-Flores G, Mosquedo-Taylor A 1993 Mandibular metastasis as the first manifestation of hepatocellular carcinoma: report of a case and review of the literature. J Oral Maillofac Surg 51:318–321

Bennett J, Thomas G, Evans A W et al 2000 Osteosarcoma of the jaws: a 30-year retrospective review. Oral Surg Oral Med Oral Pathol Oral Radiol Endod 90:323–333

Bunel K, Sindet-Pedersen S 1993 Central hemangioma of the mandible. Oral Surg Oral Med Oral Pathol 75:565–570

Cawson R A, Binnie W H, Barrett A W, Wright J M 2001 *Oral disease*, 3rd Edn. Mosby-Wolfe, London

Cawson R A, Binnie W H, Barrett A W, Wright J M 1998 *Lucas's Pathology of tumors of the oral tissues*. Churchill Livingstone, Edinburgh

Cawson R A, Langdon J D, Eveson J W 1996 *Surgical pathology of the mouth and jaws*. Wright, Oxford

Dagenais M, Pharoah M J, Sikorski P A 1992 The radiographic characteristics of histiocytosis X. A study of 29 cases that involve the jaws. Oral Surg Oral Med Oral Pathol 74:230–236

Emile J-F, Wechsler J, Brousse N et al 1995 Langerhans cell histiocytosis. Definitive diagnosis with the use of monoclonal antibody O10 on routinely paraffin-embedded samples. Am J Surg Pathol 19:636–641

Epstein J B, Voss N J S, Stevenson-Moore P 1984 Maxillofacial manifestations of multiple myeloma. An unusual case and review of the literature. Oral Surg Oral Med Oral Pathol 57:267–271

Fartarsch M, Vigneswaran N, Diepgen T L, Hornstein O P 1990 Immunohistochemical and ultrastructural study of histiocytosis X and non-X histiocytoses. J Am Acad Dermatol 23:885–892

Favara B E, Jaffe R 1994 The histopathology of Langerhans' cell histiocytosis. Br J Cancer 70(Suppl. XXIII):S17–S23

Fechner R E, Mills S E 1992 Tumors of the bones and joints. *Atlas of tumor pathology*. Third series. Fascicle 8. Armed Forces Institute of Pathology, Washington DC

Flick W G, Lawrence F R Oral amyloidosis as initial symptom of multiple myeloma. Oral Surg Oral Med Oral Pathol 49:18–20

Furutani M, Ohnishi M, Tanaka Y 1994 Mandibular involvement in patients with multiple myeloma. J Oral Maxillofac Surg 52:23–25

Garrington G E, Collett W K 1988 Chondrosarcoma. I. A selected literature review. J Oral Pathol 17:1–11

Garrington G E, Scofield H H, Cornyn J, Hooker S P 1967 Osteosarcoma of the jaws. Analysis of 56 cases. Cancer 20:377–391

Garrington G E, Collett W K 1988 Chondrosarcoma. II. Chondrosarcoma of the jaws: analysis of 37 cases. J Oral Pathol 17:12–20

Hackney F L, Aragon S B, Aufdemorte T B, Holt R G, Sickels J E V 1991 Chondrosarcoma of the jaws: clinical findings, histopathology and treatment. Oral Surg Oral Pathol Oral Med 71:139–143

Harris M 1993 Central giant cell granulomas regress with calcitonin therapy. Br J Oral Maxillofac Surg 31:89–94

Thongngarm T, Lynch C, McMurray R W 2000 Primary non-Hodgkin's lymphoma of bone. J Rheumatol 27:2923-2924

Hartman K S 1980 Histiocytosis X. A review of 114 cases with oral involvement. Oral Surg Oral Med Oral Pathol 49:38–54

Hawkins P N 1994 Amyloidosis. Medicine Int 22:76–82

Henry C H, Granite E L, Rafetto L K 1992 Osteochondroma of the mandibular condyle: report of a case and review of the literature. J Oral Maxillofac Surg 50:1102–1108

Hirshberg A, Leibovich P, Buchner A 1994 Metastatic tumors to the jaw bones: analysis of 390 cases. J Oral Pathol Med 23:337–341

Kanazawa H, Shoji A, Yokoe H, Midorikawa S, Takamiya Y 1993 Solitary plasmacytoma of the mandible, Case report and review of the literature. J Cranio Max Fac Surg 21:202–206

Kilpatrick S E, Wenger D E, Gilchrist G S, Shives T C, Woolan P C 1995 Langerhans' cell histiocytosis (Histiocytosis X) of bone. A clinicopathologic analysis of 263 pediatric and adult cases. Cancer 76:2471–2484

Kyle R A 2000 The role of bisphosphonates in multiple myeloma. Ann Intern Med 132:734–736

Lambertenghi-Delilliers G, Bruno E, Cortelezzi A, Fumagalli L, Morosini A 1988 Incidence of jaw lesions in 193 patients with multiple myeloma. Oral Surg Oral Med Oral Pathol 65:533–537

Lieberman P H, Jones C R, Steinman R M et al 1996 Langerhans' cell (eosinophilic) granulomatosis. A clinicopathologic study encompassing 50 years. Am J Surg Pathol 20:519–552

Lucas D R, Unni K K, McLeod R A, O'Connor M I, Sim F H 1994 Osteoblastoma: a clinicopathologic study of 306 cases. Hum Pathol 25:117–134

Millar B G, Browne R M, Flood T R 1990 Juxtacortical osteosarcoma of the jaws. Br J Oral Maxillofac Surg 28:73–79

Mintz G A, Abrams A M, Carlsen G D, Melrose R J, Fister H W 1981 Primary malignant giant cell tumor of the mandible. Report of a case. Oral Surg Oral Med Oral Pathol 51:164–171

Mosby E L, Lowe M W, Cobb C M, Ennis R L 1992 Melanotic neuroectodermal tumor of infancy: review of the literature and report of a case. J Oral Maxillofac Surg 50:886–894

Ormiston I W, Piette E, Tideman H, Wu P C 1994 Chondrosarcoma of the mandible presenting as periodontal lesions: report of 2 cases. J Cranio Max Fac Surg 22:231–235

Regezi J A, Zarbo R J, McClatchey K D, Courtney R M, Crissman J D 1987 Osteosarcomas and chondrosarcomas of the jaws: immunohistochemical correlations. Oral Surg Oral Med Oral Pathol 64:302–307

Reinish E I, Raviv M, Srolovitz H, Gornitsky M 1994 Tongue, primary amyloidosis and multiple myeloma. Oral Surg Oral Med Oral Pathol 77:121–125

Whitaker S B, Waldron C A 1993 Central giant cell lesions of the jaws. A clinical, radiologic and histopathologic study. Oral Surg Oral Med Oral Pathol 75:199–208

Willman C L, Busque L, Griffith B B, Favara B E, McClain K L, Duncan M H et al 1994 Langerhans'-cell histiocytosis (histiocytosis X) — a clonal proliferative disease. N Engl J Med 331:154–160

Wood R E, Nortje C J, Hesseling P, Grotepass F 1990 Ewing's tumor of the jaw. Oral Surg Oral Med Oral Pathol 69:120–127

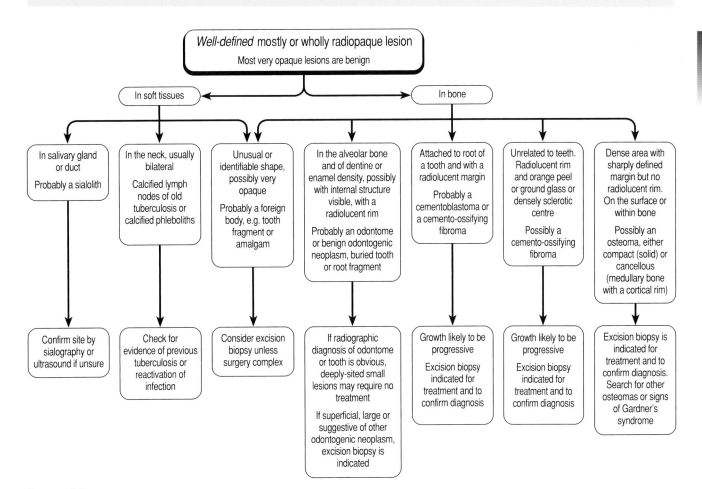

Summary 9.1 Differential diagnosis of a well-defined radio-opaque lesion in the jaws.

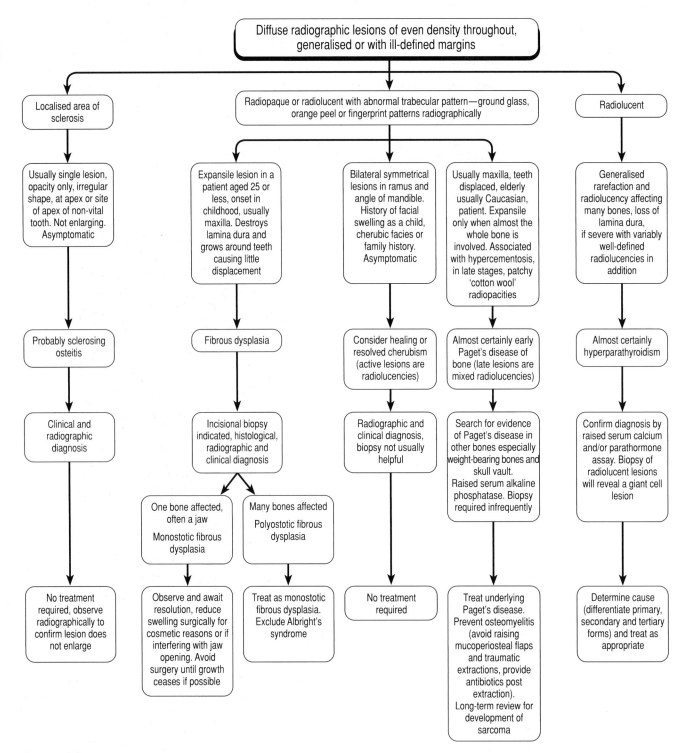

Summary 9.2 Differential diagnosis of an ill-defined or diffuse radiographic lesion in the jaws.

Genetic, metabolic and other non-neoplastic bone diseases

GENETIC DISEASES OF BONE

Osteogenesis imperfecta (brittle bone syndrome)

The term *brittle bone syndrome* should not be confused with the considerably more common disease of osteoporosis which is frequently termed *brittle bone disease*. In osteogenesis imperfecta, which is usually transmitted as an autosomal dominant trait, the bones are excessively fragile. Defects in genes for procollagen alpha helix prevent polymerisation into normal collagen and its mineralisation. As a result, biosynthesis of type I collagen is defective, so that osteoblasts fail to form bone in adequate amounts, leading to fractures and abnormal dentine (Fig. 10.1).

The bones are thin and lack the usual cortex of compact bone but development of epiphyseal cartilages is unimpaired so that

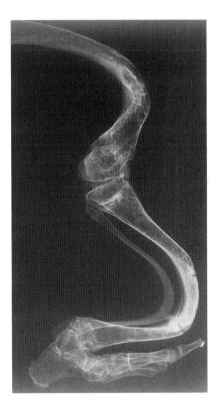

Fig. 10.2 Osteogenesis imperfecta. Leg of an infant with a severe type of osteogenesis imperfecta showing severe bending as a result of multiple fractures under body weight.

bones can grow to their normal length. Nevertheless, they may become so distorted by multiple fractures as to cause dwarfism. The most severe cases (Type II) usually die at birth or soon after: mild cases (Type V) may have little disability. In the more common form (Type I), the many fractures can cause severe deformities (Figs 10.2 and 10.3). The sclera of the eyes may also appear blue (their thinness allows the pigment layer to show through), deafness also develops. Obvious dentinogenesis imperfecta is sometimes associated but all patients have some degree of abnormality of the dentine (Ch. 2).

There is no effective treatment but it is essential to protect the child from even minor injuries and to minimise deformity by attending to fractures. Care must be taken during dental extractions, but fractures of the jaws are uncommon in this disease.

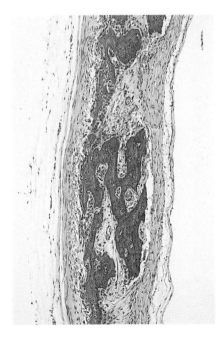

Fig. 10.1 Osteogenesis imperfecta. A section from the vault of the skull of a stillborn infant with type III disease; the most severe form of osteogenesis imperfecta shows that the bone is small in amount, primitive (woven) in character and shows no attempt at differentiation into cortical plates and medullary space.

153

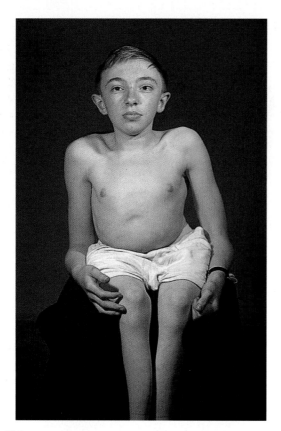

Fig. 10.3 Clinical appearance of a severely affected child with osteogenesis imperfecta type III in which there is progressive deformity.

Key features are summarised in Table 10.1.

Table 10.1 Osteogenesis imperfecta: key features
● Thin fragile bones due to inadequate type I collagen formation ● Usually inherited as an autosomal dominant trait ● Multiple fractures typically lead to gross deformities ● Variable degrees of dentinogenesis imperfecta associated ● Jaw fractures are uncommon

Osteopetrosis — marble bone disease

Osteopetrosis is a rare genetic disease in which the bones become solidified and dense (Fig. 10.4) but brittle. There is inactivity of osteoclasts and absence of normal modelling resorption. Medullary spaces are minute (Fig. 10.5), and the epipyseal ends of the bones are club-shaped. In the skull there may be compression of cranial nerve canals and deficits or pain can result. Because of the deficiency of marrow space, the liver and spleen take on blood-cell formation, but anaemia is common. Osteomyelitis is a recognised complication and prevention of dental infections is important. There is no effective treatment apart from marrow transplantation. Key features are summarised in Table 10.2.

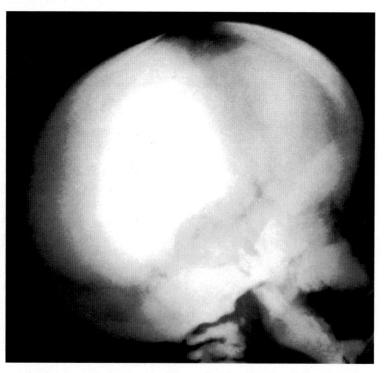

Fig. 10.4 Osteopetrosis. In contrast to osteogenesis imperfecta the bone is excessively thick and dense as a result of defective resorption.

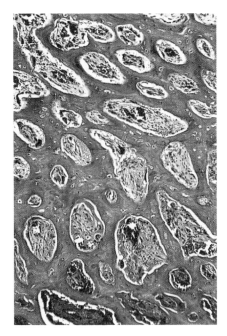

Fig. 10.5 Osteopetrosis. Almost solid bone with only small lacunae has replaced the medullary space.

Table 10.2 **Osteopetrosis: key features**

- Rare genetic defect of osteoclastic activity
- Bones lack medullary cavities but are fragile
- Extramedullary haemopoiesis in liver and spleen but anemia common
- Osteomyelitis a recognised complication
- Bone marrow transplantation offers the main hope

Achondroplasia

Achondroplasia is the most common type of genetic skeletal disorder and manifests itself as short-limbed dwarfs who traditionally became circus clowns. The essential defect is failure of normal cartilage proliferation in the epiphyses and base of the skull. The limbs are therefore excessively short in relation to the trunk, while the head, which is normal in size, appears disproportionately large. Defective growth at the base of the skull causes the middle third of the face to be retrusive and the profile to be concave. The mandible is often protrusive, and as a result of the disparity of growth of the jaws, there is usually severe malocclusion. There is no effective treatment, but the occlusion may be improved by orthodontic treatment.

Key features are summarised in Table 10.3.

Table 10.3 **Achondroplasia: key features**

- A common type of genetic dwarfism
- Failure of proliferation of cartilage in epiphyses and base of skull
- Short limbs but normal sized skull
- Middle third of face retrusive due to deficient growth of skull base
- Malocclusion may need correction

Cleidocranial dysplasia

In this rare familial disorder there is defective formation of the clavicles, delayed closure of fontanelles and sometimes retrusion of the maxilla. Partial or complete absence of clavicles allows the patient to bring the shoulders together in front of the chest (Fig. 10.6). This disorder is one of the few recognisable causes of delayed eruption of the permanent dentition. Many permanent teeth may remain embedded in the jaw (Fig. 10.7) and frequently become enveloped in dentigerous cysts (Ch. 7). Key features are summarised in Table 10.4.

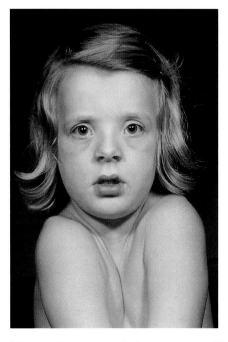

Fig. 10.6 Cleidocranial dysplasia. Defective development of the clavicles allows this abnormal mobility of the shoulders. Other members of the family were also affected.

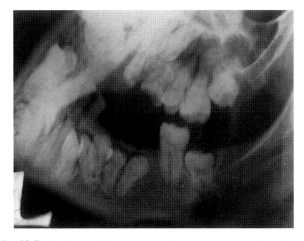

Fig. 10.7 Cleidocranial dysplasia. A radiograph of the jaw of the father of the patient in Figure 10.6. There are many additional teeth but widespread failure of eruption.

Table 10.4 Cleidocranial dysplasia: key features

- Rare genetic disorder causing defective formation of clavicles, delayed closure of fontanelles and other defects
- Many or most permanent teeth typically remain embedded in the jaw
- Many additional unerupted teeth also present
- Sometimes many dentigerous cysts

Cherubism

Cherubism is inherited as an autosomal dominant trait, but as a result of weaker penetrance of the trait in females, the phenotype is approximately twice as common in males. The gene for cherubism maps to chromosome 4p16.3. Like other genetic diseases, many non-familial cases are seen as a result of new mutations. Usually, only isolated cases are encountered, but a family with no fewer than 20 affected members has been reported. The disorder may be seen almost worldwide, but appears to be rare in Japan.

The onset is typically between the ages of 6 months to 7 years, but rarely is delayed until late teenage or after puberty. Typically, symmetrical swellings are noticed at the age of 2 to 4 years in the region of the angles of the mandibles and, in severe cases, in the maxillae. The symmetrical mandibular swellings give the face an excessively chubby appearance (Fig. 10.8). The alveolar ridges are expanded and the mandibular swellings may sometimes be so gross lingually as to interfere with speech, swallowing or even breathing, but the rapidity of progress is variable. Teeth are frequently displaced and may be loosened.

Maxillary involvement is usually associated with widespread mandibular disease and is uncommon. Extensive maxillary lesions cause the eyes to appear to be turned heavenward; this together with the plumpness of the face, is the reason for these patients being likened to cherubs. The appearance of the eyes is due to such factors as the maxillary masses pushing the floors of the orbits and eyes upwards and also exposing the sclera below the pupils. Expansion of the maxillae may also cause stretching of the skin and some retraction of the lower lids. Rarely, destruction of the infra-orbital ridges weakens support for the lower lid. Maxillary involvement can also cause the palate to assume an inverted V shape.

Despite lack of inflammation, there is frequently cervical lymphadenopathy, due to reactive hyperplasia and fibrosis. This is typically seen in the early stages and may completely subside by puberty.

Radiographic changes may be seen considerably earlier than clinical signs, and are usually more extensive than the clinical swelling. The angles of the mandible are particularly involved but the process extends towards the coronoid notch and sometimes also forwards along the body (Fig. 10.9). The lesions simulate multilocular cysts as a result of fine bony septa extending between the soft tissue masses. Panoramic radiographs help to determine the extent of the disease but it is more clearly visualised by CT scanning.

Maxillary involvement is shown by diffuse rarefaction of the bone, but spread of lesions can cause opacity of the sinuses. A distinctive radiographic sign is exposure of the posterior part of the hard palate in lateral skull films, as a result of forward displacement of the teeth. Even after complete clinical resolution of the facial swelling, bone defects may persist radiographically. Growth is rapid for a few years, then slows down until puberty is reached. There is then slow regression until, by adulthood, normal facial contour is typically completely restored. However, radiolucent areas may persist longer.

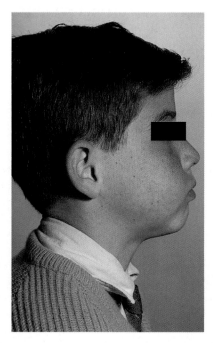

Fig. 10.8 Cherubism. The typical 'cherubic' bulging of the cheeks can be seen.

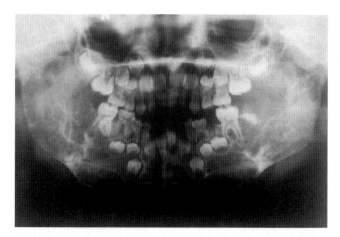

Fig. 10.9 Cherubism. Both rami, much of the body of the mandible and the posterior maxillae are expanded by multilocular radiolucent lesions which have displaced and destroyed developing teeth.

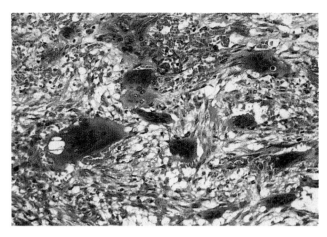

Fig. 10.10 Cherubism. An early lesion showing multinucleate giant cells lying in haemorrhagic oedematous fibrous tissue. The appearances are indistinguishable histologically from giant cell granuloma.

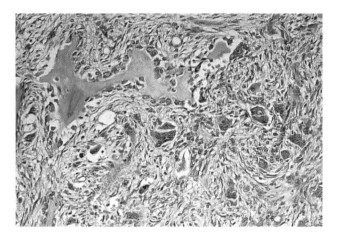

Fig. 10.11 Cherubism. In a late lesion there is formation of woven bone by the fibrous tissue and giant cells are less numerous. Eventually bone remodelling will restore the contour and quality of the bone.

Pathology

The lesions consist of multinucleated giant cells (Fig. 10.10) and resemble giant cell granulomas or hyperparathyroidism. With the passage of time, giant cells become fewer and there is bony repair of the defect (Fig. 10.11).

Management

Because of natural regression of the disease, treatment can usually be avoided. If disfigurement is severe the lesions respond to curettage or to paring down of excessive tissue but, in the early stages particularly, will recur.

Key features are summarised in Table 10.5.

Hypophosphatasia

Hypophosphatasia is an uncommon recessive genetic disorder. The early-onset type causes rickets-like skeletal disease with defective mineralisation. Defective cementogenesis results in

Table 10.5 Cherubism: key features
● Inherited as autosomal dominant trait
● Jaw swellings appear in infancy
● Angle regions of mandible affected symmetrically giving typical chubby face
● Symmetrical involvement of maxillae also in more severe cases
● Radiographically, lesions appear as multilocular cyst-like areas
● Histologically, lesions consist of giant cells in vascular connective tissue
● Lesions regress with skeletal maturation and normal facial contour restored

premature loss of teeth, and this is sometimes the only sign of the disease (see Fig. 2.28). Plasma alkaline phosphatase levels are low but urinary phosphoethanolamine excretion is raised. Late-onset hypophosphatasia is sometimes a dominant trait, and its main manifestation is fragility of the bones.

Sickle cell anaemia and thalassaemia major

Bone changes are uncommon but when severe, these diseases (Ch. 25), particularly thalassaemia, can cause bony malformations of the maxillofacial region. In particular, expanded erythropoiesis causes thickening but osteoporosis of the bones of the skull. In sickle cell anaemia infarcts in the jaws are painful. Symptomatically and radiographically they can mimic osteomyelitis. Bone infarcts may appear relatively radiolucent at first, but become sclerotic, and opaque areas in the skull or jaws are left by earlier infarcts.

In thalassaemia the diploic spaces of the skull are enlarged due to marrow expansion and have a hair-on-end appearance radiographically and a thin cortex. The maxillae may also be expanded causing severe malocclusion. The zygomatic bones are pushed outwards and the nasal bridge depressed in severe cases.

METABOLIC BONE DISEASE

Rickets

Vitamin D is essential for the absorption and metabolism of calcium and phosphorus. Deficiency during the period of bone development causes rickets with defective calcification and development of the skeleton, but rarely of the teeth (Ch. 30).

Defective calcium and phosphorus metabolism may also result from chronic renal disease (either hereditary or inflammatory) causing abnormal excretion of these minerals. Defective development of bone (renal rickets) can result.

The onset of rickets is usually in infancy. The main defects are broadening of the growing ends of bones and prominent costochondral junctions due to the epiphyseal defects (Fig. 10.12). The weakened bones bend readily. Typical changes in the skulls are wide fontanelles, bossing of the frontal and

157

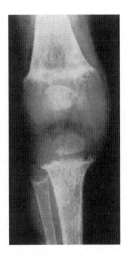

Fig. 10.12 Rickets. Overgrowth of cartilage (as shown in the section in Figure 10.13) causes the epiphyseal plate to be broad, thick and irregular, and the ends of the bone become splayed. The growing end of the bone is ill-defined and calcification defective.

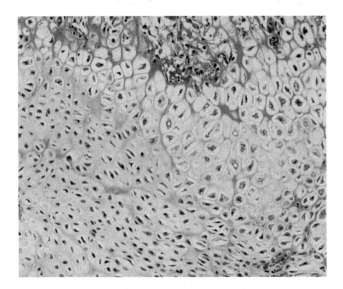

Fig. 10.13 Rickets. Microscopically the epiphyseal plate has become disorganised with loss of the well-drilled lines of chondrocytes. There is also fibrous proliferation, but no calcification.

parietal eminences and thinning of the back of the skull. Radiographs show the wide, thick epiphyses and deformities (Fig. 10.13). There are usually normal serum calcium but low phosphorus levels, or either may be depressed. The alkaline phosphatase level is raised.

Pathology

Throughout the bone, but especially at the ends of the shafts, trabeculae become surrounded by newly formed, uncalcified osteoid matrix. In the zone of provisional calcification, mineralisation of cartilage fails, and the cartilage cells continue to proliferate until the epiphyseal plate becomes greatly thickened, wide and highly cellular. Blood vessels invade and

branch irregularly among the proliferating cartilage cells. They are accompanied by connective tissue which further disorganises the epiphysis.

Dental changes. Teeth have a priority over the skeleton for minerals, and dental defects rarely result from rickets. Hypo-calcification of dentine, with a wide band of predentine and excessive interglobular spaces, may be seen in unusually severe rickets. Eruption of teeth may also be delayed. Rachitic children are not abnormally susceptible to dental caries, and 'shortage of calcium' as a cause of dental caries is a myth.

Treatment

Vitamin D, the equivalent of 2000 to 3000 i.u. daily, should be given. The diet should also be adequate in other components. Orthopaedic treatment may be needed to correct deformities.

Scurvy

Scurvy, caused by vitamin C deficiency, leads to defective formation of collagen and osteoid matrix; such matrix as forms is well calcified. Infantile scurvy, with skeletal defects, is largely of historical interest in Britain but has been described, for instance, in an infant whose mother had eccentric ideas about diet. A case with gingival bleeding was described in 2000.

The amount of osteoid matrix formed is small but highly calcified so that the ends of the long bones are sharply defined radiologically. Weakness of the connective tissue and the hae-morrhagic tendency (purpura) cause detachment of the periosteum by bleeding and bone pain. The haematoma becomes calcified as shown in the radiograph (Fig. 10.14).

Severe scurvy also causes swollen, bleeding gingivae (Ch. 5) and early tooth loss (see Ch. 30).

Hyperparathyroidism

Primary hyperparathyroidism is usually caused by hyperplasia or adenoma of the parathyroids but is uncommon. Over-production of parathormone (PTH) mobilises calcium and raises the plasma calcium level.

Post-menopausal women are mainly affected. The major symptoms result from renal damage which leads to hyper-tension or other cardiovascular disease. Peptic ulcer symptoms or mere malaise are also common. Bone disease is rarely seen now, because of earlier treatment, but small lesions may be detectable radiographically. Among dental patients a cyst-like swelling of the jaw with the histological features of a giant-cell lesion is the classical way by which hyperparathyroidism has been detected, but is rare. It is essential not to miss this diag-nosis, because of the risk of irreversible renal damage in the absence of treatment. The possibility of secondary hyperpara-thyroidism (see below) should also be excluded.

Radiographically, the main effects are thinning of bone trabeculae, subperiosteal resorption of the bone of the fingers

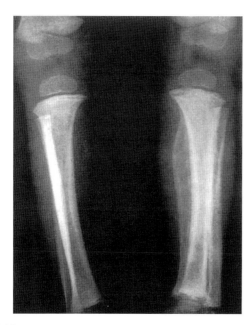

Fig. 10.14 Scurvy. In contrast to rickets, calcification is unimpeded and there is a thick layer of calcified cartilage at the end of the bone. Osteoid formation, on the other hand, is poor, so that little bone can be formed. The attachment of the periosteum to the bone is weak, so that it is easily separated; haemorrhage beneath it (as here) is due to scorbutic purpura, and this becomes calcified.

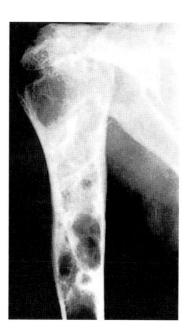

Fig. 10.16 Hyperparathyroidism. Osteitis fibrosa cystica in the humerus of the same patient with a parathyroid adenoma. Note also the loss of trabecular pattern and cortex.

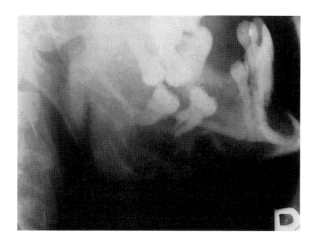

Fig. 10.15 Hyperparathyroidism. A patient of 51 with hyperparathyroidism as a result of a parathyroid adenoma. There is an area of bone destruction simulating a multilocular cyst.

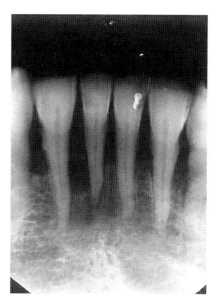

Fig. 10.17 Hyperparathyroidism. A periapical view reveals the relative radiolucency of the bone. There is loss of lamina dura around the roots, loss of trabeculae centrally and coarsening of the trabecular pattern elsewhere.

and resorption of the terminal phalangeal tufts. In severe disease, radiolucent cyst-like areas (osteitis fibrosa cystica) often with a multiloculated appearance are a typical but rare finding (Figs 10.15 and 10.16). Alveolar bone may also be resorbed but re-forms with treatment (Figs 10.17 and 10.18).

Pathology

Histologically, the cyst-like areas are foci of osteoclasts in a highly vascular stroma (Fig. 10.19). Extensive haemosiderin deposits cause the lesion to appear as a brown tumour.

These foci are indistinguishable from giant-cell granulomas of the jaws. Unlike the latter, there are characteristic changes in blood chemistry (Table 10.6) and sometimes multifocal involvement of other bones. Occasionally, bone lesions cause pathological fractures. The increased excretion of calcium leads ultimately to renal calcinosis or stone formation and renal damage. Other clinical features also result from the hyper-calcaemia. Blood chemistry examination is essential in patients

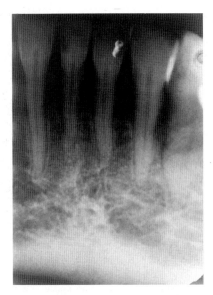

Fig. 10.18 Hyperparathyroidism. The same patient after treatment shows improved bone density and reformation of the lamina dura and cortex.

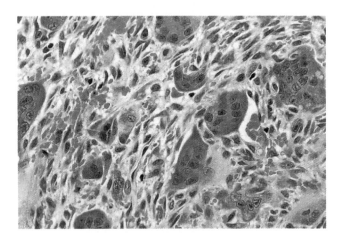

Fig. 10.19 Hyperparathyroidism. Multinucleate osteoclast-like giant cells are lying in a haemorrhagic fibrous tissue. The appearances are indistinguishable from giant cell granuloma histologically.

Table 10.6 Biochemical findings in primary hyperparathyroidism

- Raised plasma calcium (2.8 mmol/l or more)
- Low plasma phosphorus (less than 0.8 mmol/l)
- Raised plasma parathyroid hormone levels
- Raised plasma alkaline phosphatase (over 100 IU/l)

found to have giant-cell lesions of the jaws, especially adults of middle age or over.

Secondary hyperparathyroidism results from prolonged stimulation of the parathyroids by a persistently depressed plasma calcium. The most common cause is chronic renal failure.

Secondary hyperparathyroidism is now a more frequent cause of osteolytic bone lesions than primary but shows the

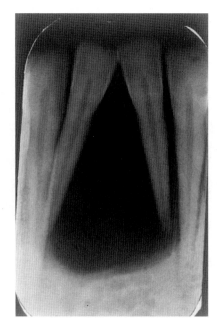

Fig. 10.20 Hyperparathyroidism. In this patient with hyperparathyroidism as a result of rejection of a kidney graft there is a well-defined area of bone loss.

same histological picture of osteoclastic proliferation. Such lesions may also be a sign of rejection of a renal transplant (Fig. 10.20).

Hyperparathyroidism is also present in 95% of patients with type 1 multiple endocrine adenoma (MEN 1) syndrome as discussed in Chapter 31.

Management

In primary hyperparathyroidism, surgical removal of the parathyroids is curative. For secondary hyperparathyroidism the renal failure should be treated if possible. Bone lesions may respond to oral administration of vitamin D, whose metabolism is abnormal as a result of the renal disease. If hypercalcaemia is of very long-standing, parathyroid hyperplasia may be irreversible (so called tertiary hyperparathyroidism) and need to be treated by parathyroidectomy.

Key features are summarised in Table 10.7.

Table 10.7 Hyperparathyroidism: key features

- Overproduction of parathyroid hormone due to hyperplasia or adenoma of parathyroid glands leads to mobilisation of bone calcium
- Significant bone disease now uncommon
- Common effects are malaise, hypertension, or peptic ulcer
- Jaw lesions are rare, but appear radiographically as multilocular cyst-like areas sometimes with multifocal involvement of other bones
- Histologically, bone lesions consist of vascular foci of giant cells, indistinguishable from giant cell granulomas
- Diagnosis confirmed by raised serum calcium, parathyroid hormone and alkaline phosphatase but low serum phosphorus

Gigantism and acromegaly

Overproduction of pituitary growth hormone, usually by an adenoma, before the epiphyses fuse, gives rise to *gigantism* with overgrowth of the whole skeleton. After fusion of the eiphyses, overproduction of growth hormone gives rise to *acromegaly*. The main features are continued growth at the mandibular condyle, causing gross prognathism, macroglossia, thickening of the facial soft tissues and overgrowth of the hands and feet (see Ch. 31).

Fluorosis

Excessive amounts of fluorides in the drinking water, as in certain parts of Northern India, cause severe mottling of the teeth and also sclerosis of the skeleton. The intervertebral ligaments and muscle insertions calcify, causing stiffness (particularly of the back) and pain. Histologically the bone changes are somewhat similar to those of Paget's disease.

BONE DISEASES OF UNKNOWN CAUSE

Paget's disease of bone (osteitis deformans)

Paget's disease causes bone distortion and weakening, particularly in the elderly. Patients past middle age are affected most severely. In Britain, up to 3% of people over 40 may have radiographic signs of Paget's disease, but clinical disease is less common. The cause is unknown but intranuclear inclusions compatible with a paramyxo- or other virus have been demonstrated in both osteoblasts and osteoclasts. A genetic factor may also be involved.

Bones most frequently affected are sacrum, spine, skull, femora and pelvis. The disease may be widespread and is usually symmetrical, but sometimes a single bone is affected. In the uncommon severe form, the main features are an enlarged head, thickening of long bones, which bend under stress, and tenderness or aching pain which can be severe and almost intractable. The vault of the skull is more often affected than the facial skeleton, and the maxilla considerably more frequently than the mandible (Fig. 10.21). Narrowing of foramina can occasionally cause cranial nerve deficits.

When the jaws are affected the alveolar process becomes symmetrically and grossly enlarged (Figs 10.22 and 10.23). There may also be gross and irregular hypercementosis of teeth, which may become fused to sclerotic areas of the bone. Attempts to extract affected teeth may succeed only by tearing away a large mass of bone. Severe bleeding or osteomyelitis of ischaemic bone may follow.

The main radiographic features are lower density of the bone in the early stages and sclerosis in the later stages. Changes are patchily distributed and loss of normal trabeculation causes the bone to have a characteristic cotton-wool appearance.

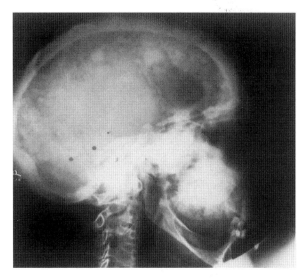

Fig. 10.21 Paget's disease of the skull and maxilla. The thickening of the bone and the irregular areas of sclerosis and resorption, which give it a fluffy appearance, are in striking contrast to the unaffected mandible.

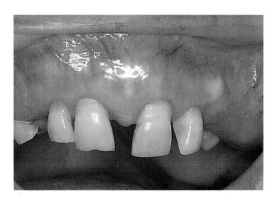

Fig. 10.22 Paget's disease of bone. Characteristic features of the involved maxilla are the broadening and deepening of the alveolar process, generalised enlargement and spacing of the teeth.

Pathology

Bone resorption and replacement becomes rapid, irregular, exaggerated and purposeless. The changes progress erratically but the ultimate result is thickening of affected bones without localised swellings.

In the early stages there is typically resorption which is later followed by sclerosis, but since closely adjacent parts of the bone may show different stages of the disease, a common result is patchy area of osteoporosis and of sclerosis

Destruction and new bone formation may alternate rapidly, and the change in bony activity is marked histologically by blue-staining reversal lines. Their irregular pattern characteristically produces a jigsaw puzzle ('mosaic'*) appearance in the bone (Figs 10.24 and 10.25).

*The traditional description of a 'mosaic' pattern to the reversal lines in Paget's disease seems particularly inept. Mosaics are composed of tiny, regular cubes of ceramics.

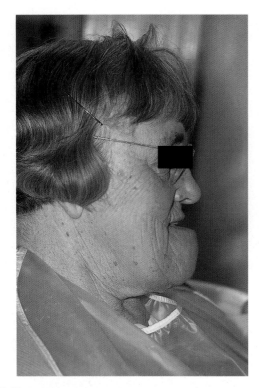

Fig. 10.23 Paget's disease. A rare example of severe mandibular involvement.

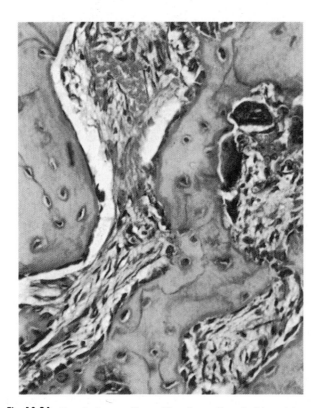

Fig. 10.24 Paget's disease of bone. There is a well-marked 'mosaic' pattern of the bone due to repeated alternation of resorption and apposition. The marrow has been replaced by fibrous tissue and there are many osteoblasts and osteoclasts lining the surface of the bone.

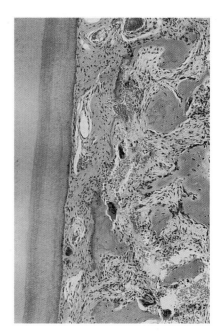

Fig. 10.25 Paget's disease affecting the jaw results in destruction of the lamina dura surrounding the teeth and, at a later stage, causes hypercementosis and sometimes ankylosis.

The main histological changes are the irregular pattern of reversal lines, many osteoblasts and osteoclasts (often abnormally large), fibrosis of the marrow spaces and increased vascularity. In the late stages, affected bones are thick, the cortex and medulla are obliterated and the whole bone is spongy in texture.

Serum calcium and phosphorus levels are usually normal, but the alkaline phosphatase level is particularly high and may reach 700 iu/l. The development of osteosarcoma is a recognised but rare complication of Paget's disease and virtually never affects the jaws. Many patients live to an advanced age in spite of their disabilities.

Treatment is with calcitonin or bisphosphonates, or both. Calcitonins, such as salcatonin, have to be given by injection and are more effective for reducing bone pain and osteolysis, but can cause nausea and an unpleasant taste. Calcitonin is also given preoperatively to reduce bleeding from the highly vascular bone and may help to relieve cranial nerve deficits. Bisphosphonates (such as sodium etidronate) can be given orally and depress bone turnover by slowing both the dissolution and growth of hydroxyapatite crystals.

Key features are summarised in Table 10.8.

Fibro-osseous lesions

This term is used for disorders ranging from fibrous dysplasia to the circumscribed lesions of cemento-ossifying fibroma and the cemental dysplasias (Table 10.9), because they share histological features. Cherubism is sometimes included but has been described earlier. Behaviour varies but growth in early life with spontaneous arrest and increasing ossification, roughly

Table 10.8   Paget's disease: key features

- Persons past middle age affected
- Common radiographic finding. Less common as clinical disease
- Enlargement of skull, thickening but weakness of long bones and bone pain are typical of severe disease
- Maxilla occasionally, but mandible rarely affected
- Teeth may show gross irregular hypercementosis
- Radiographically, patchy sclerosis and resorption give a cottonwool appearance
- Histologically, irregular resorption and apposition leaves jigsaw puzzle ('mosaic') pattern of reversal lines
- Serum alkaline phosphatase up to 700 u/l

Table 10.9   Fibro-osseous lesions

- Fibrous dysplasia
  Monostotic
  Polyostotic
- Cemento-osseous dysplasias (Ch. 8)
  Periapical cemental dysplasia
  Focal cemento-osseous dysplasia
  Florid cemento-osseous dysplasia
- Fibro-osseous neoplasms
  Cemento-ossifying fibroma (Ch. 8)

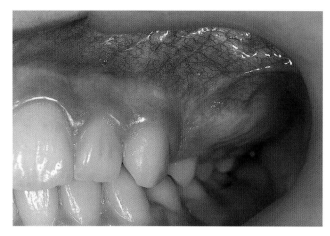

Fig. 10.26 Fibrous dysplasia. Typical presentation with a poorly-defined, rounded expansion of the maxilla with displacement of teeth and intact overlying mucosa.

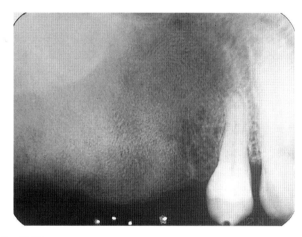

Fig. 10.27 Fibrous dysplasia. This is a well-established lesion with a rounded swelling which merges imperceptibly with normal bone surrounding the canine. There is loss of lamina dura and cortex in the affected area and the fine trabecular pattern produces an orange-peel or thumb-print appearance.

coinciding with skeletal maturation is typical of non-neoplastic fibro-osseous lesions. Because of their histological similarities, the diagnosis depends greatly on the clinical and radiographic findings.

Fibrous dysplasia

Monostotic fibrous dysplasia gives rise to a bony swelling caused by a poorly circumscribed area of fibro-osseous proliferation. This typically starts in childhood but usually undergoes arrest in adulthood. The jaws are the most frequent sites in the head and neck region. Males and females are almost equally frequently affected.

Clinically, a painless, smoothly rounded swelling, usually of the maxilla, is typical (Fig. 10.26). The mass may become large enough to disturb function and cause malocclusion by displacing teeth.

Radiographically, there is typically an area of weak radiopacity, with a fine orange-peel texture and an eggshell-thin cortex of expanded bone (Fig. 10.27). The degree of radiopacity depends on the amount of lesional bone which may give a predominantly radiolucent or more sclerotic appearance. The key feature is that the margins merge imperceptibly with the surrounding normal bone.

Polyostotic fibrous dysplasia is rare but shows histologically similar lesions in several bones, skin pigmentation and endocrine abnormalities. Females are affected in the ratio of 3 to 1 and the disease may be seen in childhood. *Albright's syndrome* comprises polyostotic fibrous dysplasia, skin pigmentation and sexual precocity.

Polyostotic fibrous dysplasia involves the head and neck region in up to 50% of cases. A jaw lesion may then be the most conspicuous feature and polystotic disease may not be suspected initially. In a young girl in particular, investigation for other skeletal lesions and pigmentation may therefore be indicated. Skin pigmentation consists of brownish macules which frequently overlie affected bones and appear especially on the back of the neck, trunk, buttocks, or thighs, but hardly ever on the oral mucosa.

Pathology

The lesions consist of loose cellular fibrous tissue containing slender trabeculae of woven bone of variable shape which merge imperceptibly into surrounding normal bone (Figs 10.28 and 10.29).

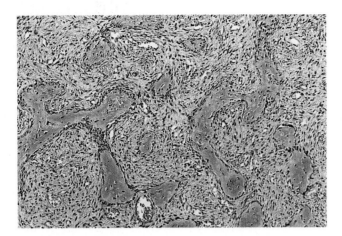

Fig. 10.28 Fibrous dysplasia. Slender trabeculae of woven bone, said to resemble Chinese characters in shape, lying in a very cellular fibrous tissue. With maturation there is progressively more bone formation.

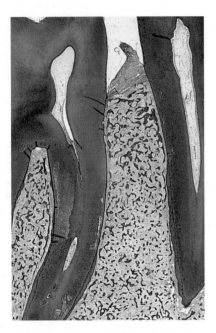

Fig. 10.29 Fibrous dysplasia. There is loss of lamina dura around the teeth and its replacement by lesional bone. These numerous small trabeculae give rise to the ground-glass and orange-peel appearances radiographically.

Osteoblasts are scattered throughout the substance of the trabeculae rather than surrounding them. Some lamellar bone or calcified spherules and occasional loose foci of giant cells can also be seen.

Treatment

The disease is self-limiting, but grossly disfiguring lesions may need to be excised. This should be delayed if possible until the process has become inactive. There is a small risk of sarcomatous change, particularly in the polyostotic variant.

Key features are summarised in Table 10.10.

Table 10.10   Monostotic fibrous dysplasia: key features
● Persons under 20 years mainly affected
● Localised swelling usually of maxilla
● Radiographically, normal bone trabeculation replaced by ground glass or orange-peel pattern
● Lesions merge imperceptibly with normal bone at the margins
● Histologically, normal bone replaced by fibrous connective tissue containing slender trabeculae of bone
● Usually becomes inactive with skeletal maturation

Cemento-osseous dysplasias

These are of periodontal ligament origin and discussed in Chapter 8. They involve the same pathological processes but differ mainly in their extent and radiographic appearances.

Solitary and aneurysmal bone cysts

These lesions, despite their names, are not cysts, and are merely cyst-like in appearance, radiographically. They are skeletal diseases and involve the jaws less frequently than other bones.

Solitary (simple) bone cyst

Solitary bone cysts are mostly seen in teenagers, and uncommon after the age of 25. They form painless swellings or are chance radiographic findings. The mandible is mainly affected. Females are affected more often in a ratio of about 3:2.

Radiographically, these cavities form rounded, radiolucent areas which generally tend to be less sharply defined than odontogenic cysts, and have two unusual features. First, the area of radiolucency is typically much larger than the size of the swelling suggests. Second, the cavity arches up between the roots of the teeth and may as a consequence be first seen on a bite-wing radiograph (Figs 10.30 and 10.31).

Pathogenesis and pathology. Solitary bone cysts used to be known as 'haemorrhagic' or 'traumatic' bone cysts and postulated to result from injury to, and haemorrhage within, the bone of the jaw. This was then supposed to be followed by failure of organisation of the clot and of repair of the bone. However, there is little evidence to support this theory. Blood-filled bone cavities form in the jaws as a consequence of enucleation of true cysts, but solitary bone cysts do not arise as a result. Further, a common form of treatment is to open solitary bone cysts to allow bleeding into the cavity. Normal healing then follows. It seems hardly likely that intrabony haemorrhage can both cause and cure these lesions. Futile speculation about these lesions should not obscure the fact that their cause remains unknown. The cavity has a rough bony wall. There may be a thin connective tissue lining or only a few red cells, blood pigment or giant cells adhering to the bone surface (Fig. 10.32). There are often no cyst contents but there may sometimes be a little fluid.

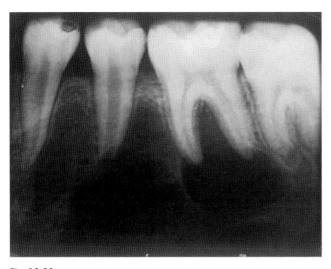

Fig. 10.30 Solitary bone cyst. Typical appearance showing a moderately well-defined but non-corticated radiolucency extending up between the roots of the teeth.

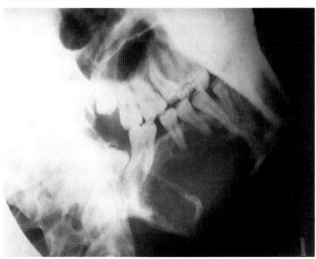

Fig. 10.31 Solitary bone cyst. Oblique lateral view showing a large rounded expansile radiolucent lesion extending from the first premolar to the angle. This cyst is more expansile than is usual and shows the variability of presentation of a solitary bone cyst.

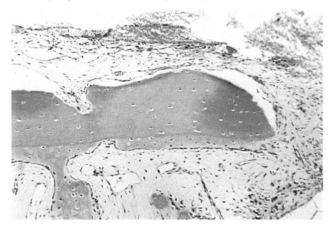

Fig. 10.32 Solitary bone cyst. The scanty cyst lining comprises bone and a thin layer of fibrous tissue. Epithelium is not present and in some cases even the fibrous lining is lacking.

Table 10.11 Solitary bone cysts: key features
● Often chance radiographic findings. Rarely expand the jaw
● Are of unknown aetiology
● Have no epithelial lining. Appear empty at operation or contain pale fluid
● Diagnosis suggested by radiographic features (especially extension between tooth roots) and findings at operation
● Histology confirms the lack of epithelial lining
● Resolve after surgical opening and closure, or occasionally spontaneously

Key features of solitary bone cysts are summarised in Table 10.11.

Management. Solitary bone cysts are not seen in elderly patients, and in those that have refused surgery, so that it is apparent that these lesions resolve spontaneously. It may be necessary, however, to open the cavity, if only to confirm the diagnosis. The characteristic lack of cyst fluid and the unlined bony wall are usually enough to provide a diagnosis, but it is preferable, if possible, to remove any connective tissue lining for histological examination. Opening of the cavity is followed by healing, probably as a result of bleeding. Alternatively, healing after opening of the cavity is merely coincidental. Natural regression, if permitted, seems probable and reparative changes have been seen in excised specimens.

Aneurysmal bone cyst

Aneurysmal bone cysts are exceedingly rare in the jaws. Little is known of their pathogenesis and the most likely possibility is that they are vascular malformations.

Clinical features. Most patients are between 10 and 20 years of age, and there appears to be no strong predilection for either sex. The mandible is usually affected. The main manifestation is usually a painless swelling and a radiolucent area, which may be balloon-like or occasionally show a suggestion of trabeculation or loculation.

Key features of aneurysmal bone cysts are summarised in Table 10.12.

Table 10.12 Aneurysmal bone cyst: key features
● Rare in the jaws
● Jaw lesions are usually in the mandibular ramus and angle
● Affect patients usually between 10 and 20 years
● Are of unknown aetiology
● Form very expansile soap-bubble radiolucencies which may be mistaken clinically and radiographically for ameloblastoma or odontogenic keratocyst
● Histologically consist of a mass of blood-filled spaces with scattered giant cells
● Are treated by curettage but sometimes recur

CHAPTER
10

Pathology. The aneurysmal bone cyst is in no sense a cyst except in its radiographic appearance. Histologically, there is a highly cellular mass of blood-filled spaces which has been likened to a blood-filled sponge (Fig. 10.33). The extreme cellularity, mitotic activity and frequent presence of many giant cells may lead to confusion with a sarcoma. It is essential that this mistake should not be made and the patient subjected, as a consequence, to unnecessarily radical and possibly hazardous treatment. Treatment consists of thorough curettage which may need to be repeated, as the lesion occasionally recurs.

Table 10.13 **Aspects of bone diseases of dental significance**

- Osteogenesis imperfecta – associated dentinogenesis imperfecta
- Osteopetrosis – anaemia and risk of osteomyelitis
- Cleidocranial dysplasia – multiple unerupted teeth
- Cherubism – cyst-like giant cell lesions
- Rickets – hypocalcification of teeth in severe cases
- Scurvy – purpura, swollen, bleeding gingivae
- Hyperparathyroidism – 'cyst-like' giant cell lesions
- Paget's disease – overgrowth of maxilla sometimes
- Fibrous dysplasia – typically, hard swelling of maxilla
- Solitary bone cyst – cyst-like radiolucency
- Aneurysmal bone cyst – cyst-like radiolucency

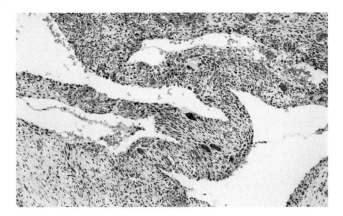

Fig. 10.33 Aneurysmal bone cyst. Cyst wall composed of loose fibrous tissue containing occasional giant cells and large blood-filled spaces.

SUGGESTED FURTHER READING

Cawson R A, Binnie W H, Barrett A W, Wright J M 2001 *Oral disease.* 3rd Edn. Mosby-Wolfe, London

Cawson R A, Langdon J D, Eveson J W 1996 *Surgical pathology of the mouth and jaws.* Wright, Oxford

Chindia M L, Ocholla T J, Imalingat B 1991 Osteopetrosis presenting with paroxysmal trigeminal neuralgia. A case report. Int J Oral Maxillofac Surg 20:199–200

Cornelius E A, McClendon J L 1969 Cherubism — hereditary fibrous dysplasia of the jaw. Roentgenographic features. Am J Roentgenol 106:136–143

Droz-Desprez D, Azou C, Bordigoni P, Bonnaure-Mallet M 1992 Infantile osteopetrosis: a case report on dental findings. J Oral Pathol Med 21:422–425

Ebata K, Usami T, Tohnai I, Kaneda T 1992 Chondrosarcoma and osteosarcoma arising in polyostotic fibrous dysplasia. J Oral Maxillofac Surg 50:761–764

Freemont A J 1996 The pathology of osteogenesis imperfecta. J Clin Pathol 49:618–619

Frohberg U, Tiner B D 1995 Surgical correction of facial deformities in a patient with cleidocranial dysplasia. J Craniofac Surg 6:49–53

Hitomi G, Nishide N, Mitsui K 1996 Cherubism: diagnostic imaging and review of the literature in Japan. Oral Surg Oral Med Oral Pathol Radiol Endod 81:623–628

Koury M E, Regezi J A, Perrott D H, Kaban L B 1995 'Atypical' fibro-osseous lesions: diagnostic challenges and treatment concepts. Int J Oral Maxillofac Surg 24:162–169

Lala R, Matarazzo P, Bertelloni S et al 2000 Pamidronate treatment of bone fibrous dysplasia in nine children with McCune-Albright syndrome. Acta Paediatr 89:188–193

Mangion J, Rahman N, Edkins S et al 1999 The gene for cherubism maps to chromosome 4p16.3. Am J Hum Genet 65:151–157

Melrose R J, Abrams A M, Mills B G 1976 Florid osseous dysplasia. A clinicopathologic study of thirty-four cases. Oral Surg Oral Med Oral Pathol 41:62–68

Peters W J N 1979 Cherubism: a study of twenty cases in one family. Oral Surg Oral Med Oral Pathol 47:307–311

Ruggieri P, Sim F H, Bond J R, Unni K K 1994 Malignancies in fibrous dysplasia. Cancer 73:1411–1424

Shapiro F 1993 Osteopetrosis. Current clinical considerations. Clin Orthop Rel Res 294:34–44

Schneider L C, Mesa M L 1990 Differences between florid osseous dysplasia and chronic diffuse sclerosing osteomyelitis. Oral Surg Oral Med Oral Pathol 70:308–312

Summerlin D-J, Tomich O E 1994 Focal cemento-osseous dysplasia: a clinicopathological study of 221 cases. Oral Surg Oral Med Oral Pathol 78:611–620

Talley D B 1952 Familial fibrous dysplasia of the jaws. Oral Surg 5:1012–1019

Tamura Y, Welch D C, Zic J A et al 2000 Scurvy presenting as painful gait with bruising in a young boy. Arch Pediatr Adolesc Med 154:732–735

Waldron C A 1993 Fibro-osseous lesions of the jaws. J Oral Maxillofac Surg 51:828–835

Williams H K, Mangham C, Speight P M 1999 Juvenile ossifying fibroma. An analysis of eight cases and a comparison with other fibro-osseous lesions. J Oral Pathol Med 29:13–18

von Wovern N 2000 Cherubism: a 36 year follow-up of 2 generations in different families and review of the literature. Oral Surg Oral Med Oral Pathol Radiol Endod 90:765–772

Younai F, Eisenbud L, Sciubba J J 1988 Osteopetrosis: a case report including gross and microscopic findings in the mandible at autopsy. Oral Surg Oral Med Oral Pathol 65:214–221

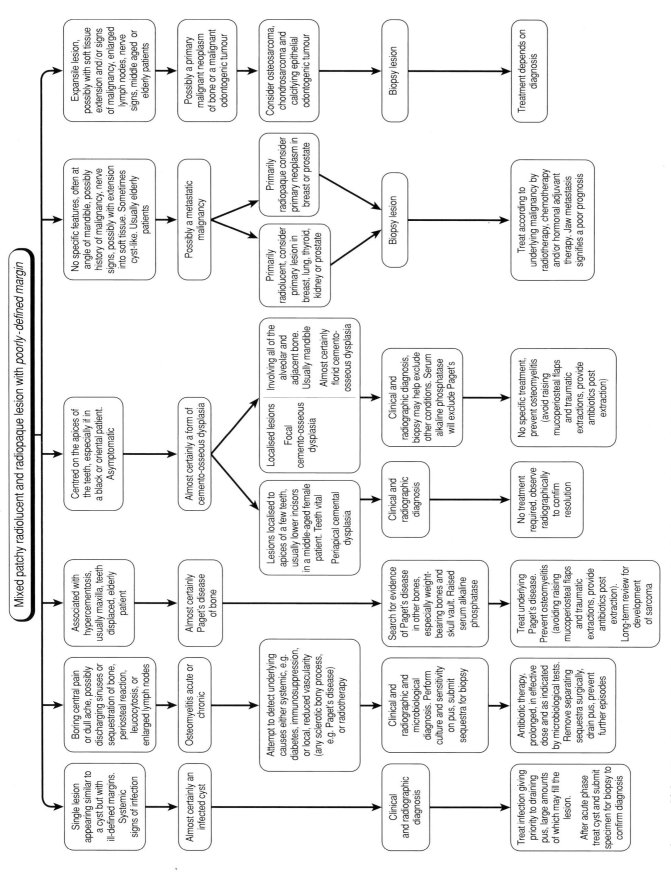

Summary 10.1 Differential diagnosis and management of a poorly-defined mixed radiolucency in the jaws.

Disorders of the temporomandibular joints and periarticular tissues

Temporomandibular joint disorders can cause various combinations of limitation of movement of the jaw, pain, locking or clicking sounds. Pain in particular is a frequent cause of limitation of movement. These complaints are rarely due to organic disease of the joint and many are due to trauma. However, these functional disorders must be considered in the differential diagnosis. Important causes of limitation of mandibular movement are summarised in Tables 11.1 and 11.3.

Trismus may be defined as inability to open the mouth due to muscle spasm, but the term is usually used for limited movement of the jaw from any cause and usually refers to temporary limitation of movement. The term *ankylosis* usually refers to persistent limitation of movement and can be either bony or fibrous. However, the term trismus is sometimes loosely used to mean ankylosis. Inability to open the mouth fully is usually temporary and causes are summarised below.

Table 11.1 **Causes of limitation of mandibular movement**

- ● Intracapsular causes*
  - Infective arthritis
  - Juvenile arthritis
  - Traumatic arthritis and disk damage
  - Intracapsular condylar fracture
- ● Pericapsular causes*
  - Irradiation and other causes of fibrosis
  - Dislocation
  - Condylar neck fracture
  - Infection and inflammation in adjacent tissues
- ● Muscular
  - TMJ dysfunction syndrome
  - Myalgia caused by bruxism
  - Haematoma from ID block
  - Tetanus
- ● Other
  - Oral submucous fibrosis
  - Systemic sclerosis
  - Zygomatic and maxillary fractures
  - Drugs
  - Craniofacial anomalies involving the joint

*Apart from irradiation, intracapsular and periarticular causes may be acute and reversible or, alternatively, lead to fibrous ankylosis of the joint. Infection and trauma are the most common causes

TEMPORARY LIMITATION OF MOVEMENT (TRISMUS)

Infection and inflammation in or near the joint

The main cause is acute pericoronitis with associated muscle spasm. Mumps can also cause transient and unnoticed limitation of movement. Rare causes include suppurative arthritis, osteo-myelitis, cellulitis and suppurative parotitis. Submasseteric abscess results in profound trismus, and infection in the pterygoid, lateral pharyngeal or submandibular spaces may also cause varying degrees of trismus.

Mandibular block injections may cause inflammation of the muscles around the joint and oedema, either because of irritation by the local anaesthetic or by introduction of infection, but rarely do so.

Injuries

Unilateral condylar neck fracture usually produces only mild limitation of opening with deviation of the jaw to the affected side, but closing into intercuspal occlusion may be difficult. Bilateral displaced condylar fractures cause an anterior open bite with limited movement. Rarely, a fall on the chin can result in unilateral or bilateral dislocation of the condylar head into the middle cranial fossa and severe restriction of all movements. Less severe injuries frequently result in an effusion into the temporomandibular joint; both wide opening and complete closure are then obstructed.

Any unstable mandibular fracture causes protective muscle spasm and limitation of movement. Patients suffering from displaced Le Fort II or III fractures often complain of limited opening whereas in reality they are fully open with the jaws wedged apart by the displaced middle third. Reduction of the fracture allows closure.

Tetanus and tetany

These are rare causes of masticatory muscle spasm. Trismus (lockjaw) is a classical early sign of tetanus which, though rare, must be excluded because of its high mortality. This possibility should be considered whenever a patient develops acute severe limitation of movement of the jaw without local cause but has had a penetrating wound, even if small, elsewhere.

Tetany is most likely to be seen as a result of anxiety and hyperventilation syndrome.

Temporomandibular pain dysfunction syndrome

Pain dysfunction syndrome is one of the most common causes of temporary limitation of movement of the temporomandibular joint as discussed later.

Hysterical trismus

Inability to open the mouth is occasionally the main symptom in disturbed patients.

Drugs

Phenothiazine neuroleptics can cause tardive dyskinesia with uncontrollable, involuntary grimacing or chewing movements. Tardive dyskinesia is typically a result of long-term treatment: unlike drug-related Parkinsonism, there is little response to treatment. Metoclopramide, which has phenothiazine-like properties, can cause limitation of movement of the jaw.

Management

In all these conditions the essential measure is to relieve the underlying cause.

DISLOCATION

The temporomandibular joint may become fixed in the open position by anterior dislocation; this is due to forcible opening of the mouth by a blow on the jaw, or during dental extractions under general anaesthesia. In the latter case, the condition should be noticed immediately. It must be corrected before the patient recovers consciousness, by pressing downwards and backwards on the lower posterior teeth. Occasionally a patient will dislocate spontaneously whilst yawning. Epileptic patients sometimes also dislocate during fits.

Occasionally, the dislocation remains unnoticed and, surprisingly, a patient may tolerate the disability and discomfort for weeks or even months (Fig 11.1–11.3). In these cases, effusion into the joint, following injury, becomes organised to form fibrous adhesions. When this happens, manual reduction may be impossible and open reduction, with division of adhesions, must be carried out.

Recurrent dislocation

Recurrent dislocation of the temporomandibular joint is more common and is typically seen in adolescent girls and young adults. It is a typical feature of floppy joint syndromes, notably

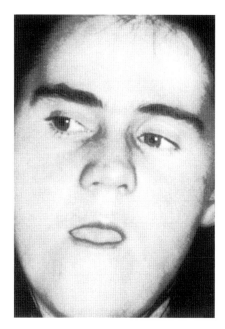

Fig. 11.1 Long-standing dislocation of the jaw: the teeth had been extracted about a month previously; in spite of the patient's inability to close her mouth and the distorted appearance, the dislocation remained unrecognised. (Taken before the advent of colour photography.)

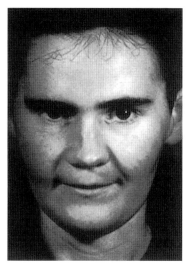

Fig. 11.2 Reduction of the dislocation (performed by open operation because of development of fibrous adhesions) restores the patient's normal appearance and movements of the jaw.

Ehlers–Danlos and Marfan's syndromes, or there may be no underlying systemic disorder.

Augmentation of the eminence by bone graft or down-fracture of the eminence are overall the most successful procedures.

PERSISTENT LIMITATION OF MOVEMENT

Management of ankylosis depends on its aetiology and can be classified for surgical purposes as shown in Table 11.2.

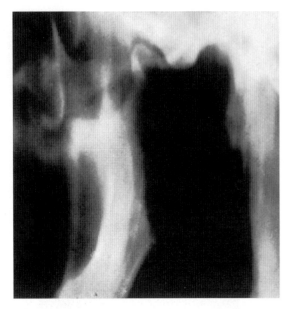

Fig. 11.3 Dislocation of the jaw. Radiography of a temporomandibular joint of the same patient showed complete dislocation of the condyle in front of the eminentia articularis. (Figures 11.3–11.5 by courtesy of the late Professor I Curson).

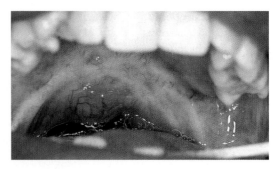

Fig. 11.4 Oral submucous fibrosis. Typical appearance in a relatively advanced case with pale fibrotic bands of scarring running across the soft palate and down the anterior pillar of the fauces. Similar fibrous bands were present in the buccal mucosa bilaterally.

Oral submucous fibrosis

Oral submucous fibrosis is a disease which causes changes somewhat similar to those of scleroderma but limited to the oral tissues. The disease is virtually only seen in those from the Indian subcontinent.

The cause is unknown but the main contributor is thought to be the chewing of a preparation (*pan*) which typically consists of areca nut, tobacco and lime wrapped in betel leaf. Experimentally, an alkaloid component of the areca nut, arecoline, can induce fibroblast proliferation and collagen synthesis experimentally, and may penetrate the oral mucosa to cause progressive cross-linking of collagen fibres. Chewing areca nut alone can also cause oral submucous fibrosis. Susceptibility to submucous fibrosis also appears to be related to specific HLA types.

Clinically, symmetrical fibrosis of such sites as the buccal mucosa, soft palate or inner aspects of the lips is characteristic. The overlying mucosa may be normal or there may be a vesiculating stomatitis. Fibrosis causes extreme pallor of the affected area which becomes so hard that it cannot be indented with the finger (Fig. 11.4). Ultimately, opening the mouth may become so limited that eating and dental treatment become increasingly difficult and tube feeding may become necessary.

Histologically, the subepithelial connective tissue becomes thickened, hyaline and avascular, and there may be infiltration by modest numbers of chronic inflammatory cells. The epithelium usually becomes thinned and may show atypia. Underlying muscle fibres undergo progressive atrophy (Fig. 11.5).

Management

In patients from the Indian subcontient, with this clinical picture, the diagnosis can rarely in doubt. Scleroderma should be readily differentiated by the dermal and visceral involvement, the less severe oral changes and its autoantibody profile.

Treatment is unsatisfactory. Patients must stop the habit of betel chewing and intralesional injections of corticosteroids may be tried in association with muscle stretching exercises to prevent further limitation of opening, but the benefit is not great. Wide surgical excision of the affected tissues including the underlying buccinator muscle together with skin grafting

---

Table 11.2 Management of ankylosis

Mechanical interference with opening ('pseudo-ankylosis') Causes include:
- Trauma: depressed fracture of the zygomatic bone or arch
- Hyperplasia: developmental overgrowth of the coronoid process
- Neoplasms: osteochondroma, osteoma, osteosarcoma of the coronoid process
- Miscellaneous: myositis ossificans, congenital anomalies

Extracapsular ankylosis ('false ankylosis') Causes include:
- Trauma: Periarticular fibrosis (wounds/burns). Posterior or superior dislocation. Long-standing anterior dislocation
- Infection: Chronic periarticular suppuration
- Neoplasia: Fibrosarcoma of the capsule. Chondroma or chondrosarcoma
- Periarticular fibrosis
  Irradiation
  Oral submucous fibrosis
  Progressive systemic sclerosis

Irradiation

The penetrating power of modern sources such as cobalt 60 or linear accelerators are such that high doses can damage deep tissues without a superficial burn. Radiation involving the region of the masticatory muscles, for the treatment of a maxillary tumour for instance, often leads to fibrosis of muscle and adhesions to the surrounding fascial layers, causing fibrous ankylosis.

Treatment is difficult and may involve division of muscle attachments from the jaw or section of the angle or body of the mandible to produce a false joint. Bone surgery is complicated by the risk of osteoradionecrosis and infection (see Ch. 6).

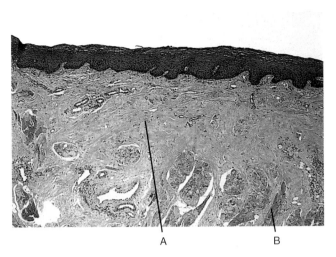

Fig. 11.5 Oral submucous fibrosis. There is fibrosis (A) extending from the epithelium down into the underlying muscle (B), which is replaced by hyalinised fibrous tissue.

can be carried out, but is likely to be followed by relapse. However, no form of treatment is more than palliative and in some cases operative treatment may become unavoidable. The most important measure is prevention and that use of *pan* should be forbidden in patients. This may be initially effective but fibrosis often recurs even though the patient complies. Regular follow-up is important because malignant change is reported to be about 5–8%.

Progressive systemic sclerosis (scleroderma)

Systemic sclerosis is an uncommon connective tissue disease characterized by widespread subcutaneous and submucous fibrosis. Though the most obvious feature is the progressive stiffening of the skin, the gastrointestinal tract, lungs, heart and kidneys can also be affected.

Systemic sclerosis is a connective tissue (collagen vascular) disease associated with a variety of autoantibodies (see Ch. 25).

Clinically, women between the ages of 30 and 50 are predominantly affected. Raynaud's phenomenon is the most common early manifestation, often associated with arthralgia. A hallmark of the disease is involvement of the hands causing such changes as atrophy of or ischaemic damage to the tips of the fingers and contractures preventing straightening of the fingers (see Fig. 1.3).

The skin becomes thinned, stiff, tethered, pigmented and marked by telangiectases. The head and neck region is involved in over 75% and in a minority, symptoms start there. Narrowing of the eyes and taut, mask-like limitation of movement (Mona Lisa face) can give rise to a characteristic appearance. The lips may be constricted (fish mouth) or become pursed with radiating furrows. Occasionally, involvement of the periarticular tissues of the temporomandibular joint together with the microstomia may greatly limit opening of the mouth, but this is typically much less frequent and severe than in the case of oral submucous fibrosis. Involvement of the oral submucosa may cause the tongue to become stiff and narrowed (chicken tongue)

but the clinical effects on the oral tissues are typically relatively minor compared with those seen in oral submucous fibrosis. Widening of the periodontal ligament space is another abnormality characteristic of systemic sclerosis but seen in fewer than 10% of cases. The mandibular angle may be resorbed or rarely there is gross extensive resorption of the jaw. Sjögren's syndrome also develops in a significant minority.

Histologically, there is great thickening of the subepithelial connective tissue, degeneration of muscle fibres and atrophy of minor glands. The collagen fibres are swollen and eosinophilic. There are scattered infiltrates of chronic inflammatory cells which are frequently perivascular and arterioles typically show fibrointimal thickening of their walls.

Complications and prognosis. The main disabilities caused by systemic sclerosis are dysphagia and pulmonary, cardiac or renal involvement. Visceral disease, particularly dysphagia and reflux oesophagitis, are common and are sometimes the initial symptoms. Pulmonary involvement leads to impaired respiratory exchange and, eventually, dyspnoea and pulmonary hypertension. Cardiac disease can result from the latter or myocardial fibrosis. Renal disease secondary to vascular disease is typically a late effect; it leads to hypertension and is an important cause of death. The overall 5-year survival rate is 70%.

No specific treatment is available. Immunosuppressive drugs are ineffective. Penicillamine may be given to depress fibrous proliferation but can cause loss of taste, oral ulceration, lichenoid reactions and other complications. Symptomatic measures such as those described for oral submucous fibrosis can be used to prevent undue limitation of jaw movement. Complications such as renal failure are managed by conventional means.

Causes of intracapsular ankylosis are shown in Table 11.3.

Management

Once ankylosis has become established, the objectives of surgery are to establish joint movement and function, to prevent

---

Table 11.3 Important causes of intracapsular ankylosis ('true ankylosis')

- Trauma
  Intracapsular comminuted fracture of the condyle disorganises the joint. Bleeding may be followed by organisation and bone formation. Early mobilisation of such injuries should prevent bony ankylosis
  Penetrating wounds
  Forceps delivery at birth
- Infection
  Otitis media/mastoiditis
  Osteomyelitis of the jaws
  Haematogenous — pyogenic arthritis
- Systemic juvenile arthritis
  Psoriatic arthropathy
  Osteoarthritis (rarely)
  Rheumatoid arthritis (rarely)
- Neoplasms — chondroma, osteochondroma, osteoma
- Miscellaneous
  Synovial chondromatosis

relapse, to restore appearance and occlusion in the adult, and to achieve normal growth and occlusion in the child by interceptive surgery and orthodontics.

In osteoarthrectomy, a block of bone is removed and relapse is prevented by interposition of a temporalis muscle flap, silicone rubber, or metal. In the growing patient, joint reconstruction using a free costo-chondral bone graft gives better results as in many cases the graft will grow with the patient, preventing subsequent facial deformity.

ARTHRITIS AND OTHER CAUSES OF PAIN IN OR AROUND THE JOINT

The main causes are:

Injury. Dislocation, joint effusion or fractures of the neck of the condyle can cause pain of varying severity, but surprisingly often fractures in this region pass unnoticed.

Infection and inflammation. Acute pyogenic arthritis is exceedingly rare but exceedingly painful.

Rheumatoid and other arthritides. The temporomandibular joints tend to be much less severely affected than other small joints. If specifically asked, many patients with rheumatoid arthritis admit to temporomandibular joint symptoms but overall, pain is not conspicuous. Pain associated with osteoarthritis of this joint is even more uncommon.

Vascular disease. Cranial arteritis is an important cause of ischaemia and pain in the masticatory muscles while chewing.

Muscle spasm. The most common causes of pain in the region of the temporomandibular joint is so-called pain dysfunction syndrome as discussed later.

Salivary gland disease. Painful conditions of the parotids (inflammatory or neoplastic) can cause pain in this region.

Ear disease. Otitis externa, otitis media and mastoiditis are potent causes of pain referred to the temporomandibular joint.

Rheumatoid arthritis

The main feature of this common multisystem disease is chronic inflammation of many joints, pain, progressive limitation of movement, varying degrees of constitutional upset and immunological abnormalities.

Rheumatoid arthritis is the only important inflammatory disease of the temporomandibular joints, but is nevertheless, an infrequent cause of significant symptoms there.

Clinical features. Women are affected, particularly in the third and fourth decades. Loss of weight, malaise and depression are common. The smaller joints are mainly affected (particularly those of the hands), and the distribution tends to be symmetrical.

The main symptoms of temporomandibular joint involvement are crepitus and limitation of movement, but severe pain is surprisingly uncommon. The temporomandibular joints are never involved alone and the other affected joints usually dominate the picture. One large survey found 71% of patients with rheumatoid arthritis to have clinical abnormalities of the

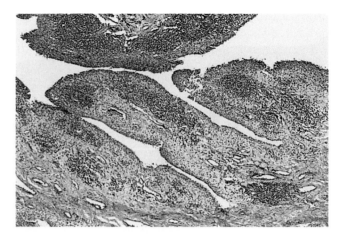

Fig. 11.6 Rheumatoid arthritis. Inflamed villi of pannus growing across the surface of a temporomandibular joint severely affected by rheumatoid arthritis. The condylar surface is destroyed.

temporomandibular joints, while 79% showed radiographic abnormalities. Despite the fact that these were middle-aged patients with long-standing disease, pain was *not* significantly more common than in control patients. The main clinical abnormalities were limitation of opening or crepitus, both of which were considerably more common than in other patients.

Radiography shows flattening of the condyles with loss of contour and irregularity of the articular surface are typical findings. The joint space may be widened by exudate in the acute phases but later narrowed. The underlying bone may be osteoporotic and the margins of the condyles may be irregular. There may be limitation of condylar movement.

Histologically, there is proliferation and hypertrophy of the synovial lining cells and infiltrations of the synovium by dense collections of lymphocytes and plasma cells (Fig. 11.6). The inflammatory cells are often arranged as focal aggregates with germinal centres. There is effusion into the synovial fluid which contains neutrophils and fibrinous exudation from the hyperaemic vessels onto the surface of the synovial membrane. A vascular, inflamed mass of granulation tissue (pannus) spreads over the surfaces of the articular cartilages from their margins and is followed by death of chondrocyes and loss of intercellular matrix. Fibrous adhesions form between the joint surfaces and the meniscus. The meniscus may eventually be destroyed and inflammatory changes in the ligaments and tendons can lead to fibrous ankylosis and loss of stability of the joint.

Management

Diagnosis is based on the clinical, radiographic and autoantibody findings. Serum IgG is usually raised and a variety of autoantibodies, particularly rheumatoid factor and antinuclear antibodies, may be detected.

Generally speaking, though rheumatoid arthritis is a common disease, specific treatment of TMJ symptoms is unlikely to be necessary. The mainstay of treatment is the use of non-steroidal anti-flammatory drugs, but any gross abnormalities of occlusion, such as overclosure, should be corrected to reduce stress on the temporomandibular joints.

Osteoarthritis

Osteoarthritis is a systemic disease, particularly of the elderly, in which there is a defect of cartilage repair exacerbated by trauma. Heavy stress, particularly on weight-bearing joints, is the main cause of pain, but frequently joints with radiographic signs of osteoarthritis are painless (Fig. 11.7).

Osteoarthritis of the temporomandibular joint is mainly a post-mortem finding in elderly patients, is occasionally seen by chance in radiographs, but is not a cause of significant symptoms. Nevertheless, the conviction that osteoarthritis is a significant cause of temporomandibular joint pain even in young persons, is widely held in the United States in particular, and surgical intervention was common. However, the tide of litigation that followed has led to more conservative measures, and an International Conference on Temporomandibular Joint Surgery commented disarmingly that 'it was noted that facts are commonly not allowed to interfere in discussions of TMJ problems'. Although some degree of consensus was reached at this conference, it was apparent that neither the pathogenesis nor the effectivenesss of surgical treatment of this condition were firmly established. More frequently now, other interventions such as intra-articular steroid injections are used.

In the rare event that a patient has pain associated with osteoarthritis of the temporomandibular joint, any factor contributing to stress on the joint should be relieved. Anti-inflammatory analgesics are the main line of treatment.

The concept of TMJ 'internal derangement' is also open to a variety of interpretations. Some regard it as an underlying cause of pain. However, internal derangements seen radiographically are frequently painless. It therefore remains too controversial a subject to discuss here.

Other types of arthritis

Many other types of arthritis can affect the temporomandibular joints but rarely do so. They include psoriatic arthritis, the juvenile arthritides, gout, ankylosing spondylitis, Lyme disease and Reiter's disease. Psoriatic arthropathy can cause ankylosis of the temporomandibular joint. Some of the variants of juvenile arthritis, such as Still's disease, are severe and disabling. Destruction of the condylar head, severely limited opening and secondary micrognathia have been reported. Management is essentially that of the underlying disease.

Cranial (giant-cell) arteritis

Cranial arteritis occasionally causes ischaemic pain in the masticatory muscles in elderly patients and should be considered in patients over middle age who complain of headache and pain on mastication.

Clinically, women, usually after the age of 55, are predominantly affected. The disease may start with malaise, weakness, low-grade fever, and loss of weight. Severe throbbing headache is the most common symptom. The temporal artery frequently becomes red, tender, firm, swollen, and tortuous. In 20% of patients there is ischaemic pain in the masticatory muscles, comparable to and often misnamed intermittent claudication (claudication is literally, *limping*). More important is involvement of the ophthalmic artery causing disturbances of vision or sudden blindness. Polymyalgia rheumatica may be associated. There is then weakness and pain of the shoulder or pelvic girdles associated with the febrile symptoms. The ESR is usually greatly raised.

Histologically, inflammation involves the arterial media and intima. The infiltration by mononuclear cells is typically associated with multinucleate cells. Intimal damage leads to formation of thrombi, which usually become organised and there may be severe damage to the internal elastic lamina, sometimes going on to complete destruction (Figs 11.8 to 11.10). Healing is by fibrosis, particularly of the media, thickening of the intima, and partial recanalisation of the thrombus. Lesions skip short lengths of an artery and a biopsy should be at least 3 cm long.

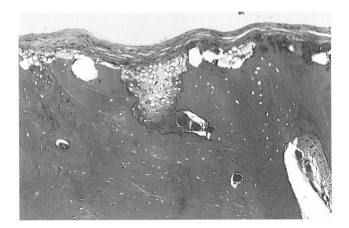

Fig. 11.7 Osteoarthritis. The fibrocartilage layer is split and the underlying bone shows resorption and repair centrally

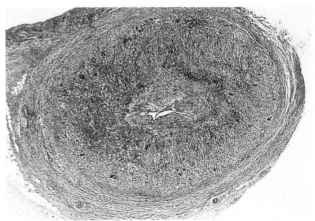

Fig. 11.8 Giant cell (temporal) arteritis. The structure of the artery is disrupted by inflammatory cells and the lumen is much reduced in size.

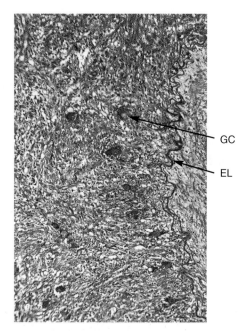

Fig. 11.9 Giant cell (temporal) arteritis. At higher power the internal elastic lamina of the artery may be seen together with giant cells, lymphocytes and neutrophils in the media. GC, giant cell; EL, elastic lamina.

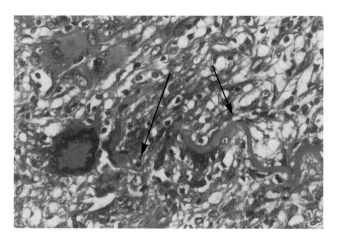

Fig. 11.10 Giant cell (temporal) arteritis. At high power multinucleate giant cells, lymphocytes and neutrophils may be seen amongst the remnants of the artery's internal elastic lamina (arrowed).

Management

The possibility of complications, particularly blindness, which develops in up to 50% of untreated patients, makes it essential to start treatment early. Systemic corticosteroids (starting with 60 mg/day) should be given on the basis of inflamed scalp vessels and a high (> 70 mm/hour) ESR. Corticosteroids are usually quickly effective and should be continued until the ESR falls to normal.

Pain dysfunction syndrome

Pain dysfunction syndrome predominantly affects young women and is characterised by pain, clicking sounds from the

Table 11.4 Typical features of pain dysfunction syndrome
● Female to male preponderance of nearly 4 to 1 ● Most patients are between 20 and 40 years ● Onset is usually gradual ● Onset occasionally ascribed violent yawning, laughing, or a similar incident ● Pain usually one-sided, rarely severe ● Typically a dull ache is made worse by mastication ● Pain typically felt in front of the ear ● Frequently also limitation of opening, or 'locking' of the jaw ● Ultimately self-limiting

joint, or limitation of movement (Table 11.4). It is overall the most common cause of complaints related to the temporomandibular joint.

The area may be tender to pressure and a clicking sound, when the mouth is opened or closed, is common. Sometimes pain is felt lower down over the ramus, occasionally at the angle of the jaw and more rarely still, other sites nearby. Defects of occlusion can often be found as in any other patients.

Aetiology

Abnormalities of occlusion, such as lack of posterior occlusal support from loss of molar teeth, are often blamed but there is no evidence that they are a cause. In spite of the problems created by dentures, for instance, edentulous patients seem rarely, if ever, to be affected. Trauma, particularly minor injuries such as may be caused by violent yawning, laughing, or dental treatment, is occasionally a possible factor but the evidence does not seem strong. Illustrative of some of the difficulties in identifying this complaint and its causes is that its prevalence reported in different surveys ranges from 12% to 86% of adults.

All the evidence suggests that pain dysfunction syndrome is of dubious aetiology that typically affects only a restricted group of the population. It is self-limiting and does not progress to permanent damage or degenerative arthritis later in life. Elderly patients are remarkably free from temporomandibular joint symptoms. Defective neuromuscular coordination, causing areas of spasm of the masticatory muscles, appears to be the main cause.

Investigation

In view of the absence of objective signs, diagnosis is largely by exclusion. Organic causes (as enumerated above) of pain or limitation of movement of the joint should be ruled out by investigation. As in all cases of pain in the region of the jaws, referred pain from the teeth should be carefully excluded.

The temporomandibular joint should be palpated for tenderness or swelling which, if present, suggest organic disease. Crepitus may be felt but is not specific and is not necessarily a sign of significant joint disease. Radiographs of the joints may be taken to make sure that movements are not excessive in either direction and are equal on both sides. However the main value of radiographs is to exclude such changes as fluid accumulation (widening of the joint space) or damage or deformity of the joint surfaces, indicating organic disease. Trigeminal neuralgia can be occasionally triggered by movement of the jaw and should be suspected in older patients, particularly when the pain is severe and paroxysmal. Response to treatment with carbamazepine is virtually diagnostic.

Management

In the US this complaint has been investigated and treated (often by surgery) so excessively vigorously that the resulting litigation has forced a search for a consensus on management. It is now accepted that the indications for active intervention, particularly surgery or 'occlusal therapy' are of questionable value. Moreover, there is a strong placebo effect in any form of treatment. The main principles of management of pain dysfunction syndrome are summarised in Table 11.5.

Any abnormal biting habits should be identified and controlled. Faulty neuromuscular control should be dealt with by exercises to correct faulty patterns of activity as shown by such abnormalities as deviations on closure.

In practice, fitting an acrylic overlay appliance is simple and usually effective. It also tends to relieve abnormal grinding habits. It should cover the occlusal surfaces of the teeth and allow free occlusion without cuspal interference. Short-term use of simple analgesics may also be helpful.

Table 11.5 Principles of management of pain dysfunction syndrome

- Reassurance
- Habit management and physical therapy
- Occlusal appliances
- Analgesics

'Costen's syndrome'

This syndrome comprises headache, ear symptoms (tinnitus or deafness) and burning pain in the tongue and throat and was ascribed to over-closure causing excessive backward movement of the head of the condyle. This syndrome does not exist but the term 'Costen's syndrome' persists in medicine and is often thought to be synonymous with pain dysfunction syndrome.

Condylar hyperplasia

Condylar hyperlasia is a rare, usually unilateral, overgrowth of the mandibular condyle. It causes facial asymmetry, deviation of the jaw to the unaffected side on opening, and a crossbite. The condition usually manifests itself after puberty and is slowly progressive. Pain in the affected joint is variable. If the condition is still active at the time of diagnosis, an intracapsular condylectomy should be performed to destroy the active growth

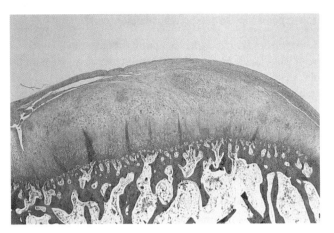

Fig. 11.11 Condylar hyperplasia. The condyle retains an immature structure with a thick cartilage layer, calcification and new bone formation, reflecting the continued growth.

centre. If the disease has stabilised — usually at the end of puberty or shortly afterwards — corrective osteotomies should restore the occlusion and facial symmetry (Fig. 11.11).

Neoplasms

Tumours of the temporomandibular joint are rare, but may arise from the condyle — either the bone or articular cartilage — or from the joint capsule. Metastatic tumours such as those from the breast, prostate and thyroid occasionally metastasise to the condylar head (see Chapter 6).

Though otherwise rare in the facial skeleton, osteochondroma (Fig. 11.12) is probably the most common tumour of the condyle or coronoid process. Osteoma and chondroma and their malignant counterparts may develop, but apart from their interference with joint function and disturbance of occlusion, their behaviour and management are the same as when they arise elsewhere in the jaws. Condylectomy may be required for a neoplasm such as an osteochondroma and an external approach is used.

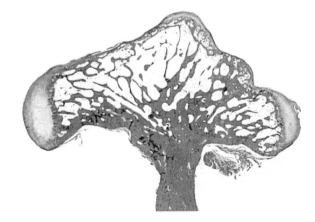

Fig. 11.12 Osteochondroma of the condyle. Two cartilage-capped exostoses arising near the condyle have grown progressively to form a distorted condylar head several centimetres across.

175

Loose bodies in the temporomandibular joints

Loose bodies are rare in the temporomandibular joints compared with other joints. Many types of loose bodies are recognised but the main causes are osteochondritis dissecans and synovial chondromatosis.

Osteochondritis dissecans

This is the main cause of loose bodies in joints, most commonly in the knee. It is believed to result from trauma causing an area of subchondral bone to undergo avascular necrosis with subsequent degenerative changes in the overlying articular cartilage. This area subsequently separates to produce one or several loose bodies. In the temporomandibular joint, the patient has discomfort and episodes of locking. The loose body may be seen on tomography, arthrography or arthroscopy. Surgical removal of the loose body, which is always in the lower joint compartment, relieves the symptoms.

Synovial chondromatosis

In this disease, foci of cartilage develop in the synovial membrane; it is thought to be a benign neoplasm. Synovial chondromatosis rarely affects the temporomandibular joint, but can cause swelling and limitation of movement, with deviation to the affected side on opening. Conventional radiographs may show radiopaque masses in the region of the joint capsule, but if no abnormality may be seen, MRI should reveal multiple cartilaginous nodules and distension of the capsule. Both upper and lower joint compartments are involved and exceptionally rarely the process may extend into the cranial cavity.

Histologically, there is proliferation and atypia of chondrocytes in the subsynovial connective tissue with formation of microscopic or larger nodules of cartilage. These nodules enlarge, may calcify and escape into the joint cavity. The appearance of the chondrocytes is such that it is possible to mistake the lesion for a chondrosarcoma if the pathologist is not made aware of the clinical history and operative findings. It has been shown immunohistochemically that most of the nuclei of the chondrocytes are inactive and that malignancy can be excluded.

Removal of the loose bodies and the whole of the affected synovium are curative. Incomplete excision can be followed by recurrence.

SUGGESTED FURTHER READING

Bjornland T, Refsum S B 1944 Histopathologic changes in the temporomandibular joint disk in patients with chronic arthritic disease. A comparison with internal derangement. Oral Surg Oral Pathol Oral Med 77:572–578

Borle R M, Borle S R 1991 Management of oral submucous fibrosis: a conservative approach. J Oral Maxillofacial Surg 49:788–791

Buckingham R B, Braun T, Harinstein D, Oral K, Bauman D H, Bartynski W, Killian P J, Bidula L P 1991 Temporomandibular joint dysfunction: a close association with systemic joint laxity (the hypermobile joint syndrome). Oral Surg Oral Med Oral Pathol 72:514–519

Cawson R A, Binnie W H, Barrett A W, Wright J M 2001 *Oral disease*, 3rd Edn. Mosby-Wolfe, London

Cawson R A, Langdon J D, Eveson J W 1996 *Surgical pathology of the mouth and jaws*. Wright, Oxford

Chalmers I M, Blair G S 1973 Rheumatoid arthritis of the temporomandibular joint. A clinical and radiological study using circular tomography. Quart J Med XLII:369–386

Denucci D J, Dionne R A, Dubner R 1996 Identifying a neurobiologic basis for drug therapy in TMDs. JADA 127:581–593

Forssell H, Happonen R-P, Forssell K, Virolainen E 1985 Osteochondroma of the mandibular condyle, report of a case and review of the literature. Br J Maxillofac Surg 23:183–189

Goldstein B H 1999 Temporomandibular disorders. A review of current understanding. Oral Surg Oral Med Oral Pathol Oral Radiol Endod 88:379–385

Goss A N 1993 Toward an international consensus on temporomandibular joint surgery. Report of the Second International Consensus Meeting, April 1992, Beunos Aires, Argentina. Int J Oral Maxillofac Surg 22:78–81

Harris M, Feinmann C, Wise M, Treasure F 1993 Temporomandibular joint and orofacial pain: clinical and medicolegal management problems. Br Dent J 174:129–136

Harris R J 1988 Lyme disease involving the temporomandibular joint. J Oral Maxillofac Surg 46:78–79

Holmlund A, Reinholt F, Bergstedt H 1992 Synovial chondromatosis of the temporomandibular joint. Report of a case. Oral Surg Oral Med Oral Pathol 73:266–268

Kaban L B, Belfer M L 1981 Temporomandibular joint dysfunction: an occasional manifestation of serious psychopathology. J Oral Surg 39:742–746

Kerscher A, Piette E, Tideman H, Wu P C 1993 Osteochondroma of the coronoid process of the mandible. Oral Surg Oral Med Oral Pathol 75:559–564

Könönen M 1992 Signs and symptoms of craniomandibular disorders in men with Reiter's disease. J Craniomandib Disord Facial Oral Pain 6:247–253

Koorbusch G F, Zeitler D L, Fotos P G, Doss J B 1991 Psoriatic arthritis of the temporomandibular joints with ankylosis. Oral Surg Oral Med Oral Pathol 71:267–274

Larheim T A, Haanaes H R 1981 Micrognathia, temporomandibular joint changes and dental occlusion in juvenile rheumatoid arthritis of adolescents and adults. Scand J Dent Res 89:329–328

Leighty S M, Spach D H, Myall R W T, Burns J L 1993 Septic arthritis of the temporomandibular joint: review of the literature and report of two cases in children. Int J Oral Maxillofac Surg 22:292–297

Lustmann J, Zeltser R 1989 Synovial chondromatosis of the temporomandibular joint. Review of the literature and case report. J Oral Maxillofac Surg 18:90–94

Maher R, Lee A J, Warnakulasuriya K A A S et al 1994 Role of areca nut in the causation of oral submucous fibrosis: a case-control study in Pakistan. J Oral Pathol Med 23:65–69

Miles D A, Kaugars G A 1991 Psoriatic involvement of the temporomandibular joint. Literature review and report of two cases. Oral Surg Oral Med Oral Pathol 71:770–774

Pillai R, Balaram P, Reddiar K S 1992 Pathogenesis of oral submucous fibrosis. Relationship to risk factors associated with oral cancer. Cancer 69:2011–2020

Rosati L A, Stevens C 1990 Synovial chondromatosis of the temporomandibular joint presenting as an intracranial mass. Arch Otolaryngol Head Neck Surg 116:1334–1337

Sun S, Helmi E, Bays R 1990 Synovial chondromatosis with intracranial extension. Oral Surg Oral Med Oral Pathol 70:5–9

White R D, Makar J, Steckler R M 1992 Synovial sarcoma of the temporomandibular joint. J Oral Maxillofac Surg 50:1127–1230

SOFT-TISSUE DISEASE

CHAPTER 12

Diseases of the oral mucosa: introduction and mucosal infections

A few mucosal diseases, such as lupus erythematosus, are important indicators of severe underlying systemic disease, and rare conditions such as acanthosis nigricans can be markers of internal malignancy. Pemphigus vulgaris is potentially lethal, as is HIV infection — which can give rise to a variety of mucosal lesions. Biopsy is mandatory, particularly in the bullous diseases, as in such cases the diagnosis can only be confirmed by microscopy. In other cases, microscopic findings can be less definite, but often (as in the case of major aphthae for example) serve to exclude more dangerous diseases. Mucosal ulceration — a break in epithelial continuity — is a frequent feature of stomatitis. Important causes are summarised in Table 12.1. However, ulceration is not a feature of all mucosal diseases as discussed below.

Table 12.1 Important causes of oral mucosal ulcers

Vesiculo-bullous diseases	Ulceration without preceding vesiculation
Infective	*Infective*
Primary herpetic stomatitis	Cytomegalovirus-associated
Herpes labialis	ulceration
Herpes zoster and chickenpox	Some acute specific fevers
Hand-foot-and-mouth disease	Tuberculosis
	Syphilis
Non-infective	
Pemphigus vulgaris	*Non-infective*
Mucous membrane pemphigoid	Traumatic
Linear IgA disease	Aphthous stomatitis
Dermatitis herpetiformis	Behçet's disease
Bullous erythema multiforme	HIV-associated mucosal ulcers
	Lichen planus
	Lupus erythematosus
	Chronic ulcerative stomatitis
	Eosinophilic ulceration
	Wegener's granulomatosis
	Some mucosal drug reactions
	Carcinoma (Chap 17)

PRIMARY HERPETIC STOMATITIS

Primary infection is caused by *Herpes simplex* virus, usually type 1, which, in the non-immune, can cause an acute vesiculating stomatitis. However, most primary infections are subclinical. Thereafter, recurrent (reactivation) infections usually take the form of *herpes labialis* (cold sores or fever blisters).

Transmission of herpes is by close contact and up to 90% of inhabitants of large, poor, urban communities, develop antibodies to herpes virus during early childhood. In many British and US cities, by contrast, approximately 70% of 20-year-olds may be non-immune, because of lack of exposure to the virus. In more affluent countries the incidence of herpetic stomatitis has declined and it is seen in adolescents or adults, rather than children. It is more common in the immunocompromised, such as HIV infection, when it can be persistent or recurrent.

Clinical features

The early lesions are vesicles which can affect any part of the oral mucosa, but the hard palate and dorsum of the tongue are favoured sites (Figs 12.1 and 12.2). The vesicles are dome-shaped and usually 2–3 mm in diameter. Rupture of vesicles leaves circular, sharply defined, shallow ulcers with yellowish or greyish floors and red margins. The ulcers are painful and may interfere with eating.

The gingival margins are frequently swollen and red, particularly in children, and the regional lymph nodes are enlarged

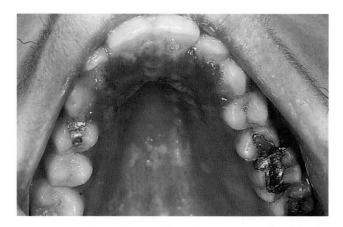

Fig. 12.1 Herpetic stomatitis. Pale vesicles and ulcers are visible on the palate and gingivae, especially anteriorly, and the gingivae are erythematous and swollen.

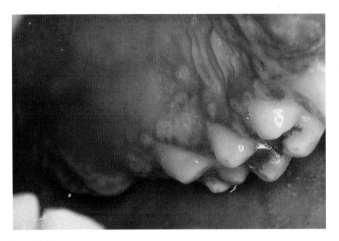

Fig. 12.2 Herpetic stomatitis. A group of recently ruptured vesicles on the hard palate, a characteristic site. The individual lesions are of remarkably uniform size but several have coalesced to form larger irregular ulcers.

and tender. There is often fever and systemic upset, sometimes severe, particularly in adults.

Oral lesions usually resolve within a week to ten days, but malaise can persist so long that an adult may not recover fully for several weeks.

Pathology

Vesicles are sharply defined and form in the upper epithelium (Fig. 12.3). Virus-damaged epithelial cells with swollen nuclei

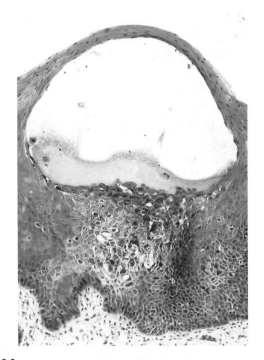

Fig. 12.3 Herpetic vesicle. The vesicle is formed by accumulation of fluid within the prickle cell layer. The virus-infected cells, identifiable by their enlarged nuclei, can be seen in the floor of the vesicle and a few are floating freely in the vesicle fluid.

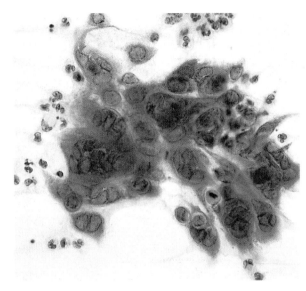

Fig. 12.4 A smear from a herpetic vesicle. The distended degenerating nuclei of the epithelial cells cluster together to give the typical mulberry appearance.

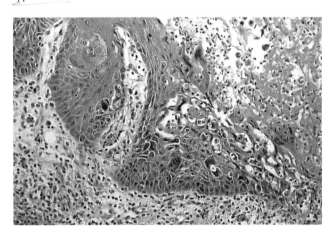

Fig. 12.5 Herpetic ulcer. The vesicle has ruptured to form an ulcer (right) and the epithelium at the margin contains enlarged, darkly staining virus-infected cells liberating free virus into the saliva.

and marginated chromatin (ballooning degeneration) are seen in the floor of the vesicle and in direct smears from early lesions (Fig. 12.4). Incomplete division leads to formation of multinucleated cells. Later, the full thickness of the epithelium is destroyed to produce a sharply defined ulcer (Fig. 12.5).

Diagnosis

The clinical picture is usually distinctive (Table 12.2). A smear showing virus-damaged cells is additional diagnostic evidence. A rising titre of antibodies reaching a peak after 2–3 weeks provides absolute but retrospective confirmation of the diagnosis.

Treatment

Aciclovir is a potent antiherpetic drug and is life-saving for potentially lethal herpetic encephalitis or disseminated infection.

Table 12.2 Typical features of herpetic stomatitis

- Usually caused by *H. simplex* virus type I
- Transmitted by close contact
- Vesicles, followed by ulcers, affect any part of the oral mucosa
- Gingivitis sometimes associated
- Lymphadenopathy and fever of variable severity
- Smears from vesicles show ballooning degeneration of viral-damaged cells
- Rising titre of antibodies to HSV confirms the diagnosis
- Aciclovir is the treatment of choice

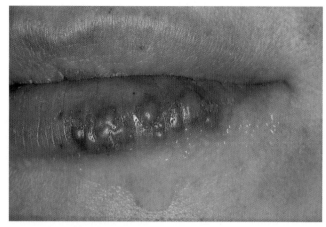

A

Aciclovir suspension used as a rinse and then swallowed should accelerate healing of severe herpetic stomatitis if used sufficiently early. Bed rest, fluids and a soft diet may sometimes be required.

In mild cases, topical tetracycline suspension, rinsed round the mouth several times a day, relieves soreness and may hasten healing by controlling secondary infection.

Unusually prolonged or severe infections or failure to respond to aciclovir (200–400 mg/day by mouth for seven days) suggest immunodeficiency, and herpetic ulceration persisting for more than a month is an AIDS-defining illness.

HERPES LABIALIS

After the primary infection, the latent virus can be reactived in 20–30% of patients to cause cold sores (fever blisters). Triggering factors include the common cold and other febrile infections, exposure to strong sunshine, menstruation or, occasionally, emotional upsets or local irritation, such as dental treatment. Neutralising antibodies produced in response to the primary infection are not protective.

Clinically, changes follow a consistent course with prodromal paraesthesia or burning sensations, then erythema at the site of the attack. Vesicles form after an hour or two, usually in clusters along the mucocutaneous junction of the lips, but can extend onto the adjacent skin (Fig. 12.6).

The vesicles enlarge, coalesce and weep exudate. After two or three days they rupture and crust over but new vesicles frequently appear for a day or two only to scab over and finally heal, usually without scarring. The whole cycle may take up to 10 days. Secondary bacterial infection may induce an impetiginous lesion which sometimes leaves scars.

Treatment

In view of the rapidity of the viral damage to the tissues, treatment must start as soon as the premonitory sensations are felt. Aciclovir cream is available without prescription and may be effective if applied at this time. This is possible because the course of the disease is consistent and patients can recognise

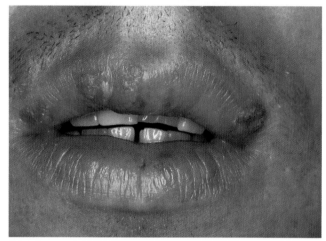

B

Fig. 12.6 Herpes labialis. **A.** Typical vesicles. **B.** Crusted ulcers affecting the vermilion borders of the lips.

the prodromal symptoms before tissue damage has started. However, penciclovir applied 2-hourly is more effective.

Herpetic cross-infections

Both primary and secondary herpetic infections are contagious. *Herpetic whitlow* (Fig. 12.7) is a recognised though surprisingly uncommon hazard to dental surgeons and their assistants. Herpetic whitlows, in turn, can infect patients and have led to outbreaks of infection in hospitals and among patients in dental practices. Now that gloves are universally worn when giving dental treatment, such cross-infections should no longer happen. In immunodeficient patients, such infections can be dangerous but aciclovir has dramatically improved the prognosis in such cases and may be given on suspicion.

Mothers applying antiherpetic drugs to children's lesions should wear gloves.

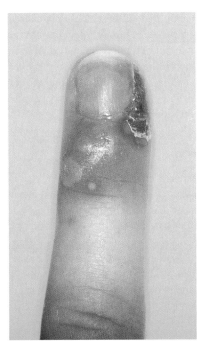

Fig. 12.7 Herpetic whitlow. This is a characteristic non-oral site for primary infection as a result of contact with infected vesicle fluid or saliva. The vesiculation and crusting are identical to those seen in herpes labialis.

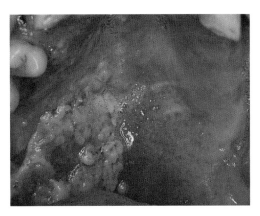

Fig. 12.8 Herpes zoster. A severe attack in an older person shows confluent ulceration on the hard and soft palate on one side.

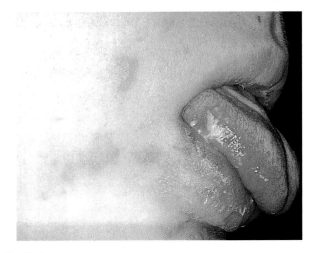

Fig. 12.9 Herpes zoster of the trigeminal nerve. There are vesicles and ulcers on one side of the tongue and facial skin supplied by the first and second divisions. The patient complained only of toothache.

HERPES ZOSTER OF THE TRIGEMINAL AREA

Zoster (shingles) is characterised by pain, a vesicular rash and stomatitis in the related dermatome. The varicella zoster virus (VZV) causes chickenpox in the non-immune (mainly children), while reactivation of the latent virus causes zoster, mainly in the elderly.

Unlike herpes labialis, repeated recurrences of zoster are very rare. Occasionally there is an underlying immuno-deficiency. Herpes zoster is a hazard in organ transplant patients and can be an early complication of some tumours, particularly Hodgkin's disease, or, increasingly, of AIDS — where it is five times more common than in HIV-negative persons and potentially lethal.

Clinical features

Herpes zoster usually affects adults of middle age or over but occasionally attacks even children. The first signs are pain and irritation or tenderness in the dermatome corresponding to the affected ganglion.

Vesicles, often confluent, form on one side of the face and in the mouth up to the midline (Figs 12.8 and 12.9). The regional lymph nodes are enlarged and tender. The acute phase usually lasts about a week. Pain continues until the lesions crust over and start to heal, but secondary infection may cause sup-puration and scarring of the skin. Malaise and fever are usually associated.

Patients are sometimes unable to distinguish the pain of trigeminal zoster from severe toothache, as in the patient shown in Figure 12.9. This has sometimes led to a demand for a dental extraction. Afterwards, the rash follows as a normal course of events and this has given rise to the myth that dental extractions can precipitate facial zoster.

Pathology

The varicella zoster virus produces similar epithelial lesions to those of herpes simplex, but also inflammation of the related posterior root ganglion.

Management

Herpes zoster is an uncommon cause of stomatitis, but readily recognisable (Table 12.3).

Table 12.3   **Herpes zoster of the trigeminal area: key features**

- Recurrence of VZV infection typically in the elderly
- Pain precedes the rash
- Facial rash accompanies the stomatitis
- Lesions localised to one side, within the distribution of any of the divisions of the trigeminal nerve
- Malaise can be severe
- Can be life-threatening in HIV disease
- Treat with systemic aciclovir, intravenously, if necessary
- Sometimes followed by post-herpetic neuralgia, particularly in the elderly

According to the severity of the attack, oral aciclovir (800 mg five times daily, usually for 7 days) should be given at the earliest possible moment, together with analgesics. The addition of prednisolone may accelerate relief of pain and healing. In immunodeficient patients, intravenous aciclovir is required and may also be justified for the elderly in whom this infection is debilitating.

Complications. Post-herpetic neuralgia mainly affects the elderly and is difficult to relieve (Ch. 34).

CYTOMEGALOVIRUS-ASSOCIATED ULCERATION

Cytomegalovirus (CMV) is a member of the herpes virus group. Up to 80% of adults show serological evidence of CMV infection without clinical effects but it is a common complication of immunodeficiency, particularly AIDS. In the latter it can be life-threatening.

Oral ulcers in which CMV has been identified are sometimes clinically indistinguishable from recurrent aphthae, others have raised, minimally rolled borders. Generally, the ulcers are large, shallow and single, and affect either the masticatory or non-masticatory mucosa. Sometimes, oral ulcers are associated with disseminated CMV infection.

Microscopically, CMV-associated ulcers are non-specific, but cells with typical owl-eye intranuclear inclusions can be seen in the inflammatory infiltrate in the ulcer floor. They are usually recognisable by light microscopy but their nature can be confirmed by immunocytochemistry (see Fig. 1.8), in-situ hybridisation or electron microscopy.

The virus present in oral lesions may merely be a passenger, but their causative role is suggested by reports of response to ganciclovir.

HAND-FOOT-AND-MOUTH DISEASE

This common, mild viral infection which often causes minor epidemics among school children, is characterised by ulceration of the mouth and a vesicular rash on the extremities.

Hand-foot-and-mouth disease is usually caused by strains of Coxsackie A virus. It is highly infectious, frequently spreads through a classroom in schools and may also infect a teacher or parent. The incubation period is probably between 3–10 days. *Foot-and-mouth disease of cattle* is a quite different, rhinovirus infection, which rarely affects humans but can also cause a mild illness with vesiculating stomatitis.

Clinical features

The small scattered oral ulcers usually cause little pain. Intact vesicles are rarely seen, and gingivitis is not a feature. Regional lymph nodes are not usually enlarged, and systemic upset is typically mild or absent.

The rash consists of vesicles, sometimes deep-seated, or occasionally bullae, mainly seen around the base of fingers or toes, but any part of the limbs may be affected (Fig. 12.10). The rash is often the main feature and such patients are unlikely to be seen by dentists. In some outbreaks either the mouth or the extremities alone may be affected.

Serological confirmation of the diagnosis is possible but rarely necessary as the history, especially of other cases, and clinical features are usually adequate. The disease typically resolves within a week. No specific treatment is available or needed but myocarditis or encephalitis are rare complications.

Key features are summarised in Table 12.4.

Table 12.4   **Hand-foot-and-mouth disease: key features**

- Caused mainly by Coxsackie A viruses
- Higly infectious
- School children predominantly affected
- Occasionally spreads to teacher or parent
- Typically mild vesiculating stomatitis and/or vesiculating rash on extremities
- Rarely severe enough for dental opinion to be sought
- Confirmation of diagnosis (if required) by serology
- No specific treatment available or needed

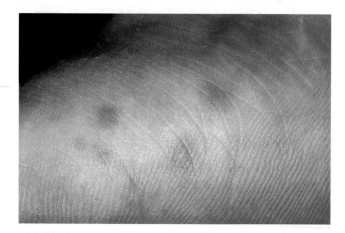

Fig. 12.10 Hand-foot-and-mouth disease. The rash consists of vesicles or bullae on the extremities; in this patient they are relatively inconspicuous.

THE ACUTE SPECIFIC FEVERS

Fevers which cause oral lesions are rarely seen in dentistry. Those which cause vesicular rashes (smallpox and chickenpox) produce the same lesions in the mouth.

In the prodromal stage of measles, Koplik's spots form on the buccal mucosa and soft palate and are pathognomonic. Palatal petechiae or ulceration, involving the fauces especially, are seen in glandular fever and are accompanied by the characteristic, usually widespread lymphadenopathy.

KAWASAKI'S DISEASE (MUCOCUTANEOUS LYMPH NODE SYNDROME)

Kawasaki's disease is endemic in Japan but uncommon in Britain. It is frequently unrecognised and has caused significant mortality. Though its epidemiology suggests that it is an infection, this has not been established.

Clinical features

Children are affected and have persistent fever, oral mucositis, ocular and cutaneous lesions, and cervical lymphadenopathy (Ch. 24). Oral lesions consist of widespread mucosal erythema with swelling of the lingual papillae (strawberry tongue) but are insignificant compared with the serious cardiac effects (Ch. 27).

TUBERCULOSIS

The recrudescence of tuberculosis in the West is partly a consequence of the AIDS epidemic. Moreover, multiply-resistant mycobacteria are becoming widespread. Oral tuberculosis is rare and a complication of pulmonary disease with infected sputum. Those with HIV infection are an important group of victims, but oral tuberculosis is occasionally seen in immunocompetent persons who are usually elderly men with pulmonary infection that has progressed unrecognised or who have neglected treatment.

The typical lesion is an ulcer on the mid-dorsum of the tongue; the lip or other parts of the mouth are infrequently affected. The ulcer is typically angular or stellate, with overhanging edges and a pale floor, but can be ragged and irregular (Fig. 12.11). It is painless in its early stages and regional lymph nodes are usually unaffected.

The diagnosis is rarely suspected until after biopsy.

Pathology

Typical tuberculous granulomas are seen in the floor of the ulcers (Fig. 12.12). *Mycobacteria* are rarely identifiable in the

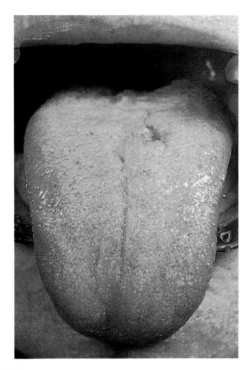

Fig. 12.11 A tuberculous ulcer of the tongue. The rather angular shape and overhanging edges of the ulcer are typical. The patient was a man of 56 with advanced but unrecognised pulmonary tuberculosis.

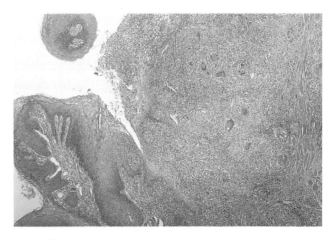

Fig. 12.12 Tuberculous ulcer. At the margin numerous granulomas are present in the ulcer bed. The darkly stained multinucleate Langhans' giant cells are visible even at this low power.

oral lesion but can be demonstrated in the sputum. Chest radiographs show advanced infection.

Tuberculosis or non-tuberculous mycobacterial infection must be considered in patients with AIDS who develop oral ulceration with histological granuloma formation.

Management

Diagnosis is confirmed by biopsy, chest radiography and a specimen of sputum. Mycobacterial infection is confirmed by culture or PCR.

Oral lesions clear up rapidly if vigorous multidrug chemotherapy is given for the pulmonary infection. No local treatment is needed.

Tuberculous cervical lymphadenopathy (see Ch. 26)

SYPHILIS

As a result of contact tracing and early treatment, fewer than 150 cases a year of primary or secondary syphilis were seen in England and Wales in the 1980s. However, since the mid-1990s the prevalence has steadily risen. This is a world-wide trend and the disease has, for example, become widespread in Eastern Europe.

Oral lesions in each stage of syphilis are clinically quite different from each other. Oral lesions have recently been reported in Britain but some may pass unrecognised.

Primary syphilis

An oral chancre appears 3–4 weeks after infection and may form on the lip, tip of the tongue or, rarely, other oral sites. It consists initially of a firm nodule about a centimetre across (Fig. 12.13). The surface breaks down after a few days, leaving a rounded ulcer with raised indurated edges. This may resemble a carcinoma, particularly if on the lip. However, the appearances vary. A chancre is typically painless but regional lymph nodes are enlarged, rubbery and discrete. A biopsy may only show non-specific inflammation but sometimes there is conspicuous perivascular infiltration.

Serological reactions are negative at first. Diagnosis therefore depends on finding *Treponema pallidum* by dark-ground illumination of a smear from the chancre, but they must be distinguished from other oral spirochaetes. Clinical recognition of oral chancres is difficult but important. They are highly infective, and treatment is most effective at this stage.

After eight or nine weeks the chancre heals, often without scarring.

Secondary syphilis

The secondary stage develops 1–4 months after infection. It typically causes mild fever with malaise, headache, sore throat and generalised lymphadenopathy, soon followed by a rash and stomatitis.

The rash is variable, but typically consists of asymptomatic pinkish (coppery) macules, symmetrically distributed and starting on the trunk. It may last for a few hours or weeks and its presence or history is a useful aid to diagnosis. Oral lesions, which rarely appear without the rash mainly affect the tonsils, lateral borders of the tongue and lips. They are usually flat ulcers covered by greyish membrane and may be irregularly linear (*snail's track ulcers*) or coalesce to form well-defined rounded areas (*mucous patches*).

Discharge from the ulcers contains many spirochaetes and saliva is highly infective. Serological reactions (see below) are positive and diagnostic at this stage, but biopsy is unlikely to be informative.

Tertiary syphilis

Late stage syphilis develops in many patients about three or more years after infection. The onset is insidious and during the latent period, the patient may appear well. A characteristic lesion is the gumma.

Clinically, a gumma, which may affect the palate, tongue or tonsils can vary from one to several inches in diameter. It begins as a swelling, sometimes with a yellowish centre which undergoes necrosis, leaving a painless indolent deep ulcer. The ulcer is rounded, with soft, punched-out edges. The floor is depressed and pale (wash-leather) in appearance. It eventually heals with severe scarring which may distort the soft palate or tongue, or perforate the hard palate (Fig. 12.14) or destroy the uvula.

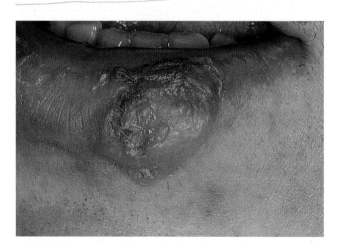

Fig. 12.13 Primary chancre. The lower lip is a typical site for extragenital chancres but they are rarely seen.

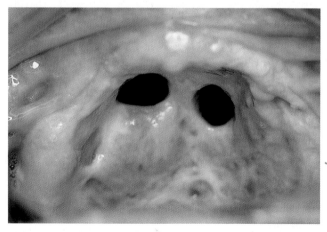

Fig. 12.14 Tertiary syphilis; gummas of the palate. Necrosis in the centre of the palate has caused perforation of the bone and two typical round punched-out holes.

Microscopically, there may be no more than a predominance of plasma cells in the inflammatory infiltrate (a common finding in oral lesions) but associated with peri- or endarteritis. Granuloma formation is rare. Also rarely, there may be diffuse chronic inflammatory infiltration of the lingual muscles or coagulative necrosis mimicking caseation. However, the appearances can be completely nonspecific. Diagnosis therefore depends on the serological findings.

Leukoplakia of the tongue may also develop during this late stage (Ch. 16), and other effects of syphilis such as aortitis, tabes or general paralysis of the insane may be associated.

Management

Serological confirmation of the infection is essential (Table 12.5). Tests are either specific (such as the FTA-ABS) or non-specific as in the VDRL. The VDRL becomes positive 4–6 weeks after infection, and becomes negative only after effective treatment, but false positives can result from several other causes. The FTA-ABS acts as a check against false positive or negative results, but remains positive despite effective treatment for the life of the individual.

Table 12.5 Interpretation of serological tests for syphilis

VDRL	FTA-ABS	*Usual interpretation*
+	–	False-positive
+	+	Active syphilis
–	+	Treated syphilis

The Rapid Plasma Reagin (RPR) titre may also be high in active syphilis but it is also a non-specific (lipoidal antigen) test. Specific tests include the *Treponema pallidum* haemagglutination assay (THPA), the fluorescent treponemal antibody absorption test (FTA-abs test), and the treponemal enzyme-linked immunosorbent assay (ELISA). Specific and non-specific tests are used in combination to distinguish active syphilis from false positives.

Antibiotics, particularly penicillin, are the mainstay of treatment, but tetracycline and erythromycin are also effective. Treatment should be by a specialist and must be continued until non-specific serological reactions (VDRL) are persistently negative.

CANDIDOSIS

Candidal infection can cause a spectrum of lesions (Table 12.6) particularly thrush, chronic white plaques (chronic hyperplastic candidosis, 'candidal leukoplakia') or erythematous areas such as denture stomatitis.

Table 12.6 Spectrum of oral candidosis

- Acute candidosis
  Thrush
  Acute antibiotic stomatitis
- Chronic candidosis
  Denture-induced stomatitis
  Chronic hyperplastic candidosis (Ch. 16)
  Chronic mucocutaneous candidosis (Ch. 15)
  Erythematous candidosis
- Angular stomatitis (common to all types of oral candidosis)

Thrush*

Thrush, a disease recognised in infants by Hippocrates, can also affect adults. In the 19th century, Trousseau called thrush a 'disease of the diseased'; this has been dramatically confirmed by its frequency in HIV disease.

Factors predisposing to candidal infection are shown in Table 12.7.

Table 12.7 Important predisposing factors for oral candidosis

- Immunodeficiency (e.g. diabetes mellitus or AIDS) or immunosuppression (including steroid inhalers)
- Anaemia
- Suppression of the normal oral flora by antibacterial drugs
- Xerostomia

Neonatal thrush results from immaturity of the immune response and infection is probably acquired during passage through the birth canal. Any adult male who develops thrush *without apparent cause* should be suspected of having HIV infection. However, any form of candidosis can be secondary to HIV infection.

Clinical features

Thrush forms soft, friable, and creamy coloured plaques on the mucosa (Fig. 12.15). The distinctive feature is that they can be easily wiped off, to expose an erythematous mucosa. Their extent varies from isolated small flecks to widespread confluent plaque. Angular stomatitis is frequently associated, as it is with any form of intra-oral candidosis.

Pathology

A Gram-stained smear shows large masses of tangled hyphae, detached epithelial cells and leucocytes (Fig. 12.16). Biopsy shows hyperplastic epithelium infiltrated by inflammatory

---

*The term *thrush* is not a nickname, as is sometimes thought, but of considerable antiquity. By contrast the pretentious alternative term 'acute pseudomembranous candidosis' is inappropriate as the plaques are not a necrotic slough.

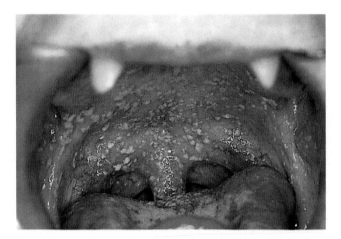

Fig. 12.15 Thrush. The lesions consist of soft, creamy patches or flecks lying superficially on an erythematous mucosa. This soft palate distribution is particularly frequent in those using steroid inhalers.

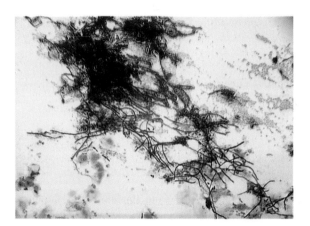

Fig. 12.16 Direct smear from thrush. The tangled mass of Gram-positive hyphae of *Candida albicans* is diagnostic. A few yeast cells may be present as well, but it is the large number of hyphae which is diagnostic.

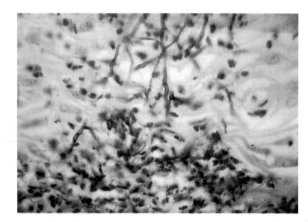

Fig. 12.17 Thrush. At high power the components of a plaque may be clearly seen. The surface layers of the epithelium are separated by inflammatory oedema and are colonised by fungal hyphae and infiltrated by neutrophils.

Table 12.8 Thrush: key features

- Acute candidosis
- Secondary to various predisposing factors (Table 12.7)
- Common in HIV infection and indicates low immunity
- Creamy soft patches, readily wiped off the mucosa
- Smear shows many Gram-positive hyphae
- Histology shows hyphae invading superficial epithelium with proliferative and inflammatory response
- Responds to topical antifungals or itraconazole

oedema and cells, predominantly neutrophils. Staining with PAS shows many candidal hyphae growing down through the epithelial cells to the junction of the plaque with the spinous cell layer (Fig. 12.17). At this level there is a concentration of inflammatory exudate and inflammatory cells. More deeply, the epithelium is hyperplastic but attenuated, with long slender processes extending down into the corium, surrounded by a light infiltrate predominantly lymphoplasmacytic.

The microscopic appearances explain both the friable nature of the plaques of thrush and their ready detachment. Key features are summarised in Table 12.8.

Management

Control of any local cause such as topical antibiotic treatment may alone cause thrush to resolve. If not, a course of nystatin or amphotericin lozenges should allow the oral microflora to return to normal. Failure of resonse to topical antifungals such as nystatin suggests immune deficiency. *HIV infection should always be suspected when thrush is seen in an adult male in whom there is no other detectable cause.* In such patients, candidosis may respond to fluconazole or itraconazole, but is typically associated with a low CD4 count and indicates a poor prognosis.

Rarely, persistent thrush is an early sign of chronic mucocutaneous candidosis such as candida-endocrinopathy syndrome (Ch. 15).

Angular stomatitis

Angular stomatitis is typically caused by leakage of candida-infected saliva at the angles of the mouth. It can be seen in infantile thrush, in denture wearers or in association with chronic hyperplastic candidosis. It is a characteristic sign of candidal infection.

Clinically, there is mild inflammation at the angles of the mouth. In elderly patients with denture-induced stomatitis, inflammation frequently extends along folds of the facial skin extending from the angles of the mouth (Fig. 12.18). These folds have frequently but unjustifiably been ascribed to 'closed bite', but in fact, are due to sagging of the facial tissues with age. Furrows at the angles of the mouth are made deeper by loss of vertical dimension and by loss of support to the upper lip by resorption of the underlying bone. Though establishment of correct vertical dimension and increasing the thickness of the

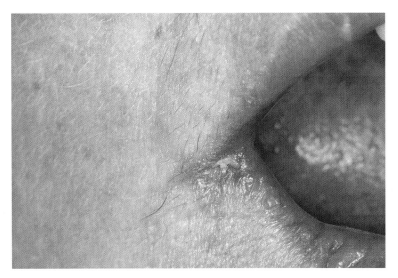

Fig. 12.18 Angular stomatitis. Cracking and erythema at the commissure is due to leakage of saliva containing *C. albicans*, constantly reinfecting the lesion.

labial flange of the upper denture can slightly lessen these furrows, they can rarely be eliminated in this way. Plastic surgery is required when patients are anxious to have these signs of age removed.

Treatment of intraoral candidal infection alone causes angular stomatitis to resolve. If there is co-infection with *S. aureus*, local application of fusidic acid cream may be required.

Denture-induced stomatitis

A well-fitting upper denture cuts off the underlying mucosa from the protective action of saliva. In susceptible patients, particularly smokers, this can promote candidosis, seen as a symptomless area of erythema. The erythema is sharply limited to the area of mucosa occluded by a well-fitting upper denture or even an orthodontic plate (Fig. 12.19). Similar inflammation

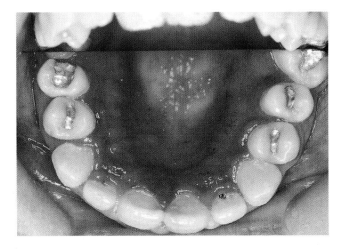

Fig. 12.19 Typical denture stomatitis. Clear demarcation between the erythema of the mucosa covered, in this instance, by an orthodontic appliance. The pallor of the palate behind the posterior margin is clearly seen.

is not seen under the more mobile lower denture which allows a relatively free flow of saliva beneath it. Angular stomatitis is frequently associated and may form the chief complaint.

Smoking also appears to increase susceptibility to this infection.

In the past, denture-induced stomatitis was ascribed to 'allergy' to denture base material but there is no foundation for this fancy. Methylmethacrylate monomer is mildly sensitising but even the rare individuals sensitised to it can wear the polymerised material without any reaction.

Pathology

Gram-stained smears show candidal hyphae and some yeast forms which have proliferated in the interface between denture base and mucosa. Histologically, there is typically mild acanthosis with prominent blood vessels superficially and a mild chronic inflammatory infiltrate. The inflammation is probably a response to enzymes such as phospholipases produced by this fungus.

Management

The clinical picture is distinctive but the diagnosis can be confirmed by finding candidal hyphae in a Gram-stained smear taken from the inflamed mucosa or the fitting surface of the denture*. The infection responds to antifungal drugs, but topical agents such as nystatin or amphotericin can only gain access to the palate if the patient leaves out the denture while the tablets are allowed to dissolve in the mouth.

---

*Quantification of candidas in the saliva is of no value as asymptomatic candidal carriage is common.

Table 12.9   Denture-induced stomatitis: key features

- Candidal infection promoted by well-fitting upper denture
- Enclosed mucosa is cut off from protective action of saliva
- Mucosal erythema sharply restricted to area covered by the denture
- Angular stomatitis frequently associated
- Hyphae proliferate in denture–mucosa interface
- Smear shows Gram-positive hyphae
- Resolves after elimination of *C. albicans* by antifungal treatment

Porous

Methylmethacrylate denture base also harbours *C. albicans* and may therefore form a reservoir which can reinfect the mucosa. Elimination of *C. albicans* from the denture base is important and can be achieved by soaking the denture in 0.1% hypochlorite or dilute chlorhexidine overnight.

A simpler alternative is to coat the fitting surface of the denture with miconazole gel or varnish while it is being worn. The denture should be removed and scrubbed clean at intervals and miconazole re-applied three times a day. This treatment should be continued until the inflammation has cleared and *C. albicans* has been eliminated. This is likely to take 1–2 weeks but patients should be warned not to continue this treatment indefinitely.

It should be noted that resistance to miconazole is growing. Also the oral gel is absorbed and, like other imidazole antifungal drugs, enhances the anticoagulant effect of warfarin.

Lack of response may be due to poor patient compliance or

to an underlying disorder, particularly iron deficiency. If candidal infection is unusually florid or associated with patches of thrush, a blood picture should be requested. Itraconazole or fluconazole orally have a systemic effect and can be used for resistant cases but topical treatment is safer, less expensive and usually satisfactory.

Key features are summarised in Table 12.9.

Acute antibiotic stomatitis

This can follow overuse or topical oral use of antibiotics, especially tetracycline, suppressing normal, competing oral flora. It is infrequently seen now. Clinically, the whole mucosa is red and sore. Flecks of thrush may be present. Resolution may follow withdrawal of the antibiotic but is accelerated by topical antifungal treatment.

Generalised candidal erythema, which is clinically similar, can also be a consequence of xerostomia which promotes candidal infection. It is a typical complication of Sjögren's syndrome. Nystatin suspension or miconazole gel held in the mouth is usually effective.

Erythematous candidosis

This term applies to patchy red mucosal macules due to *C. albicans* infection in HIV-positive patients (see Fig. 22.3). Favoured sites, in order of frequency, are the hard palate, dorsum of the tongue and soft palate.

Treatment with itraconazole is usually effective.

APPENDIX 12.1 TREATMENT OF CANDIDOSIS

Confirm diagnosis with smear (most types) or biopsy (chronic hyperplastic candidosis) unless presentation is typical					

Check history for predisposing causes which may require treatment

If candidosis is recurrent or not responsive to treatment, test for anaemia, folate and vitamin B_{12} deficiency and perform a urine test for diabetes

If a denture is worn:
  Cease night-time wear
  Check denture hygiene and advise
  Soak denture overnight in antifungal (dilute hypochlorite, chlorhexidine mouthwash) or, less effective, apply miconazole gel to denture fit surface while worn

If a steroid inhaler is used, check it is being used correctly, preferably with a spacer. Advise to rinse mouth out after use.

Drug treatments

Presentation	Generalised acute or chronic	Chronic hyperplastic form	Angular stomatitis	Immunosuppression or otherwise resistant to treatment*
Drug of choice and regime	Nystatin 100 000 units QDS for 7–10 days as suspension or pastilles *or* Amphotericin 10 mg QDS as lozenges or suspension 10–14 days.	Miconazole gel 24 mg/ml. Apply QDS	Apply miconazole gel 24 mg/ml QDS to the angles of the mouth 10–14 days or fusidic acid cream	Consider fluconazole 50 mg/day for 7–14 days (longer in immunosuppression) or itraconazole
Notes	Amphotericin is generally preferred over nystatin which has an unpleasant taste	Only effective if lesion accessible for application. For recurrent infection in white patches fluconazole may be required simultaneously	Must treat intraoral infection simultaneously. This is always present even if not evident.	Itraconazole (100 mg/day for 14 days) has a higher risk of adverse effects
Cautions	Neither has any significant unwanted effects	Significant doses may be absorbed if applied to denture fit surface. Avoid in pregnancy. Potentiates warfarin anticoagulation, numerous other but less frequent effects	No adverse effects if only small amounts are applied as described above.	Avoid in pregnancy and renal disease. Numerous drug interactions possible

If there is conspicuous papillary hyperplasia of the palate, consider treatment (cryosurgery or excision) after treatment when inflammation has subsided. The irregular surface predisposes to recurrence of candidosis.

*Candidal resistance to azole drugs is possible but failure of treatment is more likely to result from non-compliance with local measures such as denture wear and cleaning or an untreated underlying condition.

SUGGESTED FURTHER READING

Alam F, Argiriadou A S, Hodgson T A et al 2000 Primary syphilis remains a cause of oral ulceration. Br Dent J 189:352–354

Alrabiah F A, Sacks S L 1996 New antiherpesvirus agents. Their targets and therapeutic potential. Drugs 52:17–32

Cawson R A, Binnie W H, Barrett A W, Wright J 2001 *Oral disease*, 3rd Edn. Mosby-Wolfe, London

Drew W L 2000 Ganciclovir resistance: a matter of time and titre. Lancet 355:609–610

Epstein J B, Sherlock C H, Wolber R A 1993 Oral manifestations of cytomegalovirus infection. Oral Surg Oral Med Oral Pathol 75:443–451

Glesby M J, Moore R D, Chaisson R E 1995 Clinical spectrum of herpes zoster in adults infected with human immunodeficiency virus. Clin Infect Dis 21:370–375

Jones A C, Freedman P D, Phelan J A, Baughman R A, Kerpel S M 1993 Cytomegalovirus infections of the oral cavity. Oral Surg Oral Med Oral Pathol 75:76–85

Nachbar F N, Classen V, Nachbar T et al 1996 Orificial tuberculosis detection by polymerase chain reaction. Br J Dermatol 135:106–109

Regezi J A, Eversole R, Barker B F et al 1996 Herpes simplex and cytomegalovirus coinfected ulcers in HIV-positive patients. Oral Surg Oral Med Oral Pathol Oral Radiol Endod 81:55–62

Scully C 1989 Orofacial herpes simplex infections; current concepts in the epidemiology, pathogenesis and treatment, and disorders in which the virus may be implicated. Oral Surg Oral Med Oral Pathol 68:701–710

Whitley R J, Weiss H, Gnann J W 1996 Acyclovir with and without prednisone for the treatment of herpes zoster. A randomized, placebo-controlled trial. Ann Intern Med 125:376–383

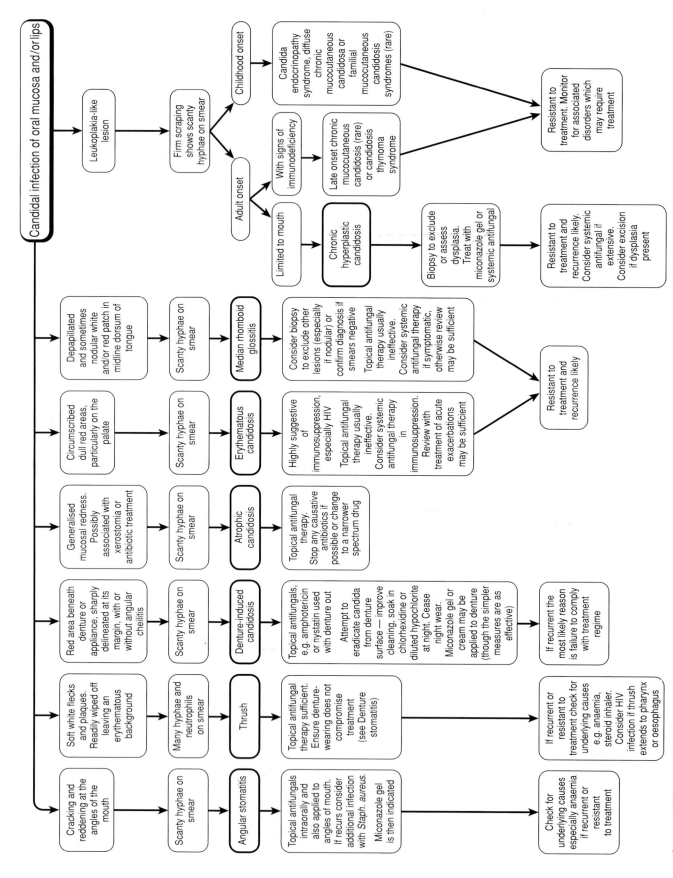

Summary 12.1 Summary of the types of oral candidal infection and their management.

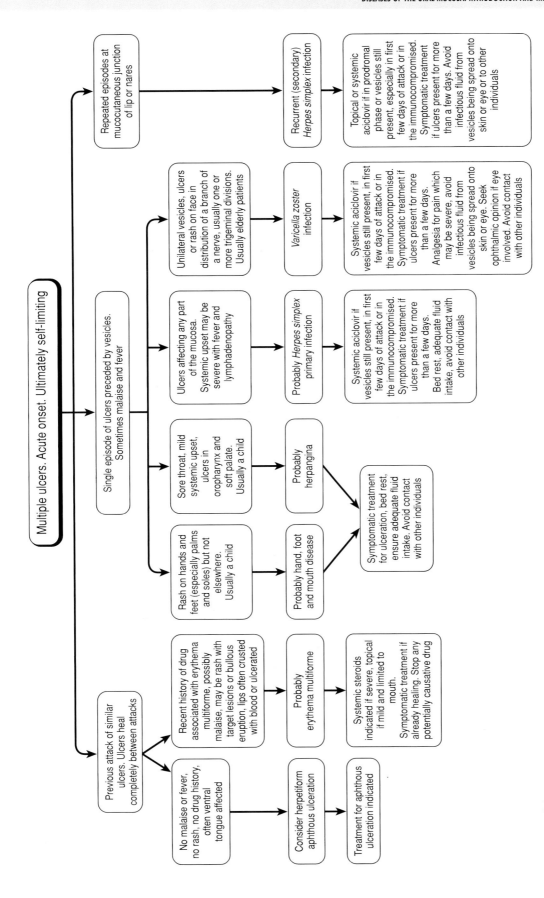

Summary 12.2 Differential diagnosis and management of the common and important causes of multiple oral ulcers with acute onset.

Diseases of the oral mucosa: Non-infective stomatitis

TRAUMATIC ULCERS

Traumatic ulcers are usually caused by a denture and often seen in the buccal or lingual sulcus. They are tender, have a yellowish floor, and red margins; there is no induration. If caused by the sharp edge of a broken-down tooth, they are usually on the tongue or buccal mucosa. Occasionally, a large ulcer is caused by biting the cheek after a dental local anaesthetic (see Fig. 33.1).

Traumatic ulcers heal a few days after elimination of the cause. If they persist for more than 7–10 days, or there is any other cause for suspicion as to the cause, biopsy should be carried out.

Factitious ulceration (self-inflicted oral lesions)

Factitious ulcers in the mouth are traumatic but considerably less common than the usual type. They are typically a consequence of a disturbed mental state ('a call for attention'). Rarely, factitious oral ulceration has been a prelude to suicide.

The most common type of self-inflicted oral injuries has been so-called self-extraction of teeth. The diagnosis of self-inflicted injuries may be difficult but suspicious features are shown in Table 13.1.

Table 13.1 Features suggestive of factitious oral lesions

- Lack of correspondence with any recognisable disease
- Bizarre configuration with sharp outlines
- Usually in an otherwise healthy mouth
- Clinical features inconsistent with the history
- In areas accessible to the patient

Investigation may be needed to exclude organic disease. Underlying emotional disturbance is typically well-concealed. Frequently the diagnosis can be confirmed only by discreet observation after admission to hospital. The patient's family doctor should be told of the need for specialist psychiatric assessment.

RECURRENT APHTHOUS STOMATITIS (RECURRENT APHTHAE)

Recurrent aphthae constitute the most common oral mucosal

disease and affect 10–25% of the population, but many cases are mild and accepted with little complaint.

Table 13.2 Possible aetiological factors for recurrent aphthae

- Genetic predisposition
- Exaggerated response to trauma
- Infections
- Immunological abnormalities
- Gastrointestinal disorders
- Haematological deficiencies
- Hormonal disturbances
- Stress

Aetiology

The main factors thought to contribute are shown in Table 13.2.

Genetic factors. There is some evidence for a genetic predisposition. The family history is sometimes positive and the disease appears to affect identical twins more frequently than non-identical. However, this probably applies to a minority. A variety of HLA associations have been reported but no one haplotype seems to be consistently associated. In the possibly related Behçet's disease (see below) the evidence for a genetic predisposition is much stronger.

Trauma. Some patients think that the ulcers result from trauma because the early symptoms simulate pricking of the mucosa by (for instance) a toothbrush bristle. Trauma may dictate the site of ulcers in patients who already have the disorder, but most aphthae are in relatively protected sites and the masticatory mucosa is generally spared.

Infections. There is no evidence that aphthae are directly due to any microbes, and there is scanty evidence that cross-reacting antigens from streptococci or L-forms play any significant role. The hypothesis that there may be defective immuno-regulation caused by herpes or other viruses is unproven.

Immunological abnormalities. Since the etiology of recurrent aphthae is unknown, there has been a facile tendency to label them as 'autoimmune'. A great variety of immunological abnormalities have been reported but there have been almost as many contrary findings and no convincing theory of immuno-pathogenesis takes into account the clinical features. It is also possible that the immunological abnormalities are as much a consequence of the ulcers as the cause. Evidence of an association with atopic (IgE-mediated) disease is unconfirmed. Circulating antibodies to crude extracts of fetal oral mucosa have been reported, but their titre is unrelated to the severity of the disease and in many patients there are no significant changes in immunoglobulin levels. Antibody-dependent cytotoxic mechanisms have been postulated but not convincingly demonstrated. The histological features of aphthae (see below) have also been invoked to support hypotheses that the disease is either an immune complex-mediated (type III) or a cell-mediated (type IV) reaction according to taste. However, others have failed to confirm the presence of circulating immune complexes, and in any case the significance of such complexes, which are sometimes detectable in the absence of disease, is notoriously difficult to interpret. Depressed circulating helper/suppressor T lymphocyte ratios have been reported, but others have found no difference between active and remittant phases of the disorder. Recurrent aphthae also lack virtually all features of and any association with typical autoimmune diseases (Ch. 23). They also fail to respond reliably to immunosuppressive drugs and become more severe in the immune deficiency state induced by HIV infection.

Gastrointestinal disease. Aphthae were previously known as 'dyspeptic ulcers' but are only rarely associated with gastrointestinal disease. Any association is usually because of a deficiency, particularly of vitamin B_{12} or folate secondary to malabsorption. An association with coeliac disease (sometimes asymptomatic) has been found in approximately 5% of patients with aphthae, but a secondary haematinic deficiency, particularly folate deficiency, is probably the cause.

Haematological deficiencies. Deficiencies of vitamin B_{12}, folate, or iron have been reported in up to 20% of patients with aphthae. Such deficiencies are probably more frequent in patients whose aphthae start or worsen in middle age or later. In many such patients, the deficiency is latent, the haemoglobin is within normal limits, and the main sign is micro- or macrocytosis of the red cells. In patients who thus prove to be vitamin B_{12} or folate deficient, remedying the deficiency may bring rapid resolution of the ulcers.

Hormonal factors. In a few women, aphthae are associated with the stressful luteal phase of the menstrual cycle, but there is no strong evidence that hormone treatment is reliably effective.

'Stress'. Some patients relate exacerbations of ulceration to times of stress, and some studies have reported a correlation. However, stress is notoriously difficult to quantify, and some studies have found no correlation.

HIV infection. Aphthous stomatitis is a recognised feature of HIV infection. Its frequency and severity are related to the degree of immune deficiency, as discussed later.

Non-smoking. It has long been established that recurrent aphthae are a disease, almost exclusively, of non-smokers. And this is one of the few consistent findings. Recurrent aphthae may also start when smoking is abandoned. The reasons are unclear but it is believed that smoking has a systemic protective action against this disease.

In brief, therefore, the aetiology of recurrent aphthae is unclear. There is no evidence that they are a form of auto-immune disease in any accepted sense, and it is uncertain whether many of the reported immunological abnormalities are cause or effect. However, in a minority of patients there is a clear association with haematological deficiencies. The latter in turn may be secondary to small-intestine disease or other cause of malabsorption.

That speculation about the cause of recurrent aphthae has continued for at least half a century, the variety of current theories and the contradictory findings, indicate how little is known.

Clinical features

Typical features of recurrent aphthae are summarised in Table 13.3.

Females are not significantly more frequently affected than males. The frequency of ulceration typically reaches a peak in early adult life or a little later, then gradually wanes. Recurrent aphthae are rare in the elderly, particularly the edentulous. However, older persons may be affected if a haematological deficiency develops. The great majority of patients are clerical, semi-professional, or professional workers and are total non-smokers. Occasionally, aphthae start when smoking is given up.

The usual history is of painful ulcers recurring at intervals of approximately 3 to 4 weeks. Occasionally they are continuously present. Unpredictable remissions of several months may be noted. Individual minor aphthae persist for 7 to 10 days then heal without scarring. Aphthae typically affect only the non-keratinised mucosa such as the buccal mucosa, sulcuses, or lateral borders of the tongue, but major aphthae can affect the masticatory mucosa. Ulcers are of three clincially distinguishable types (Table 13.4).

The pain of major aphthae can interfere with eating. Moreover, major aphthae are sometimes a feature of HIV disease and add to such patients' burdens.

Table 13.3 **Typical features of recurrent aphthae**

- Onset frequently in childhood but peak in adolescence or early adult life
- Attacks at variable but sometimes relatively regular intervals
- Most patients are otherwise healthy
- A few have haematological defects
- Most patients are non-smokers
- Usually self-limiting eventually

Pathology

There is alleged to be initial lymphocytic infiltration followed by destruction of the epithelium and infiltration of the tissues by neutrophils. Mononuclear cells may also surround blood vessels (perivascular cuffing). These changes are said to be consistent with either type III or IV reactions, but true vasculitis is not seen. Overall the appearances are non-specific (Fig. 13.5).

193

Table 13.4   Types of recurrent aphthae

- Minor aphthae
  The most common type
  Non-keratinised mucosa affected
  Ulcers are shallow, rounded, 5–7 mm across, with an
  erythematous margin and yellowish floor (Fig. 13.1)
  One or several ulcers may be present
- Major aphthae
  Uncommon
  Ulcers frequently several centimetres across (Fig. 13.2)
  Sometimes mimic a malignant ulcer
  Ulcers persist for several months
  Masticatory mucosa such as the dorsum of the tongue or
    occasionally the gingivae may be involved
  Scarring may follow healing (Fig. 13.3)
- Herpetiform aphthae
  Uncommon
  Non-keratinised mucosa affected
  Ulcers are 1–2 mm across
  Dozens or hundreds may be present
  May coalesce to form irregular ulcers (Fig. 13.4)
  Widespread bright erythema round the ulcers

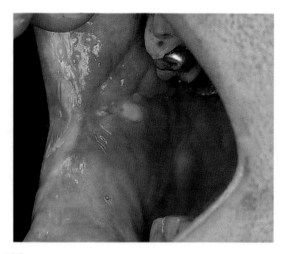

Fig. 13.3 Recurrent aphthous stomatitis, major type. The same ulcer shown in Figure 13.2 but healing. The ulcer is much smaller but there is scarring and puckering of the surrounding mucosa.

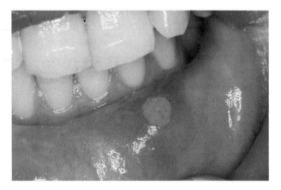

Fig. 13.1 Aphthous stomatitis, minor form. A single, relatively large shallow ulcer in a typical site. There is a narrow band of periulcer erythema. These features are non-specific and the diagnosis must be made primarily on the basis of the history.

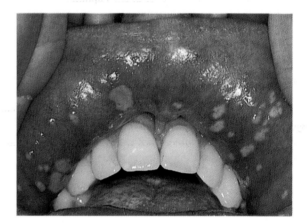

Fig. 13.4 Recurrent aphthous stomatitis, herpetiform type. There are numerous small, rounded and pinpoint ulcers, some of which are coalescing. The surrounding mucosa is lightly erythematous and the overall picture is highly suggestive of viral infection, but the attacks are recurrent and no virus can be isolated.

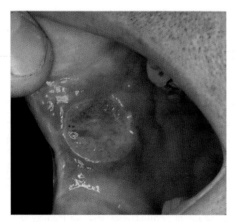

Fig. 13.2 Aphthous stomatitis, major type. This large, deep ulcer with considerable surrounding erythema has been present for several weeks.

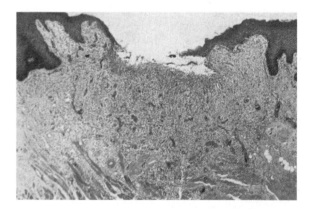

Fig. 13.5 Recurrent aphtha. Section of an early ulcer showing the break in the epithelium, the inflammatory cells in the floor and the inflammatory changes more deeply where numerous dilated vessels can be seen.

Biopsy is of no value in the diagnosis except to exclude carcinoma in the case of major aphthae. Aphthae are not preceded by vesiculation and smears readily distinguish herpetiform aphthae from herpetic ulceration.

Diagnosis and management

The most important diagnostic feature is the history of recurrences of self-healing ulcers at fairly regular intervals (Table 13.5). The only other condition with this history is Behçet's disease. Usually, increasing frequency of ulcers brings the patient to seek treatment. Otherwise most patients appear well, but haematological investigation is particularly important in older patients. Routine blood indices are informative, and usually the most important finding is an abnormal mean corpuscular volume (MCV). If macro- or microcytosis is present, further investigation is necessary to find and remedy the cause. Treatment of vitamin B_{12} deficiency or folate deficiency is sometimes sufficient to control or abolish aphthae.

Apart from the minority with underlying systemic disease, treatment is empirical and palliative only. Despite numerous clinical trials, no medication gives completely reliable relief. Patients should therefore be made to understand that the trouble may not be curable but can usually be alleviated and usually resolves eventually of its own accord.

Corticosteroids. Some patients get relief from Corlan (hydrocortisone hemisuccinate 2.5 mg) pellets allowed to dissolve in the mouth three times a day. Corticosteroids are unlikely to hasten healing of existing ulcers, but probably reduce the painful inflammation. The most rational form of

treatment is for patients to take these pellets continuously (whether or not ulcers are present) to enable the corticosteroid to act in the very early, asymptomatic stages. This regimen is only applicable to those who have frequent ulcers (at 2- or 3-week intervals or more frequently). This should be tried for 2 months then stopped for a month to assess any improvement and whether there is any deterioration without treatment.

Triamcinolone dental paste is a corticosteroid in a vehicle which sticks to the moist mucosa. When correctly applied the vehicle absorbs moisture and forms an adhesive gel which can remain in place for one or several hours but it is difficult to apply a fragment of this paste to the ulcer and to get it to adhere firmly. It is only useful for patients with infrequent ulcers, for ulcers near the front of the mouth and for patients dextrous enough to be able to follow the instructions. This gel should form a protective layer over the ulcer to help make it comfortable. The corticosteroid is slowly released and has an anti-inflammatory action. Another alternative is the use of a corticosteroid asthma spray to deposit a potent corticosteroid over the ulcer. Topical corticosteroids used as described have no systemic effect.

Tetracycline mouth rinses. Trials both in Britain and the USA showed that tetracycline rinses significantly reduced both the frequency and severity of aphthae. For herpetiform aphthae particularly, the contents of a tetracycline capsule (250 mg) can be stirred in a little water and held in the mouth for 2–3 minutes, three times daily. Some patients like to use this mouth rinse regularly for 3 days each week if they have frequent ulcers. An antifungal drug may also need to be given to patients who are susceptible to superinfection by *Candida albicans.*

Chlorhexidine. A 0.2% solution has also been used as a mouth rinse for aphthae. Used three times daily after meals and held in the mouth for at least 1 minute, it has been claimed to reduce the duration and discomfort of aphthous stomatitis. Zinc sulphate or zinc chloride solutions may also have a slight beneficial effect.

Topical salicylate preparations. Salicylates have an anti-inflammatory action and also have local effects. Preparations of choline salicylate in a gel can be applied to aphthae. These preparations, which are available over the counter, sometimes appear to be helpful.

Possible treatments for recurrent aphthae are summarised in Appendix 13.1.

Treatment of major aphthae. Major aphthae, whether or not there is underlying disease such as HIV infection, may sometimes be so painful, persistent, and resistant to conventional treatment as to be disabling. Reportedly effective treatments include azathioprine, cyclosporin, colchicine and dapsone, but thalidomide is probably most reliably effective. Their use may be justified for major aphthae even in otherwise healthy persons if they are disabled by the pain and difficulty of eating. However, thalidomide can cause severe adverse effects and is strongly teratogenic, and, like the other drugs mentioned, can only be given under specialist supervision.

Table 13.5 Check-list for diagnosis of recurrent aphthae

History	*The history is all-important* Check for: Recurrences Pattern? Minor, major or herpetiform type? Onset as child or teenager Family history Distribution only on non-keratinised mucosa Signs or symptoms of Behçet's disease (ocular, genital, skin, joint lesions) (Table 13.6)
Examination	Check for: Discrete well-defined ulcers Scarring or soft palate involvement suggesting major aphthae Exclude other diseases with specific appearances e.g. lichen planus or vesiculobullous disease
Special investigations	*Used to exclude underlying conditions,* *especially in patients with onset in later life* Check for: Anaemia, iron, red cell folate and vitamin B_{12} status History of diarrhoea, constipation or blood in stools suggesting gastrointestinal disease, e.g. coeliac disease or malabsorption

195

BEHÇET'S DISEASE

Behçet's syndrome was originally defined as a triad of oral aphthae, genital ulceration and uveitis. However, it is a multi-system disorder with varied manifestations and termed Behçet's disease. It is rare in the UK and USA but is relatively common in countries bordering the Mediterranean (Behçet was a Turk) and very common in Japan. The aetiology is unknown but is thought to be either an infection or an immunological reaction to an infectious agent.

Patients are usually young adult males between 20 and 40 years old. Patients suffer one of four patterns of disease, namely:

1. Mucocutaneous (oral and genital ulceration)
2. Arthritic (joint involvement with or without mucocutaneous involvement)
3. Neurological (with or without other features) or
4. Ocular (with or without other features). HLA-B51

The racial distribution suggests a strong genetic component and this is confirmed by the fact that each of these presentations is linked to a different HLA tissue type. HLA-B12 and/or DR2 types, for example, are linked to mucocutaneous and arthritic disease. Unfortunately these HLA associations are of no value in diagnosis but HLA-B51 is useful as a predictor of ocular lesions, which can lead to blindness. Diagnostic criteria are listed in Table 13.6.

The oral aphthae of Behçet's disease are not distinguishable from common aphthae. They are the most consistently found feature and frequently the first manifestation. Behçet's disease should therefore be considered in the differential diagnosis of aphthous stomatitis particularly in patients in an at-risk racial group, and the medical history should be checked for the features shown in Table 13.6. The frequency of other manifestations is highly variable. As a result there are no absolute criteria or reliable tests for the diagnosis, but aphthous stomatitis in combination with any two of the other major features can be regarded as adequate.

Special tests are not helpful in diagnosis, apart from the pathergy test. The test is positive if there is an exaggerated

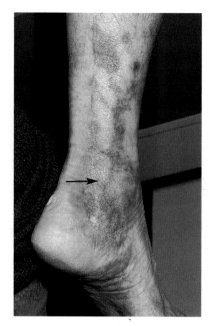

Fig. 13.6 Thrombophlebitis in Behçet's disease. Inflammation and pigmentation highlight the sites of veins (arrow) and their valves. This is only one of several possible skin manifestations.

response to a sterile needle puncture of the skin. However, the test must be interpreted by an experienced clinician and tends to be positive only in Mediterranean patients. Moreover, a positive pathergy test does not correlate with the presence of oral lesions or with the overall severity of the disease and is rarely positive in UK patients. It is also not entirely specific for Behçet's disease.

The importance of making the diagnosis is indicated by the life-threatening nature of thrombosis and the risk of blindness or brain damage.

The main pathological finding is vasculitis and anti-endothelial cell (aEC) antibodies are reportedly found in 50% of those with active disease, but their role remains uncertain. The aetiology is largely speculative but lesions may result from immune-complex mediated vasculities of small vessels which is said to be present in mucocutaneous and all types of lesion. However, microscopic evidence of vasculitis in the oral ulcers is open to question.

Treatment is difficult and requires a multidisciplinary approach. The oral ulceration may be treated in the same way as the common form. When major aphthae are severe or if there is frequent recurrence, thalidomide or colchicine, or both, are often used and are highly effective.

HIV-ASSOCIATED ORAL ULCERATION

Patients with HIV infection (Ch. 24) are susceptible to severe recurrent aphthae which are not otherwise distinguishable from

---

Table 13.6 Diagnostic criteria for Behçet's disease

Major criteria	Minor criteria
• Recurrent oral aphthae	• Arthralgia or arthritis
• Genital ulceration	• Gastrointestinal lesions
• Eye lesions (Recurrent hypopyon, iritis or iridocyclitis; chorioretinitis)	• Vascular lesions (mainly thrombotic) (Fig. 13.6)
• Skin lesions (Erythema nodosum, subcutaneous thrombophlebitis, hyperirritability of the skin)	• Central nervous system involvement

common aphthae. With declining immune function, the ulcers become more frequent and severe, and by interfering with eating may contribute to the patient's deterioration. Biopsies should be taken to exclude opportunistic infections otherwise the aetiology is unknown. Treatment with thalidomide is frequently effective, but in some cases cytomegalovirus can be seen in biopsies, and treatment with ganciclovir may be more appropriate.

Necrotising oral ulceration may also be seen.

LICHEN PLANUS

Lichen planus is a common chronic inflammatory disease of skin and mucous membranes. It mainly affects patients of middle age or over. Oral lesions have characteristic appearances and distribution.

Aetiology

In spite of histological changes which can be diagnostic, the aetiology of lichen planus remains problematical. The predominantly T-lymphocyte infiltrate suggests cell-mediated immunological damage to the epithelium and a plethora of immunological abnormalities has been reported. Though it has not been possible to demonstrate humoral or lymphocytotoxic mechanisms, the inflammatory infiltrate consists mainly of T lymphocytes. Both CD4 and CD8 cells are present but numbers of CD8 cells may rise with disease progression and they are more numerous in relation to the epithelium. Precise trigger mechanisms remain unclear but lichen planus undoubtedly appears to be a T-lymphocyte mediated disorder.

Disease indistinguishable from lichen planus, induced by drugs (notably gold and anti-malarial agents), also suggests involvement of immunological mechanisms. Oral lichen planus is also a virtually invariable feature and an early sign of graft-versus-host disease (Ch. 23) but this does not clarify any immunological mechanisms.

Clinical features

Typical features of lichen planus are summarised in Table 13.7.

The lesions' characteristic appearance and distribution should be taken into account in making the diagnosis.

Striae are most common and typically form sharply-defined snowy-white, lacy, starry, or annular patterns (Fig. 13.7). They may occasionally be interspersed with minute, white papules. Striae may not be palpable or may be firmer than the surrounding mucosa.

Atrophic areas are red areas of mucosal thinning (Fig. 13.8) and often combined with striae.

Erosions are shallow irregular areas of epithelial destruction. These also can be very persistent and may be covered by a smooth, slightly raised yellowish layer of fibrin (Fig. 13.9). The

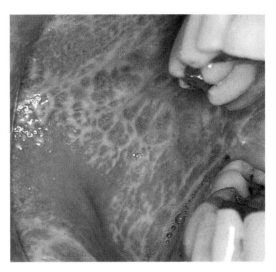

Fig. 13.7 Lichen planus, striate pattern. This is the most common site and type of lesion, a lacy network of white striae on the buccal mucosa. The lesions are usually symmetrically distributed.

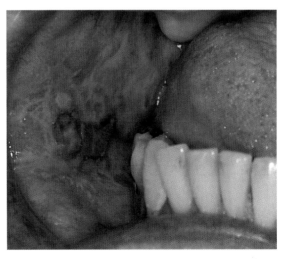

Fig. 13.8 Lichen planus, atrophic type. There are shallow irregular zones of erythema surrounded by poorly defined striae.

Table 13.7 **Oral lichen planus: typical features**

- Females account for at least 65% of patients
- Patients usually over 40 years
- Untreated disease can persist for 10 or more years
- Lesions in combination or isolation, comprise:
    Striae
    Atrophic areas
    Erosion
    Plaques
- Common sites are:
    Buccal mucosae
    Dorsum of tongue
    Gingivae (infrequently)
- Lesions usually bilateral and often symmetrical
- Cutaneous lesions only occasionally associated
- Usually, good response to corticosteroids

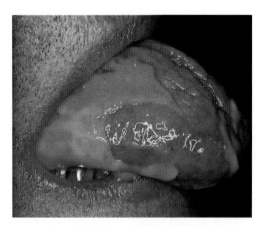

Fig. 13.9 Severe erosive lichen planus. Thick plaques of fibrin cover extensive ulcers on the dorsum of the tongue in this case.

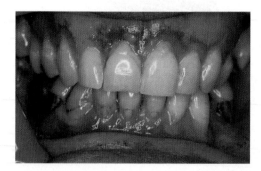

Fig. 13.11 Desquamative gingivitis caused by lichen planus. A well-defined band of patchy erythema extends across the full width of the attached gingiva around several teeth. This change may be localised or widespread. Within the red areas faint white flecks and striae are sometimes visible

margins may be slightly depressed due to fibrosis and gradual healing at the periphery. Striae may radiate from the margins of these erosions.

Plaques are occasionally seen in the early stages particularly on the dorsum of the tongue. Otherwise they may result from persistent disease and mainly affect the buccal mucosa.

Distribution

The buccal mucous membranes, particularly posteriorly, are by far the most frequently affected, but lesions may spread forward almost to the commissures. The next most common site is the tongue, either the edges or the lateral margins of the dorsum, or less frequently the centre of the dorsum. The lips and gingivae may also occasionally be affected but the floor of the mouth and palate usually escape. Lesions are very often symmetrical, sometimes strikingly so (Fig. 13.10).

Symptoms

Striae alone may be asymptomatic and unnoticed by the patient,

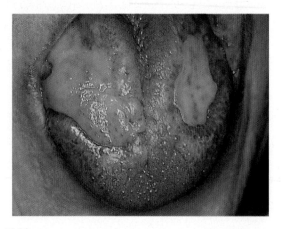

Fig. 13.10 Erosive lichen planus of the tongue. Two extensive areas of shallow ulceration have formed symmetrically on the tongue. Lingual involvement is seen, usually in severe cases where the buccal mucosa and other sites are also affected.

or cause roughness or slight stiffness of the mucosa. Atrophic lesions are sore, and erosions usually cause more severe symptoms still and may make eating difficult.

Gingival lichen planus

The gingivae are occasionally the only site of lichen planus which needs to be distinguished from other forms of gingivitis. Lesions are usually atrophic so that the gingivae appear shiny, inflamed and smooth ('desquamative gingivitis') (Fig. 13.11). Striae are uncommon but sometimes present in other parts of the mouth. Only limited segments of the gingivae may be affected.

Soreness caused by atrophic lesions makes toothbrushing difficult. Plaque accumulation and associated inflammatory changes appear to aggravate lichen planus. The contribution of local irritation to lichen planus is suggested by disappearance of the lesions when the teeth are extracted. Lichen planus of the denture-bearing area is virtually unknown.

Skin lesions

Lichen planus is a common skin disease but skin lesions are uncommon in those who complain of oral symptoms. Skin lesions typically form purplish papules, 2–3 mm across with a glistening surface marked by minute fine striae and are usually itchy. Typical sites are the flexor surface of the forearms and especially the wrists (Fig. 13.12). Skin lesions help, but are not essential, to confirm the diagnosis of oral lichen planus.

Pathology

Corresponding with their clinical features, lesions fall into three distinct histological types (Table 13.8).

Typical histological features of atrophic lesions are summarised in Table 13.9.

Erosions merely show destruction of the epithelium, leaving only the fibrin-covered, granulating connective tissue floor of the lesion. Diagnosis depends on seeing atropic lesions or striae nearby.

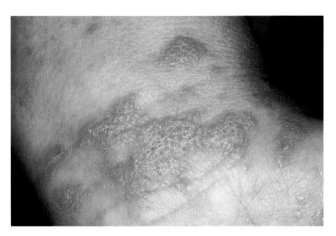

Fig. 13.12 Dermal lichen planus. This, the flexor surface of the wrists, is a characteristic site. The lesions consist of confluent papules with a pattern of minute white striae on their surface.

Table 13.8 Lichen planus: typical histological features of white lesions (striae) (Figs 13.13–13.15)

- Hyperkeratosis or parakeratosis
- Saw-tooth profile of the rete ridges sometimes
- Liquefaction degeneration of the basal cell layer
- Compact, band-like lymphoplasmacytic (predominantly T-cell) infiltrate cells hugging the epithelio-mesenchymal junction
- CD8 lymphocytes predominate in relation to the epithelium

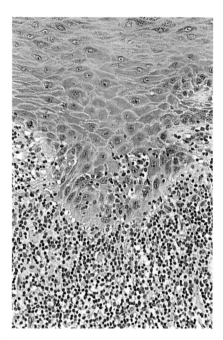

Fig. 13.14 Lichen planus. The basement membrane is thickened and lymphocytes from the dense infiltrate below emigrate into the basal cells of the epithelium where they are associated with focal basal cell degeneration.

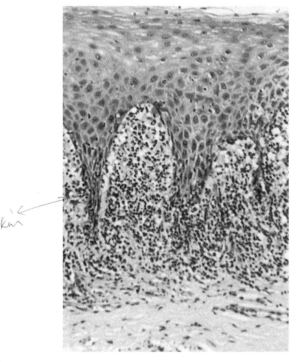

skin

Fig. 13.13 Lichen planus. The rete ridges have the characteristic pointed (saw-tooth) outline which is frequent in the skin but uncommon in mucosal lichen planus.

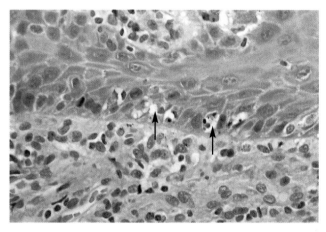

Fig. 13.15 Lichen planus. Lymphocytes infiltrating the basal cells are associated with basal cell apoptosis, loss of a prominent basal cell layer and prickle cells abutting the basement membrane. A cluster of apoptotic bodies is visible (arrows), each consisting of a shrunken bright pink cell with a condensed and fragmented nucleus.

Table 13.9 Lichen planus: typical histological features of atrophic lesions (Fig. 13.16)

- Severe thinning and flattening of the epithelium
- Destruction of basal cells
- Compact band-like, subepithelial inflammatory infiltrate hugging the epithelio-mesenchymal junction

apoptotic bodies; shrunken bright pink cell with a condensed & fragmented nucleus.

199

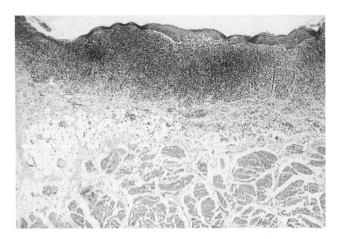

Fig. 13.16 Lichen planus. The epithelium is atrophic and greatly thinned. A well-demarcated, dense, broad band of lymphocytes extends along the superficial corium immediately below the epithelium.

Diagnosis

The diagnosis of lichen planus can usually be made on the history, the appearance of the lesions and their distribution. However, dysplastic leukoplakias occasionally have a streaky whitish appearance. A biopsy should be taken, particularly when striae are ill-defined, plaques are present or the lesions are in any other ways unusual.

Management

Patients are sometimes concerned that lichen planus is infectious and should be reassured that this is not so.

Topical application of potent anti-inflammatory corticosteroids is usually effective but monitoring is required and these preparations are suitable only for hospital use. Possible alternatives are to use similar corticosteroids (such as beclomethasone) from aerosol inhalers used for asthma. Approximately six puffs from an inhaler can be used to deliver enough of the corticosteroid to an ulcer.

Check list for management of lichen planus

Always check for drugs which might cause a lichenoid reaction. This is indistinguishable clinically but may respond to a change of medication

When inflammation worsens or symptoms become more severe consider the possibility of superinfection with candida

Biopsy lesions which appear unusual, form homogeneous plaques or are in unusual sites

Check for skin lesions which may aid diagnosis

Reassure patients that the condition is not usually of great consequence despite the fact that it can cause constant irritating soreness. Tell patients that the severity waxes and wanes unpredictably and the condition may persist for many years

Be aware that squamous carcinoma may develop in lesions, although very rarely. Follow up lesions associated with reddening, and any unusual in site, appearance or severity

---

Potent corticosteroids used topically may occasionally promote thrush as a side-effect. Triamcinolone dental paste applied to the lesions is an alternative but less effective form of treatment. Gingival lichen planus is the most difficult to treat. The first essential is to maintain rigorous oral hygiene. Corticosteroids should also be used, as already described, and in this situation triamcinolone dental paste may be useful as it can readily be applied to the affected gingivae. In unresponsive cases, tactolimus mouth-rinses may be effective. In exceptionally severe cases, if topical treatment fails, treatment with systemic corticosteroids is effective.

Lichenoid reactions

This term is given to lichen planus-like lesions caused by either systemic drug treatment or those where the histological picture is not completely diagnostic.

A very wide range of drugs can cause lichenoid reactions of the skin, mucous membranes or both (Table 13.10). The clinical features are often indistinguishable from 'true' lichen planus and usually consist only of white striae. When there is severe atrophy or ulceration, detecting a possible causative drug may aid management and a complete drug history is mandatory in all patients thought to suffer from lichen planus. Some features which suggest a drug reaction are shown in Table 13.11.

Table 13.10 Some drugs capable of causing lichenoid reactions

These are only the more common causes:
Colloidal gold
Beta-blockers
Oral hypoglycaemics
Allopurinol
Non-steroidal anti-inflammatory drugs
Antimalarials
Methyldopa
Penicillamine
Some tricyclic antidepressants
Thiazide diuretics
Captopril

Table 13.11 Features suggesting a lichenoid reaction

- Onset associated with starting a drug
- Unilateral lesions or unusual distributions
- Unusual severity
- Widespread skin lesions
- Localised lesion in contact with restoration

In practice it can be difficult or impossible to differentiate lichenoid reactions from lichen planus. Many patients are taking potentially causative drugs, sometimes more than one. However, these may not be responsible as lichen planus is so common a disease that its presence may be coincidental. Also, the drugs often cannot be stopped because of possible medical adverse effects. Changing to another drug may not be helpful as the alternative may also cause a reaction.

Proof of causation requires withdrawal and rechallenge after healing but the risk is hardly ever justified. Also, reactions may persist months or years after administration (especially after colloidal gold injection). Often a causative drug is not even suspected because it has been taken without prescription.

Biopsy can sometimes distinguish lichenoid reactions but the features are relatively subtle and not completely specific. While biopsy is of value to exclude other conditions it cannot usually distinguish lichen planus from a lichenoid reaction.

Lichenoid reactions are treated in exactly the same way as lichen planus with withdrawal of drug(s) if possible. Thus, the absolute distinction between lichen planus and lichenoid reaction is not always necessary for treatment.

Topical lichenoid reactions are most frequently responses to restorative materials, either amalgam or polymeric. The clinical appearances are similar or identical to lichen planus or lupus erythematosus but lesions are localised to mucosa in contact, not just close to, restorations.

The more sharply defined a lesion is, the more atrophic or ulcerated, and the more closely related to a restoration, the more likely it is that removal of the restoration will be effective.

Corroded amalgam restorations are more likely to trigger reactions, but which components of restorative materials are responsible remains unclear. Several metals in amalgams are haptens and patients with amalgam reactions are more likely to show hypersensitivity to metals on skin testing. Another possible cause is the tiny particles of amalgam in the mucosa, thought to be the result of removal of amalgams by air turbine. Microscopic particles are thrown from the bur with sufficient energy to penetrate the tissues but the significance is unknown.

Lichenoid reactions to restorations are confirmed when healing follows removal of the restoration. Patch testing for metal hypersensitivity and biopsy are not useful for diagnosis as the skin can react to a substance which causes no reaction in the mouth (Ch. 27). The decision whether to remove a restoration or not can therefore be a matter of trial and error.

Malignant change in lichen planus

The risk of and possible frequency of malignant change in lichen planus has long been controversial. Reportedly 1–4% of patients suffer this complication after 10 years, but there is growing controversy about such figures. Doubts about the validity of the diagnosis of lichen planus, in reports of malignant change, have been expressed — dysplastic lesions, for example, may have a streaky appearance that has been mistaken for striae. Also, because lichen planus is so common a disease, the quoted rates for malignant change would greatly exceed the actual incidence of oral cancer.

Specific risk factors have also not been identified with certainty.

LUPUS ERYTHEMATOSUS

Lupus erythematosus is a connective tissue disease which has two main forms, namely systemic and discoid. Either can give rise to oral lesions which may appear similar to those of oral lichen planus.

Systemic lupus erythematosus has varied effects (Ch. 25). Arthralgias and rashes are most common, but virtually any organ system can be affected. A great variety of autoantibodies, particularly antinuclear, is produced.

Discoid lupus is essentially a skin disease with mucocutaneous lesions indistinguishable clinically from those of systemic lupus. These may be associated with arthralgias but rarely, significant autoantibody production.

Clinically, oral lesions appear in about 20% of cases of systemic lupus, and can rarely be the presenting sign (Fig. 13.17). Typical lesions are white, often striate, areas with irregular atrophic areas or shallow erosions, but the patterns, particularly those of the striae, are typically far less sharply defined than in lichen planus. They are often patchy and unilateral and may be in the vault of the palate which lichen planus typically spares.

Lesions can form variable patterns of white and red areas. There may also be small slit-like ulcers just short of the gingival margins. In about 30% of cases, Sjögren's syndrome develops and rarely, cervical lymphadenopathy (Ch. 26) is the first sign.

Pathology

Lesions show irregular patterns of epithelial atrophy and acanthosis. Liquefaction degeneration of the basal cell layer is typical and there is PAS positive thickening of the basement membrane zone and around blood vessels due to deposition of antigen/antibody complexes (Fig. 13.18). In the corium there is

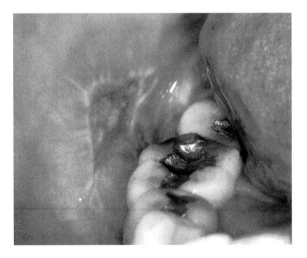

Fig. 13.17 Lupus erythematosus. The clinical presentation is often very similar to lichen planus, with ulceration, atrophy and striae. Lesions on the soft palate or with radiating striae, as here, should be investigated for lupus erythematosus.

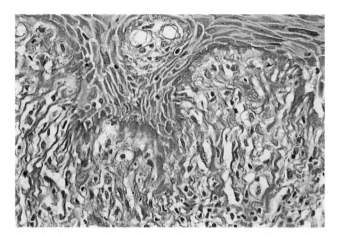

Fig. 13.18 Lupus erythematosus stained with PAS to show the thickened basement membrane.

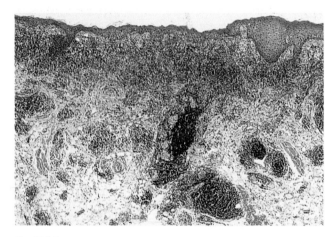

Fig. 13.19 Lupus erythematosus. The histological picture is similar to that seen in lichen planus, with a subepithelial band of lymphocytes, basal cell degeneration and epithelial atrophy. The dense perivascular infiltrates of lymphocytes in the deeper tissues are characteristic of lupus erythematosus.

oedema and often a hyaline appearance. The inflammatory infiltrate is highly variable in density, typically extends deeply into the connective tissue, and may have a perivascular distribution (Fig. 13.19).

Lupus erythematosus shows more irregular patterns of acanthosis and lacks the band-like distribution of lymphocytes in the papillary corium of lichen planus.

In frozen sections, a band of immunoglobulins and complement (C3) with a granular texture deposited along the basement membrane may be shown by immunofluorescence. This deposit also underlies normal epithelium in systemic lupus. In paraffin sections, immunoglobulin deposits may be detectable using immunoperoxidase staining. Obvious vasculitis may be seen in systemic, but not in discoid lupus erythematosus.

Diagnosis of systemic lupus erythematosus should be confirmed by the pattern of antinuclear autoantibodies. The most specific is that to double-stranded (native) DNA. Haematological findings in active SLE include a raised ESR, anaemia and, often, leukopenia or thrombocytopenia.

Oral lesions of discoid lupus erythematosus may respond in some degree to topical corticosteroids. However, oral lesions in acute systemic lupus erythematosus may not respond to doses of corticosteroids adequate to control systemic effects of the disease. Under such circumstances, palliative treatment is needed until disease activity abates.

CHRONIC ULCERATIVE STOMATITIS

This uncommon mucosal disease is associated with IgG antibodies to squamous epithelium nuclear protein.

Clinically, females over 40 years are mainly affected. Lesions are usually erosions, but sometimes lichen planus-like. Some examples have in fact, been mistaken for lichen planus clinically, so that it seems possible that antinuclear antibody chronic ulcerative stomatitis may be more common than is appreciated. Skin involvement is uncommon.

Histologically, the appearances may be similar to erosive lichen planus. However, immunofluorescence shows speckled antinuclear antibodies in the perilesional mucosa and shaggy deposits of fibrinogen in the basement membrane zone. Serum shows antinuclear antibody in high titre that reacts with guinea pig oesophagus substrate but the titre does not correspond with clinical severity. The target antigen is an epithelial nuclear protein, which has been shown to be homologous to the p53 tumour suppressor gene.

The most effective treatment appears to be with chloroquine or hydroxychloroquine, supplemented if necessary with prednisolone. However, complete clearance is not always achieved or resolution may be followed by relapses. Immunological changes also persist after clearance of the lesions. Doses of chloroquine phosphate or hydroxychloroquine sulphate should be kept below 4 mg/kg or 6.5 mg/kg respectively to minimise the risk of ocular damage. Key features of chronic ulcerative stomatitis are summarised in Table 13.12.

Table 13.12 Chronic ulcerative stomatitis: key features

- Females over 40 years mainly affected
- Lesions resemble striae or erosions of lichen planus
- Direct immunofluorescence shows speckled IgG antibodies to squamous epithelial nuclear protein
- Circulating epithelial nuclear antibodies in high titre
- Chloroquine or hydroxychloroquine moderately effective

PEMPHIGUS VULGARIS

Pemphigus is an uncommon autoimmune disease causing vesicles or bullae on skin and mucous membranes. It is usually fatal if untreated. Females usually aged 40–60 years are predominantly affected. Lesions often first appear in the mouth but spread widely on the skin. Vesicles are fragile and infrequently seen intact in the mouth. Residual erosions often have ragged edges and are superficial, painful and tender (Fig. 13.20). Gently stroking the mucosa can cause a vesicle or bulla to appear (Nikolsky's sign).

Progress of the disease is very variable. It may sometimes be fulminating with rapid development of widespread oral ulceration, spread to other sites such as the eyes within a few days, and very soon afterwards to the skin.

Skin lesions consist of vesicles or bullae varying from a few millimetres to a centimetre or so across (Fig. 13.21). The bullae at first contain clear fluid which may then become purulent

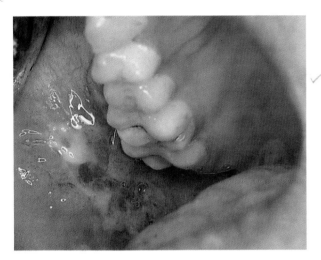

Fig. 13.20 Pemphigus vulgaris. Typical oral presentation with erythema, erosions and persistent ulcers. The surrounding epithelium is friable and disintegrates on gentle stroking.

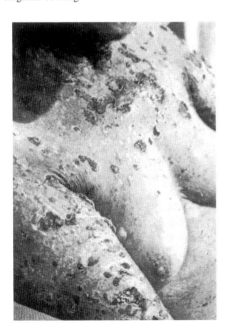

Fig. 13.21 Pemphigus vulgaris. The characteristic bullae often appear in the mouth but soon spread over the skin, forming widespread moist or crusted lesions when they rupture. (Taken before the advent of colour photography.)

or haemorrhagic. Rupture of vesicles leaves painful ragged erosions. Protein, fluid and electrolytes are lost from the raw areas and they readily become secondarily infected. Without treatment, death usually follows, but immunosuppressive treatment is usually life-saving.

Pathology

An immunopathogenesis can be more convincingly demonstrated in pemphigus vulgaris than in any other oral disease and the histological findings are summarised in Table 13.13.

The epithelial cells which lose their attachments become rounded in shape and the cytoplasm contracts around the nucleus. Small groups of these rounded-up acantholytic (*Tzanck*) cells can often be seen histologically in the contents of a vesicle or in a smear from a recently ruptured vesicle.

Pemphigus antibodies are tissue-specific and react only to the epithelial cell surface antigen, an intercellular adhesion molecule (ICAM), desmoglein 3 (Fig. 13.23). The mechanism of breakdown of intercellular attachments appears to result from synthesis of proteases by the epithelial cells.

Table 13.13 **Pemphigus vulgaris: pathology**

- Loss of intercellular adherence of suprabasal spinous cells (acantholysis)
- Formation of clefts immediately superficial to the basal cells
- Extension of clefts to form intraepithelial vesicles (Fig. 13.22)
- Rupture of vesicles to form ulcers
- High titre of circulating antibodies to epithelial 'intercellular cement substance' (desmoglein 3)
- Binding of antibodies to intercellular substance detectable by fluorescence microscopy

Management

The diagnosis must be confirmed as early as possible. Biopsy is essential and the changes are sufficiently characteristic to make a diagnosis. Immunofluorescence microscopy should be

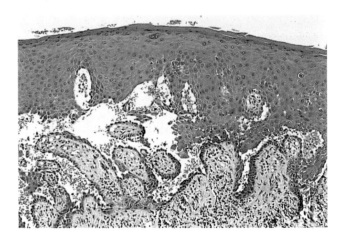

Fig. 13.22 Pemphigus. The edge of a bulla formed by separation of the epithelium just above the basal cells. There is acantholysis centrally and a layer of basal cells remains covering the dermal papillae.

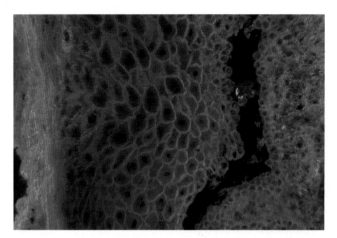

Fig. 13.23 Pemphigus vulgaris. Frozen tissue stained with fluorescent antibody to IgG shows fluorescence along the lines of the interepithelial attachments typical of pemphigus. See also Figure 1.6

used to exclude similar but less common diseases. Once the diagnosis has been confirmed, immunosuppressive treatment is required. There is little consensus about dosage but a typical regimen is 80–100 mg/day of predisolone plus azathioprine (1–1.5 mg/kg daily). Azathioprine is given to allow doses of the corticosteroid to be lowered and reduce their side-effects. Treatment can only be stopped if relapse fails to follow withdrawal and immunosuppressive treatment itself causes a significant mortality. With combined immunosuppressive treatment, the average mortality is approximately 6%. More recently mycophenolate mofetil has been used with benefit and has significantly fewer adverse effects.

The main features of the several variants of pemphigus are summarised in Appendix 13.2.

Key clinical features are summarised in Table 13.14.

Table 13.14   Pemphigus vulgaris: key clinical features

- Females predominantly affected, usually aged 40–60 years
- Lesions often first in the mouth but spread widely on the skin
- Lesions consist of fragile vesicles and bullae
- Ruptured vesicles form irregular erosions on the mucosa
- Nikolsky's sign may be positive
- Widespread skin involvement is fatal if untreated
- Good response to *prolonged* immunosuppressive treatment

MUCOUS MEMBRANE (CICATRICIAL) PEMPHIGOID

Mucous membrane pemphigoid is an uncommon chronic disease causing bullae and painful erosions (Table 13.15). Skin involvement is uncommon and often trivial. The term *cicatricial pemphigoid* is sometimes used for this group of diseases, but particularly applies to ocular involvement where scarring is prominent and impairs sight.

Lesions (Fig. 13.24) are rarely widespread and progress is very slow. 'Desquamative gingivitis' can be a manifestation

---

Table 13.15   Mucous membrane pemphigoid: typical features

- Females mainly affected and usually elderly
- Oral mucosa often the first site
- Involvement of the eyes, may cause scarring and blindness
- Skin involvement absent or minimal
- Indolent, non-fatal disease
- Oral bullae are subepithelial and frequently seen intact

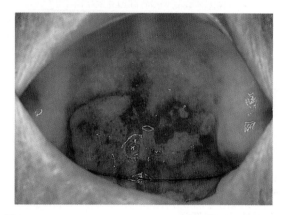

Fig. 13.24 Mucous membrane pemphigoid. Typical oral presentation with persistent erythema and ulceration of the palate. On close examination tags of epithelium are sometimes seen at the ulcer margins.

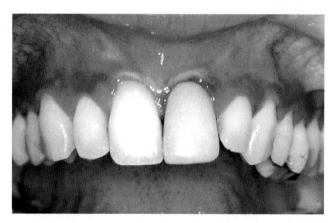

Fig. 13.25 Desquamative gingivitis as a result of mucous membrane pemphigoid. There is patchy reddening involving the attached gingivae around several teeth and in places the erythema extends to the alveolar mucosa. Unlike desquamative gingivitis caused by lichen planus, there are no flecks or striae and occasionally tags of separating epithelium may be found.

(Fig. 13.25). Nikolsky's sign is typically positive and a striking clinical finding is sometimes that the epithelium slides away underneath the edge of a sharp scalpel when a biopsy is attempted. In the mouth, bleeding into bullae can cause them to appear as blood blisters. Rupture of erosions leaves raw areas with well-defined margins. Individual erosions persist for some weeks then slowly heal. Further erosions may develop nearby and this process may persist for a year or more. Lesions may remain localised to the mouth for very long periods and may never involve other sites.

The main features of the sub-types of pemphigoid are summarised in Appendix 13.3.

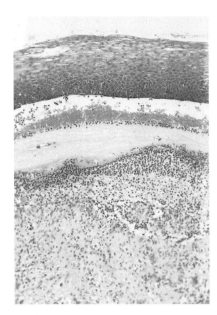

Fig. 13.26 Mucous membrane pemphigoid. The full thickness of the epithelium has separated cleanly from the underlying connective tissue to form a fluid-filled bulla. A light inflammatory infiltrate is present in the underlying connective tissue.

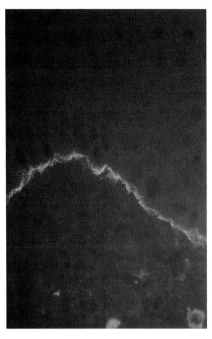

Fig. 13.27 Mucous membrane pemphigoid. Frozen tissue stained with fluorescent anti-C3 shows a line of fluorescence along the basement membrane indicating complement activation there. See also Figure 1.6.

Pathology

Histologically there is loss of attachment and separation of the full thickness of the epithelium from the connective tissue at basement membrane level. Epithelium, though separated, remains for a time intact and forms the roof of a bulla (Fig. 13.26). The floor of the bulla is formed by connective tissue alone, infiltrated with inflammatory cells. The disease is immunologically mediated, and binding of immunoglobulin or more frequently of complement components along the basement membrane zone can be demonstrated (Fig. 13.27). Circulating autoantibodies are detectable by sensitive techniques.

Management

The diagnosis is confirmed by biopsy and immunofluorescence microscopy but it is preferable to obtain an intact vesicle or bulla.

Oral mucous membrane pemphigoid can often be effectively controlled with topical corticosteroids. Doses are small and without systemic effects.

Because of the possible risk to sight, ocular examination is necessary if early changes in the eyes are suspected. If the eyes become involved, systemic corticosteroids have to be given and are effective.

'Desquamative gingivitis'

The term '*desquamative gingivitis*' is a clinical description, not a diagnosis. It is used for conditions in which the gingivae appear red or raw. Usually the whole of the attached gingiva of varying numbers of teeth is affected (see Figs 13.11 and 13.25).

Lichen planus is the most common cause. The gingivae then appear smooth, red and translucent due to the thinness of the atrophic epithelium. In older patients mucous membrane pemphigoid may cause gingival erosions. Pemphigus vulgaris is another possible cause. In all cases, the appearances are strikingly different from simple marginal gingivitis, and the diagnosis should be confirmed by biopsy.

ERYTHEMA MULTIFORME

This is a mucocutaneous disease but among dental patients oral lesions are the most prominent or the only ones present (Table 13.16).

Target lesions are red macules a centimetre or more in diameter with a bluish cyanotic centre. In severe cases skin lesions are

Table 13.16 Erythema multiforme: typical clinical features

- Occasionally triggered by herpetic infection or drugs
- Adolescents or young adults, particularly males, mainly affected
- Mild fever and systemic upset may be associated
- Lips frequently grossly swollen, split, crusted and bleeding (Fig. 13.28)
- Widespread irregular fibrin-covered erosions and erythema in the mouth (Fig. 13.29)
- Conjunctivitis may be associated
- Cutaneous lesions may consist of widespread erythema alone (Fig. 13.30), or characteristic target lesions
- Attacks may recur at intervals of several months
- Remittent but usually ultimately self-limiting

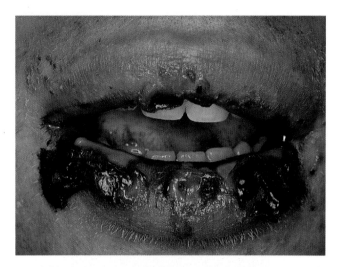

Fig. 13.28 Erythema multiforme. Ulceration of the vermilion border of the lip with bleeding, swelling and crusting is characteristic.

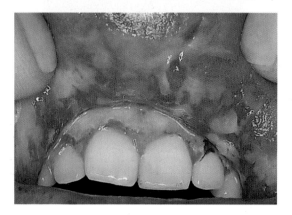

Fig. 13.29 Erythema multiforme. There is ulceration, erythema, sloughing of epithelium and a small vesicle centrally. The anterior part of the mouth and the lips are typically affected.

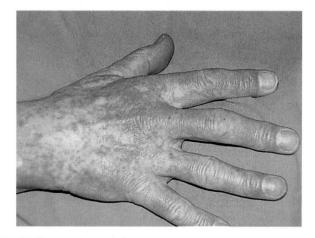

Fig. 13.30 Erythema multiforme. As the name suggests, the rash is variable and ranges from patchy erythema, as here, to the more characteristic target lesions and bullae.

bullous. The attack usually lasts for 3 or 4 weeks with new crops of lesions developing over a period of about 10 days. Recurrences, usually at intervals of several months, for a year or two are characteristic and are sometimes increasingly severe.

In the most severe cases ocular damage may impair sight and occasionally cause blindness. With widespread skin blistering this condition is known as *toxic epidermal necrolysis*. Very rarely, renal damage can be fatal.

Aetiology and pathology

The aetiology is not clear and though the disease may be reaction to a variety of causes, no convincing mechanism has been proposed. Infections, particularly herpetic, can be triggering factors. Drugs, particularly sulphonamides and barbiturates, have also been implicated, but a positive drug history is also rare. Even when drugs have been taken, coincidence cannot always be excluded and in most patients no precipitating cause can be found.

The histological appearances are variable. Widespread necrosis of keratinocytes with eosinophilic colloid change in the superficial epithelium may be conspicuous. This may progress to intraepithelial vesicle or bulla formation (Fig. 13.31). However, subepithelial vesiculation is more frequent (Fig. 13.32). Degenerative changes in the epithelium are associated with infiltration by inflammatory cells which also involve the corium and may have a perivascular distribution. Leakage of immunoglobulins from blood vessels has been reported, but vasculitis is not seen histologically.

Management

Patients should be warned of the possibility of recurrences but that the disease usually runs a limited course.

There is no specific treatment. Systemic corticosteroids may give symptomatic relief. Antibiotics are usually also given in severe cases with the idea of preventing secondary infection. Levamisole has also been reported to be effective. In some cases aciclovir is effective.

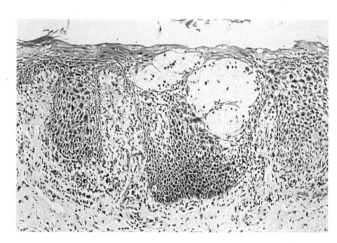

Fig. 13.31 Erythema multiforme. At higher power there is necrosis of prickle cells producing intraepithelial vescicles.

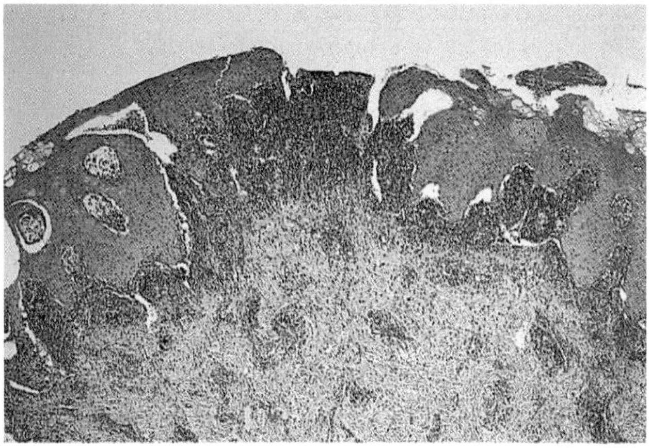

Fig. 13.32 Erythema multiforme. There is a dense inflammatory infiltrate immediately below the epithelium and around blood vessels in the deeper corium. The epithelium is separating from the connective tissue, here along the basement membrane, and there is ulceration centrally.

'Allergic' stomatitis

Many otherwise harmless substances coming into contact with the skin cause hypersensitisation in susceptible subjects. When this has happened further contact causes an inflammatory reaction. Examples are eczema or contact dermatitis caused by a wide variety of household and industrial materials. Some mucous membranes such as the eyes can also become sensitised in this way, but the different parts of the body differ widely in their response. Sulphonamide ointments, for example, are highly sensitising to the skin but cause little trouble in the eyes. The oral mucous membrane appears to show yet other differences and appears to be unable to mount reactions comparable with contact dermatitis, and there is no such condition as oral eczema. Most so-called allergic reactions of the mouth are due to direct irritation by the substance.

Even patients who are sensitised to a material such as nickel can tolerate it in the mouth; it may then cause a characteristic rash but not oral lesions. Amalgam restorations cause no trouble in patients sensitised to mercury, though the material should not be allowed to come into contact with the skin (Ch. 25). Similar considerations apply to methylmethacrylate. Those few people who are sensitised to the monomer can wear acrylic dentures with impunity. Inflammation under acrylic dentures, often in the past described as 'acrylic allergy' is usually candidal infection. Authenticated cases of contact hypersensitisation of the oral mucous membrane are so few as to make it questionable whether the oral mucosa can mount this type of reaction. If it does so it must be phenomenally rare.

MISCELLANEOUS MUCOSAL ULCERS

Eosinophilic ulcer (atypical or traumatic eosinophilic granuloma)

Tumour-like ulcerated lesions with a microscopic picture resembling that of Langerhans' cell histiocytosis, may occasionally form in the oral soft tissues, particularly the tongue, but also the gingivae and, occasionally, other sites. Sometimes there is a history of trauma and, experimentally, crush injury to muscle can induce a proliferative response with tissue eosinophilia.

Clinically, the ulcerated mass may be mistaken for a carcinoma but is typically soft: almost any age can be affected.

Pathology

There is typically a dense aggregation of eosinophils and cells which resemble histiocytes beneath the ulcerated surface. The histiocytes lack the ultrastructural features and surface markers of Langerhans' cells but are occasionally pleomorphic.

The differential diagnosis is from Langerhans' cell histiocytosis, which can be excluded by the absence of Langerhans' cells markers (Ch. 9). In practice, lesions usually heal spontaneously within 3–8 weeks, and management of an isolated soft tissue mass having these histological characteristics, should be expectant.

Ruptured blood blisters (localised oral purpura)

Rupture of blood blisters leaves painful ulcers. Bullae of mucous membrane pemphigoid sometimes fill with blood but must be distinguished from localised oral purpura or systemic purpura (Ch. 23).

Wegener's granulomatosis

Mucosal ulceration is occasionally a feature of this disease but mainly in its established stage (Ch. 28). Clinically, ulceration may be widespread but is otherwise non-specific.

Oral reactions to drugs

A great variety of drugs (Table 13.10) can cause mucosal reactions, either as local effects (Fig. 13.33) or through systemic mechanisms which are often obscure. Systemically mediated reactions include ulceration, lichenoid reactions and erythema multiforme. These reactions are discussed in more detail in Chapter 35.

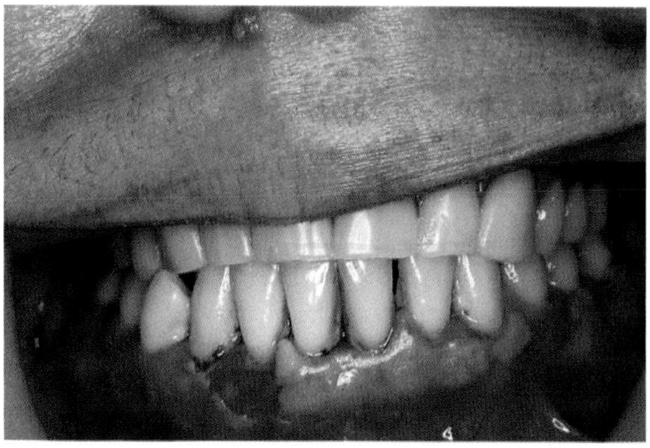

Fig. 13.33 Chemical burn. The gingivae are white and necrotic following injudicious use of a caustic agent. On the patient's right side full-thickness ulceration is present.

Some uncommon mucocutaneous diseases

In many of these conditions, the oral lesions are rare or insig-nificant in comparison with the skin disease (Table 13.17). See also pemphigus and pemphigoid variants below.

Table 13.17 Some uncommon mucosal diseases

Disease	Cause	Oral features	Treatment
Epidermolysis bullosa	Autosomal recessive — gravis type due to type VII collagen defect (junctional type usually lethal at birth)	Subepithelial bullae leading to severe intraoral scarring after minimal trauma especially in recessive types	None wholly effective. Protect against any mucosal abrasion
Pyostomatitis vegetans	Complication of inflammatory bowel disease particularly ulcerative colitis	Yellowish miliary pustules in thickened, erythematous mucosa release pus, leaving shallow ulcers. Suprabasal clefting and intraepithelial vesiculation or abscesses containing eosinophils. Sometimes intercellular Ig. Peripheral eosinophilia up to 20% of WBC	Control of inflammatory bowel disease or systemic prednisolone
Gonorrhoea	N. gonorrhoeae sexually transmitted	Oropharyngeal erythema or ulcers rarely seen	Amoxycillin, spectinomycin or a 4-quinoline
Reiter's disease	Urethritis, conjunctivitis, arthritis. Post-infective reaction	Painless circinate white lesions, histologically psoriasis-like	Oral lesions self-limiting
Leprosy	Mycobacterium leprae	Oral ulcers or nodules. Seen mainly in Asia	Dapsone
Keratosis follicularis (Darier's disease; warty dyskeratoma)	Genetic. Autosomal dominant	Intraepithelial bullae containing granulocytes and acantholytic cells Pebbly lesions mainly of palate due to hyperkeratosis, acantholysis with 'corps ronds' and 'grains' (dyskeratosis)	Oral lesions not troublesome but respond to retinoids

APPENDIX 13.1 TREATMENT FOR APHTHOUS STOMATITIS

Exclude underlying causes e.g. iron, vitamin B_{12} and folate deficiency. Treat these first		
Exclude possibility of Behçet's disease; if likely, refer to specialist centre		
Select treatments approximate to severity and patients' expectations of treatment. Patients may need to try several before they find one that works well for them		
Before drug treatment, reassure patients that RAS is common, not serious but troublesome with no significance for general health. Advise to avoid spicy, sharp and salty food and acid and carbonated drinks (or use a straw) when ulcers are present. Such reassurance and advice may be sufficient for those with only occasional ulcers.		
Select a treatment from those below. Those in the shaded boxes are not suitable for treatment in general dental practice because of the need to monitor for adverse effects but could be prescribed in conjunction with the patient's medical practitioner.		
Preparations marked* are available without prescription in the UK. Triamcinolone in Orabase can only be supplied over the counter in a 5 g tube for 5 days use		
Note that children less than 6 years old cannot rinse and expectorate effectively		
Treatment	Instructions	Indication/problems
Covering agents, e.g. carboxymethylcellulose paste (Orabase)*, carmellose sodium*	Apply QDS to dried areas around ulcer with moist finger. Allow film to hydrate before contact with adjacent mucosa. Use as required	Infrequent ulcers anteriorly in sulci, ideally single ulcers. Handling is difficult, patient must be dextrous. Unpleasant texture and taste. Symptomatic treatment only by protecting ulcer.

Treatment	Instructions	Indication/problems
Topical gels, e.g. Carbenoxolone (Bioral)*, choline salicylate (Bonjela)*, aminacrine and lignocaine (various)*	Use according to manufacturer's instructions	Ulcers must be accessible. Carbenoxolone is claimed to speed healing but the others are symptomatic treatments only. Choline salicylate is not associated with Reye's syndrome and may be used in children. Large amounts can cause salicylate poisoning in small children
Mouthwashes, e.g. obtundents (benzydamine)* or antiseptics (Chlorhexidine)*	Use according to manufacturer's instructions. Hold in mouth for 1–2 minutes for maximum effect	Infrequent ulcers or crops of ulcers (recurring > 6-weekly), useful when ulcers are widely separated around the mouth or inaccessible to pastes and gels. Benzydamine is a symptomatic treatment only. Antiseptics may shorten healing time, presumably by reducing bacterial colonisation of the ulcer surface. Benzydamine may sting and chlorhexidine has unpleasant taste and causes staining
Low potency steroid, e.g. hydrocortisone sodium succinate (Corlan) pellets 2.5 mg	Hold pellet on ulcer and allow to dissolve in contact, QDS	Single ulcers or crops of clustered ulcers. Ulcer must be accessible, usually in sulcus. No significant adverse effects, safe in children. If used regularly have slight therapeutic effect and may reduce recurrence. Very slow to dissolve
Low potency steroid paste, e.g. triamcinolone 0.1% in Orabase*	As covering agents	See covering agents. If used regularly has slight therapeutic effect and may reduce recurrence rate. Much of the symptomatic effect derives from the Orabase vehicle
Tetracycline mouthwash	Dissolve *soluble* tetracycline capsule contents (very few preparations available) 250 mg in 5–10 ml water and rinse for 2–3 minutes QDS 5 days	Particularly useful for herpetiform ulceration. Not for those aged less than 12 years. Long courses predispose to candidosis
Steroid aerosols, e.g. beclomethasone diproprionate (100 micrograms/puff)	1 puff per ulcer QDS max, maximum 8 puffs per day	Useful to deliver potent steroids to inaccessible areas, e.g. oropharynx. Spreads dose fairly widely and so more useful in widespread ulceration from lichen planus than in RAS. Risk of steroid adverse effects with prolonged use
Steroid mouthwash, e.g. betamethasone sodium phosphate	Dissolve 0.5 mg in 5 ml water and rinse for 2–3 minutes QDS from onset of prodrome and while ulcer or symptoms present. For severe ulceration may be used six times daily	Useful for widespread ulcers and when severity merits potent therapeutic treatment, e.g. crops of ulcers 6-weekly or more frequently, RAS major or severe pain. Significant risk of steroid adverse effects with prolonged use — important to spit out after use. In severe cases dose may be swallowed for a short period for additional systemic effect
Systemic drugs, e.g. steroids, azathiaprine, colchicine, thalidomide, intralesional steroid injection (major RAS only)	Various regimes	Reserved for the most severe minor RAS, major RAS and ulcers refractory to other treatments. Colchicine and Thalidomide are particularly effective in Behçet's disease and RAS major. Significant risk of adverse effects — reserved for treatment in specialist centres

APPENDIX 13.2 PEMPHIGUS VARIANTS

These may resemble pemphigus vulgaris clinically, but differ in their histological features, target antigens and response to treatment.

Paraneoplastic pemphigus

Associated particularly with lymphomas, leukaemias and Castleman's disease. Severe mucosal involvement. Varied skin lesions. Suprabasal intraepithelial acantholysis. IgG deposits on cell surfaces throughout the epithelium. IgG deposits along BMZ. Circulating IgG autoantibodies. Several target antigens including desmogleins 1 and 3. Usually resolves with removal of the tumour, but stomatitis sometimes intractable.

IgA pemphigus

Rare mucosal involvement. Skin vesicles or pustules. Neutrophil infiltration and acantholysis of epithelium. Circulating IgA autoantibodies in 50%. Usually responds to dapsone.

Pemphigus herpetiformis

Occasional mucosal involvement. Pruritic skin lesions. Eosinophilic spongiosis and intraepithelial pustules, with or without acantholysis. Target antigens, desmoglein 1 and sometimes desmoglein 3. Responds to dapsone, sometimes with immunosuppressive treatment.

Pemphigus foliaceus

No mucosal involvement. Target antigen desmoglein 1.

APPENDIX 13.3 SUB-TYPES OF PEMPHIGOID

Linear IgA disease

Predominantly cutaneous but mucosal involvement frequent; ocular disease rare. Subepithelial blistering with mixed inflammatory infiltrate including eosinophils. Linear band of IgA along BMZ. Circulating IgA autoantibodies in low titre.

Bullous pemphigoid

Skin bullae with rare oral involvement. Not histologically distinguishable from mucous membrane pemphigoid.

Anti-epiligrin pemphigoid

Mucocutaneous blistering, but rare ocular or laryngeal involvement. Intense linear IgG deposition along BMZ. Circulating IgG antibodies. Target antigen, laminin 5 and its subunits. Immunosuppressive treatment may be required.

Anti-p105 pemphigoid

Severe mucosal and skin blistering may have sudden onset. Subepithelial blistering with papillary neutrophil infiltration. Linear deposits of IgG and C3 along BMZ. Circulating IgG antibodies against a 105-kDa component of BMZ.

Note: The last two entities have been only recently recognised, so that they have not yet been fully characterised.

SUGGESTED FURTHER READING

Allen C M 1998 Is lichen planus really premalignant? Oral Surg Oral Med Oral Pathol Oral Radiol Endod 85:347

Amagai M 2000 Towards a better understanding of pemphigus autoimmunity. Brit J Dermatol 143:237–243

Calabrese L, Fleischer A B 2000 Thalidomide: current and potential clinical applications. Am J Med 108:487–495

Carson P J, Hameed A, Ahmed A R 1996 Influence of treatment on the clinical course of pemphigus vulgaris. J Am Acad Dermatol 34:645–652

Cawson R A, Binnie W H, Barrett A W, Wright J 2001 *Oral disease*, 3rd Edn. Mosby-Wolfe, London

Cervera R, Navarro M, López-Soto A, Cid M-C, Font J, Esparza J et al 1994 Antibodies to endothelial cells in Behçet's disease: cell binding activity heterogeneity and association with clinical activity. Ann Rheum Dis 53:265–267

Chan L S, Yancey K B, Hammerberg C, Soong H K, Regezi J A, Johnson K, Cooper K D 1993 Immune-mediated subepithelial blistering diseases of mucous membranes. Arch Dermatol 129:448–455

Chorzelski T P, Olszewska M, Jarzabek-Chorzelski M, Jablonsa S 1998 Is chronic ulcerative stomatitis an entity? Clinical and immunological findings in 18 cases. Eur J Dermatol 8:261–265

Church L F, Schosser R H 1992 Chronic ulcerative stomatitis associated with stratified epithelial specific antinuclear antibodies. A case report of a newly described entity. Oral Surg Oral Med Oral Pathol 73:579–582

Cribier B, Garnier C, Lausriat D, Heid E 1994 Lichen planus and hepatitis C virus infection: an epidemiologic study. J. Am Acad Dermatol 31:1070–1072

Eisen D, Ellis C N, Duell E A, Griffiths C E M, Voorhees J J 1990 Effect of topical cyclosporine rinses on oral lichen planus. A double blind analysis. N Engl J Med 323:290–294

Enk A H, Knop J 1999 Mycophenolate is effective in the treatment of pemphigus vulgaris. Arch Dermatol 135:54–56

Hietanen J, Pihlman K, Linder E, Reunala T 1987 No evidence of hypersensitivity to dental restorative materials in oral lichen planus. Scand J Dent Res 95:320–327

Ho V C, Gupta A K, Ellis C N, Nickoloff B J, Vorrhees J J 1990 Treatment of severe lichen planus with cyclosporine. J Am Acad Dermatol 22:64–68

Horie N, Shimoyama T, Kato T et al 2000 Eosinophilic ulcer of the tongue: a case report with immunohistochemical study. Oral Med Pathol 4:25–29

Huilgol S C, Bhogal B S, Black M M 1995 Immunofluorescence of the immunobullous disorders. Eur J Dermatol 5:186–195

Karjalainen T K, Tomich C E 1989 A histopathologic study of oral mucosal lupus erythematosus. Oral Surg Oral Med Oral Pathol 67:547–554

SUGGESTED FURTHER READING (*cont'd*)

Laeijendecker R, van Joost T 1994 Oral manifestations of gold allergy. J Am Acad Dermatol 30:205–209

Laine J, Kalimo K, Forssell H, Happonen R-P 1992 Resolution of oral lichenoid lesions in patients allergic to mercury compounds. Br J Dermatol 126:10–15

Lee L A, Walsh P, Prater C A et al 1999 Characterization of an autoantigen associated with chronic ulcerative stomatitis: the CUSP autoantigen is a member of the p53 family. J Invest Dermatol 133:146–151

Lee K-H, Bang D, Choi E-S et al 1999 Presence of circulating antibodies to a disease-specific antigen on cultured human dermal microvascular endothelial cells in patients with Behçet's disease. Arch Dermatol Res 291:374–381

Lozada-Nur F 2000 Oral lichen planus and oral cancer: is there enough evidence: Oral Surg Oral Med Oral Pathol Radiol Endod 89:265–266

Lozada-Nur F, Gorsky M, Silverman S 1989 Oral erythema multiforme: clinical observations and treatment of 95 patients. Oral Surg Oral Med Oral Pathol 67:36–40

MacPhail L A, Greenspan D, Feigal D W, Lennette E T, Greenspan J 1991 Recurrent aphthous ulcers in association with HIV infection. Description of ulcer types and analysis of T-lymphocyte subsets. Oral Surg Oral Med Oral Pathol 71:678–683

Porter S R, Bain S E, Scully C M 1992 Linear IgA disease manifesting as recalcitrant desquamative gingivitis. Oral Surg Oral Med Oral Pathol 74:179–182

Porter S R, Kirby A, Olsen I et al 1997 Immunologic aspects of dermal and oral lichen planus. A review. Oral Surg Oral Med Oral Pathol Oral Radiol Endod 83:358–366

Porter S R, Scully C, Flint S 1988 Hematologic status in recurrent aphthous stomatitis compared with other oral diseases. Oral Surg Oral Med Oral Pathol 66:41–44

Porter S R, Scully C, Pedersen A 1998 Recurrent aphthous stomatitis. Crit Rev Oral Biol Med 9:306–321

Rehberger A, Püspök A, Stallmeister T et al 1998 Chrohn's disease masquerading as aphthous ulcers. Eur J Dermatol 8:274–276

Sakane T, Takeno M, Suzuki N et al 1999 Behçet's disease. N Engl J Med 341:1284–1291

Scully C, de Almeida O P, Porter S R et al 1999 Pemphigus vulgaris: the manifestations and long-term management of 55 patients with oral lesions. Br J Dermatol 140:84–90

Scully C, Carrozzo M, Gandolfo S et al 1999 Update on mucous membrane pemphigoid. A heterogeneous immune-mediated subepithelial blistering entity. Oral Surg Oral Med Oral Pathol Oral Radiol Endod 88:56–68

Scully C, Porter S R 1989 Recurrent aphthous stomatitis: current concepts of etiology, pathogenesis and treatment. J Oral Pathol Med 18:21–27

van der Meij E H, Reibel J, Slootweg P J et al 1999 Interobserver and intraobserver variability in the histologic assessment of oral lichen planus. J Oral Pathol Med 28:274–277

Van der Meij E H, Schepman K P, Smeele L E et al 1999 A review of the recent literature regarding malignant transformation of oral lichen planus. Oral Surg Oral Med Oral Pathol Radiol Endod 88:307–310

Van Gestel A, Koopman R, Wijnands M, van de Putte L, van Riel P 1994 Mucocutaneous reactions to gold: a prospective study of 74 patients with rheumatoid arthritis. J Rheumatol 21:1814–1819

Vente C, Reich K, Ruuprecht R et al 1999 Erosive lichen planus: response to topical treatment with tacrolimus. Br J Dermatol 14:338–342

Vincent S D, Lilly G E, Baker K A 1993 Clinical, historic, and therapeutic features of cicatricial pemphigoid. A literature review and open therapeutic trials with corticosteroids. Oral Surg Oral Med Oral Pathol 76:453–459

Williams J V, Marks J G, Billingsley E M 2000 Use of mycophenolate mofetil in the treatment of paraneoplastic pemphigus. Br J Dermatol 142:506–509

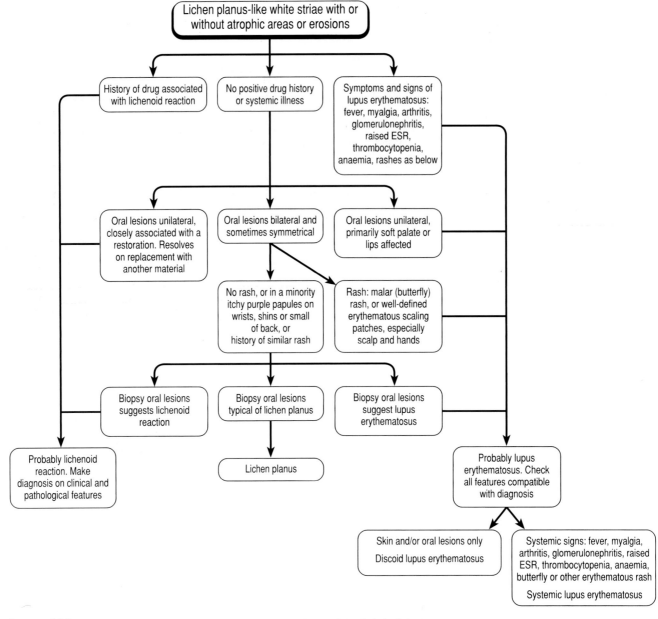

Summary 13.1 Differential diagnosis of oral lichen planus and conditions which mimic it clinically.

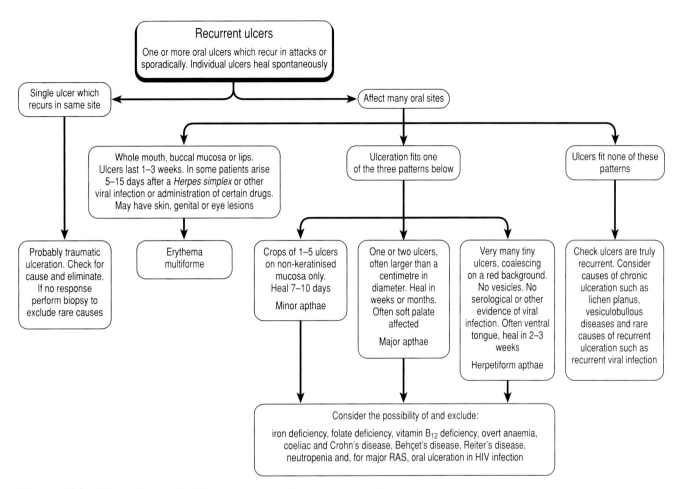

Summary 13.2 Differential diagnosis of the common causes of recurrent oral ulceration.

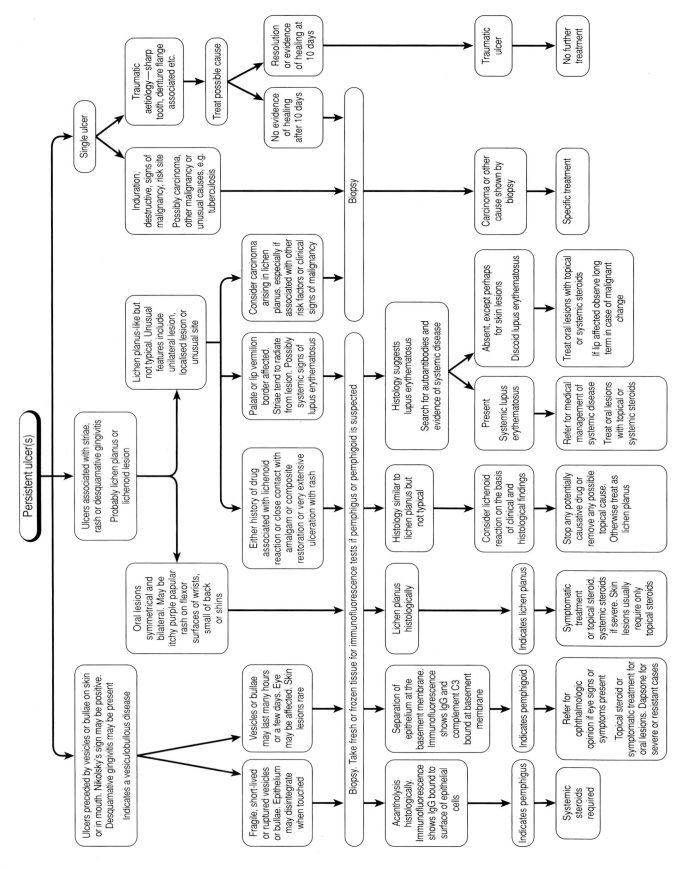

Summary 13.3 Differential diagnosis and management of persistent oral ulceration.

CHAPTER 14 Tongue disorders

The tongue can be involved in generalised stomatitis, as in herpetic stomatitis for example, and show lesions similar to those in other parts of the mouth. The tongue is also the site of lesions or the source of symptoms peculiar to itself. For unknown reasons, it can manifest the earliest symptoms of anaemia or latent defects of haemopoiesis.

Patients are also aware that doctors traditionally look at the tongue. As a result, they look at their own and as a consequence sometimes worry about insignificant changes or think normal features, such as the foliate papilla, are a cause for concern.

THE SORE TONGUE

There are several clinical types of sore tongue (Table 14.1).

Ulceration of the tongue

The tongue may be involved in, or even the predominantly affected site of, various types of stomatitis such as herpes simplex or, more frequently, lichen planus (see Fig. 13.10). The tongue may also be the site of solitary ulcers, particularly carcinoma, which when far back may be difficult to see. The lateral borders are affected and carcinoma of the dorsum of the tongue is exceptionally rare.

When there are definable lesions of these kinds, diagnosis is usually straightforward and depends on clinical examination and sometimes biopsy.

Glossitis

Glossitis is the term used for the red, smooth and sore tongue particularly characteristic of anaemia. These features are a combination of *signs* (redness and smoothness) and a *symptom*

Table 14.1 Clinical types of sore tongue

- Ulcers (of any type) involving the tongue
- Glossitis (red and sore tongue)
- The sore, physically normal tongue
- Geographical tongue (erythema migrans)

(soreness) which are not always associated. Tongues can be sore in the absence of visible changes or smooth but asymptomatic from a variety of causes (Table 14.2).

Table 14.2 Important causes of glossitis

- Anaemia
- Vitamin B group (especially B_{12}) deficiencies
- Candidosis

Iron deficiency and pernicious anaemia are the main causes (Fig. 14.1). Women are more frequently affected. Detailed haematological examination is essential. These investigations are important, as a fall in haemoglobin level may lag behind other changes. Thus there may be glossitis, haematological signs of a deficiency state, but a haemoglobin level within

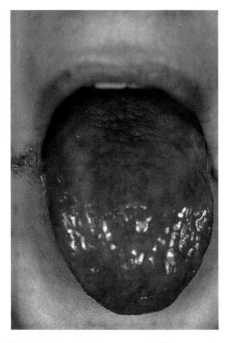

Fig. 14.1 Glossitis in iron-deficiency anaemia. The tongue is smooth due to atrophy of the papillae, and is red and sore. Anaemia is the commonest diagnosable cause of glossitis and must always be looked for by haematological examination.

215

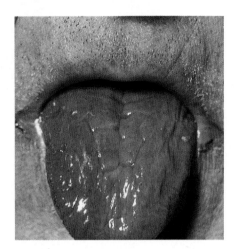

Fig. 14.2 Glossitis in antibiotic stomatitis. The tongue is red, smooth and sore as in anaemic glossitis, but the appearance is partly due to inflammatory oedema. Similar changes affect the rest of the mucosa and other features of candidosis, such as thrush, are often present.

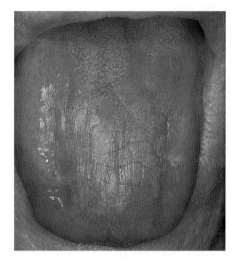

Fig. 14.3 Smooth tongue due to lichen planus. This is a late change due to longstanding disease. The tongue is smooth due to atrophy of the papillae, but has a faint silvery sheen. There are usually no symptoms at this stage.

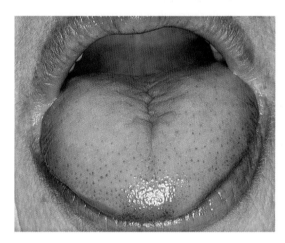

Fig. 14.4 A normal-looking but persistently sore tongue in a doctor's wife who had had repeated but inadequate haematological investigations which failed to detect early pernicious anaemia.

normal limits. Abnormalities of the red cells may be seen in a stained film, but the red cell MCV (mean corpuscular volume) is frequently a useful guide. Serum levels of iron and ferritin, B_{12} or folate (as the case may be) are depressed. When abnormalities such as these are found, specific treatment quickly relieves the symptoms.

Glossitis with angular stomatitis is characteristic of riboflavin deficiency and sometimes of nicotinic acid deficiency, but these are rare. The diagnosis of vitamin deficiency should not be made on oral signs alone in an otherwise healthy patient. These B group vitamins are frequently given in an attempt to relieve sore tongue but are virtually invariably ineffective. Their ineffectiveness makes it clear that deficiency of these vitamins is not the cause.

Candidosis can cause the tongue to be red, sore and oedematous. This is typical of acute antibiotic stomatitis (Fig. 14.2) and often then associated with angular stomatitis and other features of candidosis. This condition is rarely seen now that antibiotics are used less indiscriminately than in the past and topical oral antibiotics have now been discredited for oral infections. In Sjögren's syndrome, the tongue becomes red and acquires a cobblestone texture (see Fig. 18.11).

Lichen planus can produce a smooth tongue due to atrophy of the papillae (particularly late in long-standing disease) but there is then no soreness and typically no erythema. There is often a bluish-white sheen to the surface of the tongue, and other signs of lichen planus may be seen in other parts of the mouth (Fig. 14.3).

The sore, physically normal tongue

This type creates the most difficult problems. The symptoms are frequently psychogenic, but it is essential to exclude organic disease, particularly a haematological deficiency.

Haematological deficiencies. Soreness can precede visible, physical changes (Fig. 14.4). The haemoglobin is frequently

within normal limits but there are other abnormalities as described earlier. Treatment of the deficiency quickly relieves the symptoms.

Psychogenic disorders. Soreness of the tongue frequently appears to be psychogenic and sometimes termed 'burning mouth syndrome'. Some regard it as a variant of atypical facial pain and it is discussed in Chapter 34.

Geographical tongue (erythema migrans linguae)

In this condition there is the recurrent appearance and disappearance of red areas on the tongue. The cause is unknown but sometimes there is a clear family history of its presence in several generations. The abnormality can sometimes therefore be seen in infancy, but is probably not often noticed then. Most cases are seen in middle-aged patients. It seems improbable (but not impossible) that the condition has remained unnoticed

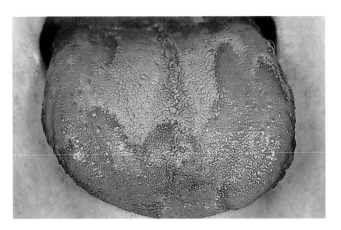

Fig. 14.5 Erythema migrans. Typical appearance with irregular depapillated patches centred on the lateral border of the tongue. Each patch has a narrow red and white rim.

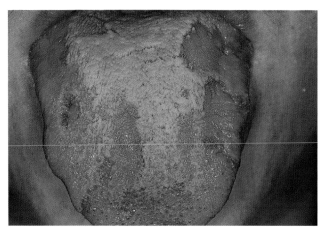

Fig. 14.6 Erythema migrans. The change of pattern can be seen, on a later occasion, in the same patient as in Fig. 14.5.

for so long. In many patients geographical tongue seems to be a developmental anomaly but there also appears to be an association with psoriasis.

Clinically, an irregular, smooth, red area appears, usually with a sharply-defined edge, where the filiform papillae stop short (Fig. 14.5). It extends for a few days, then heals, only to appear again in another area (Fig. 14.6). Sometimes the lesion is annular with a slightly raised pale margin, and several of these areas may coalesce to form a scalloped pattern. Most patients have no symptoms but some adults complain of soreness. One possible reason is that the patient has become anxious that cancer is the cause and needs to be reassured. In others, soreness may be due to an underlying haematological deficiency state, and the lesion is coincidental.

However, even children with geographical tongue sometimes complain that it is sufficiently hypersensitive to prevent them eating certain foods. The areas of epithelial thinning and inflammatory changes may therefore cause symptoms in some. Soreness in association with geographical tongue may also be psychogenic, and may then respond to appropriate treatment. Some evidence suggests a significant association between geographical tongue and emotional disturbance. However, there remains a group where no cause for the soreness can be found and no treatment seems to be effective.

Histologically, there is thinning of the epithelium in the centre of the lesion with mild hyperplasia and hyperkeratosis at the periphery (Fig. 14.7); there are chronic inflammatory cells in the underlying connective tissue. Sometimes the changes are the same as those of psoriasis.

THE FOLIATE PAPILLAE

The foliate papillae are bilateral, pinkish soft nodules on the lateral borders of the tongue at the junction of the anterior two-thirds and the posterior third (Ch. 1). They enclose lymphoid

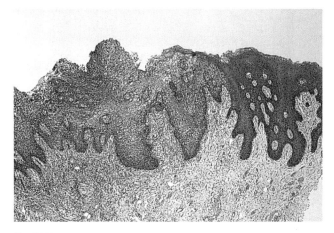

Fig. 14.7 Erythema migrans. The edge of a lesion showing normal mucosa to the right, and to the left the epithelium densely infiltrated by neutrophils. This epithelium at the advancing edge will be shed, leaving the depapillated red patch.

follicles which sometimes become hyperplastic or inflamed and sore (see Figs 1.1 and 1.2). The appearance sometimes alarms patients who need to be reassured that they are normal structures.

LINGUAL VARICOSITIES

Dilated tortuous veins may be seen along the ventral surface of the tongue and tend to become more prominent with age (Fig. 14.8). They may be noticed by patients who need to be reassured that they are not abnormal.

HAIRY TONGUE

The filiform papillae can become elongated and hair-like,

forming a thick fur on the dorsum of the tongue. The filaments may be up to half a centimetre long and pale brown to black in colour (Fig. 14.9). Adults are affected but the cause is unknown. Heavy smoking, excessive use of antiseptic mouthwashes, and defective diet have been blamed, but their effect is questionable. The discolouration is probably caused by pigment-producing bacteria and fungi but not *Candida albicans*.

Treatment is difficult. The measure most likely to succeed is to persuade the patient to scrape off the hyperplastic papillae and vigorously cleanse the dorsum of the tongue with a firm toothbrush. This removes large numbers of microorganisms mechanically and also, by removing the overgrown papillae, makes conditions less favourable for their proliferation.

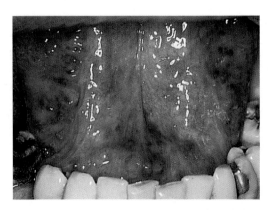

Fig. 14.8 Lingual varices. The formation of varicosities in the vessels of the undersurface of tongue and floor of mouth is a common finding with age. Occasionally such varices may be the site of thrombosis.

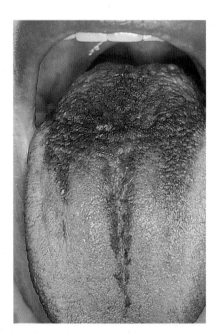

Fig. 14.9 Hairy tongue. In this patient there are numerous elongated papillae but a brown rather than black pigmentation.

Black tongue

The dorsum of the tongue may sometimes become black without overgrowth of the papillae. This may be staining due to drugs such as iron compounds used for the treatment of anaemia, but is then transient. Occasionally the sucking of antiseptic lozenges causes the tongue to become black, and this may be due to pigment-producing organisms, particularly Bacteroides strains.

Furred tongue

The tongue can become coated with desquamating cells and debris, in those who smoke heavily, in many systemic upsets, especially of the gastrointestinal tract, and infections in which the mouth becomes dry and little food is taken. A furred tongue is often seen in the childhood fevers, especially scarlet fever.

MEDIAN RHOMBOID GLOSSITIS

Median rhomboid glossitis is an abnormality in the midline of the dorsum of the tongue at the junction of the anterior two-thirds with the posterior third. The site suggests that it is developmental but it is not seen in children and no longer accepted that it results from persistence of the tuberculum impar.

Clinically, median rhomboid glossitis is seen in adults and is typically symptomless. It appears as a nodular red or pink area of depapillation (Fig. 14.10). Alternatively it may be white (Fig. 14.11).

Its chief importance is that the histological features have sometimes been mistaken for a carcinoma and treated accordingly. Quite apart from the need for proper histological assessment, carcinoma virtually never develops in this site.

Histologically, the appearances are also variable and include irregular hyperplasia with an inflammatory infiltrate (Fig. 14.12), a granular cell tumour with pseudoepitheliomatous hyperplasia (Ch. 20), or candidosis may be superimposed (the white variant).

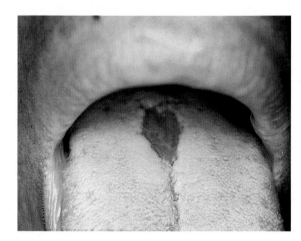

Fig. 14.10 Median rhomboid glossitis. The typical lozenge-shaped area of depapillation in the midline of the tongue.

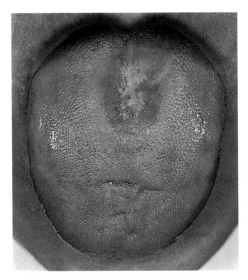

Fig. 14.11 Median rhomboid glossitis. There is a whitish patch of depapillation with sharply demarcated borders in the midline of the tongue.

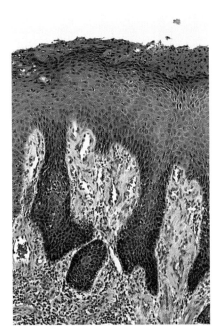

Fig. 14.12 Median rhomboid glossitis. There is hyperplasia with elongated rete processes, hyperparakeratosis and an inflammatory infiltrate of lymphocytes and plasma cells in the connective tissue. There are no signs of candidal infection.

Management

Reassurance is usually the main requirement. Candidosis can be recognised by finding hyphae in a Gram-stained smear and can be treated with an antifungal drug. However, a pink or lobulated abnormality will remain. Observation is required to detect any enlargement of the area but a need for biopsy is unlikely.

Table 14.4 Important causes of macroglossia

- Congenital haemangioma or lymphangioma (Fig. 14.13 and Ch. 20)
- Down's syndrome (Ch. 33)
- Cretinism (Ch. 31)
- Acromegaly (Ch. 31)
- Amyloidosis (Ch. 9)
- Lingual thyroid (Ch. 31)

MACROGLOSSIA

Important causes are summarised in Table 14.4.

Amyloidosis

Amyloidosis is an important cause of macroglossia since it is usually associated with life-threatening disease, particularly multiple myeloma (Ch. 9). Amyloidosis is the deposition in the tissues of an abnormal protein with characteristic staining properties. It can result from overproduction of immunoglobulin light chains, usually by multiple myeloma. In over 20% of such cases, amyloid is deposited in the mouth, particularly the tongue, to cause macroglossia or localised swellings or both (Fig. 9.24). Macroglossia due to amyloid can be so gross as to protrude from the mouth. Purpura and anaemia may be associated.

Pathology

Amyloid appears as weakly eosinophilic, hyaline homogeneous material. It is typically perivascular and stains with Congo red, which also shows a characteristic apple green birefringence under polarised light (see Fig. 9.25). There is also fluorescence with thioflavine T and a characteristic fibrillary structure by electron microscopy.

Widespread amyloidosis can cause fatal renal failure, but progress of the disease may be delayed by chemotherapy. Alternatively the patient may die from myeloma when it is the cause of amyloidosis.

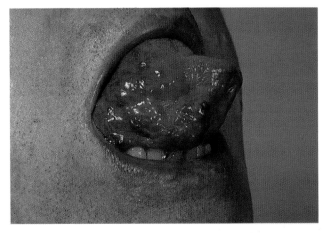

Fig. 14.13 Macroglossia due to a congenital haemangioma.

SUGGESTED FURTHER READING

Dawson T A J, Pielou W D 1967 Geographic tongue in three generations. Br J Dermatol 79:678–681

Field E A, Speechley J A, Rugman F R 1995 Oral signs and symptoms in patients with undiagnosed vitamin B_{12} deficiency. J Oral Pathol Med 24:468–470

Kleinhauz I E M, Baht R, Littner M 1994 Antecedents of burning mouth syndrome (glossodynia) — recent life events vs psychopathologic events. J Dent Res 73:567–572

Morris L F, Phillips C M, Binnie W H et al 1992 Oral lesions in patients with psoriasis. Cutis 49:339–344

O'Connor N, Bunch C 1995 Laboratory diagnosis in haematology. Medicine Int 23:489–494

Pippard M J, Heppleston A D 1996 Microcytic and macrocytic anaemias. Medicine Int 24:4–10

Rojo L, Silvestre F J, Bagan J V, De Vincente T 1994 Prevalence and psychopathology in burning mouth syndrome. Oral Surg Oral Med Oral Patol 78:312–316

Benign chronic white mucosal lesions

The appearance of most mucosal white lesions is due to hyperkeratosis; any excess keratin, becoming sodden with saliva, appears white. Apart from the lingual filiform papillae, visible keratinisation of any significant degree is abnormal in the mouth.

Chronic mucosal white plaques have sometimes been termed *leukoplakias*. This term literally means no more than a white plaque but in the past, was widely but mistakenly regarded as implying premalignancy. However, only a small minority of white patches are premalignant (Ch. 16). The majority, without malignant potential, are discussed here (Table 15.1).

Table 15.1 Important causes of benign mucosal white lesions

Prevalence	Lesion	Cause
Common	Leukoedema	Normal variation
	Frictional keratosis	Friction
	Cheek-biting	Cheek biting
	Fordyce's granules	Developmental
	Stomatitis nicotina	Pipe smoking
	Thrush	Candidal infection
Uncommon	Chemical	Caustic chemicals
	Hairy leukoplakia	Epstein–Barr virus
	White sponge naevus	Genetic
	Chronic mucocutaneous candidosis	Candidal infection/ immunodeficiency
	Psoriasis	Uncertain
	Oral keratosis of renal failure	Uncertain
	Verruciform xanthoma	Uncertain
	Skin grafts	Iatrogenic

LEUKOEDEMA

Leukoedema is a bilateral, diffuse, translucent greyish thickening, particularly of the buccal mucosa. It is a variation of normal, present in 90% of blacks and variable numbers of whites.

Histologically, there is thickening of the epithelium with intracellular oedema of the spinous layer.

Treatment is unnecessary but reassurance may be required.

FRICTIONAL KERATOSIS AND CHEEK BITING

White patches can be caused by prolonged mild abrasion of the mucous membrane by such irritants as a sharp tooth, cheek biting or dentures.

Clinical features

At first, the patches are pale and translucent (Fig. 15.1), but later become dense and white, sometimes with a rough surface. Habitual cheek biting causes an area of buccal mucosa to appear patchily red and white with a rough surface (Fig. 15.2).

Pathology

The epithelium is moderately hyperplastic with a prominent granular cell layer and thick hyperkeratosis but no dysplasia (Fig. 15.3). There are often scattered chronic inflammatory cells in the corium.

Management

Removal of the irritant causes the patch quickly to disappear. Biopsy is necessary only if the patch persists. Frictional

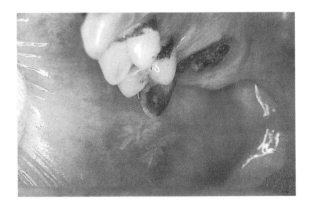

Fig. 15.1 Frictional keratosis. A poorly-defined patch of keratosis on the buccal mucosa is due to friction from the sharp buccal cusp of a grossly carious upper molar.

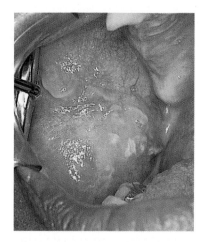

Fig. 15.2 Cheek-biting. There is whitening of the buccal mucosa and a shredded surface.

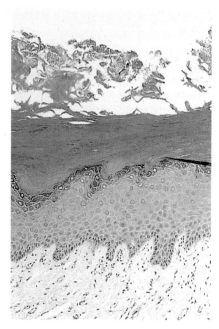

Fig. 15.3 Frictional keratosis. There is a slight hyperplasia of the basal cells and a thick layer of orthokeratin at the surface.

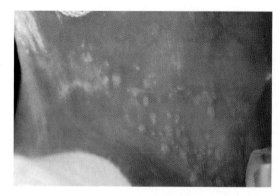

Fig. 15.4 Fordyce's spots. Clusters of creamy, slightly elevated papules on the buccal mucosa.

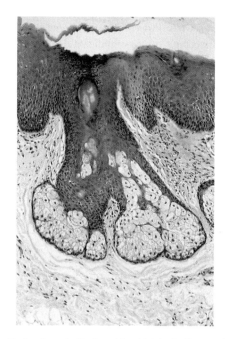

Fig. 15.5 Fordyce's spots. Each spot is a histologically normal superficial sebaceous gland without a hair follicle.

keratosis is completely benign, and there is no evidence that continued minor trauma alone has any carcinogenic potential.

FORDYCE'S GRANULES

Sebaceous glands are present in the oral mucosa in at least 80% of adults, particularly the elderly. They grow in size with age and appear in the oral mucosa as soft, symmetrically distributed, creamy spots a few millimetres in diameter, particularly in older persons (Fig. 15.4). The buccal mucosa is the main site, but sometimes the lips and rarely, even the tongue are involved.

These glands are sometimes mistaken for disease but patients can be reassured that they are of no significance. If a biopsy is carried out it shows a normal sebaceous gland with two or three lobules (Fig. 15.5).

PIPE SMOKER'S KERATOSIS ('STOMATITIS NICOTINA')

Smoker's keratosis is seen among heavy, long-term pipe smokers and some cigar smokers.

Clinical features

The appearances are distinctive in that the palate is affected, but any part protected by a denture is spared. Changes are then seen only on the soft palate.

The lesion has two components — hyperkeratosis and inflammatory swelling of minor mucous glands. Either may

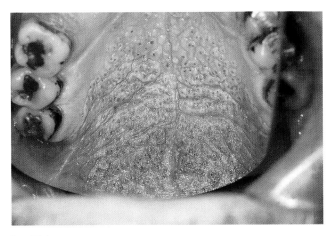

Fig. 15.6 Stomatitis nicotina (smoker's palate). There is a generalised whitening with sparing of the gingival margin. The inflamed openings of the minor salivary glands form red spots on the white background.

predominate, but typically, white thickening of the palatal mucosa is associated with small umbilicated swellings with red centres (Fig. 15.6). The white plaque is sometimes distinctly tessellated (pavement-like).

Microscopy

The white areas show hyperorthokeratosis and acanthosis with a variable inflammatory infiltrate beneath. The diagnostic feature is the swollen, inflamed mucous glands with hyperkeratosis extending up to the duct orifice (Fig. 15.7).

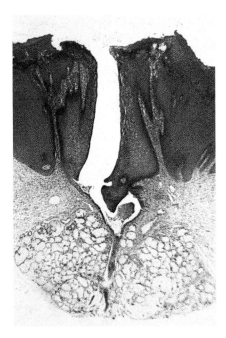

Fig. 15.7 Stomatitis nicotina (smoker's palate). The epithelium is hyperplastic and hyperkeratotic, especially around the orifice of the duct where there is a concentration of inflammatory cells.

Management

The clinical appearances, history and ease of management are so distinctive that biopsy should not be necessary. If the patient can be persuaded to stop smoking the lesion resolves within weeks. Key features are summarised in Table 15.2.

Table 15.2   Pipe smokers' keratosis ('stomatitis nicotina')
• Affects mucosa exposed to smoke (mainly the hard palate)
• Areas protected by denture unaffected
• Palate is white (keratotic) with umbilicated swellings with red centres (inflamed mucous glands)
• Responds rapidly to abstinence from pipe smoking
• Statistically, a raised risk of oral cancer but *not* in the hyperkeratinised (palatal) area (Ch. 16).

Epidemiological evidence suggests that pipe smoking raises the risk of cancer, but when oral cancer develops in association with pipe smoking it typically appears *not* in the keratotic area on the palate (one of the least common sites for cancer) but low down in the mouth, often in the lingual retromolar region. This may be the result of carcinogens pooling and having their maximal effect in drainage areas of the mouth. It also suggests that there are different causes for the hyperkeratosis and any carcinomatous change.

THRUSH

Thrush (acute candidosis, Ch. 12) is readily distinguishable from other white lesions. The patches can easily be wiped off and Gram-stained smears show a mass of long hyphae.

In a young adult, thrush in the absence of obvious predisposing cause strongly suggests HIV infection.

HIV-ASSOCIATED HAIRY LEUKOPLAKIA

Patients with HIV infection may develop a clinically and histologically distinctive white lesion. Hairy leukoplakia is an important manifestation of HIV infection and, though not entirely unique to it, is otherwise exceeding rare.

Clinical features

Hairy leukoplakia usually has a vertically corrugated or shaggy surface. The plaque is soft, usually painless and most frequently affects the lateral borders of the tongue (Fig. 15.8). Men who have sex with men are predominantly affected.

Pathology

Hairy leukoplakia shows hyperkeratosis or parakeratosis, or both, with a ridged or shaggy surface or, rarely, hair-like extensions of keratin. Secondary invasion of the surface by

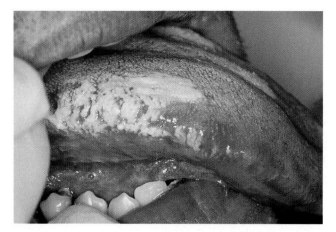

Fig. 15.8 Hairy leukoplakia in a patient with early symptomatic HIV infection. The surface of the lesion is corrugated, accentuating the normal anatomy of the lateral border of the tongue.

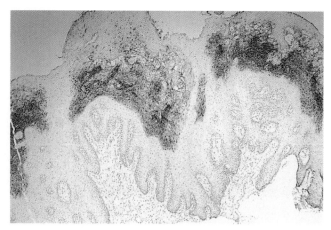

Fig. 15.10 Hairy leukoplakia. Immunocytochemical staining for Epstein–Barr virus shows positivity in the prickle cells, indicating viral infection. Details of this technique are included in Chapter 1.

candidal hyphae is relatively common but there is little or no inflammatory infiltration in the submucosa. More important is the presence of *koilocyte-like cells*, which are vacuolated and ballooned prickle cells with shrunken, dark (pyknotic) nuclei surrounded by a clear halo (Fig. 15.9).

Epstein–Barr virus (EBV) capsid antigen can be identified by in-situ hybridisation in the epithelial cell nuclei (Fig. 15.10). Viral particles resembling EBV can be seen by electron microscopy. This finding appears to be unique to hairy leukoplakia, and the likelihood that the EBV is the cause is suggested by the fact that hairy leukoplakia responds to treatment with aciclovir or its analogues.

Management

Biopsy confirmation of the diagnosis is essential. In the absence of symptoms, treatment of hairy leukoplakia is probably not justified especially as it has a remittent course and can regress

spontaneously. Hairy leukoplakia is not premalignant but it indicates advanced immunodeficiency, a more rapid progression to AIDS and a poor prognosis.

Key features are summarised in Table 15.3.

Table 15.3 Hairy leukoplakia: key features

- Usually a sign of HIV infection in male homosexuals
- Typically forms soft, corrugated, painless plaques on lateral borders of tongue
- Diagnosis by biopsy
- Histologically, koilocyte-like cells in prickle cell layer are typical
- Epstein–Barr virus antigens detectable in epithelial cell nuclei by in-situ hybridisation
- Indicates advanced immunodeficiency and poor prognosis but not premalignant
- May regress spontaneously or with HAART treatment (Ch. 24)

Hairy leukoplakia in the absence of HIV infection

Hairy leukoplakia has rarely been seen in immunodeficient, and even more rarely in immunocompetent, patients. In such patients it appears to resolve spontaneously.

WHITE SPONGE NAEVUS

White sponge naevus is a developmental anomaly inherited as an autosomal dominant trait.

Clinical features

The appearance is distinctive. The affected mucosa is white, soft and irregularly thickened (Fig. 15.11). The abnormality is usually bilateral and sometimes involves the whole oral mucosa. There are no defined borders and the edges fade imperceptibly into normal tissue. The anus and vagina can also be affected.

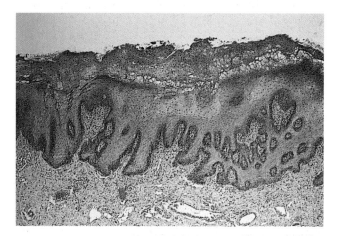

Fig. 15.9 Hairy leukoplakia. There is thickening of the epithelium and a thick superficial layer of parakeratin, below which the pale staining layer of 'koilocyte-like' cells lies. Because this patient is severely immunosuppressed there is no inflammatory reaction to the numerous candidal hyphae which are present in the surface layers of the epithelium.

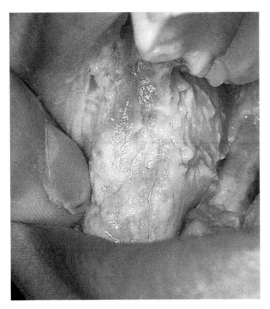

Fig. 15.11 White sponge naevus. The keratosis is irregular and folded and extends into areas which are not subject to friction.

Pathology

The epithelium is hyperplastic, with uniform acanthosis and the rete ridges have a smooth lower border. Shaggy hyperpara-keratosis and intracellular oedema with abnormally prominent epithelial cell membranes produce a so-called basket-weave appearance (Fig. 15.12). There is no dysplasia and inflammatory cells in the corium are typically absent.

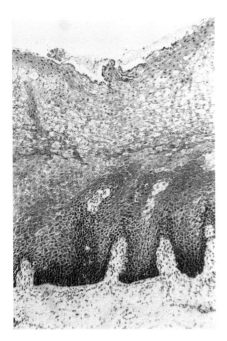

Fig. 15.12 White sponge naevus. The epithelium is acanthotic and the prickle cell layer is composed of large vacuolated cells.

Management

The appearance is readily recognised, particularly when there is widespread mucosal involvement. A positive family history is virtually confirmatory. If there is any doubt, biopsy confirms the diagnosis. The main requirement is to reassure the patient of the benign nature of the condition.

Key features are summarised in Table 15.4.

Table 15.4 White sponge naevus: key features

- Genetic — autosomal dominant trait
- Shaggy whitish thickening can involve entire oral mucosa
- White areas lack sharp borders
- Histologically, epithelial hyperplasia with basket-weave appearance
- No dysplasia or inflammation
- No treatment other than reassurance

CHRONIC MUCOCUTANEOUS CANDIDOSIS SYNDROMES

These syndromes are all rare, but difficult to manage. There are four main types (Table 15.5).

Table 15.5 Chronic mucocutaneous candidosis syndromes

- Familial (limited) type
- Diffuse type (Candida 'granuloma')
- Endocrine candidosis syndrome
- Late onset (thymoma syndrome)

Chronic mucocutaneous candidosis is sometimes classed as an immunodeficiency disease but an immune defect cannot always be found. In others it is limited to failure to respond to *C. albicans* or secondary to persistent antigenic stimulation. However, there are more profound defects in the diffuse and late onset types while the endocrine candidosis syndrome is part of an autoimmune disease.

Familial (limited) mucocutaneous candidosis

Inheritance is usually as an autosomal recessive trait. The onset is in infancy with persistent thrush in childhood. Later the oral lesions become indistinguishable from those of sporadic cases of chronic hyperplastic candidosis (Figs 15.13 and 15.14). There may be mild cutaneous involvement and sideropenia is characteristically associated.

Diffuse type mucocutaneous candidosis

Most cases are sporadic. This is the most severe type and was earlier termed 'monilial granuloma' because of the extensive, warty and often disfiguring overgrowths on the skin. Never-

225

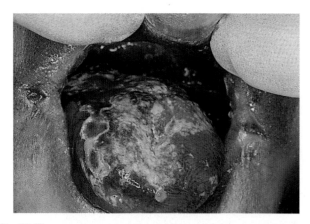

Fig. 15.13 Chronic mucocutaneous candidosis. There are extensive red and white patches affecting much of the oral mucosa and severe angular stomatitis.

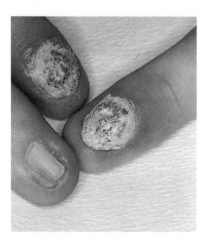

Fig. 15.14 Damage to the fingernails as seen here is typical of the more severe types of mucocutaneous candidosis.

theless, there is no granuloma formation microscopically. Instead, the lesions are produced by epithelial proliferation and an extreme expression of the same process that produces oral epithelial plaques in response to candidal invasion.

These patients are usually also abnormally susceptible to bacterial diseases, particularly pulmonary and superficial suppurative infections.

Endocrine candidosis syndrome

In this variant, chronic mucocutaneous candidosis is associated with multiple glandular deficiencies and organ-specific auto-antibody production. Nevertheless, there is no direct cause-and-effect relationship between the candidosis and the endocrine deficiency. Candidal infection can precede the onset of endocrine deficiency by as long as 15 years but occasionally this sequence is reversed. Treatment of the candidosis does not affect the endocrine deficiency and vice versa.

Endocrine-candidosis syndrome is a manifestation of type I chronic polyendocrinopathy (Ch. 31). Addison's disease and hypoparathyroidism are most frequently associated, and other

glandular deficiencies can develop, but candidosis is sometimes so mild as to pass unnoticed. Hypoplastic dental defects are frequently also present.

Adrenal failure is the main threat to life in candida-endocrinopathy syndrome but is usually now treated effectively.

Late onset mucocutaneous candidosis

This syndrome has a clear immunological basis, in that there is a persistent defect of cell-mediated immunity produced by a thyoma. In the full syndrome, myasthenia gravis and pure red cell aplasia are associated. Death from the thymoma or red cell aplasia is the main hazard.

Management of mucocutaneous candidosis syndromes

Microscopic confirmation of chronic candidosis is required (Fig. 15.15 and Ch. 16), but precise categorisation of these syndromes may have to await development of other features, such as endocrine deficiency or elucidation of a relevant family history.

Immunological investigation, apart from detection of auto-antibodies to glandular tissues in the endocrine candidosis syndrome, is not generally helpful, though detection of impaired or absent cell-mediated immunity to *C. albicans* strongly suggests that the patient has a mucocutaneous candidosis syndrome rather than limited oral hyperplastic candidosis.

The principles of management are therefore to treat the candidal infection with antifungal drugs such as itraconazole and to deal with associated disorders as appropriate. Antibacterial chemotherapy is necessary in diffuse-type chronic mucocutaneous candidosis (CMCC) and endocrine replacement is essential in endocrine candidosis.

Unlike 'idiopathic' chronic hyperplastic candidosis, chronic mucocutaneous candidosis appears to have little potential for malignant change. Key features are summarised in Table 15.6.

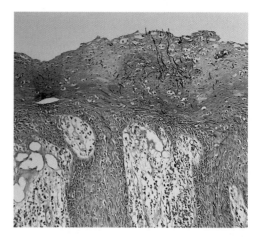

Fig. 15.15 Chronic hyperplastic candidosis. At high power the thick parakeratin layer at the surface of this lesion is seen to be invaded by numerous fungal hyphae.

Table 15.6 Chronic mucocutaneous candidosis syndromes: key features

- Onset typically in infancy as persistent thrush
- Gradual transformation into leukoplakia-like lesions
- Ungual and/or mild cutaneous candidosis sometimes associated
- Immune deficiency sometimes present
- Pulmonary and superficial suppurative infections associated in *diffuse CMCC* with gross candidal epithelial proliferation
- In *endocrine candidosis syndrome*, early-onset Addison's disease and/or hypoparathyroidism is associated but oral candidosis frequently mild
- In *late-onset CMCC*, thymoma causes defective cell-mediated immunity. Myasthenia gravis and pure red cell aplasia may be associated

PSORIASIS

Psoriasis is a common skin disease estimated to affect 2% of the population. Oral psoriatic plaques are rare but there may be an association between erythema migrans of the tongue (geographical tongue) or other mucosae, and cutaneous psoriasis.

The diagnosis should only be considered when there is cutaneous psoriasis. The appearance of the oral lesions varies from translucent plaques to that of erythema migrans. Lesions may be asymptomatic.

Diagnosis is confirmed by biopsy but the histological appearances of psoriasis and erythema migrans (Ch. 14) are sometimes very similar.

ORAL KERATOSIS OF RENAL FAILURE

Leukoplakia-like oral lesions are a rare and unexplained complication of long-standing renal failure.

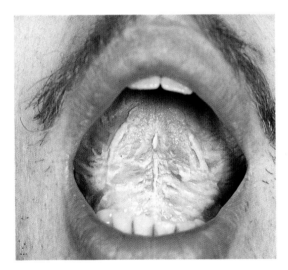

Fig. 15.16 Oral keratosis of renal failure. The white lesions are symmetrical, soft and wrinkled.

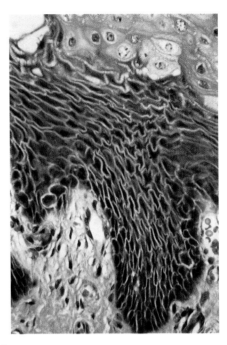

Fig. 15.17 Oral keratosis of renal failure. Microscopy shows acanthosis and a picture somewhat similar to hairy leukoplakia.

Clinically, the plaques are soft, have a crenated surface and are typically symmetrically distributed (Fig. 15.16).

Pathology

The features may not be sufficiently distinctive to allow diagnosis without knowledge of the underlying disease. There is irregular acanthosis with mild atypia of the epithelial cells and moderate parakeratosis. The appearances are somewhat similar to those of hairy leukoplakia, but Epstein–Barr virus antigen is absent. Biopsy is useful also to exclude adherent bacterial plaques, which may also develop in patients with renal failure (Fig. 15.17).

Effective dialysis or renal transplantation cause resolution of the lesion. No local treatment is necessary or likely to be effective.

VERRUCIFORM XANTHOMA

Verruciform xanthoma is a rare proliferative lesion which can have a white, hyperkeratotic surface.

Clinically, verruciform xanthoma is most common in the fifth to seventh decades. It is usually found on the gingiva but can form in almost any site in the mouth. It can be white or red in colour, be sessile or pedunculated, have a warty surface, and range in size from one to several centimetres across. It may be mistaken for a papilloma, leukoplakia or carcinoma clinically, but is readily recognisable histologically. Verruciform xanthoma is benign and has no known associations with diseases such as hyperlipidaemia or diabetes mellitus associated with cutaneous xanthoma formation.

Pathology

The warty surface is due to the much infolded epithelium which, in white variants, is hyperkeratinised or parakeratinised. In haematoxylin and eosin stained sections, the parakeratin layer stains a distinctive orange colour. The elongated rete ridges are uniformly elongated and extend to a straight, well-defined lower border (Fig. 15.18).

The diagnostic feature is the large, foamy, xanthoma cells which fill the connective tissue papillae but extend only to the lower border of the lesion (Fig. 15.19). These cells contain lipid and PAS positive granules.

Simple surgical excision is curative.

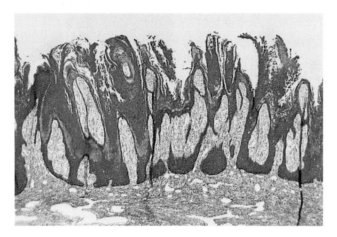

Fig. 15.18 Verruciform xanthoma. The epithelium is thin and parakeratotic and forms a series of spiky folds.

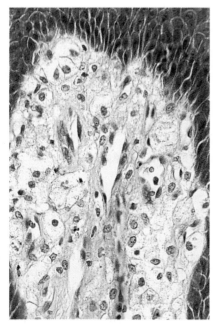

Fig. 15.19 Verruciform xanthoma. At higher power dermal papillae within the folded epithelium can be seen to contain many large rounded cells with foamy or vacuolated cytoplasm.

SKIN GRAFTS

A skin graft may be placed in the mouth to cover a raw area left after excision of, for example, a chronic white lesion.

Skin grafts typically appear sharply demarcated, smooth and paler than the surrounding mucosa and occasionally contain hairs (Fig. 15.20). However, grafts on the dorsum of the tongue may become corrugated and less easy to differentiate from a recurrence of leukoplakia (Fig.15.21).

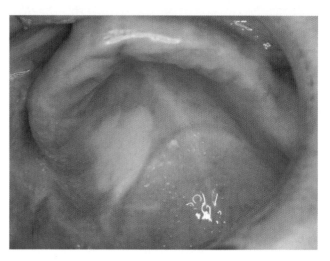

Fig. 15.20 Skin graft. A skin graft placed on the right posterior hard palate appears as a scar-like, pale patch. Hair follicles occasionally survive transplantation to the mouth.

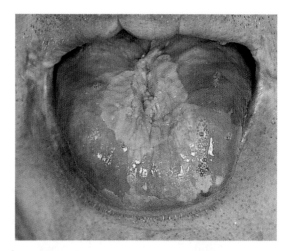

Fig. 15.21 Skin graft. This graft placed on the anterior dorsum of the tongue has contracted to produce an irregular margin and surface and might be mistaken for leukoplakia.

SUGGESTED FURTHER READING

Cawson R A, Binnie W H, Barrett A W, Wright J M 1998 *Lucas's Pathology of tumors of the oral tissues*. Churchill Livingstone, Edinburgh

Cawson R A, Binnie W H, Barrett A W, Wright J M 2001 *Oral disease*, 3rd Edn. Mosby-Wolfe, London

Cawson R A, Langdon J D, Eveson J W 1996 *Surgical pathology of the mouth and jaws*. Wright, Oxford

Epstein J B, Fatahzadeh M, Matisic J, Anderson G 1995 Exfoliative cytology and electron microscopy in the diagnosis of hairy leukoplakia. Oral Surg Oral Med Oral Pathol 79:564–569

Eisenberg E, Krutchkoff D, Yamase H 1992 Incidental oral hairy leukoplakia in immunocompetent persons. A report of two cases. Oral Surg Oral Med Oral Pathol 74:332–333

Higgs J M, Wells R S 1974 Classification of chronic muco-cutaneous candidosis. Clinical data and therapy. Hautartz 25:159–165

Ravina A, Ficarra C, Chiodo M et al 1996 Relationship of circulating CD4+ T-lymphocytes and p24 antigenemia to the risk of developing AIDS in HIV-infected subjects with hairy leukoplakia. J Oral Pathol Med 25:108–111

Oral premalignancy

Various oral mucosal lesions, particularly red lesions (erythroplasias) and some white lesions (leukoplakias), have a potential for malignant change (Table 16.1). In some of them, such as chronic hyperplastic candidosis, the risk may be very low. By contrast, the risk with erythroplasia is exceedingly high.

In general, the most common white lesions have the lowest risk of malignant transformation. Practitioners will see many oral white lesions, but few carcinomas. However, they must be able to recognise lesions at particular risk and several features help to assess the likelihood of malignant transformation. The accuracy of such predictions is low, but the process of identifying 'at risk' lesions is fundamental to diagnosis and treatment planning. Important factors are listed in Table 16.2 and information on each of these should be sought.

The best predictor of the potential for malignant transformation is the degree of dysplasia seen histologically. For this reason, and because a few lesions will already be malignant, biopsy of red and white patches is mandatory. The term *dysplasia* (literally, *abnormal growth*) is given to the cytological abnormalities seen in both malignant and premalignant cells (Table 16.3). Premalignancy is distinguished from malignancy only by the latter's invasiveness and release of metastases.

Table 16.2   Risk factors for malignant change in white lesions

History	Betel quid usage
	Tobacco smoking or snuff dipping[a]
	High alcohol intake
	Genetic disorders (see Ch. 17)
Clinical aspects	Advanced age
	Female gender[b]
	Areas of reddening in the lesion
	Areas of speckling in the lesion
	Nodular areas or ulceration
	High risk site:
	posterolateral tongue
	floor of mouth
	retromolar region
	anterior pillar of fauces
	Large lesions
	Lesions present for long periods
	Enlargement or change in character of
	pre-existing lesion
Special investigations	Degree of dysplasia on biopsy

[a]Nevertheless surveys indicate that the risk of malignant change in white lesions is higher in *non-smokers*
[b]Surveys indicate that malignant change in white lesions is more frequent in women

Table 16.1   Lesions with potential for malignant change

Lesion/condition	Aetiology	Risk of malignant change[a]	Prevalence in the UK
Dysplastic leukoplakia	Unknown	High, but can regress	Uncommon
Erythroplasia	Idiopathic/smoking	Very high	Rare
Speckled leukoplakia	Idiopathic/smoking	High	Rare
Tertiary syphilis	*Treponema pallidum*	Very high	No longer seen
Oral submucous fibrosis	'Betel' chewing	High	Uncommon
Dyskeratosis congenita	Genetic	High	Rare
Pipe smokers' keratosis	Pipe smoking	Low and not in the keratotic area	Becoming uncommon
Snuff-dippers' keratosis	Smokeless tobacco	Low	Uncommon
Chronic candidosis	*Candida albicans*	Low	Uncommon
Lichen planus	Idiopathic	Low	Common
Discoid lupus erythematosus	Autoimmune	Unclear (mainly lip)	Uncommon

[a]Risks of malignant change are difficult to determine accurately and vary with many factors discussed below. If more than 25% of lesions become malignant in 5 years this is considered an exceptionally high risk. Malignant change in 2–3% of lesions in 5 years is considered a relatively low risk. Note that the highest risk lesions are uncommon. Common lesions appear in between 1% and 5% of the population.

Table 16.3 Epithelial dysplasia: histological features

- Drop-shaped rete ridges
- Nuclear hyperchromatism
- Nuclear pleomorphism and altered nuclear/cytoplasmic ratio
- Excess mitotic activity
- Loss of polarity of cells
- Deep cell keratinisation
- Disordered or loss of differentiation
- Loss of intercellular adherence

It must be emphasised that the implications of *epithelial* dysplasia are quite different from *fibrous* dysplasia, in which there is no risk of carcinomatous change.

Nuclei stain more densely due to heavier nucleic acid content. They are variable in size, out of proportion to that of the cell, so that there may be little surrounding cytoplasm. Mitoses may be frequent and at superficial levels. Loss of polarity refers to the fact that basal cells in particular may lie higgledy-piggledy at angles to one another. Deep cell keratinisation (*dyskeratosis*) refers to individual cells which start to keratinise before the surface is reached and show eosinophilic change deeply within the epithelium. As differentiation is lost, organisation of the individual cell layers deteriorates and clearly-defined basal and spinous cell layers cannot be identified. Drop-shaped rete ridges are regarded as a particularly adverse feature. With loss of intercellular adherence, the cells become separated.

A lymphoplasmacytic infiltrate of highly variable intensity is usually present in the corium.

Dysplasia is usually graded as mild, moderate and severe as a guide to patient management (Figs 16.1–16.4). *Carcinoma-in-situ* is a controversial term sometimes used for the most severe dysplasia where the abnormalities extend throughout the thickness of the epithelium; a state sometimes graphically called 'top-to-bottom change'. In such a lesion all the cellular abnormalities characteristic of malignancy may be present; only invasion is absent. The significance of this grading is discussed below, but the histological assessment of oral epithelial dysplasia is notoriously unreliable because it is subjective and changes are not reliably correlated with behaviour.

PREMALIGNANT LESIONS AND CONDITIONS

Premalignant lesions are those lesions in which carcinoma may develop. Premalignant conditions are associated with a risk of carcinoma at some site within the mouth, not necessarily marked by a pre-existing lesion.

Erythroplasia ('erythroplakia')

Erythroplasia are red patches. The surface is frequently velvety in texture and the margin may be sharply defined. Lesions of this type typically do not from plaques (hence the term

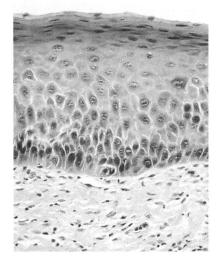

Fig. 16.1 Mild dysplasia. In this lesion there is a thin layer of parakeratin and the structure, maturation and orderly differentiation of the epithelial cells is largely unaffected. However, there is a degree of irregularity of basal cells with variation in size and hyperchromatism.

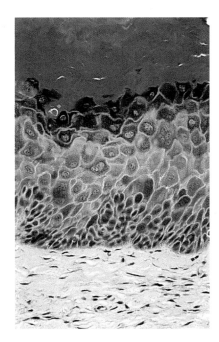

Fig. 16.2 Mild dysplasia. In this lesion there is prominent orthokeratosis and a keratohyaline layer immediately below it. Dysplasia is more prominent than in the previous figure, with enlarged hyperchromatic and bizarre cells in the basal and lower prickle cell layers.

'erythroplakia' is misleading) but, instead, they are flat or depressed below the level of the surrounding mucosa (Fig. 16.5). Erythroplasia is uncommon in the mouth but carries the highest risk of malignant transformation and lesions are often already malignant on first biopsy.

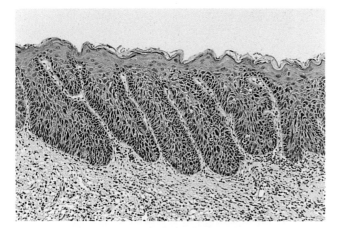

Fig. 16.3 Moderate dysplasia. The dermal papillae extend close to the surface and there are elongated rete processes, some of which are broader deeply. Enlarged and hyperchromatic cells are visible at this low power in rete processes and in most of the prickle cell layer.

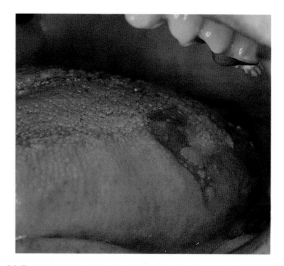

Fig. 16.5 Erythroplasia. This slightly depressed, well-defined red patch on the dorsolateral tongue showed squamous carcinoma on biopsy.

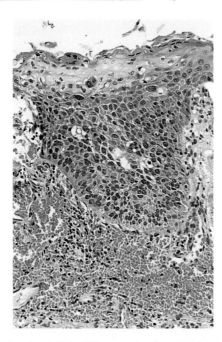

Fig. 16.4 Severe dysplasia. This rete process is composed almost entirely of cells with dark and irregularly shaped nuclei. Only the most superficial layers of cells show maturation to squamous cells and the orderly maturation and differentiation of epithelial cells has been lost.

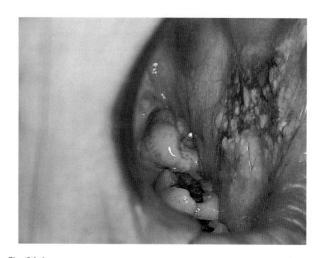

Fig. 16.6 Speckled leukoplakia. A poorly-defined speckled leukoplakia on the cheek of an elderly female. Carcinoma was present at the first biopsy.

Pathology

Erythroplastic lesions usually show epithelial dysplasia which may be severe. In other cases, there may be micro- or frankly invasive carcinoma. The epithelium is atrophic and this, together with inflammation, accounts for the red colour seen clinically.

Speckled leukoplakia

This term applies to lesions consisting of white flecks or fine nodules on an atrophic erythematous base (Figs 16.6 and 16.7). They can be regarded as a combination of or transition between

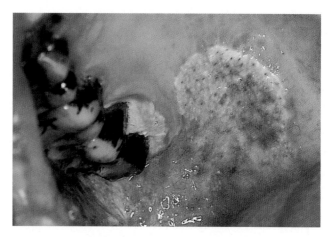

Fig. 16.7 Premalignant lesion in a betel quid chewer. The classical appearance of a speckled leukoplakia such as this is almost always associated with either severe dysplasia or invasive carcinoma. Note also the brown betel quid staining on the teeth.

leukoplakia and erythroplasia. Speckled leukoplakia also more frequently shows dysplasia than lesions with a homogeneous white surface. The histological characteristics are usually, therefore, intermediate between leukoplakia and erythroplasia.

Many cases of chronic candidosis have this appearance.

IDIOPATHIC LEUKOPLAKIA

Leukoplakia is defined as a white patch which cannot be wiped off the mucosa or ascribed to any specific disease process. Although the term is often used loosely for any white patch it should be reserved for idiopathic lesions. If investigations fail to reveal any cause, the term may be appropriate.

The most extensive follow-up studies on white patches suggest that idiopathic leukoplakia now has the highest risk of developing cancer, especially now that late stage syphilis forms a negligibly small group. Nevertheless, the malignant transformation rate of leukoplakia is relatively low, around 1–2% in 5 years, and even in smokers the vast majority of leukoplakias show no dysplasia histologically and carry no risk of malignant transformation.

Clinical features

Idiopathic leukoplakias and dysplastic lesions do not have any specific clinical appearance, but are tough and adherent and typically form plaques whose surface is slightly raised above the surrounding mucosa. The surface is usually irregular. Small and innocent-looking white patches are as likely to show epithelial dysplasia as large and irregular ones (Figs 16.8 and 16.9). However, lesions with red, nodular or verrucous areas (Fig. 16.10) should be regarded with particular suspicion. The most common sites are the posterior buccal mucosa, retromolar region, floor of mouth and tongue.

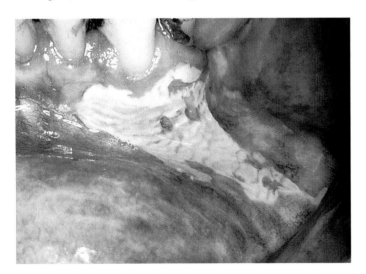

Fig. 16.8 Homogeneous leukoplakia. There is a bright, white, sharply-defined patch extending from the gingiva on to the labial mucosa. The surface has a slightly rippled appearance and no red areas are associated.

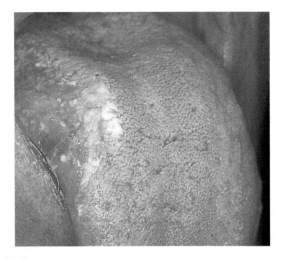

Fig. 16.9 An innocent-looking, poorly-defined inconspicuous white patch which showed dysplasia on biopsy. Despite excision, malignant transformation followed several months later.

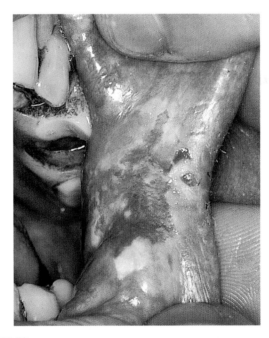

Fig. 16.10 White patch with dysplasia. This postcommissural lesion is poorly defined and comprises both red and white areas. Lesions at this site are frequently due to candidosis.

Pathology

The histopathology is highly variable but there is always parakeratosis or orthokeratosis, or both in different areas, and the two may alternate along the length of the specimen. The keratin gives the lesion its white appearance. The epithelium ranges from thinner than normal (atrophic) to much thicker (acanthotic) (see Figs 16.1 and 16.2).

Most leukoplakias show no dysplasia histologically. A minority display a range of dysplasia from mild to severe and treatment is planned partly on this basis. An inflammatory reaction of lymphocytes and plasma cells induced by the abnormal dysplastic cells is often present in the underlying connective tissue.

SUBLINGUAL KERATOSIS

The term sublingual keratosis is applied to white lesions on the floor of mouth and ventral tongue. Whether this lesion is a different entity from other leukoplakias is unclear. Malignant change was reported in an unusually high proportion of cases (30%) in one series but this has not been widely confirmed. Probably the risk of malignant transformation is less than 10% and possibly much lower.

Clinical features

Sublingual keratosis is a white, soft plaque, usually with a finely wrinkled surface, an irregular but well-defined outline and sometimes bilateral with a butterfly shape. The plaque typically extends from the anterior floor of the mouth to the undersurface of the tongue (Figs 16.11 and 16.12). There is usually no associated inflammation.

Pathology

Sublingual keratosis is not distinctive histologically and the appearances are those described above for leukoplakia.

PIPE SMOKERS' KERATOSIS

As noted earlier (Ch. 15), palatal keratosis due to pipe smoking is benign. Any carcinomas related to pipe-smoking appear in another site in the mouth and may not be preceded by keratosis.

SMOKELESS TOBACCO-RELATED KERATOSES

Hyperkeratotic mucosal lesions can result from smoking or use of smokeless tobacco ('topical tobacco' — snuff-dipping and tobacco chewing). By contrast, there is no characteristic hyperkeratotic lesion associated with the far more common habit of cigarette smoking.

Tobacco chewing and snuff-dipping (holding flavoured tobacco powder in an oral sulcus) are popular habits in the USA and some parts of Europe. Loose oral snuff appears to cause more severe changes than tobacco-chewing but not all topical tobacco habits are associated with a risk of malignant change. The use of Scandinavian-type snuff sachets appears to carry no risk and it is important to ascertain exactly what type of tobacco is used and how it is prepared. Many smokeless tobacco users also smoke and, regardless of this, all lesions is the mouths of tobacco users should be regarded with suspicion.

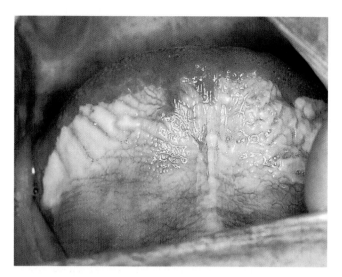

Fig. 16.11 Sublingual keratosis. This white patch involving the entire ventral tongue and floor of mouth has a uniformly wrinkled appearance. No red areas are associated but the site alone may indicate a high risk of malignant transformation.

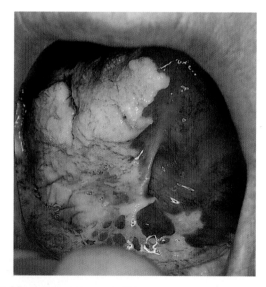

Fig. 16.12 Sublingual keratosis. This more irregular white patch is associated with some reddening in the floor of the mouth.

Clinical features

The habit of snuff-dipping or tobacco-chewing may be maintained for decades and gives rise to keratoses in the buccal or labial sulcus, where the tobacco is held. Early changes are erythema and mild, whitish thickening. Long-term use gives rise to extensive white thickening and wrinkling of the buccal mucosa. Malignant change can follow, but only after several decades of use. A high proportion of carcinomas in snuff users are verrucous in type (Ch. 17) but if they remain untreated invasive squamous carcinoma may develop.

Pathology

The main changes are thickening of the epithelium with plump or squared-off rete ridges. There are varying degrees of hyper-orthokeratosis or parakeratosis and there may be subepithelial fibrosis in the area where the tobacco is held. Dysplasia may eventually be seen.

Management

Diagnosis is based on the history of snuff use and the white lesion in the area where the tobacco is held. Biopsy is required to exclude dysplasia or early malignant change. Paradoxically, however, it appears that in snuff-dippers carcinomas appear at a later age and are better differentiated than in non-users.

Snuff-dippers' lesions will resolve on stopping the habit even after 25 years of use. This therefore is the main measure. If this fails, regular follow-up and biopsies are required.

CHRONIC HYPERPLASTIC CANDIDOSIS (CANDIDAL LEUKOPLAKIA)

Chronic oral candidosis produces a tough adherent plaque, distinguishable only by biopsy from other leukoplakias.

Clinical features

Adults, typically males of middle age or over, are affected. The usual sites are the dorsum of the tongue and the post-commissural buccal mucosa. The plaque is variable in thickness and often rough or irregular in texture, or nodular with an erythematous background (speckled). Angular stomatitis may be associated, is sometimes continuous with intra-oral plaques and suggests the candidal nature of the lesion (Figs 16.13 and 16.14).

Pathology

Unlike thrush, the plaque cannot be wiped off, but fragments can be detached by firm scraping. Gram or periodic acid–Schiff (PAS) staining then shows candidal hyphae embedded in clumps of detached epithelial cells.

Like thrush, the plaque of chronic candidosis is parakeratotic, but more coherent because it is not widely infiltrated by inflammatory exudate. In haematoxylin and eosin stained sections, hyphae form only faint tracks through the epithelium and are difficult to see. PAS stain clearly shows the hyphae growing (as in thrush) through the full thickness of the keratin to the prickle cell layer where the inflammatory cells tend to be more concentrated (Fig. 16.15).

Electron microscopy shows *Candida albicans* to be an intracellular parasite growing within the epithelial cytoplasm (Fig. 16.16). The hyphae, therefore, grow in relatively straight lines and do not follow a tortuous path along the intercellular spaces.

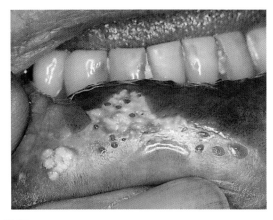

Fig. 16.13 Chronic hyperplastic candidosis. This white localised patch and its associated erythema are the result of candidal infection alone and no dysplasia was present despite the speckled clinical appearance.

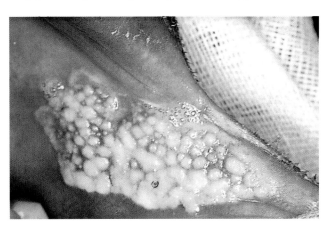

Fig. 16.14 Chronic hyperplastic candidosis. The typical site is the postcommissural buccal mucosa. This florid example is white and slightly nodular.

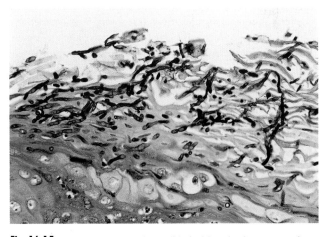

Fig. 16.15 Chronic hyperplastic candidosis. Many hyphae are growing down through the epithelial plaque. (PAS stain).

Induction of epithelial proliferation by *Candida albicans* infection has been demonstrated experimentally and in candidal plaques there is often rete hyperplasia with rounded down-growths and acanthosis. Dysplasia may be present, especially in speckled lesions.

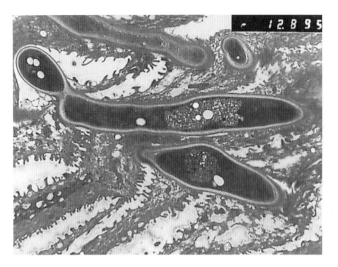

Fig. 16.16 Two candidal hyphae growing through superficial keratinocytes of the oral mucosa.

The chronic inflammatory infiltrate in the corium is variable and a fibrinous inflammatory exudate may be seen at the basement membrane.

Management

After confirmation of the diagnosis by histology, treatment should be with a systemic antifungal drug such as fluconazole, but this may have to be continued for several months. Other factors likely to perpetuate candidal infection should be controlled. Stopping the patient from smoking and elimination of candidal infection from under an upper denture are important. Any iron deficiency should also be treated.

Excision of candidal plaque alone is of little value, as the infection can recur in the same site even after skin grafting. Vigorous antifungal therapy is therefore essential, but sometimes some residual (uninfected) plaque may persist after treatment and lesions often recur and require long term intermittent antifungal therapy.

The potential for malignant change exists. The level of risk is controversial but low.

ORAL SUBMUCOUS FIBROSIS

In oral submucous fibrosis (Ch. 11) affected areas of the oral mucosa such as the palate or buccal mucosa appear almost white. The pallor is due to the underlying fibrosis and ischaemia rather than a superficial plaque, and the mucosa is typically smooth, thin and atrophic (see Figs 11.4 ad 11.5). However, erythroplasia and leukoplakia may be associated (see Fig. 16.7) and the epithelium may show dysplasia on biopsy.

Surveys suggest that oral submucous fibrosis undergoes malignant transformation in 4.5–7.6% of cases and may contribute to the high incidence of oral cancer in the Indian subcontinent and in Asian immigrant populations in other countries. Submucous fibrosis is probably premalignant because of its association with betel quid chewing.

LICHEN PLANUS

As noted in Chapter 13, it was estimated that 1–4% of patients develop carcinomas after 10 years.

However, as noted earlier, the potential of lichen planus to undergo malignant change is controversial. Rates quoted in earlier reports have been questioned, particularly because of doubts about the original diagnosis.

LUPUS ERYTHEMATOSUS

Lupus erythematosus is an uncommon connective tissue disease (Chs 12 and 23). There is a small risk of malignant change in cutaneous lupus, especially in lesions of the lower lip.

DYSKERATOSIS CONGENITA

Dyskeratosis congenita is a rare heritable recessive or dominant trait. The main features are dysplastic white or red lesions of the oral mucosa, cutaneous pigmentation, dystrophies of the nails and haematological abnormalities. Many patients may also be immunodeficient or have other abnormalities.

Causes of death include cancers of the mouth or other sites, bleeding (gastrointestinal or cerebral) but in 50% from infections, which are frequently opportunistic.

SYPHILITIC LEUKOPLAKIA

Leukoplakia of the dorsum of the tongue is a characteristic complication of tertiary syphilis but is of little more than historical interest.

Clinical features

Syphilitic leukoplakia has no distinctive features, but typically affects the dorsum of the tongue and spares the margins. The lesion has an irregular outline and surface. Cracks, small erosions or nodules may prove on histology to be foci of invasive carcinoma (Fig. 16.17). Carcinoma developing near the centre of the dorsum of the tongue is typically a sequel to syphilitic leukoplakia and, as a consequence of the great decline in late-stage syphilis, is exceedingly rare in this site now.

Pathology

In addition to hyperkeratosis and acanthosis, often with dysplasia, the characteristic late syphilitic chronic inflammatory changes,

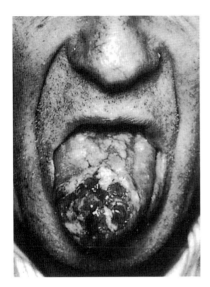

Fig. 16.17 Syphilitic leukoplakia. Carcinoma has developed in a patch of leukoplakia on the tongue of a patient who had had tertiary syphilis for many years. (Taken before the advent of colour photography.)

with plasma cells predominating, may be seen. Giant cells and, rarely, granulomas may be present. Endarteritis of small arteries is particularly characteristic. However, distinctive features of a syphilitic tissue reaction may be lacking.

Behaviour and management

The diagnosis is confirmed mainly by the serological findings. However, even if positive, biopsy is still essential, as minute areas of malignant change may be found, and the management is affected accordingly. In particular, the presence of syphilitic endarteritis, may be a contraindication to radiotherapy.

Antibiotic treatment of syphilis does not cure the leukoplakia, which persists and can undergo malignant change even after serology has become negative.

EARLY CARCINOMA

Occasionally an early carcinoma produces surface keratin and appears as a white patch (see Fig. 17.4). It should not be interpreted as malignant change in a leukoplakia.

MANAGEMENT OF DYSPLASTIC LESIONS

As noted in Chapter 17, the prognosis in oral carcinoma is good only when the diagnosis is made early and the tumour is small. Accurate assessment of the risk of malignant change in red and white patches is therefore desirable, but assessment is highly subjective. The level of risk cannot be reliably assessed from the histopathology alone and the clinical features listed in Table 16.2 should be used to help gauge the risk for an individual lesion.

The best predictor of malignant potential is the presence of dysplasia on biopsy. However, even this is rather poorly correlated with behaviour for such reasons such as inadequate sampling at biopsy and the subjective nature of assessment.

In the most extensive study based on no fewer than 782 cases of histologically unspecified oral white lesions followed for an average of 12 years, 2.4% underwent malignant change in 10 years and fewer than 5% after 20 years. However, even this low rate represents a risk of malignant change 50–100 times that in the normal mouth. It was also conspicuous, that in this and in other studies the rate of malignant change in oral leukoplakias has been up to *10 times higher in non-smokers than in smokers* and more frequent in women. Other, smaller, series have suggested rates of malignant change of 30% or more in unspecified types of white lesions, though in many cases no time scale has been indicated. The wide variation in the rate of malignant change in these different series suggests that the findings have been significantly affected by selection of cases.

It must be emphasised that these large follow-up studies have been on oral keratoses which had not been histologically assessed. Because of the rarity of dysplastic oral lesions there are very few studies, and none on a large scale, that have followed their progress for adequate periods. In a study of 45 patients with oral dysplastic lesions, followed for up to 8 years, 11% underwent malignant change in this period and up to 30% of them regressed or even ultimately disappeared spontaneously.

The principles of the management of dysplastic lesions are summarised in Table 16.4.

Table 16.4 Principles of management of dysplastic lesions

- Stop any associated habits, e.g. betel quid or smoking
- Treat candidal infection and/or iron deficiency if present
- Biopsy to assess dysplasia
- Assess risk of premalignant change on clinical and histological findings
- Consider ablation of individual lesions (see Table 16.5)
- Maintain observation for signs of malignant change

The management of dysplastic oral lesions remains controversial as their relative rarity has made it impossible as yet to accumulate enough data to make reliable predictions or evaluate treatment. It has to be assumed that dyplasia represents an early stage in the development of carcinoma and provides an opportunity to treat carcinoma at an exceptionally early, and potentially curative preinvasive stage.

Unfortunately, these assumptions are not well supported by clinical evidence. Lesions which are excised appear more likely to become frankly malignant, though this may reflect selection of the highest risk cases for surgery.

If lesions are of manageable size, it is tempting to excise them — this should presumably do no harm, but it is essentially a treatment of hope rather than certainty. An alternative approach is to observe the lesions for signs of deterioration, in the hope of detecting carcinoma as early as possible. Once carcinoma develops the treatment options are much more clear-cut.

Table 16.5 Options for management of premalignant lesions

- Observation for early detection of carcinoma
- Surgical excision with grafting, if required
- Cryotherapy
- Laser excision or vaporisation
- Topical chemotherapy
- Retinoids

A dysplastic lesion is associated with a higher risk of developing lesions elsewhere in the mouth and of developing more than one oral carcinoma. This process is sometimes described as 'field change' to convey the idea that large areas of the oral epithelium may be premalignant. Regular examination of the whole mouth is therefore essential.

Some dysplastic lesions regress spontaneously and surveys suggest that dysplastic lesions may regress as frequently as they undergo malignant change. However, disappearance of a white lesion does not necessarily indicate resolution of dysplasia and continued observation may still be indicated. Photographs or video records of lesions are an invaluable aid to long-term observation of lesions and should be used for high-risk lesions.

In practice, an attempt is usually made to remove lesions with moderate or severe dysplasia or high-risk clinical features (Table 16.5).

Surgical excision is the most common approach. It provides an excision biopsy specimen which can be examined for the extent of the dysplasia and for possible carcinoma. Unfortunately, lesions in the highest risk areas in the posterior floor of mouth are technically difficult to excise and large lesions may require grafting.

The effectiveness of other treatments has not yet been assessed on any adequate scale.

After cryotherapy ablation, the area heals rapidly to leave an apparently normal mucosa. However, there is some uncertainty about the risk of invasive carcinomas subsequently arising in these sites. Carbon dioxide laser ablation has also been advocated, but the same objections may apply. Topical chemotherapeutic agents such as bleomycin have also been used experimentally. Treatment with systemic or topical retinoids has also been tried. Topical retinoids are largely ineffective and though a proportion of white lesions resolve with systemic treatment, toxic effects are usually unacceptable. Further, lesions which resolve with treatment recur on withdrawal of the drugs.

With all such treatments the lesion is not available for histological examination and multiple biopsy before treatment is required to ensure that malignant change is not already present. They may be of value in those for whom surgery is not practical because of, for instance, unfitness for anesthesia.

In summary, frequent clinical observation, preferably with photographic records, and immediate biopsy of any areas that are suspicious or change in appearance, is generally the best option. Selected lesions with clinical features of high-risk or severe dysplasia on biopsy are probably best excised.

SUGGESTED FURTHER READING

Abbey L M, Kaugars G E, Gunsolley J C et al 1995 Interexaminer and intraexaminer reliability in the diagnosis of oral epithelial dysplasia. Oral Surg Oral Med Oral Pathol Oral Radiol Endod 80:188–191

Axell T, Pindborg J J, Smith C J et al 1996 Oral white lesions with special reference to precancerous and tobacco-related lesions: conclusions of an international symposium held in Uppsala, Sweden, May 18–21 1994. J Oral Pathol Med 25:49–54

Barnard N A, Scully C, Eveson J W, Cunningham S, Porter S R 1993 Oral cancer development in patients with oral lichen planus. Oral Pathol Med 22:421–424

Barrett A W, Kingsmill V J, Speight P M 1998 Frequency of fungal infection in biopsies of oral mucosal lesions. Oral Diseases 4:26–31

Baudet-Pommel M, Janin-Mercier A, Souteyrand P 1991 Sequential immunopathologic study of oral lichen planus treated with tretinoin and etretinate. Oral Surg Oral Med Oral Pathol 71:197–202

Borle R M, Borle S R 1991 Management of oral submucous fibrosis: a conservative approach. J Oral Maxillofacial Surg 49:788–791

Cawson R A 1966 Chronic oral candidiasis and leukoplakia. Oral Surg Oral Med Oral Pathol 22:582–591

Cawson R A 1973 Induction of epithelial hyperplasia by *Candida albicans*. Br J Dermatol 89:497–503

Cawson R A, Rajasingham K C 1972 Ultrastructural features of the invasive phase of *Candida albicans*. Br J Dermatol 87:435–443

Cawson R A, Binnie W H 1980 Candida leukoplakia and carcinoma: a possible relationship. In Mackenzie I C, Debelsteen E, Squier C A eds. *Oral premalignancy. Proceedings of the first Dow Symposium.* University of Iowa, Iowa, 59–66

Cooke B E D 1956 Leukoplakia buccalis and oral epithelial naevi. Br J Dermatol 68:151–174

Cribier B, Garnier C, Lausriat D, Heid E 1994 Lichen planus and hepatitis C virus infection: an epidemiologic study. J Am Acad Dermatol 31:1070–1072

Daniels T E, Hansen L S, Greenspan J S et al 1992 Histopathology of smokeless tobacco lesions in professional baseball players. Associations with different types of tobacco. Oral Surg Oral Med Oral Pathol 73:720–725

Davidson H R, Connor J M 1988 Dykeratosis congenita. J Med Genet 25:843–846

Einhorn J, Wersall J 1967 Incidence of oral carcinoma in patients with leukoplakia of the oral mucosa. Cancer 20:2184–2193

Eisen D, Ellis C N, Duell E A, Griffiths C E M, Voorhees J J 1990 Effect of topical cyclosporine rinses on oral lichen planus. A double blind analysis. N Engl J Med 323:290–294

Eisenberg E, Krutchkoff D, Yamase H 1992 Incidental oral hairy leukoplakia in immunocompetent persons. A report of two cases. Oral Surg Oral Med Oral Pathol 74:332–333

Epstein J B, Fatahzadeh M, Matisic J, Anderson G 1995 Exfoliative cytology and electron microscopy in the diagnosis of hairy leukoplakia. Oral Surg Oral Med Oral Pathol 79:564–569

Epstein J B, Sherlock C H, Wolber R A 1993 Hairy leukoplakia after bone marrow transplantation. Oral Surg Oral Med Oral Pathol 75:690–696

Eveson J W 1983 Oral premalignancy. Cancer Surveys 2:403–424

Field E A, Field J K, Martin M V 1989 Does candida have a role in epithelial neoplasia? J Med Vet Mycol 27:277–294

Garewal H S, Katz R V, Meyskens F et al 1999 β-carotene produces sustained remissions in patients with oral leukoplakia. Results of a multicenter prospective trial. Arch Otolaryngol Head Neck Surg 125:1305–1310

Greenspan D, Greenspan J S, Hearst N G, Li-Zhen P, Conant M A, Abrams D I, Hollander H, Levy J A 1987 Relation of oral hairy leukoplakia to infection with the human immunodeficiency virus and the risk of developing AIDS. J Infect Dis 155:475–481

Greenspan D, Greenspan J S, Conant M, Peterson V, Silverman S, DeSouza Y 1984 Oral 'hairy' leukoplakia in male homosexuals: evidence of an association with both papillomavirus and a herpes group virus. Lancet ii:831–834

Hietanen J, Pihlman K, Linder E, Reunala T 1987 No evidence of hypersensitivity to dental restorative materials in oral lichen planus. Scand J Dent Res 95:320–327

SUGGESTED FURTHER READING (cont'd)

Higgs J M, Wells R S 1974 Classification of chronic muco-cutaneous candidosis. Clinical data and therapy. Hautartz 25:159–165

Ho V C, Gupta A K, Ellis C N, Nickoloff B J, Vorrhees J J 1990 Treatment of severe lichen planus with cyclosporine. J Am Acad Dermatol 22:64–68

Holmstrup P, Thorn J J, Rindum J, Pindborg J J 1988 Malignant development of lichen planus-affected oral mucosa. J Oral Pathol Med 17:219–225

Holmstrup P 1992 The controversy of a premalignant potential of oral lichen planus is over. Oral Surg Oral Med Oral Pathol 73:704–706

Janthi V, Probert C S J, Sher K S, Mayberry J F 1992 Oral submucosal fibrosis — a preventable disease. Gut 33:4–6

Karjalainen T K, Tomich C E 1989 A histopathologic study of oral mucosal lupus erythematosus. Oral Surg Oral Med Oral Pathol 67:547–554

Kaugars G E 1992 The prevalence of oral lesions in smokeless tobacco users and an evaluation of risk factors. Cancer 70:2579–2585

Kaugars G E, Silverman S, Lovas J G L et al 1996 Use of antioxidant supplements in the treatment of human oral leukoplakia. Review of the literature and current studies. Oral Surg Oral Med Oral Pathol Oral Radiol Endod 81:5–14

Kramer I R H, El-Labban N, Lee K W 1978 The clinical features and risk of malignant transformation in sublingual keratosis. Br Dent J 144:171–176

Laine J, Kalimo K, Forssell H, Happonen R-P 1992 Resolution of oral lichenoid lesions in patients allergic to mercury compounds. Br J Dermatol 126:10–15

Larrson A, Axéll T, Andersson G 1991 Reversibility of snuff dippers' lesion in Swedish moist snuff users: a clinical and histologic study. J Oral Pathol Med 20:258–264

Laskaris G, Laskaris M, Theodoridou M 1995 Oral leukoplakia in a child with AIDS. Oral Surg Oral Med Oral Pathol 79:570–571

Lin R Y, Goodhart P 1993 The role of oral candidiasis in survival and hospitalization patterns: analysis of an inner city hospital human immunodeficiency virus/acquired immune deficiency registry. Am J Med Sci 305:345–353

Lippman S M, Batsakis J G, Toth B T, Weber R S, Lee J J, Martin J W et al 1993 Comparison of low-dose isotretinoin with beta carotene to prevent oral carcinogenesis. N Engl J Med 328:15–20

Maher R, Lee A J, Warnakulasuriya K A A S 1994 Role of areca nut in the causation of oral submucous fibrosis: a case-control study in Pakistan. J Oral Pathol Med 23:65–69

McCreary C E, Flint S R, McCartan et al 1992 Uremic stomatitis mimicking oral hairy leukoplakia. Report of a case. Oral Surg Oral Med Oral Pathol Oral Radiol Endod 83:350–353

McGrath J A 1999 Dyskeratosis congenita: new clinical and molecular insights into ribosome function. Lancet 353:1204–1205

Mincer H H, Coleman S S, Hopkins K P 1972 Observations on the clinical characteristics of oral lesions showing histologic epithelial dysplasia. Oral Surg 33:389–399

Morris L F, Phillips C M, Binnie W H, Sander H M, Silverman H K, Menter M A 1992 Oral lesions in patients with psoriasis: a controlled study. Cutis 49:339–344

Murti P R, Daftary D K, Bhonsle R B et al 1986 Malignant potential of oral lichen planus: observations in 722 patients from India. J Oral Pathol 15:71–77

Murti P R, Bhonsle R B, Pindborg J J et al 1985 Malignant transformation rate in oral submucous fibrosis over a 17-year period. Community Dent Oral Epidemiol 13:340–341

Nicholas G E et al 1990 White sponge nevus. Obstet Gynecol 76:545–548

Nowparast B, Howell F V, Rick G M 1981 Verruciform zanthoma: a clinicopathologic review and report of fity-four cases. Oral Surg Oral Med Oral Pathol 51:619–625

O'Grady J F, Reade P C 1992 Candida albicans as a promotor of oral neoplasia. Carcinogenesis 13:783–786

Pillai R, Balaram P, Reddiar K S 1992 Pathogenesis of oral submucous fibrosis. Relationship to risk factors associated with oral cancer. Cancer 69:2011–2020

Pindborg J J, Roed-Petersen B, Renstrup G 1972 Role of smoking in floor of the mouth leukoplakias. J Oral Pathol 1:22–27

Resnick L, Herbst J S, Ablashi D V et al 1988 Regression of oral hairy leukoplakia after orally administered acyclovir therapy. JAMA 259:384–388

Rhodus N L, Johnson D K 1990 The prevalence of oral manifestations of lupus erythematosus. Quintessence Int 21:461–465

Shibuya H, Amagasa T, Seto K-I, Ishibashi K, Horiuchi J-I 1986 Leukoplakia-associated multiple carcinomas in patients with tongue carcinoma. Cancer 57:843–846

Sigurgeirsson B, Lindelöf B 1991 Lichen planus and malignancy. An epidemiologic study of 2017 patients and a review of the literature. Arch Dermatol 127:1684–1688

Silverman S, Gorsky M, Lozada F 1984 Oral leukoplakia and malignant transformation. A follow-up study of 257 patients. Cancer 53:563–568

Silverman S, Bhargava R, Mani N J, Smith L W, Malaowalla A M 1976 Malignant transformation and natural history of oral leukoplakia in 57,518 industrial workers in Gujerat, India. Cancer 38:1790–1795

Sklavounou A, Laskaris G 1990 Oral psoriasis: report of a case and review of the literature. Dermatologica 180:157–159

Voute A B E, de Jong W F B, Schulten E A J M, Snow G B, van der Waal I 1992 Possible premalignant character of oral lichen planus; the Amsterdam experience. J Oral Pathol Med 21:326–329

Yavalzyilmaz E 1992 Oral-dental findings in dyskeratosis congenita. J Oral Pathol Med 21:280–284

Zain R B, Ikeda N, Gupta P C et al 1999 Oral mucosal lesions associated with betel quid, areca nut and tobacco chewing habits: consensus from a workshop held in Kuala Lumpur, Malaysia, November 25–27, 1996. J Oral Pathol Med 28:1–4

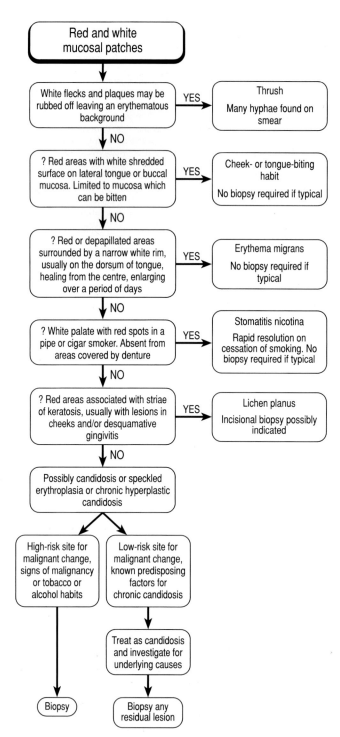

Summary 16.1 Differential diagnosis and management of the common causes of red and white patches of the oral mucosa.

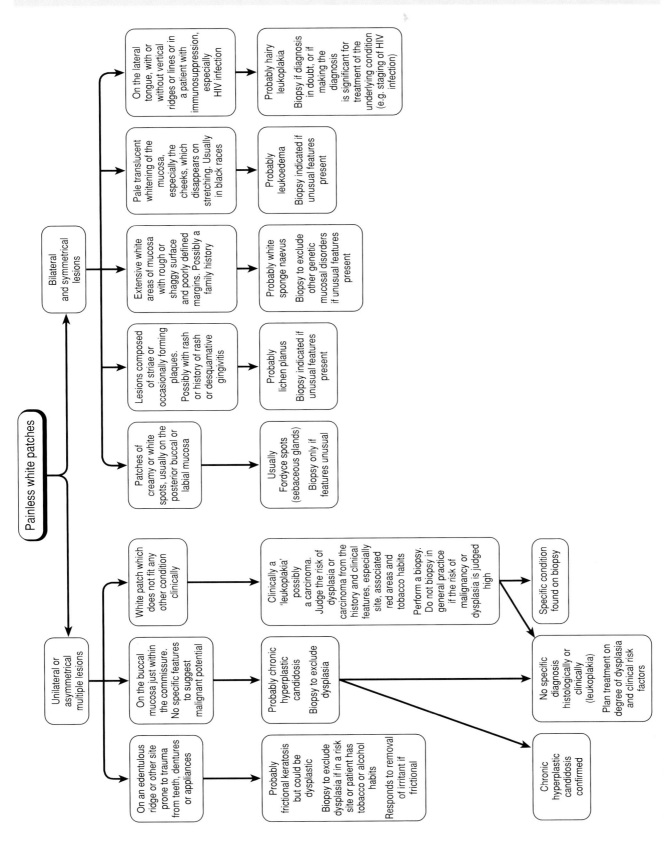

Summary 16.2 Summary of the key features of the common and important oral white patches.

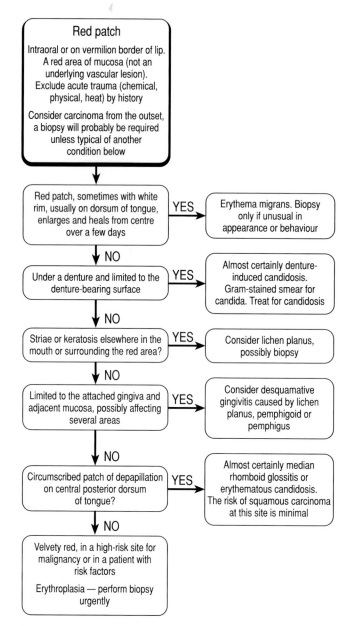

Red patch

Intraoral or on vermilion border of lip.
A red area of mucosa (not an
underlying vascular lesion).
Exclude acute trauma (chemical,
physical, heat) by history

Consider carcinoma from the outset,
a biopsy will probably be required
unless typical of another
condition below

Red patch, sometimes with white
rim, usually on dorsum of tongue,
enlarges and heals from centre
over a few days

YES → Erythema migrans. Biopsy
only if unusual in
appearance or behaviour

NO

Under a denture and limited to the
denture-bearing surface

YES → Almost certainly denture-
induced candidosis.
Gram-stained smear for
candida. Treat for candidosis

NO

Striae or keratosis elsewhere in the
mouth or surrounding the red area?

YES → Consider lichen planus,
possibly biopsy

NO

Limited to the attached gingiva and
adjacent mucosa, possibly affecting
several areas

YES → Consider desquamative
gingivitis caused by lichen
planus, pemphigoid or
pemphigus

NO

Circumscribed patch of depapillation
on central posterior dorsum
of tongue?

YES → Almost certainly median
rhomboid glossitis or
erythematous candidosis.
The risk of squamous carcinoma
at this site is minimal

NO

Velvety red, in a high-risk site for
malignancy or in a patient with
risk factors

Erythroplasia — perform biopsy
urgently

Summary 16.3 Differential diagnosis of common and important red
patches affecting the oral mucosa.

Oral cancer

Over 90% of malignant neoplasms (cancers) of the mouth are squamous cell carcinomas arising from mucosal epithelium. Most of the remainder are adenocarcinomas of minor salivary glands: only a few are undifferentiated or metastases.

EPIDEMIOLOGY

Oral carcinoma accounts for only about 2% of all malignant tumours in such countries as the United Kingdom and the United States. In most countries where reliable data are available, the incidence of cancer of the mouth, though variable, is low. India and Sri Lanka are, however, exceptional, and cancer of the mouth accounts for approximately 40% or more of all cancer there, though the incidence varies widely in different parts of this sub-continent.

Approximately 2000 cases of intraoral and lip carcinoma are registered each year in the United Kingdom. For most of this century the incidence of oral cancer has declined but though it is rare, cases are now more frequently seen in those aged 30–50.

Age and gender incidence

Oral cancer is an age-related disease, and 98% of patients are over the age of 40. While the overall incidence in the population is only about 1 in 20 000, this rises to 1 in 1100 in males of 75 and over. There is a sharp and virtually linear increase of incidence of mouth cancer with age, as with carcinoma in many other sites.

Cancer of the mouth is considerably more common in men than women in most countries, and carcinoma of the lip is at least eight times as common in men as in women in Britain. Intraoral cancer used to be several times more frequent in men than women, but the male to female ratio is overall about 3:2, and in south-east England recent figures show little difference in incidence between the genders. The change is the result of the progressive decline in oral cancer in men in former years, but a low, static rate in women.

The incidence of oral cancer rises steeply with age and with an ageing population, oral cancer will become more common.

AETIOLOGY

It has not been possible to prove conclusively a causative association between specific aetiological factors and oral cancer. This is partly because the quality of cancer statistics is very variable and partly because the aetiology of malignancy is complex and multifactorial. Causative factors operate over a long period and the process of malignant change is so slow that there is a prolonged lag period before it becomes evident. This has been shown strikingly in Japan, where cancers were still developing half a century after the radiation exposure from atomic bombs.

Significant or speculative risk factors for oral squamous cell carcinoma are summarised in Table 17.1.

Table 17.1 Possible aetiological factors for oral cancer

- Possible carcinogens
  Tobacco
  Alcohol
  Areca nut ('betel')
- Sunlight (lip only)
- Infections
  Syphilis
  Candidosis
  Viruses
- Mucosal diseases
  Oral epithelial dysplasia
  Lichen planus
  Oral submucous fibrosis
- Genetic disorders (rare)
  Dyskeratosis congenita
  Fanconi's anaemia

Tobacco use

The effects of tobacco on the mouth depend on the way it is used, and this varies in different countries. In Westernised countries, cigarette smoking predominates and pipe smoking has declined. In some countries, notably in India, the southern states of the USA and Sweden, tobacco chewing or snuff-dipping (unsmoked tobacco held in the mouth for prolonged periods) is a habit. Methods of processing tobacco before use also vary widely, so that its products released into the mouth differ considerably in their effect. This is particularly noticeable in India where, in some areas, the use of a particular type of tobacco appears to be associated with a very high incidence of cancer.

Cigarette smoking

Smoking is considered to be a major aetiological factor, particularly in association with alcohol, and its importance is that it is preventable. However, it is difficult to demonstrate a direct causal link between cigarette smoking and oral cancer. In the UK data have shown that oral cancer in males steadily *declined* over a period of more than three-quarters of a century while cigarette consumption grew steadily. Also, there is some evidence that the incidence of oral cancer in males may be rising again despite the fact that males are now smoking less.

Equally difficult to explain is the fact that mouth cancer in women has remained at a steady low level despite their widespread adoption of cigarette smoking. The escalation of their cigarette consumption is shown by the fact that the lung cancer rate in women has risen to nearly equal that of men in the USA.

Also puzzling is that, unlike pipe smoking or smokeless tobacco use, there is no specific oral lesion related to cigarette smoking.

Nevertheless, many studies have closely linked smoking, particularly in association with alcohol, to oral carcinoma. In case-control studies which take account of the amount and duration of tobacco consumption, the specific site and other factors such as alcohol, cigarette smoking has been shown to be closely associated and carry a significant relative risk. The risk of developing a second primary carcinoma is also closely linked to smoking and alcohol. Thus, smoking cigarettes infrequently appears to carry a very low risk, whereas the relative risk rises dramatically in heavy smokers.

Pipe-smoking

Epidemiological evidence has associated oral cancer with pipe-smoking but the habit has steadily declined in most Westernised countries and has never become popular with women. Pipe-smokers are also likely to develop stomatitis nicotina of the palate (Ch. 15), a white patch with no premalignant potential.

Smokeless tobacco

In the southern USA there have long been the habits of 'snuff dipping' and tobacco chewing in which either dry snuff or a plug of chewing tobacco (often with various other ingredients) is held in the lower buccal sulcus for prolonged periods. These habits cause extensive hyperkeratotic plaques and, after decades of continuous use, may lead to verrucous carcinoma (see below) as well as squamous carcinoma.

Tobacco is frequently included in betel quid (see below) and

it is significant that in these habits carcinomas tend to arise at the site in the mouth where the tobacco is habitually held.

However, in the USA it has been found that cancers developed *later* in users than in non-users. The mean age of smokeless tobacco users developing either type of carcinoma was 70.5 years and of non-users was 64.2 years. Moreover, the squamous cell carcinomas in users were overall, better differentiated than those in non-users. Any carcinogenic potential for smokeless tobacco therefore appears to be low.

Moreover, the greatest consumption of smokeless tobacco is in Sweden, where there is *no* evidence of related oral cancer development.

Alcohol

Alcohol consumption has steadily risen in Britain, particularly in the past half-century when oral cancer was declining. However, as noted above, the incidence may now be rising. In some countries, such as Denmark, there is good epidemiological evidence to link alcohol intake with oral carcinoma, and in the Bas Rhin area of France, alcohol is held to be responsible for the highest oral and pharyngeal cancer incidence in Europe. The low incidence of mouth cancer among Mormons and Seventh Day Adventists, who neither drink nor smoke, supports this idea.

It is generally considered that the combination of smoking and drinking is the most important aetiological factor for mouth cancer and, as noted above, many oral cancer patients smoke and drink heavily. The relative risks for alcohol and tobacco consumption are shown in Figure 17.1.

Alcoholic drinks are not usually allowed to reside in the mouth for long periods, and there is no specific alcohol-related oral lesion. The mechanism by which alcoholic drinks might cause carcinomas is unclear and may not be their ethanol content. Drinks with the highest content of congeners, such as raw home-brewed spirits, appear to have the closest association with carcinoma. By contrast, evidence from the USA suggests that beer-drinking is associated with a greater risk. It is also possible that alcohol might predispose to carcinoma through its action on the liver and some studies have found a correlation between mouth cancer and cirrhosis. As with smoking, the total consumption is probably a critical factor.

Concern over the possible carcinogenic effects of alcohol has led to a proposal that it should be banned from mouthwashes, some of which contain more than 25% alcohol. There is as yet no conclusive link between mouthwash use and oral carcinoma.

Viruses

Human papilloma virus DNA, particularly type 16, has been found in oral cancers. Papilloma viruses are closely associated with cervical cancer but the association with oral carcinoma remains speculative and the virus may also be found in apparently normal epithelium and papillomas. Human papilloma viruses may induce p53 gene mutation, of which there is a high frequency in oral cancer.

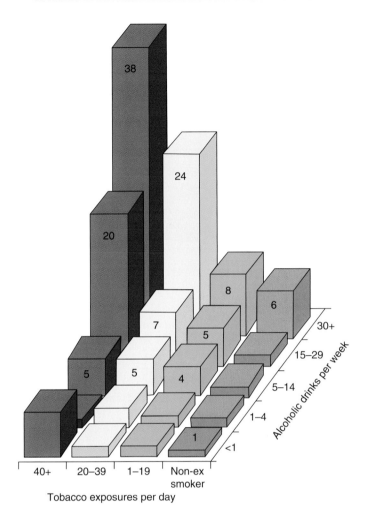

Fig. 17.1 Relative risks of developing oral cancer in consumers (males in a western population) of tobacco and alcohol. The relative risk for a non-smoker and non-alcohol consumer is taken as 1. A smoker consuming 30 cigarettes a day and 20 alcoholic drinks a week is seven times more likely to develop carcinoma.

Syphilis

Syphilitic leukoplakia, developing in late-stage disease, has a high malignant potential but is no longer a significant risk factor (Ch. 16).

Chronic candidosis

Chronic candidosis can lead to formation of hyperkeratotic plaques or speckled leukoplakias with epithelial dysplasia. There have been isolated reports of malignant change in such lesions, but, overall, this accounts for a very small proportion of cases (Ch. 16)

Malnutrition

There is a high incidence of mouth as well as oesophageal cancer in Paterson–Kelly syndrome, in which iron deficiency is a feature. However, this disease is no longer a significant risk factor.

Epidemiologically, a low vitamin A intake has been associated with oral carcinoma but deficiency of beta-carotene has now been dismissed as contributing to cancer. In India, malnutrition is widespread and may contribute, together with betel quid chewing, to the high incidence. However, there appears to be no comparably high frequency of mouth cancer in other areas, such as many parts of Africa, where malnutrition is at least as severe.

Oral sepsis

Oral sepsis has traditionally been regarded as contributing to mouth cancer. The latter is most common in low socioeconomic groups, which tend to have the most neglected mouths. Oral cancer also progressively declined in frequency in Britain, where a slow but steady improvement in oral health is well documented.

Despite such considerations the aetiological role of oral sepsis in mouth cancer remains unproven.

Betel ('pan') chewing

Use of a quid of areca nut, lime, tobacco and spices wrapped in betel leaf is a widespread habit in the Indian subcontinent and among immigrant Asian populations in the UK. The quid is held in the sulcus. Areca nut releases arecolin which, experimentally, is carcinogenic, while the tobacco contains numerous carcinogens. In South-east Asia, the quid frequently consists of areca nut with flavouring agents but no betel leaf, and is also associated with a high cancer incidence. White patches may develop where the quid is held and these have a high risk of malignant change. Betel or areca nut chewing can also cause oral submucous fibrosis which also appears to be premalignant (Ch. 11). The trismus resulting from submucous fibrosis also makes diagnosis and treatment of oral carcinoma very difficult. Betel quid chewing should be vigorously discouraged by dentists.

Sunlight

Exposure to the ultraviolet component of sunlight is a risk factor, with the result that lip cancer is predominantly a disease of outdoor workers, particularly farmers and fishermen. As with other skin cancers, fair-skinned persons are at most risk. There may be multiple lesions in the most severely affected.

The relationship between exposure to sunlight and lip cancer has been clearly shown in hot countries such as Australia and the USA with large immigrant, fair-skinned populations of European origin. In the USA, for example, the risk of lip cancer approximately doubles for every 250 miles nearer the equator the site of residence.

Dysplastic lesions caused by sunlight may precede the carcinoma and sun-damaged lip may be identified clinically by its loss of elasticity and atrophic epithelium. Changes due to sunlight are preventable and dentists should encourage the need to wear a high factor sun-block when exposed to strong sunlight.

Genetic factors

There are a few genetic disorders, notably dyskeratosis congenita (Ch. 16), of which oral cancer is a frequent feature, but such disorders are rare. Mice with a high susceptibility to oral cancer have also been bred. However, there is no other convincing evidence of any genetic trait predisposing to oral cancer in humans.

Precancerous lesions

Several premalignant lesions are recognised (Ch. 16). In general, the risk of malignant transformation in the more common white lesions is very low, but it is not known what proportion of carcinomas arise in clinically recognisable pre-malignant lesions.

Table 17.2   Cancer of the mouth: key features

- Account for approximately 2% of all cancers in the UK but one of the most common cancers in the Indian subcontinent
- Males more frequently affected
- Most patients are over 40 and incidence rises rapidly with age
- Lower lip is the most common site and related to actinic damage
- Tongue, posterolaterally, is the most common site within the mouth
- Some arise in pre-existing white or red lesions
- Heavy tobacco-smoking and alcohol consumption tend to be associated
- In the Indian subcontinent and South-east Asia, 'betel' (areca nut) chewing may be more important

SITES OF ORAL CANCER

The lower lip is the most frequent site of oral cancer overall, while the tongue is the most frequently affected site *within* the mouth. In the oral cavity, the majority of cancers are concentrated in the lower part of the mouth, particularly the lateral borders of the tongue, the adjacent floor of the mouth and lingual aspect of the alveolar margin, forming a U-shaped area extending back towards the oropharynx (Fig. 17.2). This accounts for only about 20% of the whole area of the interior of the oral cavity, but 70% of oral cancers are concentrated there. This distribution may be due to the likelihood that carcinogens could pool and concentrate in the lower mouth before swallowing. For the same reason, the hard palate and central dorsum of tongue are very rarely affected.

EARLY SQUAMOUS CELL CARCINOMA

In their earliest stages carcinomas appear as painless red, speckled or white patches and only a minority are ulcerated (Figs 17.3 and 17.4). As noted in Chapter 16, a high proportion

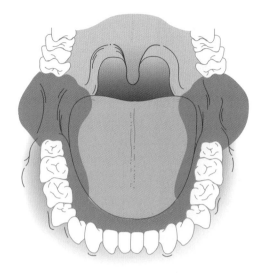

Fig. 17.2   High-risk sites for development of oral carcinoma. The shaded U-shaped area accounts for only about 20% of the whole area of the interior of the mouth but is the site of over 70% of oral cancers.

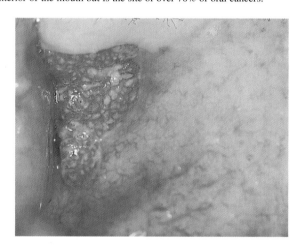

Fig. 17.3   Squamous carcinoma of the soft palate and mucosa posterior to the tuberosity appearing as a speckled leukoplakia.

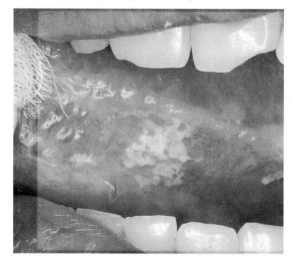

Fig. 17.4   Early squamous carcinoma. Despite its inconspicuous appearance this small white patch on the lateral border of the tongue was found to be a squamous carcinoma on biopsy.

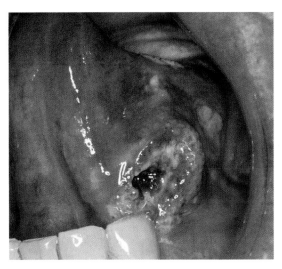

Fig. 17.5 Advanced squamous carcinoma. The classical ulcer with a rolled border and central necrosis is a late presentation. Note the surrounding areas of keratosis and erythema which had been present for many years before the carcinoma developed.

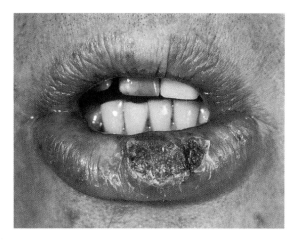

Fig. 17.6 Squamous carcinoma of lip. There is an indurated, crusted ulcer with keratosis at one margin in the centre of the lower lip.

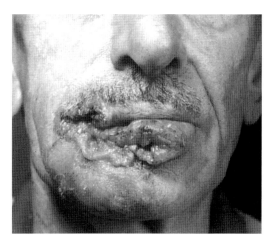

Fig. 17.7 Advanced carcinoma of lip. There is extensive ulceration and necrosis and distortion. Nowadays such extensive lesions are unusual. (Taken before the advent of colour photography.)

of erythroplasias and speckled leukoplakias are already malignant on first biopsy. The similar appearances of early carcinoma and premalignant lesions result from the processes of keratinisation and epithelial dysplasia and do not necessarily indicate that the carcinoma has arisen in a pre-existing lesion.

As a carcinoma enlarges it may develop into a raised nodule or become ulcerated. Induration results from inflammation and fibrosis and infiltration of the tissues. By the time a carcinoma has formed an indurated ulcer with the typical rolled border, it will have been present for some time (Fig. 17.5). As noted below, diagnosis at this late stage is associated with a very poor prognosis and every attempt must be made to identify carcinomas as early as possible.

Ulceration may be associated with soreness, or stinging pain when sharply flavoured food is eaten. Pain is of no value in the diagnosis of carcinoma, but is typically severe in the late stages. Bleeding, either spontaneously or to mild trauma, is also a late feature.

CARCINOMA OF THE LIP

The lip is the most common single site for oral cancer but infrequently seen in dental practice. Being visible, it is often recognised at a very early stage and so has a better prognosis than intra-oral cancer. The usual site is the vermilion border of the lower lip to one side of the midline. Men of middle age or over are predominantly affected.

An area of thickening, induration, crusting or shallow ulceration of the lip, less than a centimetre in diameter, is a common early presentation (Fig. 17.6). Advanced, neglected tumours (Fig. 17.7) are unlikely to be seen now. Spread to lymph nodes tends to be slow. The submental nodes are usually the first to be affected.

CARCINOMA OF THE TONGUE AND FLOOR OF MOUTH

The anterior part of the tongue, particularly the lateral border, and the adjacent ventral tongue and floor of mouth are frequently involved. Presentation is often late with an ulcer 2 cm or more in diameter. Approximately 60% or more patients with localised lesions less than 2 cm in diameter survive for 5 or more years after treatment. In more advanced disease the usual picture is of a typical malignant ulcer several centimetres in diameter, hard in consistency, with rolled or irregular, raised edges and a rough infected floor which bleeds readily. As growth proceeds the carcinoma becomes fixed to surrounding tissues and infiltrates the tongue, which becomes progressively stiffer and more painful. Eating, swallowing and talking become difficult. By this time pain is usually the main symptom and may radiate widely. The lymph nodes also become involved.

Affected lymph nodes are enlarged and hard, the surface becomes irregular and they become fixed to deeper tissues and

247

skin. The growth has spread beyond the tongue when the majority of patients are first seen. In such circumstances the prognosis is poor. Only one patient in six survives for 5 years or longer. In the late stages, local spread of the growth causes gross destruction of adjacent parts with widespread sloughing. The tongue becomes fixed; pain is severe and persistent; swallowing and speech are difficult. Affected lymph nodes may ulcerate through the skin. The combination of pain, infection and difficulty in eating cause loss of weight, anaemia and deterioration of general health. This state (malignant cachexia) is ultimately fatal. In other patients aspiration of septic material from the mouth causes bronchopneumonia, and, in a few haemorrhage from the growth is the cause of death.

A small, but possibly growing, proportion of patients survive treatment of the primary growth but die later from distant metastases.

CARCINOMA OF THE ALVEOLAR RIDGE, CHEEK AND PALATE

These show essentially the same features as carcinoma elsewhere. Carcinoma of the buccal mucosa is particularly associated with betel quid chewing. Carcinoma of the alveolar ridge and palate are more likely to erode bone at an earlier stage, making treatment more complex.

Pathology

The essential feature of carcinoma is the invasion of surrounding tissues by the malignant epithelial cells. The invading cells grow into the tissues, forming irregular branching processes, the tips of which are often cut off in a section to give the appearance of separate islands of tumour (Fig. 17.8). In the more infiltrative, higher grade carcinomas, single cells and small clusters of cells detach along the invasive front of the lesion. Tumour cells invade deeper tissues regardless of their nature (Fig. 17.9). Muscle, fat, nerves and eventually bone are infiltrated and destroyed. Invading cancer cells excite an inflammatory reaction and become surrounded by lymphocytes and plasma cells.

The individual cells show the features of malignancy. Large and irregularly shaped nuclei, darkly stained nuclei (hyperchromatism), frequent and sometimes abnormal mitoses and loss of the well-ordered architecture of epithelium are seen (Fig. 17.10). These are essentially the same changes as are seen in dysplastic epithelium (Ch. 16).

Squamous carcinoma is graded according to its degree of differentiation, that is the degree to which the malignant cells differentiate to form prickle cells and keratin. In well-differentiated tumours, the cells have cytoplasm which stains palely with eosin or may form concentric layers of keratin (cell-nests or keratin pearls (Fig. 17.11). In poorly-differentiated tumours the cells tend to be more irregular and darkly staining,

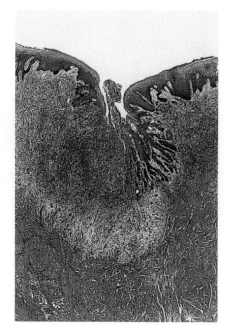

Fig. 17.8 A small squamous carcinoma. At low power the epithelium is seen to invade deeply into the connective tissue and underlying muscle. At this early stage there is no ulceration.

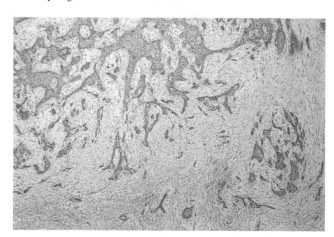

Fig. 17.9 Squamous carcinoma. Higher power shows strands of malignant epithelium invading the connective tissue.

and show little evidence of a squamous pattern. In the most poorly-differentiated carcinomas, the cells have little cytoplasm and may not be recognisable as epithelial cells by routine microscopy (Fig. 17.12). Poorly-differentiated carcinomas tend to infiltrate more widely at an early stage, are more likely to metastasise and carry a poorer prognosis.

SPREAD OF ORAL CARCINOMA

Carcinoma invades adjacent tissue by direct extension. Bone initially forms a barrier but is eventually destroyed, usually by superficial erosion, but once the cortex is breached carcinoma may invade along the medullary cavity.

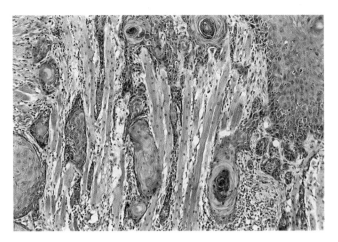

Fig. 17.10 Squamous carcinoma. At high power a group of tumour cells shows typical cytologic irregularity. Surrounding and beneath the tumour, muscle fibres are being destroyed.

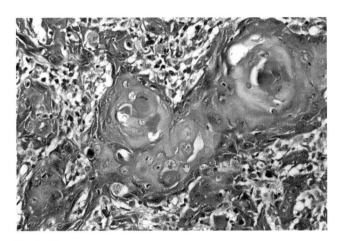

Fig. 17.11 Squamous carcinoma. In this moderately well-differentiated tumour many of the neoplastic epithelial cells are forming keratin pearls.

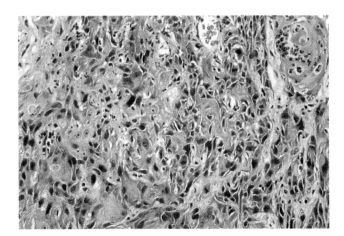

Fig. 17.12 Squamous carcinoma. In this poorly-differentiated carcinoma there is little or no keratin formation and the malignant cells show great pleomorphism with variably-sized nuclei, many of which are hyperchromatic, and frequent mitotic figures.

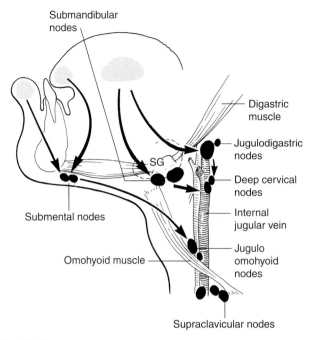

Fig. 17.13 Typical routes of lymphatic spread from lip and intra-oral squamous carcinomas (SG, Submandibular salivary gland).

Metastatic spread is primarily via the lymphatics to the regional lymph-nodes. The specific sites of metastasis depend on the drainage of the tumour site, but because most carcinomas arise posteriorly in the lower mouth, the submandibular and jugulodigastric nodes are most frequently involved. Lymphatic drainage from the tip of the tongue is to the submental nodes and then to the jugulo-omohyoid group, low down in the neck. From the dorsum and sides of the tongue, drainage is to the submandibular nodes and then to the jugulodigastric group (Fig. 17.13). Lip and floor-of-mouth carcinomas may spread bilaterally. Spread of cancer may be by an abnormal route, and all the lymph nodes of both sides of the neck must be examined.

Oral cancer spreads progressively down the jugular lymphatic chain and it is unusual for it to involve supraclavicular lymph nodes until a late stage. Perineural infiltration and vascular invasion are less common (Figs 17.14 and 17.15).

Metastatic carcinoma is initially limited to the affected node but, in time, spreads through the capsule into the tissues of the neck. Excision is then difficult and the chances of survival are diminished. This extracapsular spread is evident clinically as fixation of the node. Metastatic carcinoma forms a solid mass when small but in larger masses the central areas become necrotic and may break down so that the metastasis becomes cystic and fluctuant clinically.

Bloodstream spread is an uncommon, late feature of the disease. Key features are summarised in Table 17.3.

Management of oral carcinoma is complex and depends on the age and medical condition of the, usually elderly, patient, as well as its exact site, degree of spread (stage) and histological type. An appropriate treatment protocol must be selected for each individual case, taking these features into account.

249

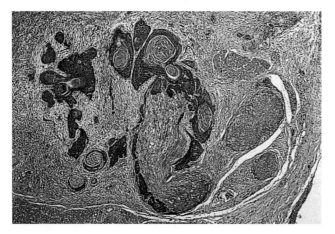

Fig. 17.14 Squamous carcinoma. In this carcinoma malignant epithelium is invading around nerve sheaths. Although this is infrequent, occasionally carcinoma may spread some distance from the main tumour mass along nerve trunks.

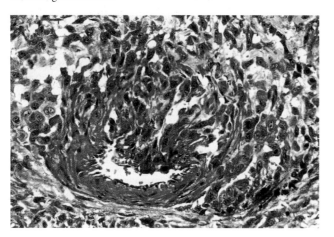

Fig. 17.15 Squamous carcinoma. Less frequent than perineural invasion is vascular invasion. Here a cluster of poorly-differentiated malignant epithelial cells have eroded the wall of the vessel and entered the circulation.

Table 17.3 Oral cancer: clinicopathological features and behaviour

- Early cancers appear as white or red patches or shallow ulcers and are painless or only slightly sore
- Later carcinomas appear as ulcers with prominent rolled edges and induration and become painful
- Over 70% or oral cancers form on the lateral borders of the tongue and adjacent alveolar ridge and floor of mouth
- Over 95% are well- or moderately well-differentiated squamous cell carcinomas
- Spread is by direct invasion of surrounding tissues and by lymphatic metastasis
- The submandibular and jugulodigastric nodes are most frequently involved
- The prognosis deteriorates sharply with local spread and nodal involvement

---

Treatment may be by surgery or radiotherapy and either may be used for cure or palliation. In practice, most intraoral carcinomas are treated by surgery combined with radiotherapy

Table 17.4 Unwanted effects of radiotherapy to the oral region

During treatment	Severe xerostomia
	Mucositis and ulceration
	Acute candidosis
	Skin erythema
Long term	Xerostomia
	Mucosal and skin atrophy
	Risk of osteomyelitis (osteoradionecrosis)
	Scarring and fibrosis of tissues
	Cataract if eye irradiated (e.g. antral carcinoma)
	Risk of late radiation-induced malignancy

('multimodality therapy'). Surgery alone is preferred for small carcinomas of the tongue which may be easily excised, for those involving bone because of the risk of later radionecrosis, and for verrucous carcinoma.

Actual and potential dental infection in the mouth must be dealt with before starting treatment, particularly if this is to be by irradiation. Dental infection or extractions may lead to extensive osteomyelitis in irradiated bone because of its poor vascularity: it is very resistant to treatment. The sockets should be healed, as nearly as possible, before radiotherapy is begun. In practice, teeth with extensive caries or periapical lesions for which rapid successful treatment cannot be guaranteed are usually extracted because of the need to start treatment quickly.

Treatment by irradiation provides a more acceptable cosmetic and functional result than major surgery but involves considerable discomfort during a long course of treatment and has unwanted effects in the long term (Table 17.4).

Radiotherapy is carried out by implantation of radioactive material into and around the neoplasm (brachytherapy), or by exposure to beams of x-rays or gamma-rays from x-ray generators or radioactive isotopes such as cobalt (teletherapy). Ionising radiation damages normal as well as neoplastic tissue, so that treatment planning is critical. The lesion is accurately localised by imaging techniques and a dose, usually in the region of 60 Gy for oral lesions, is given. Damage to surrounding tissues is limited by fractionating the dose over many visits (perhaps 30 daily fractions) and by applying external beams from many angles, but avoiding radiosensitive tissues such as the eye and bone. For teletherapy, a mask is made to fit the patient's head to allow reproducible beam angulation between visits. Radiotherapy planning and mask construction are complex and involve a short delay before treatment can start.

Surgery is mainly indicated when cancer has invaded bone or when there has been a poor response to, or recurrence after, irradiation. The aim is to excise the carcinoma with as wide a margin as possible, ideally 1 cm or more. Modern surgical methods allow excision, reconstruction, grafting or bypassing of almost any structure in the oral regions. However, a margin of more than a few millimetres is rarely achieved in practice, because the carcinoma may be too extensive and its margin may be difficult to identify at operation. Also, wider excision may make reconstruction difficult. Such a small margin is insufficient to guarantee removal of the carcinoma, which may recur at the original site.

Reconstructive surgery is normally performed at the same operation as excision, to provide a better cosmetic and functional result.

Recurrence after treatment may be at the primary site or in lymph nodes. Primary site recurrence usually signifies a poor prognosis because either a full course of radiotherapy or as large an excision as practical will already have been performed. Recurrence in lymph nodes usually appears within 2 years after treatment. The metastases probably arise from microscopic deposits of carcinoma already in the lymph nodes at the time of initial therapy (occult metastases). They may be treated surgically by block dissection or by radiotherapy and do not necessarily indicate failure of treatment. Block dissection of clinically normal cervical lymph nodes is sometimes performed to remove occult metastases, but is of controversial value.

A recent approach to treatment is photodynamic therapy. In principle, a light-sensitising drug is administered and localises to the tumour site. Exposure of the tumour to light of an appropriate wavelength triggers a photochemical reaction which should kill the cancer cells. One problem is to find a drug which allows a sufficiently selective effect and the method overall requires long-term assessment of its value.

Palliative treatment is given to patients who have advanced tumours or for treatment failures. Radiotherapy is the most practical method for palliative care but surgery is occasionally used when a large tumour compromises the airway or becomes grossly necrotic. Chemotherapy is little used in the UK, being reserved for widespread metastases or salvage therapy. It causes serious complications and there is evidence that it reduces the chances of survival.

SURVIVAL FROM ORAL CANCER

Duration of survival after treatment depends on many factors (Table 17.5). In comparison with malignant neoplasms at other body sites, oral carcinoma has a poor prognosis. The quality of life in the terminal stages is also poor.

The poorer survival of older people is probably because they are less able to withstand radiotherapy or surgery. The reason

Table 17.5 Some factors adversely affecting survival from oral cancer

- Delay in treatment
- Advanced age
- Male gender
- Tumour size
- Posterior location
- Lack of histological differentiation (high histological grade)
- Lymph node spread

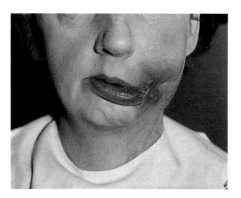

Fig. 17.16 Neglected cancer of the buccal mucosa about to ulcerate through the cheek.

for the poorer survival rates for males is uncertain, although later presentation is a possibility. Tumour stage at the start of treatment depends both on its growth rate and on delay in diagnosis. Because the stage of disease is critical to survival it is used to plan treatment and every oral carcinoma patient should be staged according to the TNM staging system (see Appendix 17.1). Each carcinoma is given a score for size (T), lymph node metastasis (N) and distant blood-borne metastasis (M). These are combined together to give a score between stage 0 (premalignancy) and IV. Unfortunately, most patients with oral carcinoma present at Stage III or IV (Fig. 17.16).

However, some small (early) carcinomas are fast-growing and aggressive, but large tumours, even if slow-growing, are more difficult to manage. In either case delay in treatment allows further tumour spread and poorer chances of long-term survival.

The highest mortality from oral cancer is in the first 2 years, the disease then continues to claim victims but at a slower rate, and those few that survive for 10 years have a reasonable chance of having been cured. As a guide to survival rates, nearly 90% of males with early-stage disease survive the first year, about 65% survive for up to 5 years, while just under 55% survive for 10 years. Of males with late-stage disease well under 45% survive the first year, about 16% survive for 5 years, and 12% survive for 10 years.

As to the site of the growth, the extremes are seen in cancer of the lip, where the 5-year survival rate for males is over 77%. For cancer of the tongue it is 26%, and in the mesopharynx it is only 17.6%. Tumours particularly of the posterior third of the tongue are not readily detectable and more difficult to excise. In general, therefore, the more posterior the tumour is, the poorer the survival.

ROLE OF THE DENTIST

Early diagnosis is critical if patients are to be cured. Small carcinomas are more easily excised, less likely to have metastasised and have the best prognosis. Unfortunately, most carcinomas present at a relatively late, incurable stage and health care workers, including dentists, frequently either fail to make the diagnosis or have actively delayed referral.

Dentists must be alert to the possibility of carcinoma even though they may encounter it only once or twice in a practising lifetime. The nature of a chronic ulcer, white or red lesion, or swelling of the mucous membrane *must* be confirmed by biopsy. Indecision about taking a biopsy or trying the effect of local measures or antibiotics can prove fatal.

The dental practitioner is likely to see more patients with white mucosal patches. As noted in Chapter 15, the vast majority of such lesions are benign and may be biopsied in a practice setting. However, it is inadvisable to perform a biopsy of a high-risk lesion (for instance an erythroplasia or speckled leukoplakia) because the practitioner may be forced into the unenviable position of having to tell the patient that they have cancer, a task for which most dentists are not trained.

Any high-risk premalignant lesion or suspected carcinoma should be referred the same day to a specialist treatment centre. An appropriately worded referral letter should state the urgent nature of the referral and the suspected malignant nature of the lesion.

Although much of a patient's treatment has to be performed in hospital, patients may continue to see their practitioner after treatment. The dental practitioner is also ideally placed for the prevention of oral cancer and can contribute in other ways (Table 17.6).

Table 17.6 Role of the dental practitioner in cancer prevention and diagnosis

- Prevention
  Actively discourage smoking and betel quid use
  Encourage moderation of alcohol intake
  Health promotion and education on oral carcinoma
  Provide check-ups for the edentulous and/or institutionalised elderly and other high risk non-attenders
- Early diagnosis
  Be vigilant and suspicious
  Always examine mucosa as well as the teeth
  Monitor low-risk premalignant lesions
  Refer all high-risk lesions on discovery
  Perform biopsy appropriately
- After treatment
  Manage simple denture problems after surgery
  Alleviate the effects of post-irradiation dry mouth, e.g. preventing caries (Chapter 3)
  Monitor for recurrence, new premalignant lesions and second primary tumours
  Monitor for cervical metastasis
  Maintain morale of and provide additional support to patients and their relatives

ORAL CANCER SCREENING

Screening is the process of applying a rapid test or examining a population to identify a group at risk from a disease. This group can then be referred for accurate and earlier diagnosis. An example is the national cervical carcinoma screening scheme using the cervical smear test. Oral carcinoma screening should be possible because the tumour is so accessible and because those at most risk (elderly persons, particularly those who smoke and drink alcohol) are readily identified. A simple effective screening test is an examination of the mouth for red and white lesions.

Because screening is not designed to be accurately diagnostic it may be performed by appropriately trained health care workers in the community. Such oral cancer screening schemes have proved successful in several countries with a high incidence. In the UK such a scheme would have the advantage that it might reach the most at-risk individuals who tend to be irregular dental attenders. It would also provide an opportunity for preventive advice to the same group.

Although a national screening scheme for the UK has been widely discussed, it has only applied on a limited scale. In the meantime, oral cancer screening continues to fall within the remit of the general dental and medical practitioner.

Tololinium chloride (toluidine blue) rinsing

Toluidine blue is a dye which binds to nuclei acids and can be used as an oral rinse in the hope of staining carcinoma and dysplastic lesions blue. The technique was extensively evaluated many years ago and is now the subject of a resurgence of interest. It may be of value when deciding which part of an extensive lesion should be biopsied or when the clinician does not feel confident about a clinical diagnosis.

However, the technique is not an accurate test for either carcinoma or premalignancy and is no more than an adjunct to clinical diagnosis. If used indiscriminately on white lesions and ulcers the technique has a high false-positive rate. Also, toluidine blue is itself mutagenic and it seems inadvisable to use it as a general screening test. The general rule should be that any suspicious lesion must be subjected to biopsy as soon as possible, regardless of the pattern of staining with toluidine blue.

Brush biopsy

This technique uses a round stiff bristle brush to collect cells from the surface and subsurface layers of a lesion by vigorous abrasion. The brush is rotated in one spot until bleeding starts, to ensure a sufficiently deep sample. The cells collected are transferred to a microscope slide and the smear is scanned in an image analyser to identify abnormal cells, which are examined

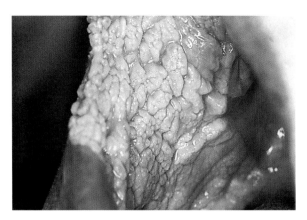

Fig. 17.17 Verrucous carcinoma. An extensive lesion covering most of the buccal mucosa and starting to involve the skin at the commissure. Such longstanding lesions are likely to develop invasive squamous carcinoma and may then metastasise. (By kind permission of Professor S J Challacombe.)

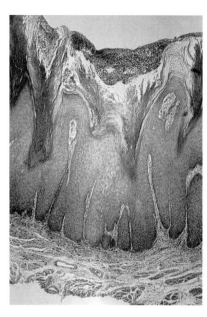

Fig. 17.18 Verrucous carcinoma. The epithelium is thickened and thrown into a series of folds with a spiky parakeratotic surface. Deeply the carcinoma retains a broad pushing front.

for diagnosis. A high degree of sensitivity and specificity for carcinoma is claimed but there is an unknown false-positive rate for identification of dysplasia. Though this technique holds great promise, it requires fuller evaluation before it can be recommended for use in primary care or for screening.

VERRUCOUS CARCINOMA

This variant of squamous cell carcinoma is a low-grade neoplasm. In the UK it is more frequent in the elderly, particularly males, and has a characteristic white, warty appearance, forming a well-circumscribed mass raised above the level of the surrounding mucosa (Fig. 17.17). If small, it may easily be mistaken for a papilloma. Verrucous carcinoma is particularly associated with the habit of snuff dipping (see above).

Pathology

Verrucous carcinoma consists of close-packed papillary masses of well-differentiated squamous epithelium which is heavily keratinised. The lower border of the lesion is well defined and formed by blunt rete processes which indent but do not invade the underlying tissues. There is typically chronic inflammation in the stroma (Fig. 17.18).

Verrucous carcinoma is slow-growing and spreads laterally rather than deeply. It can be excised relatively easily unless it is extensive. If left untreated for a period of years, a focus within verrucous carcinoma may progress to invasive squamous

carcinoma and release metastases. The neoplasm must then be treated as a conventional squamous carcinoma.

APPENDIX 17.1 THE TNM SYSTEM OF STAGING

T1   less than 2 cm greatest dimension
T2   2–4 cm greatest dimension
T3   > 4 cm greatest dimension
T4   extending to adjacent structures, e.g. bone, sinus, skin

N0   No regional lymph node metastases
N1   One ipsilateral node < 3 cm diameter
N2   Ipsilateral or contralateral nodes 3–6 cm diameter
N3   Lymph node metastasis > 6 cm diameter

M0   No distant metastases
M1   Distant metastasis (e.g. liver, lung)

Scores are compiled to designate the stage as follows:
Stage 1   T1 N0 M0
Stage 2   T2 N0 M0
Stage 3   T3 N0 M0
Stage 4   any T4
          any N2 or N3
          any M1

SUGGESTED FURTHER READING

Al-Bakkal G, Ficarra G, McNeill K et al 1999 Human papilloma virus type 16 E6 gene expression in oral exophytic epithelial lesions as detected by rtPCR. Oral Surg Oral Med Oral Pathol Oral Radiol Endod 87:197–200

Anderson D L 1971 Cause and prevention of lip cancer. J Can Dent Assoc 37:138–143

Caniff J P, Harvey W, Harris M 1986 Oral submucous fibrosis: its pathogenesis and management. Br Dent J 160:429–434

Cawson R A, Binnie W H, Barrett A W, Wright J M 2001 *Oral disease*, 3rd Edn. Mosby-Wolfe, London

Cawson R A Binnie W H, Barrett A W, Wright M 1998 *Lucas's Pathology of tumors of the oral tissues*. Churchill Livingstone, Edinburgh

Cawson R A. Langdon J D, Eveson J W 1996 *Surgical pathology of the mouth and jaws*. Wright, Oxford

Franceschi S, Munoz N, Snijders P J F 2000 How strong and how wide is the link between HPV and oropharyngeal cancer? Lancet 356:871–872

Girod S C, Pfahl M 1996 Retinoid actions and implications for prevention and therapy of cancer. Int J Oral Maxillofac Surg 25:69–73

Goldberg H I, Lockwood S A, Wyatt S W, Crosset L S 1994 Trends and differentials from cancers of the oral cavity and pharynx in the United States, 1973–1987. Cancer 74:565–572

Hogewind W F C, van der Waal I, van der Kwast W A, Snow G B 1989 The association of white lesions with oral squamous cell carcinoma. A retrospective study of 212 patients. Int J Oral Maxillofac Surg 18:163–164

Hopper C 1996 The role of photodynamic therapy in the management of oral cancer and precancer. Oral Oncol Eur J Cancer 32B:71–72

Kusama K, Okutso S, Takeda A et al 1996 p53 gene alterations and p53 protein in oral epithelial dysplasia and squamous cell carcinoma. J Pathol 178:415–421

Link J O, Kaugars G E, Burns J C 1992 Comparison of oral carcinomas in smokeless tobacco users and nonusers. J Oral Maxillofac Surg 50:452–455

Lukinmaa P-L, Hietanen J, Söderholm A-L, Lindquist C 1992 The histologic pattern of bone invasion by squamous cell carcinoma of the mandibualr region. Br J Oral Maxillofac Surg 30:2–7

Murti P R, Bhonsle R B, Pindborg J J, Daftary D K, Gupta P C, Mehta F S 1985 Malignant transformation rate in oral submucous fibrosis over a 17-year period. Community Dent Oral Epidemiol 13:340–341

Ogden G R, Kiddie R A, Lunny D P, Lane D P 1992 Assessment of p53 protein expression in normal, benign and malignant oral mucosa. J Pathol 166:389–394

Shahnavaz S A, Regezi J A, Bradley G et al 2000 p53 gene mutations in sequential oral epithelial dysplasias and squamous cell carcinomas. J Pathol 190:417–422

Warnakulasuriya A 2000 Lack of molecular markers to predict malignant potential of oral cancer. J Pathol 190:407–409

Neoplastic and non-neoplastic diseases of salivary glands

Normal function and health of the mouth depend on normal secretion of saliva by the major and minor glands. Failure of salivary secretion causes a dry mouth which is both distressing and promotes oral infections.

OBSTRUCTION

Salivary calculi

A stone can form in a salivary gland or duct. At least 80% of calculi form in the submandibular gland, about 6% in the parotid and about 2% in the sublingual and minor salivary glands.

Clinical features

Adults are mainly affected — males twice as often as females. Calculi are usually unilateral. The classical symptom is pain when the smell or taste of food stimulates salivary secretion. Alternatively, duct obstruction can lead to infection, pain and swelling of the gland.

Occasionally there are no symptoms until the stone passes forward and can be palpated in the duct or seen at the duct

orifice (Fig. 18.1). Alternatively, the stone may be seen in a radiograph. However, about 40% of parotid and 20% of submandibular stones are not radiopaque, and sialography may be needed to locate them.

Calculi are *not* a cause of dry mouth.

Pathology

Salivary calculi usually form by deposition of calcium salts around a nidus of organic material, and have a layered structure. The roughness of their surface may cause the duct lining to undergo squamous metaplasia (Fig. 18.2).

Management

If sufficiently far forward in the duct, a stone may sometimes be milked forward and manipulated out of the orifice. Otherwise the duct has to be opened. An incision, usually under local anaesthesia, is made along the line of the duct just long enough to release the mass. A temporary suture should be put through the duct behind the calculus to prevent it from slipping backwards. The papilla should be left unsutured or the margins of

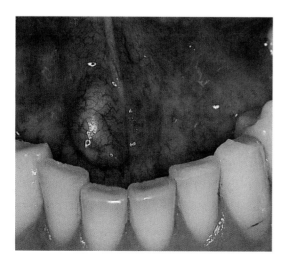

Fig. 18.1 Salivary calculus. This stone has impacted just behind the orifice of the submandibular duct forming a hard nodule. The yellow colour of the stone is visible through the thin mucosa.

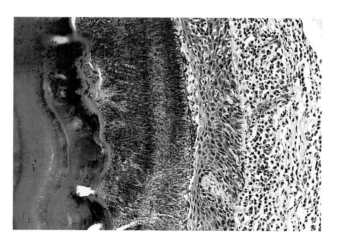

Fig. 18.2 Salivary calculus in a duct. To the left is the salivary calculus which has a lamellar structure and an irregular surface. On the surface is a thick layer of microbial flora filling the space between the stone and the epithelial lining. In the surrounding wall there is an infiltrate of lymphocytes and plasma cells and neutrophils are migrating through the duct epithelium into the lumen.

the opening are sutured to the mucosa on either side to prevent subsequent scarring and fibrous obstruction. If the gland has become damaged by recurrent infection and fibrosis, or calculi have formed within the gland itself, it may have to be excised.

Key features of salivary calculi are summarised in Table 18.1.

Table 18.1   **Salivary calculi: key features**

- Adult males mainly affected
- Usually (80%) in submandibular gland
- Usually form by accretion of calcium salts round organic nidus
- Typically cause pain by obstructing food-related surge of salivary secretion
- Occasionally asymptomatic until palpable in the mouth or seen in routine radiograph
- Do *not* cause dry mouth
- Should be removed by manipulation or incision of duct

Parotid papilla and duct strictures

The usual cause is chronic trauma (from such causes as projecting clasps, faulty restorations or sharp edges of broken teeth) leading to fibrosis. Fibrosis makes the duct papilla difficult to find and may prevent insertion of a probe.

Fibrosis and stenosis of a duct may be caused by ulceration round a calculus or result from incompetent surgery.

Sialography should show the degree of narrowing of the duct or papilla and dilatation behind. Once the cause has been removed, treatment depends on the site of the obstruction. The papilla may have to be excised and the duct lining sutured to the oral mucosa on either side. Alternatively, the duct may be dilated with bougies.

Salivary fistula

Salivary fistula, a communication between the duct system or gland with the skin or mucous membrane, is uncommon. Internal fistulae drain into the oral cavity and cause no symptoms. By contrast, parotid fistula on the skin is troublesome and often persistent. It may be the result of an injury to the cheek or a complication of surgery. Infection often becomes superimposed and persistent leakage of saliva prevents healing. The treatment is primarily by surgical repair but is difficult, especially because of the risk of damage to branches to the facial nerve.

Mucoceles and cysts

The most common type of salivary and soft-tissue cyst is the extravasation mucocele of minor glands. It is not a true cyst as it has no epithelial lining. Retention cysts are far less common. Mucoceles mainly affect the minor salivary glands, particularly of the lip. The cause is usually damage to the duct of a mucous gland. This may be caused by a blow on the lip, as might happen to a football referee holding a whistle in his mouth.

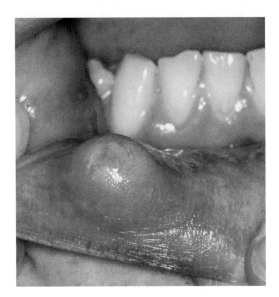

Fig. 18.3   Mucous extravasation cyst. The typical presentation at the commonest site: a rounded bluish, translucent cyst in the lower lip.

Clinical features

Mucoceles most often form in the lower lip but occasionally on the buccal mucosa or floor of the mouth (ranula). They are usually superficial and rarely larger than 1 cm in diameter. In the early stages they appear as rounded fleshy swellings. Later, they are obviously cystic, hemispherical, fluctuant and bluish due to the thin wall (Fig. 18.3). A mucocele cannot be distinguished from a retention cyst clinically, but this is of little practical importance.

Pathology

Preceding the formation of a mucocele, saliva leaking from a damaged duct into the superficial surrounding tissues excites an

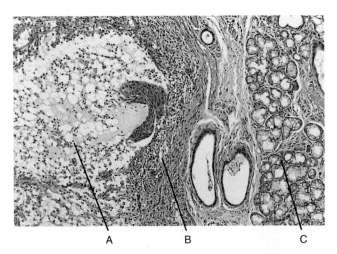

Fig. 18.4   Extravasation mucocele. To the left is a cavity of spilt mucin with the remnants of the ruptured duct lining epithelium at its edge. To the right is the associated minor mucous salivary gland. A, saliva and macrophages; B, compressed connective tissue wall; C, minor salivary gland.

inflammatory reaction (Figs 18.4 and 18.5). The pools of saliva gradually coalesce to form a rounded collection of fluid, surrounded by compressed connective tissue without an epithelial lining.

Less frequently, the duct may become obstructed but less severely damaged so that saliva does not escape into the surrounding tissues. A retention cyst thus forms with a lining of compressed duct epithelium (Fig. 18.6).

Treatment

A small superficial mucocele should be excised with the underlying gland. The latter is usually found to have been removed with the cyst but if not, recurrence is likely. Key features are summarised in Table 18.2.

Ranula

A ranula is an uncommon type of salivary cyst arising from the sublingual or submandibular salivary glands.

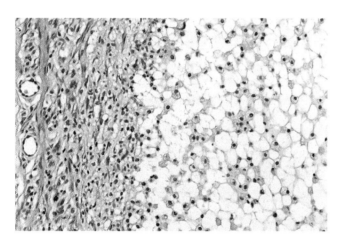

Fig. 18.5 Extravasation mucocele. Higher power showing the lining of the mucin-filled space. Macrophages are migrating into the mucin and in phagocytosing it develop a foamy or vacuolated cytoplasm.

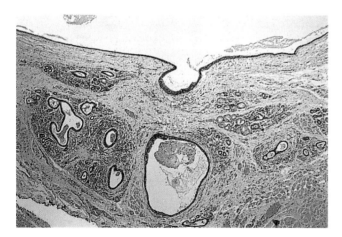

Fig. 18.6 Mucous retention cyst. Remnants of the minor mucous salivary glands are visible, together with their dilated duct, the epithelium of which is continuous with the epithelial lining of the cyst (above).

Table 18.2 Mucoceles and cysts: key features

- Most common soft tissue cyst
- Most frequently on lower lip
- Usually caused by damage to duct and extravasation of saliva
- Saliva leaking into surrounding tissues causes mild inflammation
- Saliva eventually pools up to form a mucocele with connective tissue lining
- Rarely due to duct obstruction and dilatation forming a retention cyst with epithelial lining

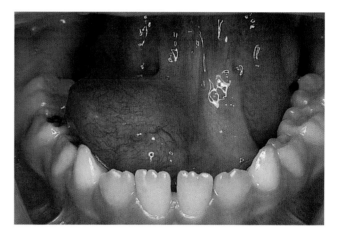

Fig. 18.7 Ranula. A large bluish, translucent swelling in the floor of the mouth caused by a mucous extravasation or retention cyst.

The structure is usually the same as other salivary retention cysts. Ranulae are usually unilateral and 2 or 3 cm in diameter (Fig. 18.7). Occasionally they extend across the whole of the floor of the mouth. They are soft, fluctuant and bluish. They are typically painless but may interfere with speech or mastication. Treatment is preferably by marsupialisation with removal of the related gland. A simple incision leads to recurrence, and enucleation is difficult because of the very thin wall.

SIALADENITIS

Mumps

Mumps is due a paramyxovirus (the mumps virus) and causes painful swelling of the parotids and sometimes other glands. It is highly infectious and is the most common cause of acute parotid swelling.

Clinical features

Children are mainly affected. An incubation period of about 21 days is followed by headache, malaise, fever and tense, painful and tender swelling of the parotids. Permanent nerve deafness or, rarely, meningitis are possible complications. Adults who contract mumps may develop orchitis or oophoritis and may have severe and prolonged malaise. After an attack immunity is long-lasting.

The diagnosis is usually obvious from the history and clinical findings, especially in a child. However, mumps may be mistaken for a dental infection or bacterial sialadenitis, if unilateral. Rarely, when the submaxillary or sublingual glands are affected, mumps may have to be differentiated from lymphadenitis. In cases of doubt a history of mumps earlier in life usually excludes this diagnosis. If necessary, the diagnosis can be confirmed by a rise in titre of complement-fixing antibodies. Afterwards, antibodies to the S antigen disappear relatively quickly, and their presence indicates recent mumps. The V antibody is persistent and indicates infection at some time previously.

With wide use of immunisation, childhood mumps should be becoming infrequent and mumps in adults may take atypical forms.

Suppurative parotitis

Suppurative parotitis traditionally affected debilitated patients, particularly postoperatively, as a result of xerostomia secondary to dehydration. Currently, suppurative parotitis is more commonly seen in ambulant patients with severe xerostomia, particularly Sjögren's syndrome, and as an uncommon complication of tricyclic antidepressant treatment. Important bacterial causes include *Staphylococcus aureus*, streptococci and anaerobes. Typical clinical features are pain in one or both parotids with swelling, redness and tenderness and often increasing malaise and fever. The regional lymph nodes are enlarged and tender, and pus exudes or can be expressed from the parotid duct (Fig. 18.8). The progress of the infection depends largely on the patient's underlying physical state.

Pathology

An intense acute inflammatory infiltrate extends along and dilates the ducts. Inflammation also extends into the periductal tissues

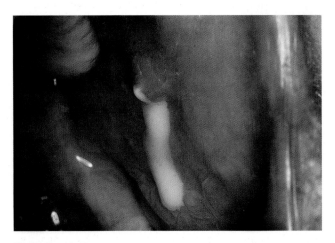

Fig. 18.8 Suppurative parotitis – pus is leaking from the parotid papilla.

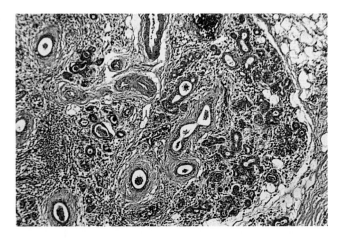

Fig. 18.9 Chronic sialadenitis resulting from obstruction. The ducts contain casts of mucin and neutrophils and are surrounded by a layer of fibrosis. There is severe acinar atrophy and the space previously occupied by acinar cells now contains infiltrates of lymphocytes and plasma cells.

and to a varying degree into acini. If neglected, abscesses form and there are varying degrees of acinar destruction.

Management

Treatment can be started with flucloxacillin, but only after pus has been obtained for culture and sensitivity testing. The antibiotic can be changed if the bacteriological findings dictate and drainage is rarely necessary.

Chronic sialadenitis

Chronic sialadenitis is usually a complication of duct obstruction. It is usually unilateral and asymptomatic or with intermittent painful swelling of the gland. Sialography may show dilatation of ducts behind the obstruction.

Pathology

There are varying degrees of destruction of acini, duct dilatation and a scattered chronic inflammatory cellular infiltrate, predominantly lymphoplasmacytic (Fig. 18.9). Extensive interstitial fibrosis, and sometimes squamous metaplasia in the duct epithelium, follow. Calculus formation may be seen in the dilated ducts.

If possible, the obstruction should be removed, but more often the gland has to be excised and the mass examined histologically to exclude a neoplasm.

DRY MOUTH (XEROSTOMIA)

Many patients with severe xerostomia make no complaint of dry mouth, though they may, for instance, admit that they have difficulty in eating dry food. Some complain of an unpleasant taste in the mouth. Conversely, some who complain of dry mouth have normal salivary flow rates on objective testing and the problem is neurotic in nature. Salivary flow studies are valuable when patients complain of dry mouth. Important causes are summarised in Table 18.3.

Table 18.3   Causes of xerostomia

- Organic causes
  Sjögren's syndrome
  Irradiation
  Mumps (transient)
  HIV infection
  HCV infection
  Sarcoidosis
  Amyloid
  Iron deposition
    (haemochromatosis,
    thalassaemia)
- Functional causes
  Dehydration
  Fluid deprivation or loss
  Haemorrhage
  Persistent diarrhoea
    and/or vomiting
  Psychogenic
    Anxiety states
    Depression
  Drugs

- Drugs
  Diuretic overdosage
  Drugs with antimuscarinic effects
    Atropine, ipratropium, hyoscine
      and other analogues
    Tricyclic and some other
      antidepressants
    Antihistamines
    Antiemetics (including
      antihistamines and
      phenothiazines)
    Neuroleptics, particularly
      phenothiazines
    Some older antihypertensives,
      (ganglion blockers and
      clonidine)
  Drugs with sympathomimetic
    actions
    'Cold cures' containing
      ephedrine, etc.
    Decongestants
    Bronchodilators
    Appetite supressants,
      particularly amphetamines

SJÖGREN'S SYNDROME

In 1933 Sjögren noticed the association of dryness of the mouth and dryness of the eyes. Later he found that there was a significant association with rheumatoid arthritis. These combinations of complaints are caused by two closely related but distinct diseases.

Primary Sjögren's syndrome comprises dry mouth and dry eyes not associated with any connective tissue disease.

Secondary Sjögren's syndrome comprises dry mouth and dry eyes associated with rheumatoid arthritis or other connective tissue disease.

Clinical features

Females are affected nearly 10 times as frequently as males. Sjögren's syndrome affects 10–15% of patients with rheumatoid arthritis, possibly 30% of patients with lupus erythematosus and a variable proportion of patients with or without other connective-tissue diseases. Sjögren's syndromes are therefore relatively common. In the absence of drug treatment or radiotherapy, they are the main cause of dry mouth but their most serious consequence is damage to the eyes and the risk of lymphoma. Primary Sjögren's syndrome tends to cause more severe oral and ocular changes and has a higher risk of lymphomatous change than secondary.

Table 18.4   Oral effects of Sjögren's syndrome

- Discomfort
- Difficulties with eating or swallowing
- Disturbed taste sensation
- Disturbed quality of speech
- Predisposition to infection

Major oral effects of Sjögren's syndrome are summarised in Table 18.4.

In the early stages, the mucosa may appear moist but salivary flow measurement shows diminished secretion. In established cases the oral mucosa is obviously dry, often red, shiny and parchment-like (Fig. 18.10). The tongue is typically red, the papillae characteristically atrophy and the dorsum becomes lobulated with a cobblestone appearance (Fig. 18.11). With diminished salivary secretion the oral flora changes and candidal infections are common. The latter are the main cause of soreness of the mouth in Sjögren's syndrome and cause

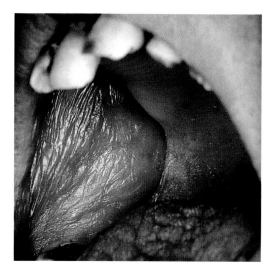

Fig. 18.10   Sjögren's syndrome. The mucosa is dry, red, atrophic and wrinkled and sticks to the fingers or mirror during examination. These changes are common to all causes of xerostomia.

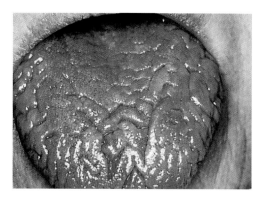

Fig. 18.11   Tongue in Sjögren's syndrome. Longstanding dry mouth and repeated candidal infection produce this depapillated but lobulated tongue.

CHAPTER 18

generalised erythema of the mucosa, often with angular stomatitis. Plaque accumulates (Fig. 18.12) and there may be rapidly progressive dental caries. The most severe infective complication is suppurative parotitis.

Swelling of the parotids is not common, but a history of swelling at some stage may be obtained in about 30% of patients. Swelling due to the syndrome itself shows no inflammation and is rarely painful (Fig. 18.13). A hot, tender parotid swelling with red, shiny overlying skin indicates suppurative parotitis. Parotid swelling appearing years after the onset strongly suggests lymphomatous change.

Sjögren's syndrome can have serious ocular effects (Table 18.5).

Aetiology and pathology

Sjögren's syndrome is an autoimmune (connective tissue) disease which shows a corresponding variety of immunological abnormalities (Table 18.6).

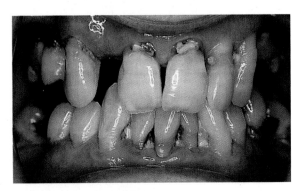

Fig. 18.12 Sjögren's syndrome. Extensive cervical caries is a frequent complication of dry mouth. In addition to the lack of saliva, patients may attempt to stimulate salivary flow with sweets or chewing gums.

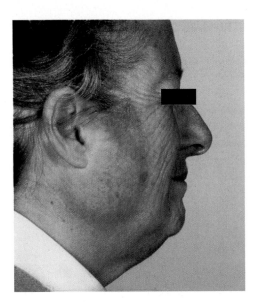

Fig. 18.13 Salivary gland swelling in primary Sjögren's syndrome. The outline of the parotid gland is clearly demarcated.

Table 18.5 Ocular effects of Sjögren's syndrome

- Failure of tear secretion
- Failure of clearance of foreign particles from the cornea and conjunctiva (*keratoconjunctivitis sicca*)
- Gritty sensation in the eyes and inflammation
- Risk of impairment or loss of sight

Table 18.6 Typical patterns of autoantibodies in primary and secondary Sjögren's syndromes

Autoantibodies	Primary SS	Secondary SS
Salivary duct antibody	10–36%	67–70%
Rheumatoid factor	50%±	90%±
SS-A (Ro) antibodies	5–10%	50–80%
SS-B (La) antibodies	50–75%	2–5%
Rheumatoid arthritis precipitin	5%±	75%±

A retrovirus or other virus is as yet unconfirmed as a cause. Histological changes are shown in Table 18.7.

Table 18.7 Histological changes in salivary glands in Sjögren's syndrome

- Polyclonal infiltration mainly by CD4 lymphocytes
- Infiltrate initially periductal
- Progressive spread of infiltrate through the glandular tissue
- Progressive destruction of secretory acini
- Proliferation of some duct tissue as epimyoepithelial islands

The final result is replacement of the whole gland by a dense lymphocytic infiltrate (Figs 18.14 and 18.15). However the infiltrate remains confined within the gland capsule and does not cross the intraglandular septa.

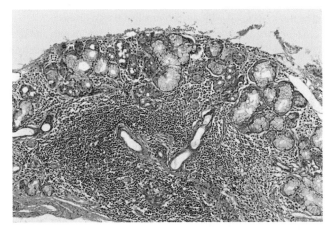

Fig. 18.14 Sjögren's syndrome. The histological appearance is typical. Dense, well-defined foci of lymphocytes surround the larger ducts in the centre of the lobules. In the area occupied by the lymphocytes there is complete acinar atrophy and a rim of residual salivary parenchyma remains around the periphery of the lobule.

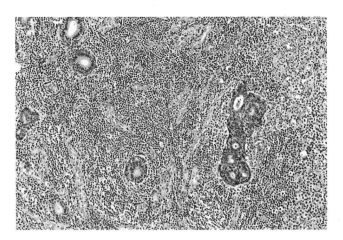

Fig. 18.15 Sjögren's syndrome. In late disease no salivary acini remain and the gland is replaced by a confluent infiltrate of lymphocytes. A few ducts remain and proliferate to form the epimyoepithelial islands. Such extensive changes sometimes suggest that there has been progression to a low-grade lymphoma.

Diagnosis

Other causes of xerostomia must be excluded (see Table 18.3). Diagnostic tests in Sjögren's syndrome are summarised in Table 18.8.

Table 18.8 Diagnostic tests in Sjögren's syndrome
• Diminished total salivary flow rate
• Labial salivary gland biopsy showing periductal lymphocytic infiltrate
• Antibody screen, especially rheumatoid factor and SS-A and SS-B
• Sialectasis on sialography
• Diminished tear secretion

Normal salivary flow is between 1 and 2 ml per minute but may be reduced to 0.5 ml/min or less. Pathological changes in labial salivary glands correlate closely with those in the parotids and lip biopsy avoids the risks of damage to the facial nerve or a parotid fistula inherent in parotid gland biopsy. A snowstorm appearance on sialography (so-called sialectasis) is due to leakage of contrast material through the duct walls (Fig. 18.16). However, in a patient who is not taking xerostomia-inducing drugs, but with rheumatoid arthritis or other connective tissue disease and objectively confirmed diminished salivary flow, further investigation seems hard to justify.

Management

Many aspects need to be taken into account (Table 18.9), but the combination of painful arthritis and dryness of the mouth in secondary Sjögren's syndrome can reduce life to prolonged misery.

Ophthalmological examination is particularly important to exclude keratoconjunctivitis sicca, which is symptomless in its early stages. Anaemia should be excluded, particularly when there is rheumatoid arthritis.

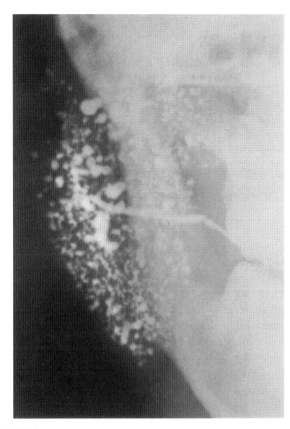

Fig. 18.16 Sjögren's syndrome. The sialogram shows the typical snowstorm appearance of blobs of contrast medium that have leaked from the duct system. Emptying and clearance of the contrast medium are also much delayed because of the reduced salivary flow.

Table 18.9 Principles of management of Sjögren's syndrome
• Salivary gland damage is irreversible
• Give reassurance and help with dry mouth
• Ophthalmological investigation for *keratoconjunctivitis sicca*
• Refer to specialist if connective tissue disease is untreated
• Check for any associated drug treatment contributing to dry mouth

• Alleviate dry mouth
  Frequent small sips of water
  Prescribe saliva substitutes

• Control caries in dentate patients
  Avoid sweets (e.g. lemon drops)
  Suggest sugar-free gum
  Check diet for excess sugary foods
  Maintain good oral hygiene
  Fluoride applications
  Chlorhexidine (0.2%) rinses

• Monitor for mucosal candidosis   Give antifungal mixtures (not tablets) as necessary
• Treat difficulties with dentures symptomatically
• Observe regularly for possible development of ascending parotitis or lymphoma

Dryness of the mouth can be relieved to some degree by providing artificial saliva (Table 18.10). Cholinesterase inhibitors such as pilocarpine are sometimes recommended to stimulate

Table 18.10 Types of artificial saliva currently available

- Glandosane spray. Carmellose (carboxymethyl cellulose) solution with sorbitol and electrolytes: neutral, lemon or peppermint flavoured
- Luborant spray. Carmellose solution with electrolytes and preservatives
- Oralbalance gel. Lactoperoxidase, glucose oxidase and xylitol
- Saliva Orthana spray. Gastric mucin, xylitol, sodium fluoride with preservatives and flavouring
- Saliva Orthana lozenges. Mucin with xylitol in sorbitol bases
- Salivace spray. Carmellose with xylitol, electrolytes and preservative
- Salivix pastilles. Sugar-free. Contain gum acacia and malic acid

salivary secretion but any benefits may be counterbalanced by side-effects such as nausea, diarrhoea and bradycardia.

Dryness of the eyes is treated with artificial tears such as methyl cellulose solution. In dentate patients, sweet-eating should be prohibited, a high standard of oral hygiene maintained and frequent dental checks are necessary. Topical fluorides should be applied regularly and 0.2% chlorhexidine mouth rinses may help to reduce plaque formation. Soreness of the mouth, due to infection by *Candida albicans*, can be treated with nystatin or amphotericin mixture, *not* tablets. Ascending parotitis should be treated as described earlier.

In view of the risk of malignant lymphoma, immunosuppressive treatment or irradiation, to reduce the size of swollen glands is contraindicated. In any case, such measures have no lasting benefit in Sjögren's syndrome. Key features are summarised in Table 18.11.

Table 18.11 Sjögren's syndromes: key features

- Middle-aged or elderly women mainly affected
- Rheumatoid arthritis or other connective tissue disease associated in secondary Sjögren's syndrome
- Dry mouth
- Dry eyes
- Polyclonal infiltration of salivary glands by CD4 lymphocytes with acinar destruction
- Multiple autoantibodies particularly Ro (SS-A) and La (SS-B)
- Significant risk of salivary gland and extrasalivary lymphomas

Salivary lymphoepithelial lesion (benign lymphoepithelial lesion, myoepithelial sialadenitis etc.)

Benign lymphoepithelial lesion is a term that has been used to describe salivary gland swelling with the histological features of Sjögren's syndrome. Other features of Sjögren's syndrome were thought to be absent but this appears to have been due to inadequate investigation. Benign lymphoepithelial lesion is a misleading term, which should be avoided as there is a high risk of lymphomatous change and it is probably not a separate entity from Sjögren's syndrome.

IRRADIATION DAMAGE

Salivary tissue is highly sensitive to ionising radiation. Irreversible destruction of acini and fibrous replacement can result from therapeutic radiation of the head and neck. Troublesome xerostomia with its attendant complications, such as rampant dental caries, is the typical result.

The management of dry mouth is as described earlier. However, it is especially important to control dental caries and its sequelae because of the danger of irradiation-associated osteomyelitis (Ch. 6) secondary to periapical infection or extractions.

HIV-ASSOCIATED SALIVARY GLAND DISEASE

Chronic parotitis in children is said to be almost pathognomonic of HIV infection. In adults, xerostomia, sometimes with cystic parotid gland swellings, may develop and be associated with generalised lymphadenopathy (Ch. 22). Young males are predominantly affected.

Pathology

The histological features are essentially similar to those of Sjögren's syndrome, apart from gross cyst formation. Also, the infiltrate is by CD8 lymphocytes and autoantibodies typical of Sjögren's syndrome are lacking. As in Sjögren's syndrome, lymphomatous change is a hazard.

HIV salivary gland cysts respond to highly-active retroviral therapy.

SJÖGREN-LIKE SYNDROME IN GRAFT-VERSUS-HOST DISEASE

A disease similar to primary Sjögren's syndrome develops in about a third of all cases of graft-versus-host disease, particularly when severe. The histological changes in lip biopsies are the same as in Sjögren's syndrome and serve to distinguish GVHD from salivary gland damage secondary to irradiation used for immunosuppression before marrow transplantation.

HYPERSALIVATION (PTYALISM)

True ptyalism is not a significant complaint as any excess of saliva can readily be swallowed. 'False ptyalism' is more common and is either delusional (a disturbed patient may suddenly become alarmed at 'water' continually appearing in the mouth) or due to faulty neuromuscular control that leads to drooling despite normal salivary flow (Table 18.12).

Table 18.12 Causes of ptyalism

- Local reflexes
  Oral infections (e.g. acute necrotising ulcerative gingivitis)
  Oral wounds
  Dental procedures
  New dentures
- Systemic
  Nausea
  Acid regurgition (reflux oesophagitis)
- Toxic
  Iodine. Heavy metal poisoning
- 'False ptyalism' (drooling)
  Psychogenic
  Bell's palsy
  Parkinson's disease
  Stroke

SALIVARY GLAND NEOPLASMS

Salivary gland tumours comprise a significant proportion of oral tumours, and are the next most common neoplasms of the mouth after squamous cell carcinoma. However, tumours of the minor intraoral salivary glands are less common than in the parotids. The incidence of salivary gland cancers in Europe is estimated to be about 1.2 per 100 000 and in England and Wales, about 600 salivary gland cancers are registered each year. However, over 75% of salivary gland tumours are benign,

so that the total number (benign and malignant) seen annually in Britain may be approximately 2400. Women are slightly more frequently affected. About 70% of salivary gland tumours develop in the parotid and a few affect the submandibular glands. Tumours in the sublingual glands are a rarity but usually malignant (Fig. 18.17).

Little is known of the aetiology of salivary gland tumours except that they can result from irradiation to the head area. In survivors of the atomic blasts at Hiroshima and Nagasaki there has been an excess of salivary gland tumours. Similarly, these tumours can follow therapeutic irradiation of, for example, the thyroid and, it is suggested, multiple dental diagnostic radiographs.

Classification

The World Health Organization 1972 classification of salivary gland tumours is still widely used and a modified version is summarised in Table 18.13.

The 1990 WHO typing of salivary gland tumours includes no fewer than 32 types of epithelial tumours, but of these only polymorphous low grade adenocarcinoma and epithelial-myoepithelial carcinoma are included in the following discussion.

General clinical features of salivary gland tumours

Adults are predominantly affected. The usual intraoral site is the palate, often at the junction of the hard and soft palate (Fig.

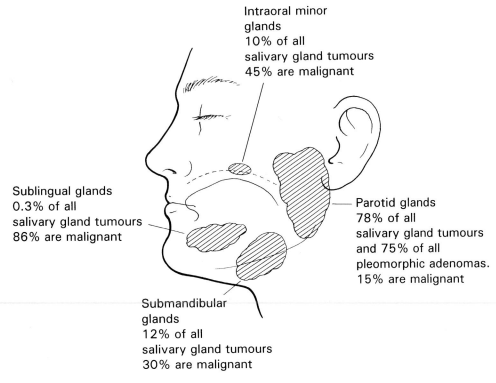

Fig. 18.17 The distribution of salivary gland neoplasms showing the approximate overall frequency of tumours in different sites and the relevant frequency of benign and malignant tumours by site.

Table 18.13 Salivary gland neoplasms (modified 1972 classification)

- Epithelial tumours
    Adenomas
        Pleomorphic adenoma ('mixed tumour')
        Monomorphic adenomas
            Warthin's tumour, Oxyphilic adenoma etc.
    Carcinomas
        Mucoepidermoid carcinoma
        Acinic cell carcinoma
        Adenoid cystic carcinoma
        Adenocarcinoma
        Epidermoid carcinoma
        Undifferentiated carcinoma
        Carcinoma in pleomorphic adenoma (malignant mixed tumour)
- Non-epithelial tumours
    Lymphomas
    Sarcomas

18.18), or occasionally the cheek or lip. Typical clinical features of benign and malignant salivary gland tumours are shown in Table 18.14. However, in their early stages, benign and malignant salivary gland tumours cannot be distinguished clinically.

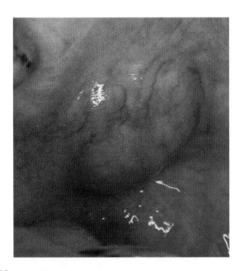

Fig. 18.18 Pleomorphic adenoma. The junction of hard and soft palates is a common intraoral site; the tumour usually feels rubbery and lobulated on palpation.

Table 18.14 Typical clinical features of salivary gland tumours

Benign salivary gland tumours	Malignant salivary gland tumours
Slow-growing	Sometimes fast-growing and painful
Soft or rubbery consistency	Sometimes hard consistency
Comprise 85% of parotid tumours	Comprise 45% of minor gland tumours
Do not ulcerate	May ulcerate and invade bone
No associated nerve signs	May cause cranial nerve palsies*

*Malignant parotid tumours can cause facial palsy in particular. Adenoid cystic carcinoma can cause multiple cranial nerve lesions especially lingual, facial or hypoglossal.

Pleomorphic adenoma

Pleomorphic adenomas ('mixed tumours') account for about 75% of parotid tumours (Fig. 18.19) but a lower proportion of intraoral salivary gland tumours. They arise mainly from duct epithelium or myoepithelial cells. A wide variety of structures may be seen (Table 18.15).

Table 18.15 Important histological features of pleomorphic adenomas

- Capsule — never complete
- Ducts
- Sheets or strands of dark-staining epithelial cells
- Squamous metaplasia and foci of keratin
- Fibrous and elastic tissue
- Myxoid tissue
- Cartilage, sometimes calcified. Rarely, true bone formation

These varied tissues are completely disordered in arrangement and the proportions of the different components also vary widely (Figs 18.20–18.23). The fibrous, myxoid, or cartilaginous mesenchymal elements are due to the pluripotential properties of myoepithelial cells. Some tumours are predominantly myxoid and can burst at operation if not gently handled, and then recur. Myoepithelial cells cannot be identified by light microscopy and can appear dark and angular, spindle-shaped or resemble plasma cells. However, immunohistochemistry shows their typical double staining with epithelial (cytokeratin) markers and mesenchymal markers, particularly S-100 protein, vimentin and actin. Myoepithelial cells may occasionally predominate or are the only cells present. Such a tumour is termed a *myoepithelioma*.

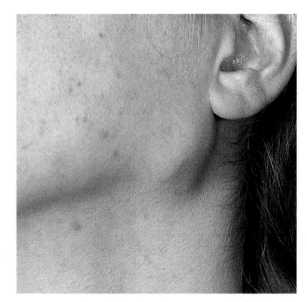

Fig. 18.19 Pleomorphic adenoma. This slowly enlarging lump in the lower pole of the parotid gland is caused by a pleomorphic adenoma but the appearance is not specific and any benign and some low-grade malignant neoplasms could appear the same.

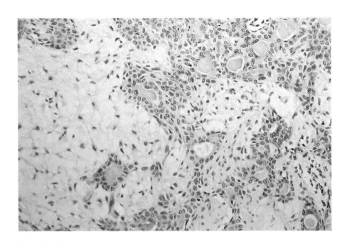

Fig. 18.20 Pleomorphic adenoma. The histological appearances are very varied. In this typical area there are clusters of ducts containing eosinophilic material surrounded by stellate cells lying in a mucinous stroma.

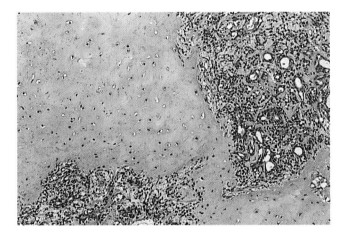

Fig. 18.21 Pleomorphic adenoma. In this area there has been maturation of the mucinous stroma to form a cartilage-like material within which there are more cellular islands with ducts.

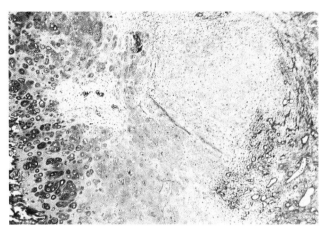

Fig. 18.22 Plemorphic adenoma. In this lesion there is formation of true cartilage which is undergoing calcification.

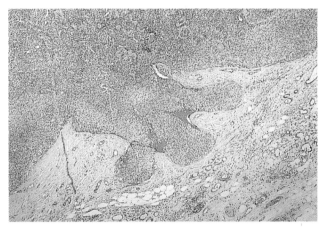

Fig. 18.23 Plemorphic adenoma. At the margins of pleomorphic adenomas there are often extensions of the tumour into and beyond the capsule, rendering enucleation an ineffective treatment.

Growth of pleomorphic adenomas is slow and may take several years to reach an inch in diameter. They form rubbery, often lobulated swellings (Fig. 18.24). When close under the mucosa, the tumour may appear bluish. The swelling is typically attached to the overlying mucosa but mobile on the deeper tissues. If neglected, pleomorphic adenomas can grow to a great size and occasionally undergo malignant change.

Treatment is by wide excision: recurrence is otherwise inevitable. The reputation of the pleomorphic adenoma for recurrence is due to the great surgical difficulties of complete removal of tumours from the parotid (the common site), where the facial nerve, in particular, makes dissection hazardous. Pleomorphic adenomas have an unusually strong tendency to seed and recur in the incision scar if opened at operation or if incompletely excised. In the case of parotid tumours, therefore, recurrences are prevented only by removing the gland with the tumour intact. The recurrence rate is low in skilled hands, but recurrences are typically multifocal and difficult to eradicate.

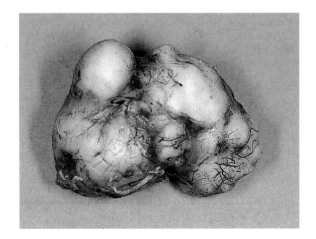

Fig. 18.24 This excised pleomorphic adenoma is 3 cm across and the lobular shape is clearly seen.

Warthin's tumour (adenolymphoma)

Warthin's tumour arises in the parotid glands and accounts for about 9% of tumours there. It has a highly characteristic histological appearance consisting of tall, eosinophilic columnar cells which form a much-folded layer covering dense lymphoid tissue, including many germinal centres (Fig. 18.25). These structures line and form papillary projections into cystic spaces (Fig. 18.26).

Warthin's tumour is benign and responds to enucleation but is sometimes multiple.

Oncocytoma

Oncocytoma is a rare benign tumour that virtually only affects the parotids, particularly in the elderly. It consists of large eosinophilic cells with small compact nuclei ('oncocytes'), which are typically arranged in solid cords.

Oncocytosis is the term given to replacement or transformation of acinar cells of the parotid (or rarely other glands)

by cells having the same appearance as those of an oncocytoma but without loss of the normal lobular architecture. Oncocytosis is usually an age-related change and when widespread the gland becomes swollen and soft.

Other adenomas

Other adenomas lack the connective-tissue components of the pleomorphic adenoma and may have a uniform cellular structure, often with a tubular or trabecular pattern. Canalicular adenomas particularly affect the upper lip and consist of small darkly-staining cells in a tubular or trabecular pattern but sometimes resembling an adenoid cystic carcinoma.

Adenomas other than pleomorphic adenoma respond to enucleation or simple excision.

MALIGNANT SALIVARY GLAND TUMOURS

Mucoepidermoid carcinoma

Mucoepidermoid carcinomas account for between 3% and 9% of salivary gland neoplasms.

Histologically, they consist of two cell types, namely large, pale mucus-secreting cells surrounded by epidermoid (squamous) cells. Either may be predominant. If mainly mucoid, the tumour tends to be cystic; if mainly epidermoid, the tumour is solid and often then more aggressive (Figs 18.27 and 18.28). There is no well-defined capsule, but the tumour usually grows slowly.

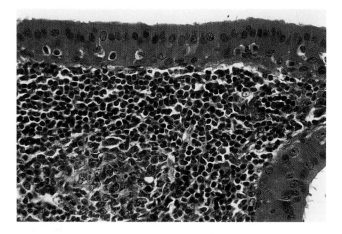

Fig. 18.25 Warthin's tumour. At higher power the tall columnar epithelial cells are readily identified and beneath them the lymphoid tissue.

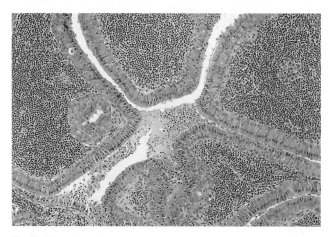

Fig. 18.26 Warthin's tumour. Tall columnar cells surround lymphoid tissue and line a convoluted cystic space.

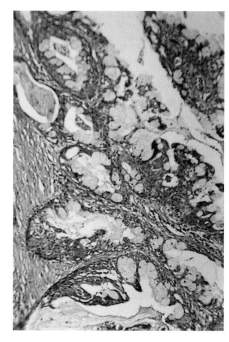

Fig. 18.27 Mucoepidermoid carcinoma. The mucous cells surround microcysts. Underlying the mucous cells are the epidermoid (squamous) cells.

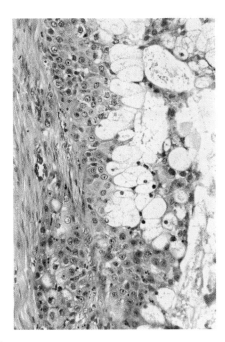

Fig. 18.28 Mucoepidermoid carcinoma. At higher power the finely granular mucous cells are seen to the right with the underlying epidermoid cells to the left.

Despite benign cytological appearances, mucoepidermoid carcinomas can be invasive and occasionally metastasise. Those which are obviously malignant microscopically are uncommon but more likely to metastasise.

Treatment is by wide excision but the tumour may recur.

Acinic cell carcinoma

Acinic cell carcinomas are rare and account for about 1% of salivary gland tumours. Their behaviour is also unpredictable from their histological appearance.

Histologically they show an almost uniform pattern of large cells, similar to serous cells, with granular basophilic cyto-

plasm, often in an acinar arrangement (Fig. 18.29). A characteristic feature is scattered round 'holes', thought to be entrapped secretion. Sometimes these are so numerous as to give the tumour a lace-like appearance.

Despite apparently benign histological appearances, acinic cell carcinomas can be invasive and occasionally metastasise. More obviously malignant variants with nuclear pleomorphism and hyperchromatism are also occasionally seen microscopically.

Adenoid cystic carcinoma

Adenoid cystic carcinoma usually has a highly characteristic histological pattern consisting of rounded groups of small darkly-staining cells of almost uniform size, surrounding multiple small clear spaces (cribriform or 'Swiss cheese' pattern) (Figs 18.30 and 18.31). Adenoid cystic carcinomas usually grow relatively slowly but tend to infiltrate along nerve sheaths. When they reach and spread along bony canals their extent is considerably greater than radiographs show. Metastases usually appear late. The prognosis is poor unless the tumour is

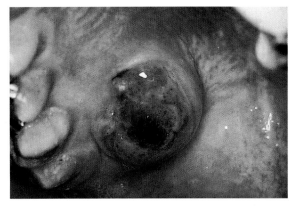

Fig. 18.30 Adenoid cystic carcinoma. There is an ulcerated mass arising from a minor gland in the palate. The clinical appearance would be the same with other malignant salivary neoplasms.

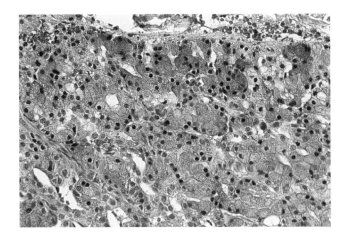

Fig. 18.29 Acinic cell carcinoma. The tumour is composed of granular acinar-type cells, sometimes arranged in acinus-like clusters and sometimes forming irregular sheets. Cytological atypia is uncommon.

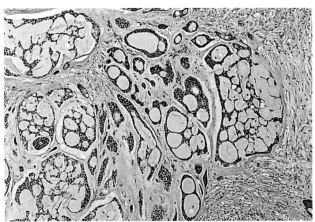

Fig. 18.31 Adenoid cystic carcinoma. The small darkly staining cells of the adenoid cystic carcinoma form cribriform islands with large holes which have been likened, rather inappropriately, to Swiss cheese.

vigorously treated by early wide excision at the earliest possible stage, often combined with radiotherapy.

Adenocarcinomas

Adenocarcinomas of the salivary glands show a variety of appearances. A few show attempts at duct formation typical of adenocarcinomas, while others have a papillary cystic pattern. Some are so poorly differentiated that their glandular origin is difficult to discern.

Polymorphous low-grade adenocarcinoma

Polymorphous low-grade adenocarcinoma arises in minor glands, particularly of the palate. It consists of cytologically benign-looking pale-staining cells in lobular, papillary or papillary cystic, cribriform or trabecular configurations (Fig. 18.32). It is invasive and can spread along nerve sheaths but rarely metastasises.

Epithelial-myoepithelial carcinoma

Epithelial-myoepithelial carcinoma is a tumour of major glands. It consists of ducts or trabeculae of benign-looking dark-staining cells with an outer layer of clear cells. The latter sometimes predominate and the tumour has to be distinguished from other clear cell tumours, most of which are malignant.

Squamous cell carcinoma

This can also affect salivary glands by metaplasia of glandular cells, as seen in pleomorphic adenoma, but is rare. It does not differ from a mucosal carcinoma histologically.

Undifferentiated carcinomas

These usually consists of closely set, small, darkly-staining cells with little cytoplasm. Rapid spread and metastasis is typical.

Malignant change in pleomorphic adenoma

Pleomorphic adenoma is one of the few benign tumours that can undergo malignant change. Clinically this is sometimes

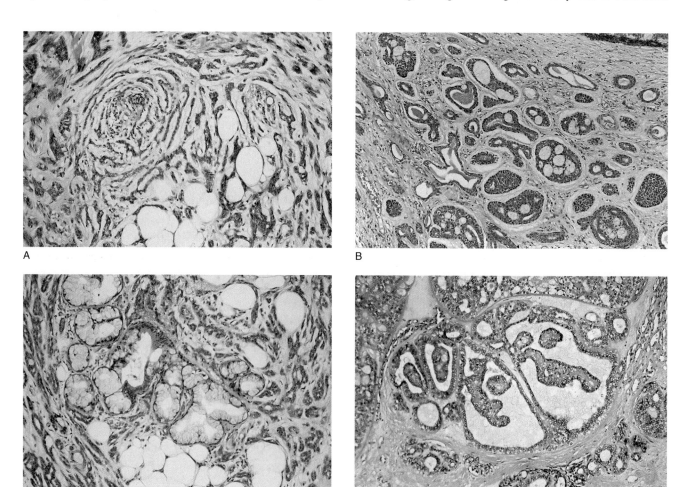

A   B

C   D

Fig. 18.32   Polymorphous low-grade adenocarcinoma. **A.** Targetoid pattern; **B.** cribriform area; **C.** surviving acini inside the tumour; **D.** papillary cystic area.

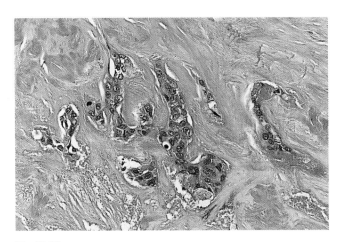

Fig. 18.33 Carcinoma arising in a pleomorphic adenoma. In longstanding pleomorphic adenomas the stroma may become hyalinised, dense and acellular. In such tumours there is a risk of transformation to carcinoma, as shown here by clusters of cells showing cytological atypia.

suggested by a sudden spurt in growth or development of pain or facial palsy.

Histologically, malignant change in pleomorphic adenoma is shown by obviously carcinomatous features adjacent to the benign cellular picture of the remainder of the tumour (Fig. 18.33). This is typically a late phenomenon, usually only after the tumour has been present for many years or in recurrences after inadequate excision.

Secondary tumours

Carcinomas and occasionally other tumours can metastasise to the salivary glands, particularly the parotid. Such secondaries can sometimes resemble primary salivary gland carcinomas: renal cell carcinoma metastases in particular can closely resemble epithelial-myoepithelial carcinoma. Diagnosis may depend on finding a primary elsewhere but usually the prognosis is almost hopeless in view of the dissemination of the tumour.

Non-epithelial tumours

The most common non-epithelial tumours of salivary glands are lymphomas. Some of these arise as a complication of Sjögren's syndrome or salivary lymphoepithelial lesion. In other cases salivary gland lymphoma is the first sign of widespread disease. Such a possibility must always be investigated since the prognosis is heavily dependent on the tumour's stage.

Juvenile haemangioma of the parotids

Juvenile haemangioma is a rare tumour which may be present at birth or first seen in childhood. Girls are more frequently affected. It forms a soft, sometimes bluish, swelling.

Histologically, the parotid structure is largely replaced by angiomatous tissue among which glandular elements can be

found. This angiomatous proliferation may occasionally be so vast as to form an arteriovenous fistula.

Sometimes these tumours regress spontaneously but if this has not happened by the age of 10 years, excision is required. Corticosteroids may delay tumour growth and facilitate later surgery.

Intraosseous salivary gland tumours

Ectopic salivary gland tissue is occasionally present in the mandible either in a cavity in the bone near the angle (Stafne bone cavity) or occasionally in other sites. Rarely, salivary gland tumours of any type can develop within the jaw (presumably from this ectopic salivary tissue) and may be mistaken by an unsuspecting pathologist for odontogenic tumours. However, they are most frequently mucoepidermoid carcinomas.

Radiographically, intraosseous salivary tumours produce cyst-like or poorly circumscribed areas of radiolucency. The diagnosis can only be made histologically. Wide excision is required.

TUMOUR-LIKE SALIVARY SWELLINGS

Necrotising sialometaplasia

This tumour-like lesion mainly affects the minor glands of the palate. It is of unknown cause. Middle-aged males are predominantly affected and are often cigarette smokers.

Typically, a relatively painless, ulcerated swelling 15–20 mm in diameter, forms on the hard palate often in the first molar region (Fig. 18.34). The margins are irregular and heaped-up or everted. Clinically, it resembles a carcinoma, for which it has sometimes also been mistaken histologically.

Pathology

There is chronic inflammation of minor salivary glands and necrosis of acini. The duct tissue undergoes squamous meta-

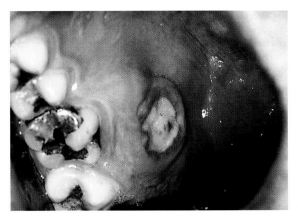

Fig. 18.34 Necrotising sialometaplasia. The clinical appearances are similar to those of a malignant salivary neoplasm.

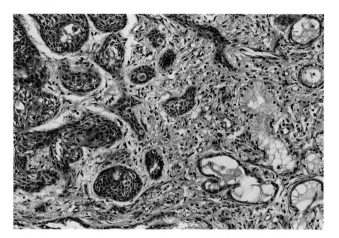

Fig. 18.35 Necrotising sialometaplasia. The histological features may also be mistaken for malignancy. There is necrosis of all the acinar cells, and only hyperplastic ducts showing squamous metaplasia remain.

plasia and proliferates to produce a pseudo-carcinomatous appearance (Fig. 18.35).

Necrotising sialometaplasia is often excised for diagnosis, but usually heals spontaneously after 8–10 weeks.

SIALADENOSIS

Sialadenosis is a non-neoplastic, non-inflammatory enlargement of salivary glands, most noticeably of the parotids, due to a variety of causes (Fig. 18.36 and Table 18.16). Histologically, there is hypertrophy of serous acini and oedema of interstitial connective tissue.

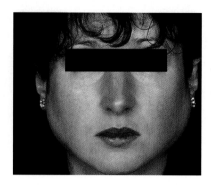

Fig. 18.36 Sialadenosis. In this case of idiopathic sialadenosis there is conspicuous swelling of the parotid glands producing a characteristic appearance.

Table 18.16 Important causes of sialadenosis

- Alcoholism
- Diabetes mellitus
- Other endocrine diseases
- Pregnancy
- Drugs (e.g. sympathomimetics)
- Bulimia
- Idiopathic

SUGGESTED FURTHER READING

Barnes L, Rao U, Krause J, Contis L, Schwartz A, Scalamonga P 1994 Salivary duct carcinoma. Part I. A clinicopathologic evaluation and DNA analysis of 13 cases with review of the literature. Oral Surg Oral Med Oral Pathol 78:64–73

Brook I 1992 Diagnosis and management of parotitis. Arch Otolaryngol Head Neck Surg 118:469–471

Brookstone M S, Huvos A G 1992 Central salivary gland tumors of the maxilla and mandible: a clinicopathologic study of 11 cases with an analysis of the literature. J Oral Maxillofac Surg 50:229–236

Callender D L, Frankenthaler R A, Luna M A, Lee S S, Goepfert H 1992 Salivary gland neoplasms in children. Arch Otolaryngol Head Neck Surg 118:472–476

Cawson R A, Binnie W H, Barrett A W, Wright J M 1998 *Lucas's Pathology of tumors of the oral tissues*. Churchill Livingstone, Edinburgh

Cawson R A, Binnie W H, Barrett A W, Wright J M 2001 *Oral disease*, 3rd Edn. Mosby-Wolfe, London

Cawson R A, Langdon J D, Eveson J W 1996 *Surgical pathology of the mouth and jaws*. Wright, Oxford

Delgado R, Vuitch F, Albores-Saavedra J 1993 Salivary duct carcinoma. Cancer 72:1503–1512

Ellis G L, Corio R L 1983 Acinic cell adenocarcinoma. A clinicopathologic analysis of 294 cases. Cancer 52:542–549

Epstein J B, Scully C 1992 The role of saliva in oral health and the causes and effects of xerostomia. Can Dent Assoc J 58:217–221

Epstein J B, Stevenson-Moore P, Scully C 1992 Management of xerostomia. Can Dent Assoc J 58:140–143

Eveson J W, Cawson R A 1986 Warthin's tumor (cystadenolymphoma) of salivary glands. A clinicopathologic investigation of 278 cases. Oral Surg Oral Med Oral Pathol 61:256–262

Falzon M, Isaacson P G 1991 The natural history of benign lymphoepithelial lesion of the salivary gland in which there is a monoclonal population of B cells. A report of two cases. Am J Surg Pathol 15:59–65

Gleeson M J, Cawson R A, Bennett M H 1986 Benign lymphoepithelial lesion: a less than benign disease. Clin Otolaryngol 11:47–51

Gleeson M J, Bennett M H, Cawson R A 1986 Lymphomas of salivary glands. Cancer 58:699–704

Hamper K, Brugmann M, Koppermann R et al 1989 Epithelial-myoepithelial duct carcinoma of salivary glands: a follow-up and cytophotometric study of 21 cases. J Oral Pathol Med 18:299–304

Hamper K, Lazar F, Dietel M, Caselitz J, Berger J, Arps H, Falkmer U, Auer G, Seifert G 1990 Prognostic factors for adenoid cystic carcinoma of the head and neck: a retrospective evaluation of 96 cases. J Oral Pathol Med 19:101–107

Hickman R E, Cawson R A, Duffy S W 1984 The prognosis of specific types of salivary gland tumors. Cancer 54:1620–1624

Holliday R A, Cohen W A, Schinella R A et al 1988 Benign lymphoepithelial parotid cysts and hyperplastic cervical lymphadenopathy in AIDS-risk patients: a new CT appearance. Radiology 168:439–441

Labrouyie E, Merlio J P H, Beylot-Barry M, Deloid B, Vergier B, Brossard G et al 1993 Human immunodeficiency virus type I replication within cystic lymphoepithelial lesion of salivary glands. Am J Clin Pathol 100:41–46

Lewis J E, Olsen K D, Weiland L H 1991 Acinic cell carcinoma. Clinicopathologic review. Cancer 68:172–179

McCluggage G, Sloan J, Cameron S, Hamilton P, Toner P 1995 Basal cell adenocarcinoma of the submandibular gland. Oral Surg Oral Med Oral Pathol 79:342–350

SUGGESTED FURTHER READING (*cont'd*)

O'Connell J E, George M K, Speculand G B, Pahor A L 1993 Mycobacterial infection of the parotid gland: an unusual cause of parotid swelling. J Laryngol Otol 107:560–564

Qureshi A A, Gitelis A, Templeton A A, Piasecki P A 1994 'Benign' metastasizing pleomorphic adenoma. A case report and review of the literature. Clin Orthopaed Rel Res 308:192–198

Raad I I, Sabbagh M F, Caranasos G J 1990 Acute bacterial sialadenitis: a study of 29 cases and review. Rev Infect Dis 12:591–601

Seifert G, Brocheriou C, Cardesa A, Eveson J W 1990 WHO International Histological Classification of Tumours. Path Res Pract 186:555–581

Seifert G, Miehlke A, Haubrich J, Chilla R 1986 *Diseases of the salivary glands*. Georg Thieme Verlag, Stuttgart

Takeichi N, Hirose F, Yamamoto H, Ezaki H, Fujikura T 1983 Salivary gland tumors in atomic bomb survivors, Hiroshima, Japan. II Pathologic study and supplementary epidemiologic observations. Cancer 52:377–385

Thackray A C, Lucas R B 1974 Tumors of the major salivary glands. *Atlas of tumor pathology*. Second Series. Fascicle 10. Washington: Armed Forces Institute of Pathology

Toynton S C, Wilkins M J, Cook H T, Stafford N D S 1994 True malignant mixed tumour of a minor salivary gland. J Laryngol Otol 108:76–79

Van der Wal J E, Snow G B, van der Waal I 1990 Intraoral adenoid cystic carcinoma. The presence of perineural spread in relation to site, size, local extension and metastatic spread in 22 cases. Cancer 66:2031–2033

Vincent S D, Hammond H L, Finkelstein M W 1994 Clinical and therapeutic features of polymorphous low-grade adenocarcinoma. Oral Surg Oral Med Oral Pathol 77:41–47

Waldron C A, Koh M L 1990 Central mucoepidermoid carcinoma of the jaws: report of four cases with analysis of the literature and discussion of the relationship to mucoepidermoid, sialodontogenic and glandular odontogenic cysts. J Oral Maxillofac Surg 48:871–877

Wolvius E B, van der Valk P, van der Wal J E, van Diest P J, Huijgens P C, van der Waal I, Snow G B 1996 Primary non-Hodgkin lymphoma of the salivary glands. An analysis of 22 cases. J Oral Pathol Med 25:177–181

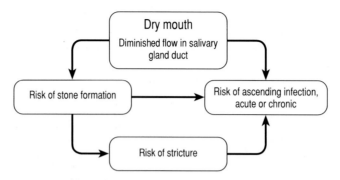

Summary 18.1 Inter-relationships between dry mouth, calculi and their complications. Note: dry mouth may promote stone formation but stones do not cause dry mouth.

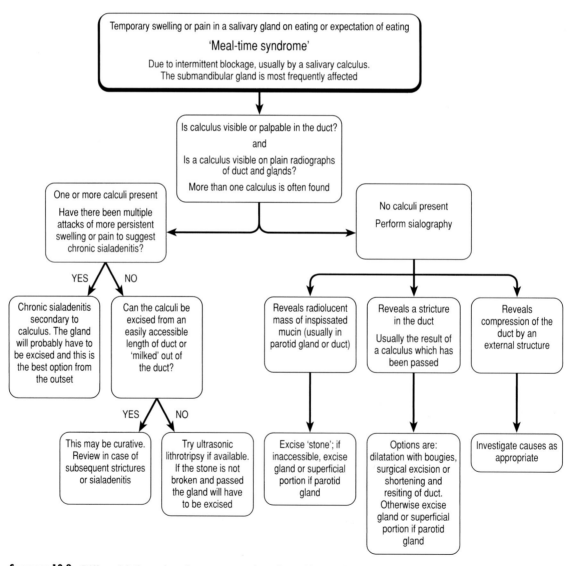

Summary 18.2 Differential diagnosis and management of a patient with 'mealtime syndrome'.

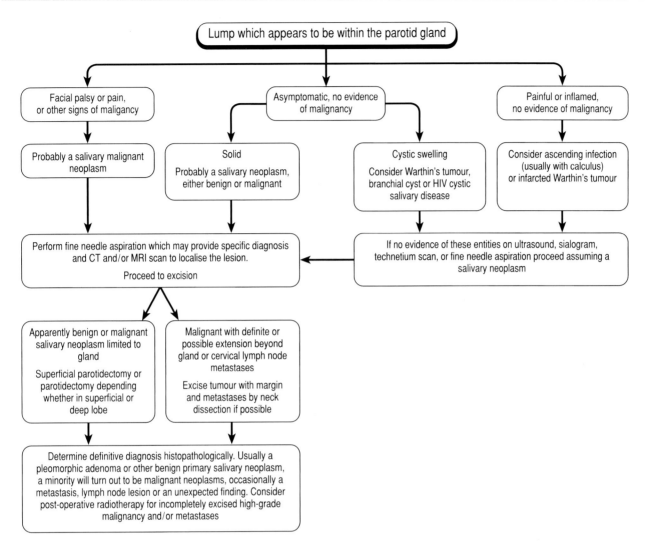

Summary 18.3 Management decisions and treatment for a lump in the parotid gland.

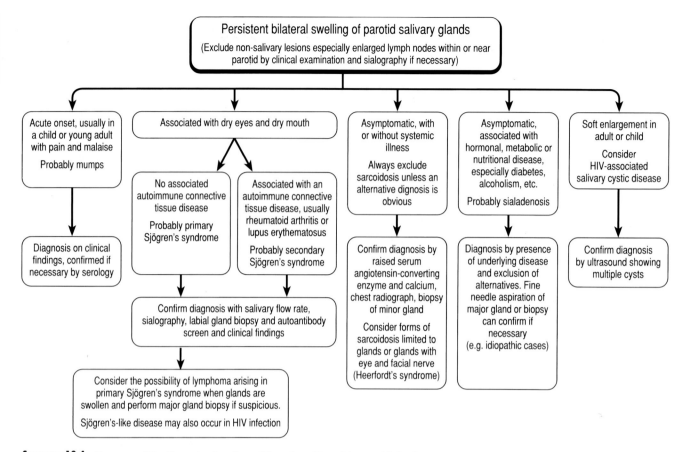

Summary 18.4   Summary of the diagnosis of persistent bilateral swelling of the parotid glands.

Common benign mucosal swellings

FIBROUS POLYPS, EPULIDES AND DENTURE-INDUCED GRANULOMAS

Fibrous nodules are the most common soft-tissue swellings of the mouth. They are not neoplasms but hyperplastic swellings that develop in sites subject to chronic minor injury and/or low-grade infection (Table 19.1). Fibromas are not recognised as an entity and in any case cannot be distinguished from fibrous hyperplasia. The term *epulis* (literally, 'on the gingiva') refers only to the site. It has no implications for the histology but in practice most epulides are fibrous.

Irritation of the gingival margin by the sharp edge of a carious cavity or by calculus may lead to the formation of a fibrous epulis; irritation of alveolar or palatal mucosa by a rough area on a denture may provoke development of a denture granuloma. Though different names are given to these lesions they are similar in origin and structure.

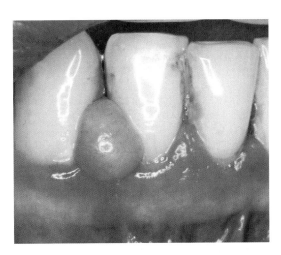

Fig. 19.1   Fibrous epulis. This lesion arising from the gingival margin between the lower central incisors is firm, pink and not ulcerated.

Table 19.1   **Fibrous nodules: practical points**

- The most common oral tumour-like swellings
- Most frequently form at gingival margins (fibrous epulis) or in relation to a denture
- They are hyperplastic responses to chronic irritation
- Should be excised complete and sent for histological examination

Clinical features

A fibrous epulis is most common near the front of the mouth on the gingiva between two teeth (Fig. 19.1). Fibrous polyps can also form on the buccal mucosa (Fig. 19.2). Denture-induced hyperplasias ('denture granulomas') often form at the edge of dentures (Fig. 19.3). These swellings are pale and firm but may be abraded and ulcerated, and then inflamed.

'*Leaf fibroma*' is another fibrous overgrowth which forms under a denture but has become flattened against the palate (Fig. 19.4). It may be difficult to see until lifted away from its bed.

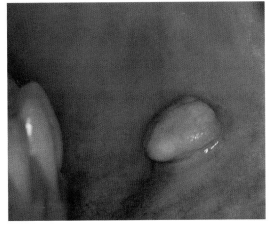

Fig. 19.2   Fibrous polyp. This lesion on the buccal mucosa has arisen as a result of cheek biting and is a firm, painless polyp covered by mucosa of normal appearance.

Pathology

These nodules consist of irregular interlacing connective tissue fibres without encapsulation but covered by epithelium, which is usually hyperplastic (Fig. 19.5).

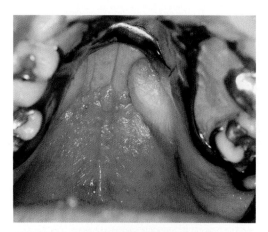

Fig. 19.3 Denture-induced granuloma. Fibrous hyperplasia at the posterior border of this upper partial denture has resulted in a firm mucosal swelling moulded to fit the denture.

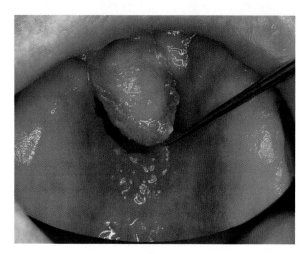

Fig. 19.4 'Leaf fibroma'. Flat lesions formed between the denture and mucosa are often termed leaf fibromas because of their shape. Raising this example with a probe reveals its pedunculated shape.

Bone formation is sometimes seen in a fibrous epulis (Fig. 19.6). In American texts a fibrous epulis containing bone is termed (in an apparent desire to cause confusion) a 'peripheral ossifying fibroma' even though it has no relation to the ossifying fibroma of bone and is not a fibroma.

Fibrous nodules should be excised together with the small base of normal tissue from which they arise. In the case of a fibrous epulis the underlying bone should be curetted. There should be no recurrence if this is done thoroughly and the source of irritation is removed.

Histological examination is needed to confirm that an epulis is fibrous and not a giant-cell lesion, pyogenic granuloma or a malignant tumour, which can very rarely form on the gingival margin and simulate a non-neoplastic epulis.

Giant-cell fibroma

This variant is distinguished microscopically by large, mono-nucleate, stellate, darkly-staining cells (quite unlike the multi-

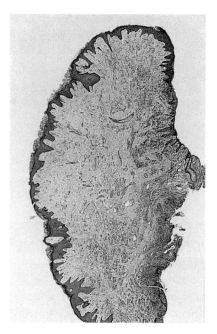

Fig. 19.5 Fibrous polyp. The lesion is composed of mature fibrous tissue covered by hyperplastic epithelium with spiky rete processes. A few inflammatory cells are present near the base.

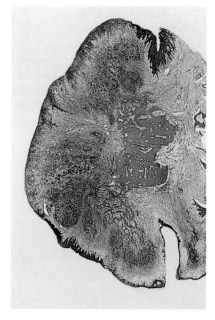

Fig. 19.6 Fibrous epulis with ossification. Much of the surface of this pedunculated nodule is ulcerated and hyperplastic epithelium covers the margins. Centrally the lesion is very cellular, partly as a result of inflammatory infiltrate, and trabeculae of woven bone are being deposited and maturing into lamellar bone. The presence of bone in a fibrous epulis appears to be of no clinical significance.

nucleate cells of a giant-cell granuloma) and less conspicuous multinucleate cells, scattered between short, coarse fibrous tissue bundles. Clinically, giant-cell fibromas are typically pedunculated and usually arise from the gingivae. The surface is frequently verrucous.

The treatment is the same as for a fibrous epulis.

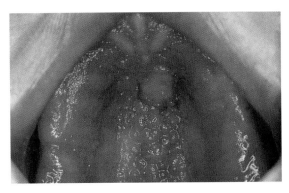

Fig. 19.7 Papillary hyperplasia of the palate. A small leaf fibroma is also present in the anterior palate.

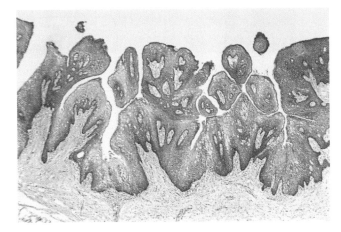

Fig. 19.8 Papillary hyperplasia. The mucosa is thrown into a series of convoluted folds covered by hyperplastic epithelium. Inflammatory change is greater when candidal infection is present.

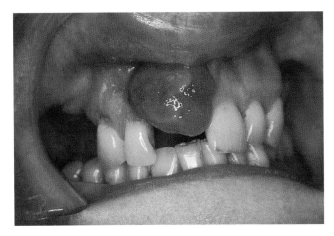

Fig. 19.9 Pyogenic granuloma. A bright red polypoid swelling. The gingiva is a common site.

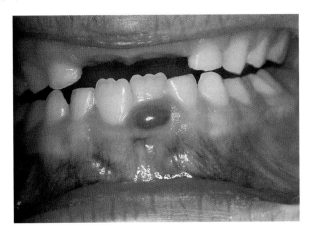

Fig. 19.10 Giant cell epulis. Typical lesion in a child showing the bluish or maroon colour of the gingival nodule. (By kind permission of Mrs H Pitt-Ford.)

PAPILLARY HYPERPLASIA OF THE PALATE

Nodular overgrowth of the palatal mucosa is occasionally seen, particularly under dentures in older persons in whom low-grade trauma or infection exacerbates the proliferation (Fig. 19.7). Candidosis is sometimes superimposed but is not the cause. Mild palatal papillary hyperplasia is also occasionally seen in non-denture wearers.

Histologically, palatal papillary hyperplasia shows close-set nodules of vascular fibrous tissue with a variable chronic inflammatory infiltrate and a covering of hyperplastic epithelium (Fig. 19.8).

There is no justification for stripping palatal papillary hyperplasia. Dentures should be kept clean and not worn overnight. Any superimposed candidal infection should be treated with an antifungal drug.

PYOGENIC GRANULOMA AND PREGNANCY EPULIS

Pyogenic granuloma is relatively uncommon. *Clinically*, it is usually red and relatively soft (Fig. 19.9). *Microsopically*, it consists of many dilated blood vessels in a loose oedematous connective tissue stroma. There is typically a dense acute inflammatory infiltrate but this may be scanty or absent. A pregnancy epulis has the same histological appearances and can only be distinguished by the nature of the patient and usually, an associated pregnancy gingivitis (see also Fig. 31.9).

GIANT-CELL EPULIS

The giant-cell epulis, like the fibrous epulis, is probably hyperplastic, but less common.

Clinically, a giant cell epulis is usually found on the gingival margin between teeth anterior to the permanent molars. Its development may therefore be related to the resorption of deciduous teeth. The swelling is rounded, soft, and typically maroon or purplish (Fig. 19.10).

Histologically, numerous multinucleate cells lie in a vascular stroma of plump spindle-shaped cells. The appearance is similar

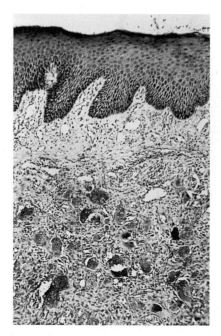

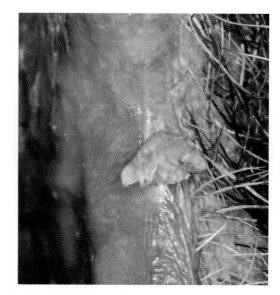

Fig. 19.12 Papilloma arising at the commissure.

Fig. 19.11 Giant cell epulis. At high magnification clusters of giant cells in vascular fibrous tissue may be seen lying immediately below the covering epithelium.

to that of a giant-cell granuloma of the jaw, but for the fact that the epulis has a covering of stratified squamous epithelium (Fig. 19.11). Very rarely a giant cell epulis is a manifestation of hyperparathyroidism, in which case changes in blood chemistry confirm the diagnosis (Ch. 10).

A giant cell epulis should be excised, together with its gingival base, and the underlying bone curetted. Adjacent teeth need not be extracted if they are healthy, and if treatment is thorough there should be no recurrence.

BENIGN EPITHELIAL TUMOURS AND TUMOUR-LIKE LESIONS

Squamous cell papilloma

Papillomas mainly affect adults and have a distinctive, clinically recognisable, cauliflower-like or branched structure of finger-like processes (Fig. 19.12).

Histologically, the papillae consist of stratified squamous epithelium supported by a vascular connective tissue core (Fig. 19.13). When keratinised, they appear white.

Human papilloma virus (HPV) of various subtypes is associated, but no inclusion bodies or other signs of viral infection are histologically evident. Oral papillomas appear to have no potential for malignant change and respond to local excision.

Infective warts (verruca vulgaris)

Oral warts are uncommon but seen particularly in children and frequently result from autoinoculation from warts on the hands.

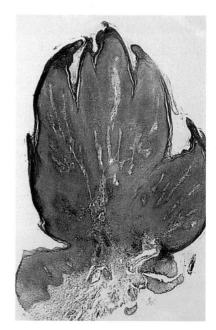

Fig. 19.13 Papilloma. The lesion consists of thickened fingers of epithelium. Slender vascular cores of connective tissue support each frond.

Histologically, the structure is generally similar to that of papillomas but there are typically large clear cells (koilocytes) with pyknotic nuclei and prominent keratohyaline granules in the superficial layers of the prickle cells. There is also positive staining of the nuclei with peroxidase-labelled antiserum to HPV.

Oral warts are occasionally multiple but if numerous or confluent, HIV infection or other cause of immunodeficiency should be suspected.

Adenoma

Intraoral adenomas arise from minor salivary glands. They typically form smooth, round or lobulated, painless firm swellings and are most frequently found on the palate (Ch. 18).

Other benign neoplasms

Benign neoplasms such as neurofibroma and lipoma which are occasionally found in the mouth are discussed in the following chapter.

SUGGESTED FURTHER READING

Abbey L M. Page D G, Sawyer D R 1980 The clinical and histopathologic features of a series of 464 oral squamous cell papillomas. Oral Surg 49:419–427

Anneroth G, Sigurdson A 1983 Hyperplastic lesions of the gingiva and alveolar mucosa. A study of 175 cases. Acta Odontol Scand 41:75–86

Cawson R A, Binnie W H, Barrett A W, Wright J M 1998 *Lucas's Pathology of tumors of the oral tissues*. Churchill Livingstone, Edinburgh

Cawson R A, Binnie W H, Barrett A W, Wright J M 2001 *Oral disease*, 3rd Edn. Mosby-Wolfe, London

Cawson R A, Langdon J D, Eveson J W 1996 *Surgical pathology of the mouth and jaws*. Wright, Oxford

Ellis G L, Jensen J L, Reingold I M, Barr R J 1977 Malignant neoplasms metastatic to the gingivae. Oral Surg Oral Med Oral Pathol 44:238–245

Giansanti J S, Waldron C A 1969 Peripheral giant cell granuloma: Review of 720 cases. J Oral Surg 27:787–791

Hirshberg A, Leibovich P, Buchner A 1993 Metastases to the oral mucosa: analysis of 157 cases. J Oral Pathol Med 22:385–390

Houston G D 1982 The giant cell fibroma. A review of 464 cases. Oral Surg 53:582–587

Zain R B, Fei Y J 1990 Fibrous lesions of the gingiva: a histopathologic analysis of 204 cases. Oral Surg Oral Med Oral Pathol 70:466–470

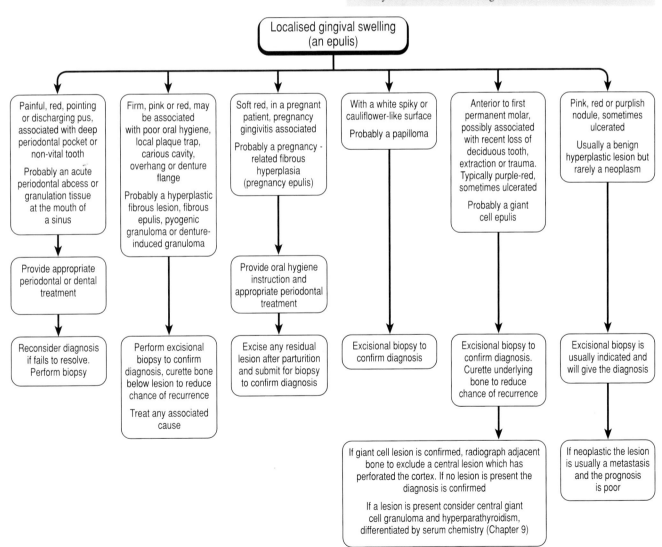

Summary 19.1 Differential diagnosis and management of the common localised gingival swellings.

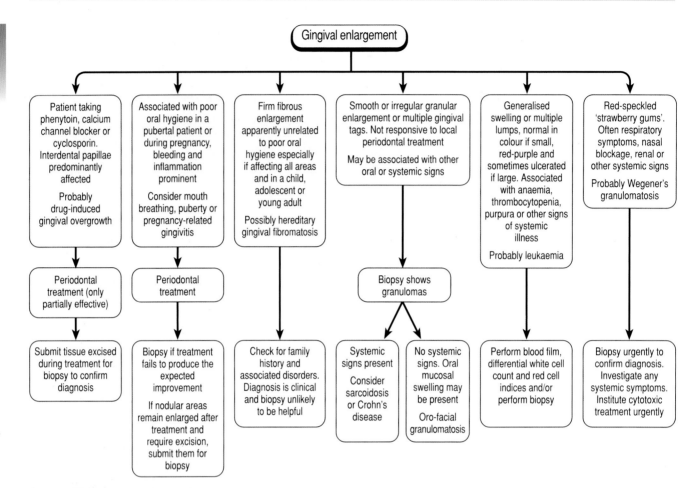

Summary 19.2 Differential diagnosis of common and important causes of gingival enlargement.

Soft tissue (mesenchymal) neoplasms

The common benign soft tissue swellings in the mouth are mostly hyperplastic and have been discussed in the previous chapter.

BENIGN NEOPLASMS

Neurofibromas

These uncommon tumours arise from nerve sheaths. They form smooth, painless lumps but are particularly rare in the mouth. When seen in the mouth, neurofibromatosis should be suspected. Also, in multiple endocrine adenoma syndrome type 2 (MEN 2) neurofibromas along the lateral borders of the tongue are a typical feature. Medullary carcinoma of the thyroid in 95%, phaeochromocytoma in 50% and hyperparathyroidism in 15% are associated (see Ch. 31). Since phaeochromocytoma in particular is life-threatening, screening for MEN 2 should be carried out if these oral neurofibromas are found.

Histologically, neurofibromas are cellular with plump nuclei separated by fine, sinuous collagen fibres, among which mast cells can usually be found. Excision is curative.

Neurilemmomas

Neurilemmomas arise from axon sheaths and, though uncommon, are more frequently found in the mouth than neurofibromas. They also form painless smooth swellings.

Histologically, the appearance is distinctive with multiple rounded masses of elongated spindle cells with palisaded nuclei (Antoni A tissue — Fig. 20.1). There is also a variable amount of unorganised loose connective tissue with scanty pleomorphic nuclei (Antoni B tissue). Excision is curative.

Lipoma and fibrolipoma

Lipomas can occasionally grow, particularly from the buccal fat pad, as soft, sometimes yellowish, swellings, which may be pedunculated (Fig. 20.2). They grow slowly and cause no symptoms unless bitten, or become conspicuous because of their size.

Histologically, lipomas consist of globules of fat supported

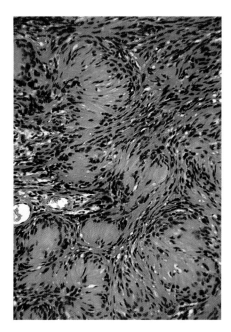

Fig. 20.1 Neurilemmoma. Antoni A tissue showing striking palisading of nuclei.

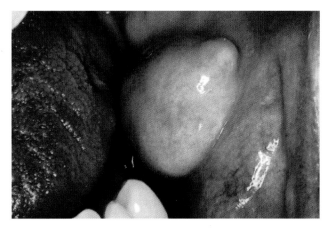

Fig. 20.2 Lipoma of the cheek. The tumour forms a pale, very soft yellowish swelling.

by areolar tissue (Fig. 20.3). Sometimes, fibrous tissue forms a large part of the tumour (fibrolipoma). They should be excised.

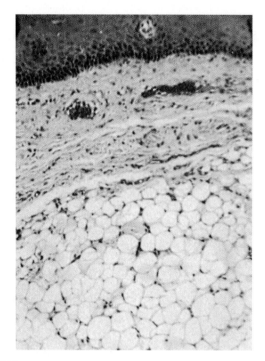

Fig. 20.3 Lipoma. The fat cells are closely packed between septa of fibrous tissue and often only partially encapsulated at the margin.

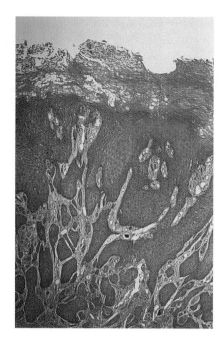

Fig. 20.4 Granular cell tumour. The irregular proliferation of the epithelium (pseudoepitheliomatous hyperplasia) may mimic a squamous carcinoma in superficial biopsy specimens.

Granular cell tumour

Clinically, granular cell tumours typically form painless smooth swellings. The tongue is the most common site.

Pathology. Large granular cells form the bulk of the lesion but pseudoepitheliomatous hyperplasia of the overlying epithelium may be conspicuous (Fig. 20.4). Electron microscopy suggests that the granular cells originate from Schwann cells. However, the presence of all stages of apparent transition of striped muscle cells into granular cells is a striking histological feature (Fig. 20.5). Elsewhere, the granular cells are large, with clearly-defined cell membranes and filled with eosinophilic granules.

The pseudoepitheliomatous hyperplasia is such that granular cell tumours have been mistaken histologically for carcinomas with resulting overtreatment. Simple excision should, however, be curative.

Congenital (granular cell) epulis

The rare congenital epulis is typically present at birth as a smooth but prominent soft nodule, usually on the alveolar ridge (Fig. 20.6). Females are predominantly affected and occasionally the mass is so large as to obstruct respiration.

Histologically, large pale granular cells with sharply-defined cell membranes are covered by epithelium which lacks pseudo-epitheliomatous hyperplasia. Immunohistochemistry suggests that the origin is myogenous.

Excision is curative but spontaneous regression is also seen.

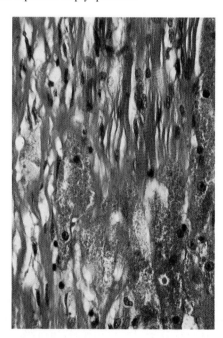

Fig. 20.5 Granular cell tumour. At high power the granular cells apparently merging with muscle fibres are characteristic and indicate the diagnosis.

Haemangiomas

Haemangiomas are mostly vascular malformations. Vascular neoplasms (apart from Kaposi's sarcoma in patients with HIV disease) are rare.

Haemangiomas may be localised but are occasionally diffuse and associated with similarly affected areas of the face. Rarely, the meninges are also involved, causing epilepsy and mental

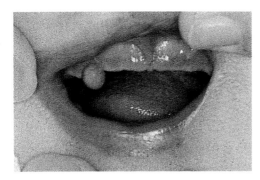

Fig. 20.6 Congenital epulis. A firm pink non-ulcerated nodule on the alveolar ridge of a neonate is the typical presentation.

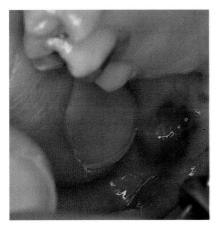

Fig. 20.7 Cavernous haemangioma of the cheek. The colour is deep purple and the structure, a mass of thin-walled blood sinuses is visible through the thin epithelium. A mass engorged with blood and as prominent as this is liable to be bitten and bleed profusely.

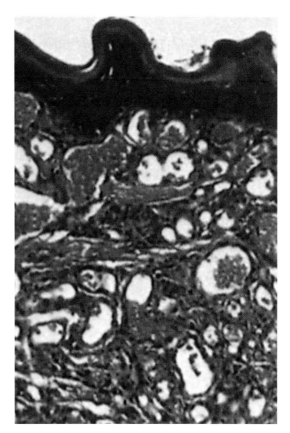

Fig. 20.8 Capillary haemangioma. Numerous large and small closely packed capillary vessels extend from the epithelium into the deeper tissues.

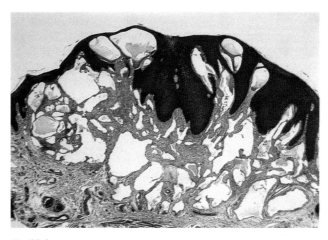

Fig. 20.9 Lymphangioma. There is a localised aggregation of cavernous lymphatics which formed a pale superficial swelling. Bleeding into these lesions causes them suddenly to become purple or almost black.

defect (Sturge–Weber syndrome). Isolated haemangiomas form purple, flat or nodular lesions which blanch on pressure (Fig. 20.7).

Histologically, haemangiomas are either capillary, cavernous or mixed. The capillary type consists of innumerable minute blood vessels and vasoformative tissue — mere rosettes of endothelial cells (Fig. 20.8). The cavernous type consists of large blood-filled sinusoids.

Excision of mucosal haemangiomas should be avoided unless trauma causes repeated episodes of bleeding. If necessary, cryosurgery may allow removal of a haemangioma without excessive bleeding.

Lymphangioma

These uncommon tumours usually form pale, translucent, smooth or nodular elevations of the mucosa. However, they may be noticed because they suddenly swell and become dark purple due to bleeding into the lymphatic spaces. Rarely, lymph-angiomas are diffuse and extensive, and cause generalised enlargement of the tongue (macroglossia) or lip.

Histologically, lymphangiomas consist of thin-walled vascular spaces sometimes containing pinkish amorphous material as a result of fixation of lymph (Fig. 20.9).

Localised lymphangiomas can be excised but this is more difficult in the diffuse type where the operation may have to be done in stages.

MALIGNANT CONNECTIVE-TISSUE TUMOURS

Sarcomas of virtually any type can affect the oral soft tissue, but most are rare. Kaposi's sarcoma has become the most common type, but among HIV-negative persons, rhabdomyosarcoma is the most common. Sarcomas tend to affect a considerably younger age group than carcinomas, and rhabdomyosarcomas are the most common oral sarcomas in children.

Sarcomas grow rapidly, are invasive, destroy surrounding tissues, and usually spread by the bloodstream. Many sarcomas are clinically indistinguishable from one another, but some, such as Kaposi's sarcoma and malignant melanoma, are pigmented and must be differentiated from benign pigmented lesions.

Rhabdomyosarcoma

Rhabdomyosarcomas can affect children or young adults and form rapidly growing soft swellings.

Histologically, several types are recognised. The embryonal type, which more frequently affects children, consists of cells of variable shape and size. Some are strap or tadpole-shaped, while muscle-like cells with cross striations may be difficult to find. The alveolar type consists of slit-like spaces into which hang tear-shaped, darkly-staining cells attached to the walls. These alveoli are separated by a fibrous stroma.

Treatment is by excision and combination chemotherapy but the prognosis is poor.

Fibrosarcoma

Fibrosarcomas consist of broad interlacing bands of fibroblasts with a streaming or herring-bone pattern (Fig. 20.10). Some produce abundant collagen, others are highly cellular with close-packed nuclei, among which there are often mitoses.

Treatment is by radical excision. Local recurrence and spread are common but metastasis is rare.

Kaposi's sarcoma

Since the outbreak of AIDS, Kaposi's sarcoma has become the most common type of intraoral sarcoma. It mainly affects men who have sex with men, who have HIV infection.

Within the mouth, the palate is the most frequent site and the tumour appears as a purplish area or nodule which bleeds readily (Fig. 20.11). In any male below the age of about 50, with such a lesion, Kaposi's sarcoma must be excluded since (in the absence of immunosuppressive treatment) it is pathognomonic of HIV disease. Kaposi's sarcoma is occasionally the first manifestation of HIV infection but is usually associated with a low CD4 count and opportunistic infections. Human herpes virus 8 (HHV-8) DNA can be found in Kaposi's sarcoma cells, and patients with both HIV and HHV-8 infection have a high risk of developing Kaposi's sarcoma. However the mode of transmission is unclear; although anal intercourse was sus-

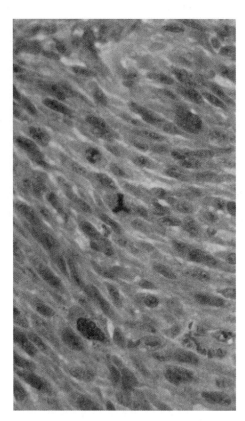

Fig. 20.10 Fibrosarcoma of the tongue. There are streams of neoplastic fibroblasts, but the striking feature is the spindle-shaped, darkly staining nuclei and their variation in size and mitoses.

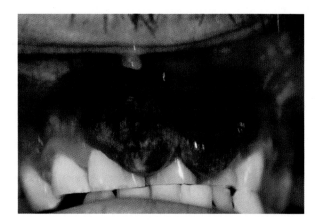

Fig. 20.11 Kaposi's sarcoma. Lesions are red, maroon or bluish and highly vascular. They may be flat or form tumour masses and the gingivae or palate are characteristic sites. (By kind permission of Professor W H Binnie.)

pected as the route, it appears that HHV-8, like the closely related Epstein–Barr virus, is mainly found in oral secretions.

Histologically, Kaposi's sarcoma is a vascular tumour in which factor VIII antigen (a marker for endothelial cells) can be identified but is not the most sensitive marker. Immunoreactivity for CD34 antigen is also positive in most spindle cells and in cells lining vascular spaces or inconspicuous vascular slits in small lesions, and in endothelium of surrounding

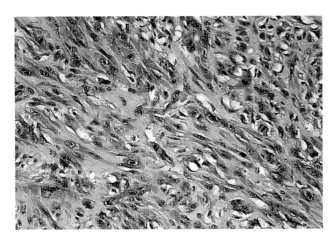

Fig. 20.12 Kaposi's sarcoma. The tumour is composed of spindled and plump cells with cytological atypia and frequent mitoses. Many of the small holes visible are the result of formation of capillaries.

vessels. CD34 reactivity appears to be the most reliable marker of endothelial progenitor cells and is valuable in the diagnosis of Kaposi's sarcoma.

The early 'pre-sarcomatous' lesion consists of a mass of capillary-size blood vessels, sometimes with mononuclear cell cuffing. It resembles granulation tissue, particularly in the mouth, where superficial lesions can be traumatised and become secondarily inflamed. Later, there is increasingly widespread angiomatous proliferation, and in some areas the vessels may be slit-shaped when obliquely sectioned. There is also proliferation of angular or spindle-shaped interstitial cells (Fig. 20.12). Ultimately, the latter predominate and show increasing numbers of mitoses. Central necrosis may develop and extravasation of red cells can leave deposits of haemosiderin.

Associated HIV infection is usually suggested by other clinical manifestations (such as opportunistic infections) and lymphopenia in the blood picture.

Kaposi's sarcoma must be distinguished from AIDS-associated thrombocytopenic purpura and bacillary angiomatosis, which may appear similar clinically. However, purpura may be seen earlier and is distinguishable by haematological testing. Key features are summarised in Table 20.1.

Table 20.1   Kaposi's sarcoma: key features

- The most common type of oral sarcoma
- Most common in male homosexuals with HIV disease
- Appears clinically as a flat or nodular purplish area
- Consists histologically of minute, proliferating blood vessels
- Good response to highly active antiretroviral therapy
- May be widely disseminated when oral lesions appear
- Death more frequently from associated opportunistic infections

Management

Various measures have been used to deal with Kaposi's sarcoma but in HIV disease highly active antiretroviral therapy (HAART) will bring resolution (Ch. 22).

Other sarcomas of oral soft tissues

Neurofibrosarcomas, liposarcomas, leiomyosarcomas and even soft-tissue osteosarcomas and chondrosarcomas may be seen, but all are rare.

LYMPHOMAS

Lymphomas can arise from any type of lymphocyte, but more frequently from B cells. They are all malignant. They comprise Hodgkin's disease and the more common non-Hodgkin lymphoma. Lymphomas relatively frequently involve the cervical lymph nodes but are rare in the mouth. However, in AIDS, lymphomas may account for 2% of oral neoplasms. They are discussed in Chapter 22.

SUGGESTED FURTHER READING

Cawson R A, Binnie W H, Barrett A W, Wright J M 2001 *Color atlas of oral disease*, 3rd Edn. Mosby-Wolfe, London

Cawson R A, Langdon J D, Eveson J W 1996 *Surgical pathology of the mouth and jaws*. Wright, Oxford

Chen S-Y, Thakur A, miller A S, Harwick R D 1995 Rhabdomyosarcoma of the oral cavity. Report of four cases. Oral Surg Oral Med Oral Pathol Oral Radiol Endod 80:192–201

Damm D D, Cibull M L, Geissler R H et al 1993 Investigation into the histogenesis of congenital epulis of the newborn. Oral Surg Oral Med Oral Pathol 76:202–212

DiCerbo M, Sciubba J J, Sordill W C, DeLuke D M 1992 Malignant schwannoma of the palate: a case report and review of the literature. J Oral Maxillofac Surg 50:1217–1221

El Naggar A K, Batsakis J G, Ordonez N G et al 1993 Rhadomyosarcoma of the adult head and neck: a clinicopathological and DNA ploidy study. J Laryngol Otol 107:716–720

Enzinger F M, Weiss S W 1995 *Soft tissue tumors*, 3rd Edn. Mosby, St Louis

Geist J R, Gander D L, Stefanac S J 1992 Oral manifestations of neurofibromatosis types I and II. Oral Surg Oral Med Oral Pathol 73:376–382

Greager J A, Reichard K, Campana J P, Das Gupta T K 1994 Fibrosarcoma of the head and neck. Am J Surg 167:437–439

Hajdu S I 1993 Peripheral nerve sheath tumours. Histogenesis, classification and prognosis. Cancer 72:3549–3552

Herdier B G, Kaplan L D, McGrath M S 1994 Pathogenesis of AIDS lymphomas. AIDS 8:1025–1049

Hirshberg A, Leibovich P, Buchner A 1993 Metastases to the oral mucosa: analysis of 157 cases. J Oral Pathol Med 22:385–390

Kraus D H, Dubner S, Harrison L B, Strong E W, Hajdu S T, Kher U et al 1994 Prognostic factors for recurrence and survival in head and neck soft tissue sarcomas. Cancer 74:697–702

Mark R J, Sercarz J A, Tran L, Selch M, Calcaterra T C 1991 Fibrosarcoma of the head and neck. Arch Otolaryngol Head Neck Surg 117:396–401

Meehan S, Davis V, Brahim J S 1994 Embryonal rhabdomyosarcoma of the floor of the mouth. A case report. Oral Surg Oral Med Oral Pathol 78:603–606

Noel J-C, Hermans P, Andre J et al 1996 Herpesvirus-like DNA sequences in Kaposi's sarcoma. Cancer 77:2132–2136

Peszkowski M J, Larsson A 1990 Extraosseous and intraosseous oral traumatic neuromas and their association with tooth extraction. J Oral Maxillofac Surg 48:963–967

Regezi J A, MacPhail L A, Daniels T E, Greenspan J S, Greenspan D, Dodd C L et al 1993 Oral Kaposi's sarcoma: a 10-year retrospective histopathologic study. J Oral Pathol Med 11:292–297

Shapiro S D, Abramovitch K, Van Dis M L 1984 Neurofibromatosis: oral and radiographic manifestations. Oral Surg Oral Med Oral Pathol 58:493–498

Stewart C M, Watson R E, Eversole L R et al 1988 Oral granular cell tumors: a clinicopathologic and immunocytochemical study. Oral Surg Oral Med Oral Pathol 65:427–435

Tran L M, Mark R, Meier R, Calcaterra T C, Parker R G 1992 Sarcomas of the head and neck. Cancer 70:160–177

Wang M B, Strasnick B, Zimmerman M C 1992 Extranodal Burkitt's lymphoma of the head and neck. Arch Otolaryngol Head Neck Surg 118:193–199

Wolvius E B, van der Valk P, van der Wal J E et al 1994 Primary extranodal non-Hodgkin lymphoma of the oral cavity. An analysis of 34 cases. Oral Oncol Eur J Cancer 30B:121–125

Zuker R M, Buenchea R 1993 Congenital epulis: review of the literature and report of a case. J Oral Maxillofac Surg 51:1040–1043

CHAPTER 21

Melanoma and other pigmented lesions

Melanoma is a highly malignant oral tumour. It usually appears as a pigmented patch which must be distinguished from many other pigmentations. Table 21.1 refers to localised pigmented lesions, many of which may have to be distinguished from melanomas.

Table 21.1   Oral pigmented lesions

Usually brown or black	Typically purple or red
Malignant melanoma	Amelanotic melanomas
Pigmented naevi	Erythroplasia (Ch. 16)
Amalgam tattoo	Haemangiomas (Ch. 20)
Addison's disease (Ch. 31)	Kaposi's sarcoma (Ch. 20)
Peutz–Jeghers syndrome	Purpura (Ch. 26)
Racial pigmentation	Other blood blisters
Lichen planus rarely (Ch. 13)	Telangiectases
	Lingual varices (Ch. 14)
	Pyogenic granuloma (Ch. 19)
	Pregnancy epulis (Ch. 19)
	Giant-cell epulis (Ch. 19)
	Geographical tongue (Ch. 14)
	Erythematous candidosis (Ch. 12)
	Median rhomboid glossitis (Ch. 14)

Racial pigmentation

This is the most common cause of oral pigmentation. The gingivae are particularly affected (Fig. 21.1). The inner aspect of the lips is typically spared.

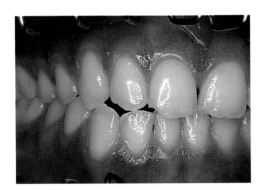

Fig. 21.1 Racial pigmentation. The distribution of melanotic mucosa around the gingival margin is characteristic.

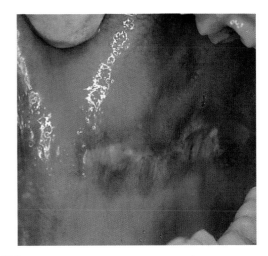

Fig. 21.2 Pigmented lichen planus. Inflammatory conditions may become pigmented, especially in dark skinned races. Here melanin delineates mucosa affected by lichen planus.

Lesions of lichen planus can also become pigmented, often intensely, in association with racial pigmentation (Fig. 21.2).

Amalgam tattoo

Fragments of amalgam frequently become embedded in the oral mucosa and form the most common pigmented patches which may simulate melanomas clinically. They are usually close to the dental arch and typically 5 mm or more across (Fig. 21.3). Dense tattoos may be radiopaque.

Pathology

Amalgam is seen as brown or black granules deposited particularly along collagen bundles and around small blood vessels (Fig. 21.4). There may be no inflammatory reaction or there may be a foreign body reaction with amalgam granules in the macrophages or giant cells.

Excision is necessary to exclude a melanoma.

Peutz–Jeghers syndrome

This autosomal dominant syndrome comprises intestinal

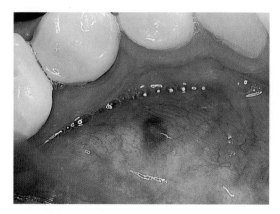

Fig. 21.3 Amalgam tattoo. Typical appearance and site; however, the lower second premolar from which the amalgam probably originated has been crowned.

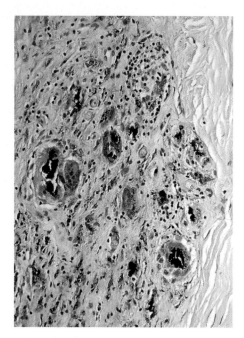

Fig. 21.4 Amalgam tattoo. There are large fragments of amalgam surrounded by foreign body giant cells and macrophages and smaller particles dispersed in fibrous tissue. Silver leaching from the smaller fragments has stained the adjacent collagen brown.

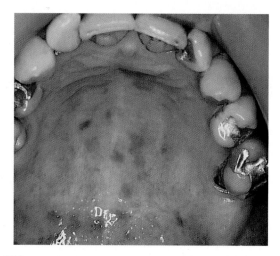

Fig. 21.5 Peutz–Jehgers syndrome. There are multiple flat, pigmented patches on the palate. Those on the lips are most characteristic but fade with age.

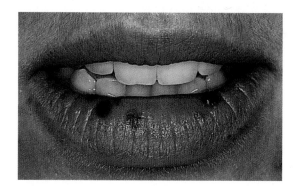

Fig. 21.6 Melanocytic naevi. These flat, pigmented patches are occasionally found on the lip and intraorally.

Oral melanotic naevi

Pigmented naevi are benign lesions of melanocytes which form circumscribed brown to black patches about 5 or 6 mm across (Fig. 21.6). They are asymptomatic but should be excised and sent for microscopy to exclude early malignant melanoma.

Pathology

The main features are modest numbers of pigmented melanocytes in the basal cell layer but many clumps of melanocytes in the corium (Fig. 21.7). Rarely, intraepithelial foci of proliferating melanocytes project into the corium and appear to be dropping off the basal layer (junctional activity). Equally rarely, junctional activity is associated with circumscribed nests of melanocytes in a limited area of the upper corium (compound naevus).

Blue naevus

The epithelium is normal, but beneath and separate from it is a focus of spindle-shaped pigmented melanocytes.

polyposis and melanotic macules, particularly of the face and mouth.

There are multiple freckles on the lips and oral mucosa. Facial pigmentation (mainly around the mouth, eyes and nose) usually fades after puberty, but mucosal pigmentation persists (Fig. 21.5).

Polyps may be present throughout the gastrointestinal tract (Ch. 29). Colon cancer is a possible hazard but the risk for breast and gynecological cancers is particularly high. Multiple oral melanotic macules may therefore indicate the need for cancer screening.

Microscopy of the macules shows increased melanin in the basal keratinocytes.

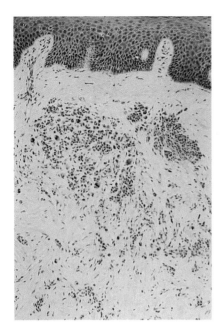

Fig. 21.7 Intramucosal naevus. A cluster of naevus cells lies in the connective tissue separated from the epithelium by a layer of normal fibrous tissue.

All these types of naevi should be excised and sent for histology.

ORAL MELANOTIC MACULES ASSOCIATED WITH HIV INFECTION

Oral and labial melanotic macules may be seen in up to 6% of patients with HIV infection. This is approximately twice the frequency seen in HIV negative persons. Also, oral melanotic macules appear to become more numerous as HIV infection advances. Increasing numbers of oral melanotic macules may appear long before HIV infection is detected.

Histologically, there is vacuolation of the spinous cells which are either in large clusters or spread throughout the epithelium. Excess melanin deposition is present in the basal cell layer and upper part of the lamina propria.

Behavior and management

Excision biopsy of melanotic macules is necessary for diagnosis but, unlike those in HIV-negative persons, these macules are more likely to enlarge and to recur after excision. Oral melanotic macules which enlarge or recur after excision may therefore be a sign of HIV infection.

MALIGNANT MELANOMA

Intraoral melanomas are rare in the US and UK. They are

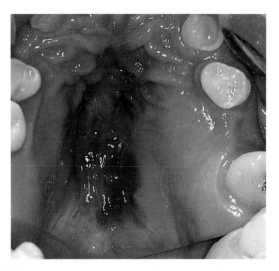

Fig. 21.8 Melanotic patch. There is poorly-demarcated pigmentation of varying density in the palate. All pigmented lesions such as this should be treated with the utmost suspicion and biopsied to exclude melanoma.

usually dark brown or black but 15% of oral melanomas are non-pigmented and typically, red. The peak age incidence is between 40 and 60. They are macular or nodular and may ulcerate: the palate is most frequently affected (Fig. 21.8). They are typically firm and rubbery but asymptomatic at first. Hence melanomas may remain unnoticed until they cause soreness, bleeding, or a neck mass, unless noticed by chance.

Melanomas of the superficial spreading type are rare in the mouth and are usually invasive unless recognised unusually early. Early diagnosis by biopsy is essential.

Pathology

Melanomas consist of neoplastic melanocytes often surrounded by clear halos, both within the epithelium and invading deeper tissues. These cells are round to spindle-shaped and typically speckled or intensely pigmented with melanin (Figs 21.9 and 21.10). However, in amelanotic melanomas, the absence of pigment makes these cells more difficult to recognise.

Diagnosis is greatly helped by immunohistochemistry. Melanomas are typically S-100, MMA (melanoma-associated antigen) positive, but HMB-45 and NKI/C3 are currently regarded as being more specific. However, a clinicopathologic and immunohistochemical analysis of oral malignant melanomas found that each of them individually showed features of each type of cutaneous melanoma, but reacted variably with the usual histochemical markers. It may therefore be that oral malignant melanomas should be regarded as a separate entity from cutaneous melanomas.

Key features are summarised in Table 21.2.

Management

The prognosis of intraoral melanomas is poor as they are frequently unrecognised until there are symptoms or involvement

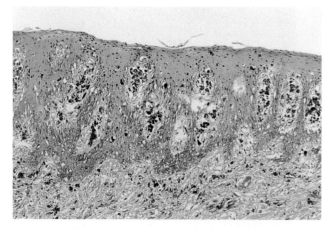

Fig. 21.9 Superficial spreading melanoma. Numerous pigmented and atypical melanocytes form nests and clusters along the basement membrane and are present within the epithelium and superficial connective tissue.

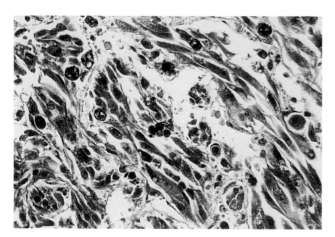

Fig. 21.10 Melanoma. Malignant spindled and round melanocytes, often with bizarre nuclei and some with melanin pigment, invading deep tissue.

Table 21.2 Malignant melanoma: key features

- Peak incidence between 40 and 60 years
- Usually appear as black or brown patches
- Amelanotic melanomas appear red
- Later cause soreness and bleeding
- Histologically consist of neoplastic melanocytes often surrounded by clear halos, within the epithelium and invading deeper tissues
- Neoplastic melanocytes are round to spindle-shaped and typically speckled or intensely pigmented with melanin
- Should be widely excised but median survival probably not longer than 2 years

---

of lymph nodes. Distant spread is to the lungs, liver, bones and other organs. *All pigmented patches in the mouth should therefore be biopsied to exclude malignant melanoma.*

Treatment is by radical excision and usually chemotherapy or radiotherapy or both. In a recent series the median survival for mucosal melanomas was less than 2 years.

Melanotic neuroectodermal tumour of infancy

One of these tumours (Ch. 9) may rarely show through the palatal mucosa as an ill-defined pigmented area in a neonate or infant.

DIFFUSE MUCOSAL PIGMENTATIONS

The most important of these is Addison's disease (Ch. 31) but is rare. Racial pigmentation is common and though most obvious on the gingivae is typically widespread. Other rare causes are drugs (such as chlorhexidine and phenothiazines, but many others) and cancer of the lung can occasionally cause pigmentation of the soft palate.

SUGGESTED FURTHER READING

Barrett A W, Bennett J H, Speight P M 1995 A clinicopathological and immunohistochemical analysis of primary oral malignant melanoma. Oral Oncol Eur J Cancer 31B:100–115

Boardman L A, Thibodeau S N, Schaid D J et al 1998 Increased risk for cancer in patients with the Peutz-Jeghers syndrome. Ann Intern Med 128:896–899

Buchner A, Hansen L S 1980 Amalgam pigmentation (amalgam tattoo) of the oral mucosa: a clinicopathological study of 268 cases. Oral Surg Oral Med Oral Pathol 49:139–147

Buchner A, Hansen L S 1987 Pigmented nevi of the oral mucosa: a clinicopathologic study of 36 cases and review of 155 cases from the literature. Oral Surg Oral Med Oral Pathol 63:566–572

Cawson R A, Binnie W H, Barrett A W, Wright J M 2001 *Color atlas of oral disease*, 3rd Edn. Mosby-Wolfe, London

Cawson R A, Langdon J D, Eveson J W 1996 *Surgical pathology of the mouth and jaws*. Wright, Oxford

Eisen D, Voorhees J J 1991 Oral melanoma and other pigmented lesions of the oral cavity. J Am Acad Dermatol 24:527–537

Ficarra G, Shillitoe E J, Adler-Storthz K et al 1990 Oral melanotic macules associated with HIV. Oral Surg Oral Med Pathol 70:301–307

Gazit D, Daniels T E 1994 Oral melanocytic lesions: differences in expression of HMB-45 and S-100 antigens in round and spindle cells of malignant and benign lesions. J Oral Pathol Med 23:60–64

Kaugars G E, Heise A P, Riley W T, Abbey L M, Svirsky J A 1993 Oral melanotic macules. A review of 353 cases. Oral Surg Oral Med Oral Pathol 76:59–61

Langford A, Pohle H D, Gelderblom H et al 1989 Oral hyperpigmentation in HIV-infected patients. Oral Surg Oral Med Oral Pathol 67:301–307

Patton L L, Brahim J S, Baker A R 1994 Metastatic malignant melanoma of the oral cavity. A retrospective study. Oral Surg Oral Med Oral Pathol 78:51–56

Strauss J E, Strauss S I 1994 Oral malignant melanoma: a case report and review of literature. J Oral Maxillofac Surg 52:972–976

Umeda M, Shimada K 1994 Primary malignant melanoma of the oral cavity — its histological classification and treatment. Br J Oral Maxillofac Surg 32:39–47

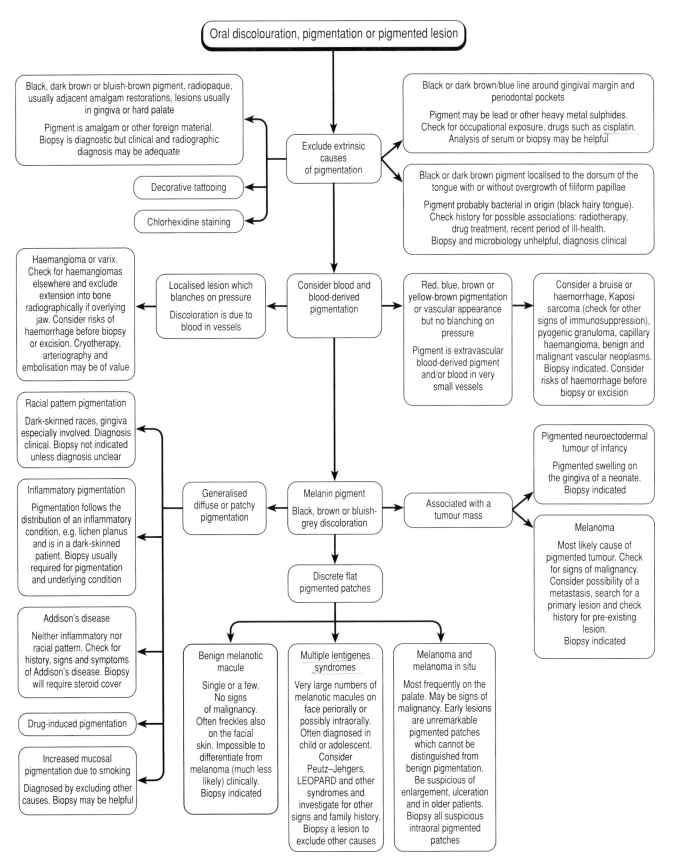

Summary 21.1 The common causes of oral pigmented lesions.

THE MEDICALLY-COMPROMISED PATIENT

Anaemias, leukaemias and lymphomas

Haematological disease is common and can cause serious complications or oral symptoms (Table 22.1).

Haemoglobin estimation and routine indices are informative and should be carried out when any patient has suspicious signs in the mouth or has to undergo oral surgery.

Table 22.1   Important effects of haematological diseases

- Anaesthetic complications
- Oral infections
- Prolonged bleeding
- Mucosal lesions

Anaemia

Causes and important types are summarised in Table 22.2.

Iron deficiency (microcytic) anaemia is the most common type and usually results from chronic menstrual blood loss. Women of child-bearing age or over, or men with peptic ulcer or haemorrhoids are mainly affected.

Table 22.2   Types and features of important anaemias

Type of anaemia	Causes or effects
1. Iron deficiency (microcytic, hypochromic anaemia)	Usually due to chronic blood loss
2. Folate deficiency (macrocytic)	Pregnancy, malabsorption, alcohol*, phenytoin-induced etc.
3. Vitamin B_{12} deficiency (macrocytic anaemia)	Usually due to pernicious anaemia, occasionally to malabsorption
4. Leukaemia and aplastic anaemia (normochromic normocytic)	Raised susceptibility to infection and bleeding tendency often associated
5. Sickle cell disease (normocytic anaemia)	Genetic. Sickle cells seen in special preparations
6. Beta-thalassaemia (hypochromic, microcytic)	Genetic. Many misshapen red cells
7. Chronic inflammatory disease (normochromic, normocytic)	Rheumatoid arthritis is a common cause
8. Liver disease (usually normocytic)	Haemorrhagic tendency may be associated

*Alcoholism should always be excluded when macrocytosis in the absence of anaemia is found — it is a characteristic sign of alcoholism.

Pernicious anaemia chiefly affects women of middle age or over and is the main cause of macrocytic anaemia. Unlike other anaemias it can cause neurological disease, particularly subacute combined degeneration of the spinal cord.

Folate deficiency also causes a macrocytic anaemia, often in younger patients, particularly in pregnancy. It must be firmly differentiated from pernicious anaemia because administration of folate to the latter can worsen neurological disease.

Leukaemia is an uncommon but frequently lethal cause of normocytic anaemia, but should be suspected in an anaemic child.

Sickle cell trait is most common in immigrants from the West Indies. Sickle cell anaemia is relatively uncommon.

Thalassaemia is mainly seen in immigrants from the Mediterranean area.

Clinical features

Anaemia, irrespective of cause, produces essentially the same clinical features (Table 22.3), particularly if severe, but some anaemias have distinctive features.

Table 22.3   General clinical features of anaemia

- Pallor
- Fatigue and lassitude
- Breathlessness
- Tachycardia and palpitations
- Glossitis or other mucosal lesions

The complexion is a poor indicator of pallor. The conjunctiva of the lower eyelid, the nail beds, and sometimes the oral mucosa, are more reliable. Cardiovascular signs (tachycardia or oedema of the ankles) result from severe anaemia. Glossitis and other mucosal diseases (Table 22.4) by contrast, can be the earliest signs as discussed below.

Mucosal disease

Glossitis

Anaemia is the most important, though not the most common, cause of a sore tongue. Soreness *can precede a fall in haemo-globin levels*, particularly when resulting from vitamin B_{12} or

Table 22.4 Features of anaemia important in dentistry

- Mucosal disease
  Glossitis
  Angular stomatitis
  Recurrent aphthae
  Infection, particularly candidosis
- Risks from general anaesthesia
  Shortage of oxygen can be dangerous
- Lowered resistance to infection
  Apart from candidosis, this is seen only in severe anaemia or when due to leukaemia

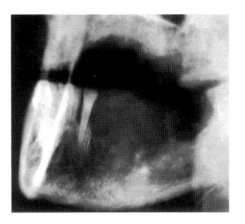

Fig. 22.2 Acute osteomyelitis in an anaemic patient. Widespread bone destruction followed straightforward extraction of the posterior teeth. The patient was found to have a haemoglobin level of 4 g/dl.

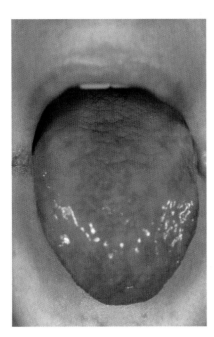

Fig. 22.1 Iron deficiency anaemia. The tongue is slightly reddened, smooth and depapillated. There is also angular cheilitis as a result of candidal infection.

folate deficiency, and can be their first sign. Later there may be obvious inflammation and atrophy of the filiform papillae (Fig. 22.1). Variants of sore tongue have been discussed in Chapter 14, but it is emphasised again that this symptom always requires careful haematological investigation, initially by means of a haemoglobin level and routine indices. Serum iron, ferritin and red cell folate levels may be required. Even though the haemoglobin may be within normal limits, enlarged erythrocytes [mean corpuscular volume (MCV) > 96 fl] frequently indicates pernicious anaemia. If any deficiency is found, the underlying cause, such as gastrointestinal disease, must be investigated.

Recurrent aphthae

Aphthae are sometimes secondary to haematological deficiency, particularly of vitamin B$_{12}$ or folate, in patients whose aphthae start or worsen late in life.

Candidosis and angular stomatitis

Iron deficiency, in particular, is a predisposing factor for candidosis (Ch. 12). Angular stomatitis is also a classical sign of iron deficiency anaemia and due to candidosis.

Dangers of general anaesthesia

Any reduction of oxygenation can precipitate irreparable brain damage or myocardial infarction when there is significant anaemia. General anaesthesia should therefore be given in hospital. The dangers are particularly great in sickle cell disease, as discussed later.

Lowered resistance to infection

Oral candidosis is the main example but, in the past particularly, osteomyelitis could follow extractions in severe anaemia (Fig. 22.2). Currently, sickle cell disease is more important in this context.

SICKLE CELL DISEASE AND SICKLE CELL TRAIT

Sickle cell anaemia mainly affects people of African, Afro-Caribbean, Indian, Mediterranean, or Middle Eastern origin. About 5000 persons in Britain are estimated to have sickle cell disease (homozygotes), but many more have sickle cell trait (heterozygotes). The defect in sickle cell disease is an abnormal haemoglobin (HbS) with the risk of haemolysis, anaemia and other effects. In heterozygotes, sufficient normal haemoglobin (HbA) is formed to allow normal life with only rare complications.

Sickle cell disease. The complications arise from polymerisation of deoxygenated HbS, which is less soluble than HbA. This forms long fibres which deform the red cells into sickle shapes and makes them vulnerable to haemolysis. Chronic

Table 22.5 Factors that can precipitate sickling crises

- Hypoxia, particularly from poorly conducted anaesthesia
- Dehydration
- Infections (including dental)
- Acidosis and fever

Table 22.6 The main types of sickling crises

- Painful crises
- Aplastic crises
- Sequestration crises

haemolysis causes chronic anaemia, but patients, under normal circumstances, typically feel well, as HbS more readily releases its oxygen content to the tissues than HbA. Exacerbation of sickling raises blood viscosity, causing blocking of capillaries and sickling crises (Tables 22.5 and 22.6).

These patients are also abnormally susceptible to infection, particularly pneumococcal or meningococcal, and osteomyelitis.

Painful crises are caused by blockage of blood vessels and bone marrow infarcts. Painful crises can effect the jaws, particularly the mandible, and mimic acute osteomyelitis clinically and radiographically. The infarcted tissue forms a focus susceptible to infection, and Salmonella osteomyelitis is a recognised hazard.

Aplastic crises are caused by human parvovirus B19 infection and require immediate transfusion.

Sequestration crises result from sickle cells pooling in the spleen, liver or lungs. An acute chest syndrome, with pain, fever and leucocytosis, is the most common cause of death.

Dental aspects of sickle cell trait and disease

Sickling trait should be suspected, particularly in those of Afro-Caribbean origin, and investigated if anaesthesia is anticipated. If the haemoglobin is less than 10 g/dl the patient is probably a homozygote with sickle cell disease. Screening tests depend on the lower solubility of HbS which produces turbidity when a reducing agent is added. Confirmation is by electrophoresis.

In those with sickle cell trait the main precaution is that general anaesthesia should be carried out with full oxygenation. In sickle cell disease the oral mucosa may be pale or yellowish due to haemolytic jaundice. Radiographic changes can be seen in the skull and sometimes the jaws (Ch. 10).

Occasionally, crises may be precipitated by dental infections such as acute pericoronitis. Prompt antibiotic treatment is therefore important. Painful bone infarcts should be treated with non-steroidal anti-inflammatory analgesics, and fluid intake should be increased. Admission to hospital is required for severe painful crises not responsive to analgesics. Rigorous routine dental care is necessary because of the susceptibility to infection.

THE THALASSAEMIAS

Alpha-thalassaemias mainly affect Asians, Africans and Afro-Caribbeans, while beta-thalassaemias mainly affect those from the Mediterranean littoral such as Greeks (thalassaemia — literally, 'sea in the blood').

Thalassaemias result from diminished synthesis of one or more of the globin chains of haemoglobin. The resulting relative excess of either the alpha or beta globin chains, which are unstable, causes them to precipitate in the red cells. Haemolysis can result.

The severity of the disease depends on the numbers of alpha or beta globin genes affected. In simplified terms, the diseases are *thalassaemia minor* in heterozygotes and *thalassaemia major* in homozygotes.

Thalassaemia minor causes mild but persistent microcytic anaemia but is otherwise asymptomatic apart sometimes from splenomegaly. Iron therapy is ineffective and leads to iron deposition in the tissues.

Thalassaemia major (usually homozygous beta-thalassaemia) causes severe hypochromic, microcytic anaemia, great enlargement of liver and spleen and skeletal abnormalities (Ch. 10) due to marrow expansion. There is failure to thrive and early death if regular transfusions are not given. They are life-saving, prevent the development of bony deformities, but lead to progressive iron deposition in the tissues. Haemosiderosis is the main cause of complications in survivors and leads to dysfunction of glands and other organs. Xerostomia can result from iron deposition in the salivary glands. Desferrioxamine, a chelating agent, may lessen the effects of iron overload, and folic acid treatment may ameliorate the haemolytic anaemia.

LEUKAEMIA

The effect of leukaemic overproduction of white cells is to suppress other cell lines of the marrow (Table 22.7). Leukaemia can affect virtually any of the white cell series but different types of acute leukaemia cannot be distinguished clinically.

Table 22.7 Major effects of acute leukaemia

- Anaemia due to suppression of erythrocyte production
- Raised susceptibility to infection due to deficiency or abnormalities of granulocytes
- Bleeding tendency (purpura) due to suppression of platelet production

Acute leukaemia

Acute lymphoblastic leukaemia is the most common leukaemia in children (usually between 3 and 5 years), while acute myeloblastic anaemia is the most common type in adults.

Table 22.8 Oral and perioral effects of acute leukaemia

- Gingival swelling
- Mucosal ulceration
- Leukaemic deposits
- Purpura
- Anaemia
- Cervical lymphadenopathy

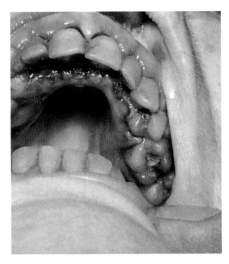

Fig. 22.3 Acute myelocytic leukaemia. The gingivae are grossly swollen and purplish; in addition there is ulceration along the palatal aspect of the anterior teeth resulting from the increased susceptibility to infection.

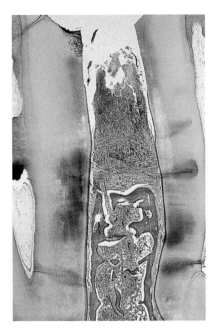

Fig. 22.4 Acute leukaemia. The gingivae and bone marrow of the interdental bone contain a confluent infiltrate of leukaemic cells.

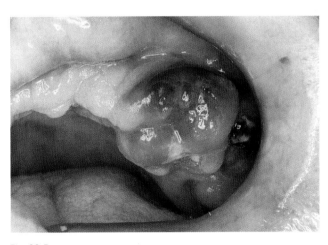

Fig. 22.5 Myeloid leukaemia. An ulcerated tumour mass formed by leukaemic cells emigrating into the tissues.

Splenomegaly or hepatomegaly, or both, and lymphadenopathy, particularly in lymphoblastic leukaemia, are usually associated. Mucosal pallor or abnormal gingival bleeding, particularly in a child, strongly suggest acute leukaemia (Table 22.8). Diagnosis depends on the peripheral blood picture and marrow biopsy.

Gingival swelling results from lack of healthy, mature white cells to counter low-grade gingival infection. The gingivae become packed and swollen with leukaemic cells, particularly in acute myelogenous leukaemia in adults. The gingivae are often purplish and may become necrotic and ulcerate (Figs 22.3 and 22.4).

Mucosal ulceration is often a combined effect of immunodeficiency and cytotoxic drugs such as methotrexate. Herpetic infections and thrush are common, and ulceration may be caused by a variety of opportunistic microbes. Also as a result of the immunodeficiency, the first sign of acute leukaemia may occasionally be an infection such as acute osteomyelitis following routine extractions.

Leukaemic deposits are tumour-like masses of leukaemic cells which may occasionally form in the mouth or salivary glands (Fig. 22.5).

Purpura can appear as excessive gingival bleeding, purplish mucosal patches, blood blisters, or prolonged bleeding after surgery. Leukaemic infiltration of an extraction socket can delay healing (Fig. 22.6).

Anaemia can cause mucosal pallor and is an important sign in children among whom anaemia is otherwise uncommon.

Cervical lymphadenopathy is particularly common in lymphocytic leukaemia but may be seen in other types or be secondary to opportunistic infections in the mouth.

Management

Biopsy of gingival swelling unresponsive to conventional treatment may lead to the diagnosis of leukaemia.

Ideally, patients with leukaemia or any others having cytotoxic treatment, should have meticulous oral hygiene to control

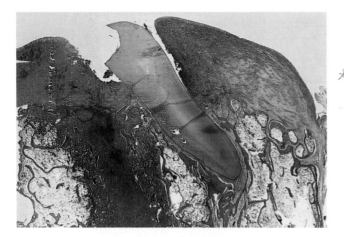

Fig. 22.6 Acute myelogenous leukaemia. Leukaemic cells have densely infiltrated the swollen gingiva and the extraction socket, which has been prevented from healing.

the bacterial population, *before* complications develop (see Fig. 5.35).

Mouth rinses (0.2% chlorhexidine or tetracycline and amphotericin) will often control severe gingival changes and superficial infections. Mucosal ulceration by Gram-negative bacilli or anaerobes may need specific antibiotic therapy, which is also necessary for systemic spread of infection.

Oral ulceration caused by methotrexate may be controlled by giving folinic acid. Extractions should be avoided because of the risks of severe infections, bleeding, or anaemia. If unavoidable, blood transfusion and generous antibiotic cover are required.

Chronic leukaemia

Chronic leukaemia is a slowly progressive disease of adults. Chronic lymphocytic leukaemia can be completely asymptomatic and may not even shorten life.

Oral manifestations (Table 22.9) are relatively uncommon or mild.

Table 22.9 Possible oral effects of chronic leukaemia

- Mucosal pallor
- Gingival or palatal swelling
- Purpura
- Oral ulceration (ulceration may be due to infection or cytotoxic drugs or both)

Management

Routine dentistry can usually be carried out with normal care. If there is significant anaemia, bleeding tendencies, or susceptibility to infection, similar precautions need to be taken to those for acute leukaemia.

LYMPHOMAS

Lymphomas, unlike leukaemias, are solid tumours, though lymphocytic lymphoma can be accompanied by lymphocytic leukaemia.

Lymphomas can arise from any type of lymphocyte, but more frequently from B cells. They are all malignant. They comprise Hodgkin's disease and the more common non-Hodgkin lymphoma.

Lymphomas involve the cervical lymph nodes relatively frequently, but are rare in the mouth. However, in AIDS, lymphomas may account for 2% of oral neoplasms.

Non-Hodgkin lymphomas

The risk of developing a lymphoma is raised in the following conditions:

1. some of the primary immunodeficiency diseases
2. cytotoxic immunosuppressive treatment
3. AIDS
4. connective tissue diseases, especially rheumatoid arthritis and Sjögren's syndrome.

Adults are predominantly affected, and, within the mouth, lymphomas form nondescript, usually soft, painless swellings, which may become ulcerated by trauma.

Histologically, lymphomas frequently present difficulties of precise diagnosis. Non-Hodgkin lymphomas may be *diffuse* and appear as solid sheets of lymphocytes which may be predominantly small or large. Alternatively they may have a *follicular* pattern. Most follicular lymphomas are low grade and have a better prognosis. The neoplastic lymphocytes show varying degrees of differentiation from mature small cells to large immunoblasts which may resemble histiocytes (Fig. 22.7). Most are of B-cell origin (Fig. 22.8).

Invasion of adjacent tissues may be seen and helps to confirm the malignant nature of these tumours (Fig. 22.9). If traumatised, inflammatory cells can obscure the lymphomatous nature of the tumour. However, lymphoma cells are monoclonal and this can be recognised by immunohistochemistry by production of kappa or lambda light chains only (Ch. 1).

Management

As well as biopsy, staging is necessary to determine the extent of spread. In general, localised disease is treated by irradiation while disseminated disease (the majority of patients) is treated by combination chemotherapy. Oral complications of treatment, such as ulceration and infection, are common.

Burkitt's lymphoma

This was the first lymphoma where an association with the Epstein–Barr virus (EBV) was shown. It is predominantly

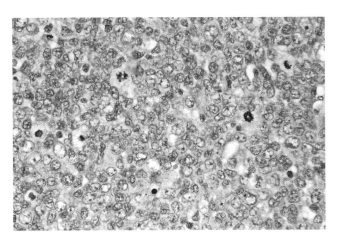

Fig. 22.7 High-grade non-Hodgkin lymphoma. Neoplastic lymphocytes with large vesicular nuclei are packed in confluent sheets. Mitotic figures are numerous.

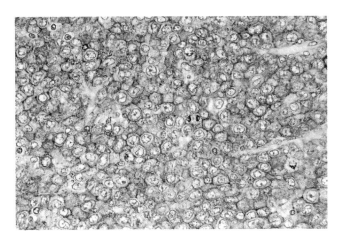

Fig. 22.8 High-grade lymphoma. Immunocytochemistry for a B cell marker produces a ring of positive brown stain on the membrane of virtually every tumour cell, indicating its B cell origin.

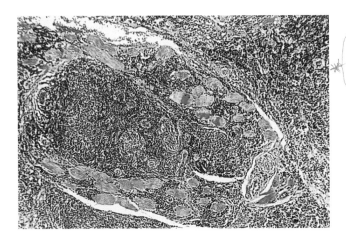

Fig. 22.9 High-grade non-Hodgkin lyphoma. Small darkly staining lymphoma cells infiltrating through muscle and fat.

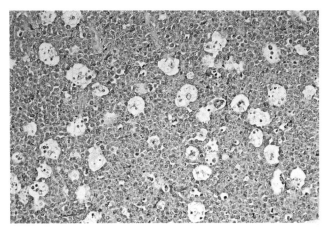

Fig. 22.10 Burkitt's lymphoma. Small darkly staining neoplastic lymphocytes form sheets in which the macrophages containing cellular debris form round, pale holes (starry sky appearance).

extranodal. It is unusual in that its onset is in childhood and is endemic in East Africa. It is also unusual in that the jaw is the single most common initial site, and spread to the parotid glands is common. Over 95% of cases respond completely to single-dose chemotherapy.

Histologically, Burkitt's lymphoma is a small-cell lymphoma containing scattered pale histiocytes which give the dark sheets of cells a so-called 'starry sky' appearance (Fig. 22.10). Lymphomas resembling Burkitt's lymphoma microscopically can also be a complication of immunosuppressive treatment or AIDS but do not behave like African Burkitt's lymphoma.

Nasopharyngeal (T-cell and NK-cell) lymphomas

These are rare causes of midline granuloma syndrome. *In their early stages they can be indistinguishable clinically from Wegener's granulomatosis* (Ch. 28).

Extension of the disease through the palate can cause swelling and ulceration as a presenting feature (Fig. 22.11). A small ulcer may extend until the whole of the palate becomes necrotic. A deep biopsy is necessary to obtain lesional tissue not obscured by necrosis.

Histological diagnosis is difficult as these lymphomas are cellularly pleomorphic. They attack blood vessels, and thus simulate vasculitis (Fig. 22.12). Secondary inflammation may also obscure the lymphoma cells, so that several biopsies may be required.

In the past, death could result from infection secondary to massive facial necrosis. Usually now, death results from dissemination of the lymphoma, but this may be delayed by radiotherapy. Key features are summarised in Table 22.10.

Hodgkin's disease

The cervical lymph nodes are frequently affected but lesions are exceptionally uncommon in the mouth. They are not clinically distinguishable from non-Hodgkin lymphoma.

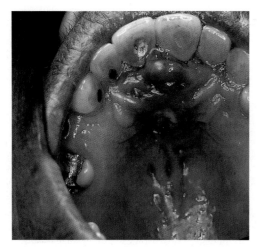

Fig. 22.11 Nasopharyngeal lymphoma. Typical slight anterior swelling and ulcer due to perforation of the palate by the tumour.

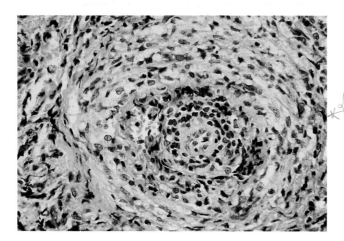

Fig. 22.12 Nasopharyngeal lymphoma. Neoplastic infiltration of a vessel wall simulating vasculitis.

Table 22.10   Key features of nasopharyneal T-cell lymphoma

- Onset typically indistinguishable from Wegener's granulomatosis
- Downward extension may cause central ulceration or necrosis of the palate enabling early diagnosis
- Histologically, the cellular picture is pleomorphic but damage to blood vessels mimics vasculitis
- T-cell or NK-cell markers confirm the diagnosis
- Spread of disease is similar to that of other lymphomas and usually, a fatal outcome
- Spread may be limited or delayed by radiotherapy

Histologically, the characteristic features are the mixed cellular picture and occasional Reed–Sternberg giant cells with paired (mirror-image) nuclei.

Permanent cure of some types of Hodgkin's disease is possible as a result of irradiation of localised disease or combined chemotherapy, and the overall 5-year survival rate may be up to 80%.

LEUCOPENIA AND AGRANULOCYTOSIS

Leucopenia is a deficiency of white cells (fewer than 5000/L with many possible causes (Table 22.11). It is a peripheral blood manifestation of actual or incipient immunodeficiency.

Leucopenia can be a chance haematological finding and may cause no symptoms until it becomes so severe as to impair defences against infection. Thus lymphopenia in an apparently healthy person may be a sign of HIV infection.

Table 22.11   Important causes of leucopenia

- Leukaemia
- Aplastic anaemia
- Drugs (Table 22.12)
- Autoimmune
- HIV infection

Agranulocytosis

Agranulocytosis is the term given to the clinical effects of severe neutropenia, namely fever, prostration and mucosal ulceration, particularly of the gingivae and pharynx.

Drug-induced leucopenia

Table 22.12   Important causes of drug-induced leukopenia

- Analgesics, especially phenylbutazone*
- Antibacterial drugs, especially chloramphenicol or (rarely) co-trimoxazole
- Phenothiazine antipsychotic drugs
- Antithyroid drugs such as thiouracil
- Cytotoxic drugs

*Use now restricted as a consequence.

Management (Table 22.13)

Aplastic anaemia

Aplastic anaemia is failure of production of all bone marrow cells (pancytopenia). The systemic and oral effects are not unlike those of acute leukaemia (purpura, anaemia and susceptibility to infection). Aplastic anaemia may be of unknown cause but is probably autoimmune. Otherwise drugs (Table 22.12) are the main cause.

The management is to stop any drugs that may be responsible and to give antibiotics and transfusions. Nevertheless approximately 50% of patients die within 6 months, usually from infection or haemorrhage, but marrow transplantation has occasionally been successful. Dental management is as for acute leukaemia.

Table 22.13 Leukopenia: principles of general and dental management

- General
  Stop any drug which may be causative
  Give antibiotics
  Give blood transfusions if necessary
- Dental
  Optimise oral hygiene
  Control oral infections (as for acute leukaemia)
  Avoid extractions
  Antibiotic cover and transfusions if necessary if surgery is unavoidable

Cyclic neutropenia

In cyclic neutropenia there is a fall in the number of circulating neutrophils at regular intervals of 3–4 weeks. There have been only about 40 reported cases in 70 years and undue emphasis has been placed on the fact that cyclic neutropenia occasionally, but not necessarily, causes oral ulceration or rapidly progressive periodontitis.

SUGGESTED FURTHER READING

Banerjee A K, Layton D M, Rennie J A et al 1991 Safe surgery in sickle cell disease. Br J Surg 78:516–519

Cranfield T, Bunch C 1995 Acute leukaemias. Medicine (UK) 23:503–509

Field E A, Speechley J A, Rugman F R 1995 Oral signs and symptoms in patients with undiagnosed vitamin B_{12} deficiency. J Oral Pathol Med 24:468–470

Gregory G, Olujohungbe A 1994 Mandibular nerve neuropathy in sickle cell disease. Local factors. Oral Surg Oral Med Oral Pathol 77:66–69

Hatton C, Mackie P H 1996 Haemoglobinopathies and other congenital haemolytic anaemias. Medicine Int 24:14–19

Higgs D R 1993 The thalassaemia syndromes. Q J Med 86:559–564

Luker J, Scully C, Oakhill A 1991 Gingival swelling as a manifestation of aplastic anaemia. Oral Surg Oral Med Oral Pathol 70:55–56

O'Connor N, Bunch C 1995 Laboratory diagnosis in haematology. Medicine Int 23:489–494

O'Rourke C, Mitropoulous C 1990 Orofacial pain in patients with sickle cell disease. Br Dent J 169:130–132

Pippard M J, Heppleston A D 1996 Microcytic and macrocytic anaemias. Medicine International 24:4–10

Podlesh S W, Boyden D K 1996 Diagnosis of acute bone/bone marrow infarction of the mandible in sickle haemoglobinopathy. Report of a case. Oral Surg Oral Med Oral Pathol Radiol Endod 81:547–549

Sansevere J J, Miles M 1993 Management of the oral and maxillofacial patient with sickle cell disease and related haemoglobinopathies. J Oral Maxillofac Surg 51:912–916

Haemorrhagic diseases

Purpura (usually platelet defects) and clotting defects are the main causes of haemorrhagic disorders.

Investigation of a history of excessive bleeding

A careful history (Table 23.1) is absolutely essential. Most of the severe haemorrhagic diseases such as haemophilia are hereditary and a positive family history should be carefully investigated. Bleeding for up to 24 hours after an extraction is usually due to local causes or a minor defect of haemostasis manageable by local measures. More prolonged bleeding is significant. Even a *mild* haemophiliac can bleed for weeks after a simple extraction.

Table 23.1   **Information required about haemorrhagic tendencies**

1. Results of previous dental operations. Have simple extractions led to prolonged bleeding?
2. Has bleeding persisted for more than 24 hours?
3. Has admission to hospital ever been necessary for dental bleeding?
4. Have other operations or injuries caused prolonged bleeding?
5. Is there a family history of prolonged bleeding?
6. Are anticoagulants or other drugs being taken?
7. Is there any medical cause such as leukaemia or liver disease?
8. Does the patient carry a warning card or hospital letter about bleeding tendencies?

Clinical examination

Signs of anaemia and purpura should be looked for. Examination of the mouth shows how any operation should be planned. In the case of haemophilia, all essential extractions should, if possible, be carried out at a single operation with factor VIII cover. Radiographs should be taken to anticipate possible difficulties in the extractions.

Laboratory investigations

Details of investigations are decided by the haematologist, but summarised in Table 23.2.

Table 23.2   **Important investigations in haemophilia**

- Haemoglobin level and blood picture
- Assessment of haemostatic function, particularly the:
    Bleeding time
    Prothrombin time (expressed as the INR)
    Activated partial thromboplastin time
    Thrombin time
- Blood grouping and cross-matching

It is important to look for anaemia. It is an almost inevitable result of repeated bleeding and worsened by any further bleeding as a result of surgery. Anemia increases the risks of general anaesthesia and should be treated before any surgery. Anaemia is also an essential feature of some haemorrhagic diseases, particularly acute leukaemia.

Blood grouping is required as transfusions may be needed before operation to improve haemostasis or afterwards, if blood loss is severe.

PURPURA

Purpura is typically the result of platelet disorders (Table 23.3) and relatively rarely caused by vascular defects. The bleeding time is prolonged but clotting function is normal. An exception is von Willebrand's disease, where there is an associated deficiency of a clotting factor.

General features of purpura

Purpura (bleeding into the skin or mucous membranes, causing petechiae, ecchymoses or 'spontaneous' bruising) also causes prolonged bleeding after injury or surgery. Unlike haemophilia, haemorrhage immediately follows the trauma but, usually, bleeding in purpura ultimately stops spontaneously as a result of normal coagulation.

Many women will say that they bruise easily, but such bruises are usually only a few millimetres across. The most informative test of platelet function is the *bleeding time*, supplemented as necessary by tests of platelet aggregation and adhesion.

Table 23.3 Causes of purpura

- Platelet disorders
  Idiopathic thrombocytopenic purpura
  Connective tissue diseases (especially systemic lupus erythematosus)
  Acute leukaemias
  Drug-associated
  HIV infection
- Vascular disorders
  von Willebrand's disease
  Corticosteroid treatment
  Ehlers–Danlos syndrome
  Infective

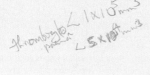

Deficiency of platelets (fewer than 100 000 mm^3), is termed thrombocytopenia, but spontaneous bleeding is uncommon until the count falls below 50 000 mm^3.

A typical site of oral purpura is the palate where the posterior border of a denture presses into the mucosa. Excessive gingival bleeding or blood blisters are other signs (Figs 23.1 and 23.2).

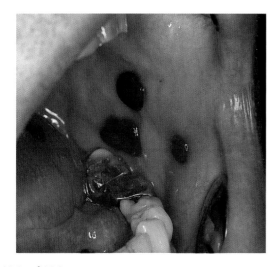

Fig. 23.1 and 23.2 Systemic purpura. The lesions are due to spontaneous bleeding into the tissues and often form at sites of trauma.

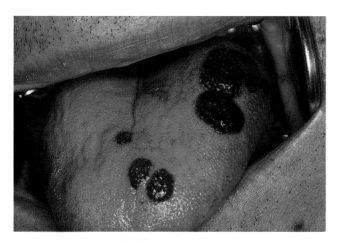

Fig. 23.2 Systemic purpura.

Idiopathic thrombocytopenic purpura

The immediate cause is IgG autoantibodies which bind to platelets. The number of platelets in the peripheral blood is low.

The disease may affect children or young adult women, and the first sign may be profuse gingival bleeding or post-extraction haemorrhage. More often there is spontaneous bleeding into the skin ('bruising').

Management

Thrombocytopenic purpura frequently responds, at least in the short-term, to corticosteroids, which can be used for urgently needed surgery. Long-term use of corticosteroids is associated with their usual hazards. Some cases resolve spontaneously but persistent cases may respond to splenectomy. However, 10–20% of cases are unresponsive to any form of treatment, and, now that haemophilia is a manageable disease, such cases have become one of the most troublesome of the haemorrhagic diseases. For operative treatment, transfusions of platelet concentrates can be given, but immunosuppressive drugs may also have to be given to prevent platelet destruction by antibodies. As with other platelet disorders, aspirin and other anti-inflammatory analgesics should be avoided.

HIV-associated purpura

Autoimmune thrombocytopenia can complicate HIV infection and can be an early sign. Purpuric patches in the mouth, particularly in a young male, should suggest this possibility and also need to be distinguished from oral Kaposi's sarcoma by tests of haemostasis and if necessary, biopsy.

Drug-associated purpura

Many drugs, particularly aspirin, interfere with platelet function (Table 23.4). Others act as haptens and cause immune destruction of platelets or suppress marrow function causing pancytopenia (aplastic anaemia) of which purpura is typically an early sign. The most frequent cause of aplastic anaemia in Britain has been phenylbutazone.

If purpura develops, the drug should be stopped, but in the case of aplastic anaemia the process may be irreversible and fatal.

Table 23.4 Important causes of drug-associated thrombocytopenia

- Chloramphenicol
- Phenylbutazone
- Indomethacin
- Thiazide diuretics
- Quinine and quinidine

Localised oral purpura

Blood blisters occasionally appear in the oral mucosa after minor or unnoticed trauma, but there is no systemic haemostatic defect. Such blisters may form in the throat and cause a choking sensation ('angina bullosa haemorrhagica'). Rupture of a blood blister leaves an ulcer (Figs 23.3–23.5).

Systemic purpura should be excluded by haematological examination, and the patient can be reassured.

von Willebrand's disease

Von Willebrand's disease is characterised both by a prolonged bleeding time and deficiency of factor VIII. It is usually inherited as an autosomal dominant — both males and females are therefore affected.

The deficiency of factor VIII is usually mild compared with the platelet defect, so that purpura is the more common manifestation. However, some patients have factor VIII levels low enough to cause a significant clotting defect. The platelet defect is usually correctable with desmopressin, which may also be

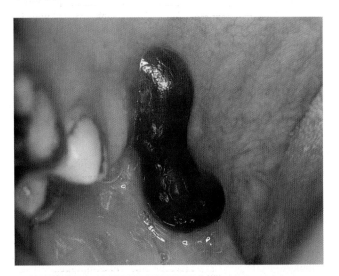

Fig. 23.3 Localised oral purpura. An intact blood blister on the soft palate and fauces.

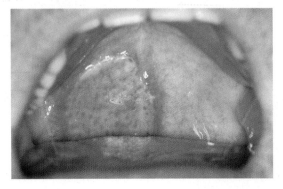

Fig. 23.4 Localised oral purpura. A ruptured blood blister has formed a large ulcer on the soft palate

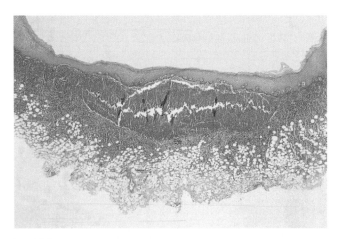

Fig. 23.5 Localised oral purpura. A blood-filled space lies immediately below the epithelium in this intact bulla.

sufficient to correct any significant factor VIII deficiency. In unusually severe cases the deficiency of factor VIII is such that surgery has to be managed as for haemophilia A. However, factor VIII remains active in the blood for a considerably longer period.

CLOTTING DISORDERS

Important causes are shown in Table 23.5.

Table 23.5 Important causes of coagulation defects

- Heritable deficiencies of plasma factors
  Haemophilia A (far the most important cause)
  Haemophilia B
  von Willebrand's disease with low factor VIII levels
- Acquired clotting defects
  Vitamin K deficiency
  Anticoagulant treatment
  Liver disease

Haemophilia A

Haemophilia is the most common and severe clotting disorder. Haemophilia A (factor VIII deficiency) affects approximately 6 per 100 000 of the population and is about 10 times as common as haemophilia B (Christmas disease, factor IX deficiency). In the past, extractions in haemophiliacs have been fatal, and extractions are still common emergencies or occasions when haemophiliacs need specific treatment.

Severe haemophilia typically causes effects in childhood, usually as a result of bleeding into muscles or joints after minor injuries. By contrast, mild haemophilia (factor VIII level over 25%) may cause no symptoms until an injury, surgery or a dental extraction precipitates prolonged bleeding. This may not happen until adult life. Severe and prolonged bleeding deeply into the

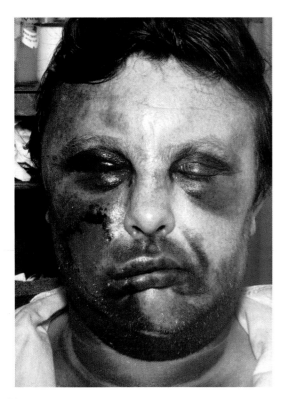

Fig. 23.6 Haemophilia. This was a mild and unsuspected haemophiliac who had never had any previous serious bleeding episodes. This enormous haematoma developed after a submucous injection for extirpation of an incisor pulp. (By kind permission of Mr A J Bridge.)

soft tissues can also follow local anaesthetic injections. Inferior dental blocks are most dangerous because of the rich plexus of veins in this area from which blood can leak down to the glottis. Even a submucous infiltration can occasionally have severe consequences (Fig. 23.6).

Clinical features

As mentioned earlier, a positive family history is always significant. However, over 30% of haemophiliacs have a negative family history, and occasionally haemophilia is discovered only as a result of postextraction haemorrhage. By contrast, it is certain that a patient who has had extractions or tonsillectomy without serious bleeding is not haemophiliac.

Typically, bleeding starts after a short delay as a result of normal platelet and vascular responses which provide the initial phase of haemostasis. There is then persistent bleeding which, if untreated, can continue for weeks or until the patient dies. Pressure packs, suturing, or local application of haemostatics are ineffective.

Haemarthroses are a well-recognised complication of uncontrolled haemophilia, but most dangerous is intracranial haemorrhage. Deep tissue bleeding can also occasionally spread down from the neck and obstruct the airway. Many haemophiliacs are carriers of HBV, HCV or HIV infection as a result of having received untreated blood products. Formation of antibodies to factor VIII is another complication.

Table 23.6 Principles of dental management of haemophilia

- History
- Laboratory findings (see also Table 23.2)
  Prolonged activated partial thromboplastin time
  Normal prothrombin time
  Normal bleeding time
  Low factor VIII levels
- Regular meticulous dental care to avoid the need for extractions
- Preoperative planning of unavoidable extractions or other surgery
- Preoperative replacement therapy
- Postoperative precautions

Principles of management (Table 23.6)

Before surgery, radiographs should be taken to forestall any complications resulting from unsuspected disease and to decide whether any other extractions are necessary. Arrangements must usually be made for admission to hospital. The number of occasions when replacement therapy has to be given should be kept to a minimum. When replacement therapy has been given, as much surgical work as possible should be done in that session. It is always wise to plan treatment with the possibility in mind that the next time the patient needs surgery may be in a place where replacement therapy is unobtainable or the patient may have developed antibodies to factor VIII.

A factor VIII level between 50% and 75% is necessary for dental extractions, and factor VIII requirement depends on the serum level and the expected severity of the surgical trauma. It is usual also to give tranexamic acid or desmopressin to reduce the amount of factor VIII needed.

Postoperatively, an antibiotic such as oral penicillin (250 mg four times a day for 7 days) is usually given to reduce the chance of wound infection and secondary haemorrhage. The risks of bleeding are greatest on the day of operation and again from 4 to 10 days postoperatively. If bleeding starts at any time after the operation, factor VIII must be given or may be given prophylactically on the fourth or fifth postoperative day. Administration of tranexamic acid is usually continued for 10 days. Aspirin and related analgesics should be avoided.

For routine dentistry, relative analgesia is preferable for sedation, to avoid the risk from accidental damage to a vein. Now that haemophiliacs *should* have a personal stock of factor VIII for use in emergencies, these problems have greatly declined. However, it may be necessary to check that the factor VIII has been taken.

Extractions in mild haemophilia may be managed by giving antifibrinolytic drugs, particularly tranexamic acid or desmopressin rather than factor VIII. For those with antibodies to factor VIII, Factor VIII inhibitor bypassing fraction may be given.

Christmas disease (haemophilia B)

Christmas disease is inherited in the same way as, and is clinically identical to, haemophilia A. However, factor IX is more stable than factor VIII. Dried factor IX fraction is given for replacement.

Factor IX remains active in the blood for more than 2 days, so that replacement therapy can be given at longer intervals than for haemophilia A. All other aspects of management haemophilia A and B are the same.

Acquired clotting defects

Overall, these are more common than the inherited defects (Table 23.7).

Table 23.7 Important acquired clotting disorders
● Vitamin K deficiency ● Anticoagulants ● Liver disease

Vitamin K deficiency

Causes include obstructive jaundice, or, less commonly, malabsorption. Important causes of obstructive jaundice are hepatitis, gall stones and carcinoma of the pancreas.

Extractions or other surgery should preferably be delayed until haemostasis recovers. In an emergency, vitamin K can be given, preferably by mouth, and its effectiveness checked by the prothrombin time. If the latter does not return to normal within 48 hours there is probably parenchymal liver disease.

Anticoagulant treatment

Coumarin anticoagulants, particularly warfarin, are used for thromboembolic disease, which can complicate atrial fibrillation or insertion of prosthetic heart valves. The underlying condition may therefore influence dental management more than the treatment. Anticoagulation should be checked regularly to maintain the prothrombin time. This is reported as the INR (international normalised ratio), at 2–3 in most cases but at 3–4.5 for those with prosthetic valves. Dental extractions can usually be carried out safely with an INR of 2–3 but the INR, alone, is not a completely reliable guide to haemostatic function.

As a precaution, only a few teeth should be extracted at one session, trauma should be minimal, and the sockets can be sutured over a layer of oxidised cellulose. Because of the risk of rebound thrombosis, anticoagulation should not be stopped. For more major surgery, anticoagulant treatment may have to be stopped if the physician agrees. If serious bleeding starts, tranexamic acid can be given, but, if otherwise uncontrollable, vitamin K may be needed.

Short-term anticoagulation with heparin is given before renal dialysis. Heparin is effective only for about 6 hours. Extractions or surgery can therefore be delayed for 12–24 hours after the last dose of heparin, when the benefits of dialysis are also maximal.

Liver disease

Haemorrhagic tendencies can result either from obstructive jaundice (infective hepatitis also has an obstructive component) or from extensive liver damage. In obstructive jaundice, vitamin K absorption may be severely impaired. Viral hepatitis or alcoholism are important causes of liver failure which results in inability to metabolise vitamin K and to produce most clotting factors. Haemorrhage can be severe and difficult to control. In mild liver disease, vitamin K may be effective. In more severe cases it is valueless, but tranexamic acid and fresh plasma infusions may control bleeding.

MANAGEMENT OF PROLONGED DENTAL BLEEDING

Patients returning with prolonged bleeding from an extraction socket are a relatively common problem. It is not usually a real emergency, except in so far as the patient and friends or relatives are alarmed. Only a little blood diluted with saliva can give the impression of significant blood loss.

The essential measures are to reassure the patient and accompanying persons, who should be coaxed out of the surgery. The patient should then be given a local anaesthetic and the mouth cleaned up to identify the source of bleeding. Any rough edges of the socket should be tidied up, the margins squeezed together and the soft tissue margins neatly sutured over it. A small piece of Surgicel or fibrin gauze can be put in the socket mouth beforehand, but suturing is the essential measure.

When all is calm, enquiry should be made into any family history of bleeding tendencies, or any other cause of haemorrhagic disease as discussed earlier.

The patient should be kept under observation to make sure that bleeding has been completely controlled. But continued oozing of blood from beneath the sutured tissues suggests some haemorrhagic disease and this, or a family history of this, are indications for referring the patient to hospital, as prolonged dental bleeding is a recognised way in which haemophilia is sometimes first recognised.

CHAPTER 23

SUGGESTED FURTHER READING

Ascher L F, Ord R A 1992 Pseudothrombocytopenia in maxillofacial surgery patients: a report of two cases. J Oral Maxillofac Surg 50:1108–1110

Association of Haemophilia Clinic Directors of Canada 1995 Haemophilia and von Willebrand's disease: 2. Management. Can Med Ass J 153:147–157

Beatty C 1995 The patient with easy bruising and bleeding. Medicine UK 23:514–517

Capitano A M, Sacco R, Mannucci P M 1991 Pseudopathologies of haemostasis and dental surgery. Oral Surg Oral Med Oral Pathol 71:184–186

Chesterman C N, Chong B H 1995 Acquired haemostatic failure. Medicine UK 23:518–524

Durham T M, Hodges E D, Harper J et al 1993 Management of traumatic oral-facial traumatic injury in the hemophiliac patient with inhibitor. Pediatr Dent 15:282–287

Giles A R, Lillicrap D P 1995 Haemophilia A and related disorders. Medicine Int 23:525–530

Lethagen S R 1995 Pathogenesis, clinical picture and treatment of von Willbrand's disease. Annals Med 27:641–651

Ludlam C A, Steel C M 1993 Haemostasis: von Willebrand's variants. Lancet 341:997

Manabe M, Tsujimaki M, Kakuta S, Nagumo M 1993 Acquired factor X deficiency: an experience with multiple tooth extraction. J Oral Maxillofac Surg 51:922–924

Marshall D A S, Berry C, Brewer A 1993 Fatal disseminated intravascular coagulation complicating dental extraction. Br J Oral Maxillofac Surg 31:178–179

McLaughlin P, Chen S, Phillips J G 1994 Disseminated intravascular coagulation presenting as perioral haemorrhage. Br J Oral Maxillofac Surg 32:94–95

Morrison A E, Ludlam C A 1994 Acquired haemophilia and its management. Br J Haematol 89:231–236

Rakocz M, Mazar A, Varon D et al 1993 Dental extractions with bleeding disorders: the use of fibrin glue. Oral Surg Oral Med Oral Pathol 75:280–282

Saulnier J, Marey A, Horellou M-H et al 1994 Evaluation of desmopressin for dental extractions in patients with haemostatic disorders. Oral Surg Oral Med Oral Pathol 77:6–12

Steinberg M J, Moores J F 1995 Use of INR to assess degree of anticoagulation in patients who have dental procedures. Oral Surg Oral Med Oral Pathol Oral Radiol Endod 80:175–177

Todd D, Galbraith D 1993 Management of an orthognathic surgery patient with factor XI deficiency: review and case report. J Oral Maxillofac Surg 51:417–420

Wahl M J, Howell J 1996 Altering anticoagulant therapy: a survey of physicians. JADA 127:625–638

Wood G D, Deeble T 1993 Warfarin: dangers with antibiotics. Dent Update October:350–353

Immunodeficiencies and HIV disease

Immune deficiencies can be primary or acquired (Table 24.1) and affect B or T lymphocytes, or both. T lymphocytes regulate B lymphocyte activity; T cell defects may therefore impair antibody production as well as cell-mediated immunity. There can also be failures of production of individual immunoglobulins such as IgA, or of complement components.

Table 24.1 Important causes of immunodeficiency

- Primary (genetic)
    T or B lymphocyte defects (Swiss type agammaglobulinaemia, Di George's syndrome, etc.)
    IgA deficiency
    Complement component deficiencies
    Down's syndrome (multiple defects)
- Secondary (acquired)
    Infections (HIV, other severe viral or bacterial infections, malaria, etc.)
    Drug-induced (immunosuppressive and anticancer treatment)
    Malnutrition (worldwide a major cause)
    Cancer (particularly lymphoreticular)
    Diabetes mellitus

Any patient who develops recurrent infections, particularly if they respond poorly to treatment or are caused by otherwise harmless microbes (opportunistic infections), is likely to be immunodeficient (Fig. 24.1).

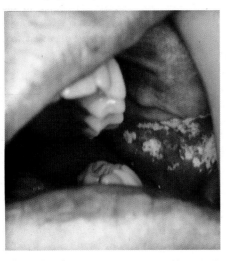

Fig. 24.1 White patches of thrush and erythema in a patient on long-term immunosuppressive treatment.

The main causes of *severe* immunodeficiency are HIV infection and immunosuppressive treatment, particularly for organ transplants. Many cancer patients are also severely immunodeficient as a result of both the neoplasm and cytotoxic drugs used for treatment. The severe primary immunodeficiencies are rare and, unless a marrow transplant can be given, are usually fatal in childhood.

Oral manifestations of immunodeficiencies

The main effect, as mentioned earlier, is abnormal susceptibility to infections, particularly candidosis or viral infections such as herpes zoster as in AIDS (see below).

SELECTIVE IgA DEFICIENCY

Selective IgA deficiency is common and potentially relevant for the mouth, as IgA is the only immunoglobulin secreted in the saliva. Selective IgA deficiency may affect about 1 in 600 of the population and has varied possible effects (Table 24.2).

Table 24.2 Possible effects of selective IgA deficiency

- Normal health
- Enhanced susceptibility especially to respiratory tract infections
- Atopic disease
- Connective tissue disease, especially lupus erythematosus

Susceptibility to oral infections

Evidence regarding the effect of IgA deficiency on dental caries and periodontal disease is conflicting. Both high and low prevalences of dental caries have been reported. Compensatory secretion of other immunoglobulins into the mouth may explain these variable findings. Gingivitis may be less severe than normal, but even this may be the result of antibiotic treatment for respiratory infections. There is no clear evidence of any significant association between oral mucosal infection and IgA deficiency.

Atopic disease. IgA deficiency may facilitate absorption of allergens. Asthma, eczema or any of the related diseases may be the first sign. However, this has no oral effects unless allergic angio-oedema involves the floor of mouth or lips.

C1 ESTERASE INHIBITOR DEFICIENCY

The familial form of this disease, *hereditary angio-oedema*, is, pedantically speaking, an immunodeficiency but there is no abnormal susceptibility to infection. There is also a rare acquired type associated mainly with lymphoproliferative diseases. They are discussed in Chapter 25, together with allergic angio-oedema, which it simulates clinically.

BONE MARROW TRANSPLANTATION

Bone marrow transplantation is used, if suitable donors can be found, for such conditions as some severe primary immuno-deficiency diseases, some leukaemias, aplastic anaemia, and some lymphomas and other neoplasms. Preoperatively, total immunosuppression by cytotoxic chemotherapy and, sometimes, total body irradiation is required to prevent graft rejection.

Oral sources of infection should be eliminated and the mouth brought to as near perfect health as possible. Elimination of oral infection (particularly periodontal disease) has a significant effect on lessening post-transplant complications and also lessens the need for dental treatment during the difficult post-transplant period.

Possible complications after transplantation are numerous (Table 24.3), particularly during the initial intensive phase of immunosuppression.

Table 24.3 **Possible complications of bone marrow transplantation**

- Oral complications
  Mucositis, mucosal ulceration, infections, haemorrhage, dry mouth, parotitis
  Gingival hyperplasia if cyclosporin is used
  In children, dental hypoplastic defects may develop
- Graft-versus-host disease
- Systemic infections (sometimes by oral bacteria). These are the chief cause of death

---

Graft-versus-host disease

This results from an attack on an immunosuppressed host by transplanted immunocompetent cells. It is, in effect, a graft rejection reaction in reverse. It most frequently follows bone marrow transplantation both because of the deep immuno-suppression and because of the many immunologically active cells in the implanted marrow.

The oral effects of graft-versus-host disease are lichen planus, a Sjögren-like syndrome with xerostomia, and a condition resembling systemic sclerosis (Ch. 23) with limited oral opening.

Graft-versus-host disease can be acute and self-limiting or responsive to treatment, or chronic. The last is the chief cause of morbidity and mortality.

Post-transplant management

The main considerations are maintenance of meticulous oral hygiene, use of fluorides to control caries, and prompt treatment of any infections that develop.

In successful cases, deep immunosuppression is maintained for up to a year post-transplantation. The implanted marrow then takes over normal haematological and immune functions. Any oral surgery should preferably be postponed until this happens.

OTHER ORGAN TRANSPLANTS

Transplantation of other organs, most frequently kidneys, is associated with similar complications to those of bone marrow transplantation. The main differences are that immunosuppression is less complete but has to be maintained indefinitely.

The chief problems are therefore the enhanced susceptibility to infections and the greater risk of lymphomas. Gingival hyperplasia due to cyclosporin may be difficult to control and can lead to accelerated periodontal destruction.

THE ACQUIRED IMMUNE DEFICIENCY SYNDROME (AIDS)

A great variety of oral diseases can arise in the acquired immune deficiency syndrome (see Table 24.6). They sometimes form the first sign of the disease and some of them herald rapid deterioration and sometimes, early death.

HIV disease has spread worldwide and is epidemic in parts of the USA and, particularly, Africa. As of December 2000, more than 36 million adults, worldwide, are estimated to be infected, and nearly 22 million people have died from AIDS. The pandemic is most severe in sub-Saharan Africa where 25 million adults, approximately 9% of the population, are infected.

By June 1994 more than 22 000 cases of HIV infection, and over 14 000 deaths from AIDS had been reported in Britain, despite the fact that the infection rate is the lowest in Europe. By contrast, cases have risen to 700 000, a jump of nearly 70% in one year, in the former Soviet Union, where it is predicted that one million Russions will have become infected within two or three years.

AIDS is transmissible to health care personnel, particularly surgeons, dental surgeons and nurses, via needles or other sharp instruments. However, the risk of acquiring HIV infection by such means is considerably smaller than that of hepatitis B.

Aetiology

AIDS is caused by a retrovirus, the human immunodeficiency virus (HIV), mainly HIV-1. HIV-2 is as yet only widely prevalent in West Africa.

The chief mode of transmission is by men who have sex with men; these account for over 70% of cases in Britain. Intravenous drug abusers are also a high-risk group. Heterosexual transmission is far less common in the Western World than in Africa. Nevertheless as a result of spread of the virus in the population, heterosexual transmission has become more frequent. In some cases this is the result of women coming from, or who have acquired the infection in, high-risk areas. Also, it appears that an unexpectedly high proportion of women indulge in, or submit to, anal intercourse. Once infected, pregnant women can transmit the infection to the fetus. Many haemophiliacs have acquired the disease from infected blood products but heat-treatment of clotting factor concentrates should have eliminated this risk.

The incubation period of AIDS is highly variable. In men who have sex with men, it averages approximately 5 years, but is sometimes as long as 10 years. Testing of infected persons also shows deterioration of immune function long before clinically apparent disease and it is still not clear whether all those who have become infected will develop the full, lethal syndrome.

In 5–15% of cases, HIV infection shows no clinical progress for periods up to 10 years, possibly because of variations in pathogenicity of HIV strains, or stronger host immune responses.

Immunology

The human immunodeficiency virus directly infects lymphocytes and other cells, such as some macrophages, which carry the CD4 marker. However, the virus appears only to be able to fuse with and enter CD4 cells as a result of interaction between the gp120 envelope proteins and a CD4 binding site by means of a family of co-receptors. The virus kills T helper (CD4) cells and reverses the ratio of helper to suppressor lymphocytes.

Antibody is produced in response to the virus but is not protective. Antibodies to HIV indicate only that infection has been acquired and all seropositive persons must be assumed to be capable of transmitting it. Detection of these antibodies is often misnamed 'the AIDS test', but it cannot predict the development of symptomatic disease. It has been useful for detecting HIV-infected persons, particularly among blood donors.

Detection of viral antigens, such as p24 protein, in the blood provides a more direct and reliable indicator of infection. HIV DNA can be quantified, and several commercial assays are available. These may use such methods as reverse transcription

polymerase chain reaction analysis. Haematological markers indicating progression to AIDS, include viral antigens in the serum, high beta-2 microglobulin levels and failure of or greatly depressed antigen-induced interferon gamma production. T helper (CD4) lymphocytes counts of less than 0.2×10^9/L or a total lymphocyte count of less than 1×10^9/L represent advanced disease.

Clinical indicators of a poor prognosis are oral thrush, herpes zoster or other persistent or recurrent infections, hairy leukoplakia, unexplained constitutional symptoms, cutaneous anergy and lymphadenopathy. Approximately 20–70% of such patients can be expected to deteriorate within less than 5 years.

The main effect of depletion of T helper cells is deepening depression of cell-mediated immunity. Thus there are declining responses of lymphocytes to antigens in vitro, and impaired or absent delayed hypersensitivity responses, long before any clinical signs of the disease appear. Apparently paradoxically, there is also polyclonal B lymphocyte activation resulting in hypergammaglobulinaemia and autoantibody production. The main effect of the immunodeficiency and chief cause of death is infection by a great variety of microbes.

The human immunodeficiency virus also attacks the central nervous system, cells of which carry receptors for the virus.

Clinical aspects

Possible major events after infection by HIV are shown in Figure 24.2 but, as mentioned earlier, it is still uncertain whether any symptomless carriers will ultimately remain healthy.

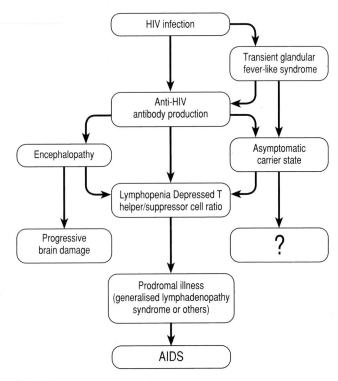

Fig. 24.2 Outcomes of HIV infection. The fate of currently asymptomatic carriers is unknown.

Usually there is a latent period for several years before signs of immunodeficiency appear. Within 10 years, approximately 50% of infected persons will probably have developed AIDS and the remainder will usually have prodromal disease or laboratory markers of immune deficiency. Severe infectious complications are to be expected and are usually the chief cause of death.

The earliest clinical manifestation of HIV infection can be a transient illness resembling glandular fever, associated with antibody production. Thereafter, in progressive cases, markers of declining cell-mediated immunity eventually become detectable and, later, various clinical syndromes.

Generalised lymphadenopathy syndrome (GLS), with widespread persistent enlargement of lymph nodes, is a typical early sign. However, the course of AIDS is highly variable and none of the prodromal symptoms appear to be inevitable.

The full syndrome of AIDS is characterised by multiple infections by bacteria, fungi, parasites and viruses. Many of these infections, such as *Pneumocystis carinii* pneumonia, are opportunistic and almost unknown in immunocompetent persons.

Though infections are the main cause of death, there is also a greatly raised incidence of tumours, particularly Kaposi's sarcoma and lymphomas, which frequently affect the oral or perioral tissues. In normal persons these tumours are not merely uncommon or rare, but particularly rare in the mouth.

Sometimes the first clinical sign of AIDS can be *Pneumocystis carinii* pneumonia or Kaposi's sarcoma.

Neuropsychiatric disease in AIDS can range from depression, to dementia and death. Opportunistic infections or tumours can also involve the central nervous system. These neurological disorders may be associated with, but can develop in the absence of, immunodeficiency.

A lesser manifestation of AIDS in some patients is autoimmune disease, particularly, thrombocytopenic purpura or less frequently a lupus erythematosus-like disease.

Once AIDS has developed, the outcome is usually fatal within 2–3 years, though the course of the disease can be modified by highly active antiretroviral therapy (HAART).

In the terminal stages of AIDS, the patient may be emaciated, with persistent diarrhoea, suffering a multiplicity of infections, disfigured by skin disease, breathless from *Pneumocystis carinii* pneumonia, frequently with a malignant tumour, and sometimes also blind and demented.

HIV assessment and staging

Staging of HIV infection is important for selecting patients for treatment and assessing prognosis, and for epidemiological studies. The Centers for Disease Control/World Health Organization classification (Table 24.4) takes both clinical and laboratory findings into account.

General aspects of dental management

The possibility of transmitting HIV infection during dental treatment inevitably causes anxiety but the risk is considerably

Table 24.4 CDC definition of AIDS in patients with laboratory evidence of HIV

A definite diagnosis of:
1. Bacterial infections, multiple or recurrent in a child < 13 years
2. Disseminated coccidioidomycosis
3. HIV encephalopathy (HIV dementia or subacute encephalitis)
4. Disseminated histoplasmosis
5. Isosporiasis with diarrhoea for > 1 month
6. Kaposi's sarcoma
7. Lymphoma of the brain (primary)
8. Non-Hodgkin's lymphoma of B cell or unknown immunological phenotype and one of several specified types
9. Disseminated mycobacterial disease (other than *Mycobacterium tuberculosis*)
10. Extrapulmonary *Mycobacterium tuberculosis* involving at least one site outside the lungs
11. Recurrent *Salmonella* (non-typhoid) septicaemia
12. HIV wasting syndrome

Or a presumptive diagnosis of:
1. Candidosis of the oesophagus
2. Cytomegalovirus retinitis with loss of vision
3. Kaposi's sarcoma
4. Lymphoid interstitial pneumonia and/or pulmonary lymphoid hyperplasia in a child ≤ 13 years of age
5. Disseminated mycobacterial disease
6. *Pneumocystis carinii* pneumonia
7. Toxoplasmosis of the brain in a patient ≥ 1 month of age

The following conditions, in the presence of HIV infection, have been added to the definition of AIDS:
1. Cervical cancer
2. Two episodes of bacterial pneumonia in 12 months
3. Pulmonary tuberculosis

CDC/WHO laboratory classification of HIV infection

CD4 cells/μl	or Total lymphocyte count/μl	Clinical Category A	B	C
[1] > 500	> 2000	A1	B1	C1
[2] 200–499	1000–1999	A2	B2	C2
[3] < 0.2	< 1000	A3	B3	C3

lower than that of acquiring viral hepatitis. Oral infections and other features of AIDS or its prodromes may enable patients to be recognised. A young adult male who develops thrush for no apparent reason is likely to have HIV disease, but if he has oral Kaposi's sarcoma, it is virtually pathognomonic. However, there are many more patients with nothing to suggest that they are infective. At the time of writing there are tens of thousands of antibody-positive, potentially infective persons in Britain, and the number rises each month.

Highly active antiretroviral therapy

The prognosis for AIDS has greatly improved with the introduction of highly active antiretroviral therapy (HAART). The latter is the term given to the use of combinations of antiretroviral drugs, such as two nucleoside reverse transcriptase inhibitors (nRTIs) plus one or two protease inhibitors, or two nRTIs plus non-nucleoside transcriptase inhibitor. All these drugs are capable of causing a wide variety of adverse effects and compliance may be unpredictable. Some important oral adverse effects from the drugs mentioned in Table 24.5 are indicated in brackets.

Table 24.5 Antiretroviral drugs used for HAART

- Nucleoside reverse transcriptase inhibitors
  Abacavir (Stevens–Johnson syndrome)
  Didanosine (dry mouth)
  Zalcitabine (oral ulcers)
  Stavudine
  Lamivudine
  Zidovudine
- Non-nucleoside reverse transcriptase inhibitors
  Nevirapine (Stevens–Johnson syndrome)
  Efavirenz (Stevens–Johnson syndrome)
- Protease inhibitors
  Indinavir (dry mouth, taste disturbance)
  Nelfinavir
  Ritonavir (taste disturbance, circumoral paraesthesia)
  Saquinavir (oral ulceration)

However, new drugs are constantly being introduced and it is not yet clear whether one combination of these drugs is more effective than another.

The benefits of highly active antiretroviral therapy are that levels of cirulating virions may be lowered to undetectable levels and that variable levels of immune recovery may be evident. The result can be a striking fall in the incidence of opportunistic infections and regression of Kaposi's sarcoma. CMV retinitis (causing blindness) has hitherto resisted treatment, but has responded well to HAART. In Britain the mortality from AIDS has fallen by more than 40% since 1996.

A controversial issue in the application of HAART is whether treatment should start early or late after acquisition of HIV infection. In the UK, to minimise toxic effects in longer-term treatment, unlike the US and most of Europe, the policy has been to delay treatment until after the CD4 count falls below 350 cells/mm^3, in an attempt also to delay the rising tide of drug-resistance due to long-term treatment. However, administration of HAART within 180 days of infection raises levels of HIV-specific CD4 cells, and patients can stop treatment for up to a year and still suppress HIV levels in the blood.

Despite initial optimism, the long-term toxicity of these regimens is as yet unknown, compliance may be difficult to maintain and their cost is such that they are available only in more affluent communities.

Worse is the finding that even the most vigorous of such treatments does not completely control HIV replication, even when there is a clear decline in morbidity and mortality. It is estimated that HAART fails in up to 50% of recipients each year, partly at least due to poor compliance with this demanding form of treatment.

Other problems are that resistance to HAART is developing and there has been a considerable rise in new cases of multidrug-resistant HIV over the past 5 years. One consequence is that patients receiving HAART may feel that they

are non-infective and transmit the disease to others. There are also as yet inaccessible reservoirs of infection. The latter are mainly inactive B-cells which contain dormant HIV DNA. Key features of AIDS are summarised in Table 24.6.

Table 24.6 AIDS: key features

- Caused by a retrovirus — usually HIV-1
- Transmitted sexually or by intravenous drug abuse, and by blood or blood products
- Progressive deterioration mainly of cell-mediated immunity
- Immunodeficiency leads to opportunistic infections such as *Pneumocystis carinii* pneumonia
- Common oral lesions include candidosis and hairy leukoplakia
- Greatly increased frequency of Kaposi's sarcoma and lymphomas, often in oral regions
- Neurological and psychological disorders may be associated
- Deaths mainly due to opportunistic infections

ORAL LESIONS IN HIV DISEASE

More than 75% of patients with AIDS have orofacial disease (Table 24.7). Before the introduction of HAART, among 2235 HIV-positive, homosexual or bisexual men in San Francisco, the most frequent oral lesions were hairy leukoplakia (18.7%), thrush (6.6%) or erythematous candidosis (2.1%), Kaposi's sarcoma (1.6%) and oral ulcers (2%). However, the frequency of such lesions varies in other groups. Kaposi's sarcoma and hairy leukoplakia, for example, are disproportionately frequent in men who have sex with men.

With the use of HAART, the frequency of HIV-related oral lesions is declining.

Oral candidosis

Oral thrush or other forms of candidosis may be seen in over 70% of patients at some stage. It indicates declining immunity and that other infections may be associated or are likely to follow. Approximately 50% of patients with HIV-associated thrush are likely to develop AIDS within 5 years.

Most other types of candidosis, such as angular stomatitis, palatal erythema or hyperplastic candidosis, may also be seen in AIDS patients (Fig. 24.3).

Viral mucosal infections

Herpetic stomatitis is less common than might be expected but can cause atypical or chronic ulceration (Fig. 24.4). Severe orofacial zoster may indicate a poor prognosis.

Cytomegalovirus can be found in some oral ulcers and the Epstein–Barr virus is the cause of hairy leukoplakia.

Papillomaviruses have been isolated from proliferative lesions, such as verruca vulgaris, condyloma acuminatum and focal epithelial hyperplasia.

Table 24.7 Oral disease in HIV infection

More common diseases	Less common

Infections
● Fungal
   Thrush and other forms of
   candidosis
 	
● Viral
   Herpes simplex
   Varicella zoster
   EB virus, including hairy
   leukoplakia
● Bacterial
   HIV-associated gingivitis
   and periodontitis
   Necrotising gingivitis
	Infections
	● Deep mycoses
	   Cryptococcosis
	   Histoplasmosis
	   Aspergillosis
	   Geotrichosis
	● Viral
	   Human papilloma virus
	   Cytomegalovirus
	
	● Bacterial
	   M. tuberculosis and
	   non-tuberculous ('atypical')
	   mycobacterioses
	   Klebsiella pneumonia
	   S. enteritidis, E. coli and
	   E. cloacae infections
	   Sinusitis
	   Exacerbations of apical
	   periodontitis
	   Submandibular cellulitis

Tumours
Kaposi's sarcoma
 	
Lymphadenopathy
	● *Tumours*
	   Non-Hodgkin lymphoma
	   (squamous cell carcinoma)
	● *Neurological disease*
	   Paraesthesiae
	   Hyperaesthesia
	   Facial palsy
	   Dysphagia
	● *Miscellaneous*
	   Recurrent aphthae
	   Progressive necrotising
	   ulceration
	   Delayed wound healing
	   Purpura
	   Pigmentation

Bacterial infections

Infections by bacteria which rarely involve the oral tissues, such as *Klebsiella pneumoniae, Enterobacter cloacae*, and *Escherichia coli*, can develop. In the later stages, there may be oral lesions secondary to systemic infections, particularly mycobacterial ulcers.

Bacillary angiomatosis

Bacillary angiomatosis is a vascular proliferative disease caused by *Bartonella henselae* and should respond to antimicrobial therapy. However, it can mimic Kaposi's sarcoma clinically and, to some extent, histologically. It affects the skin more frequently than the oral cavity. Biopsy is essential to exclude Kaposi's sarcoma.

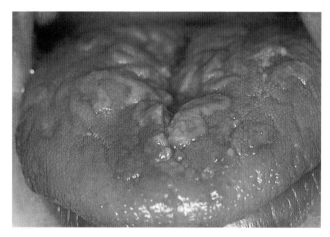

Fig. 24.4 Herpes simplex ulceration in immunodeficiency. There is extensive ulceration along the midline of the dorsal tongue and separate ulcers towards the lateral margins. In immunodeficiency the ulcers may be chronic and their clinical appearance may not suggest viral infection. Biopsy may be required for diagnosis.

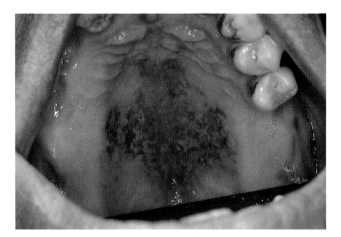

Fig. 24.3 Erythematous candidosis. An extensive red patch on the palate without white flecks which appears as denture stomatitis but without any denture being worn. Such a presentation is characteristic of immunodeficiency.

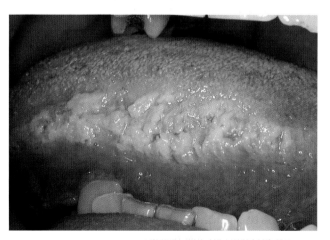

Fig. 24.5 Hairy leukoplakia. Close-up view shows the corrugated surface and suggests the soft texture of the lesion.

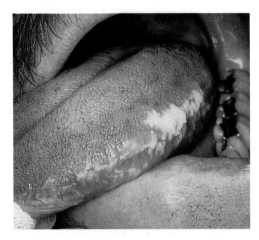

Fig. 24.6 Hairy leukoplakia. The characteristic appearance on the lateral margin of the tongue. Posteriorly the vertical ridging pattern of the lateral tongue is enhanced. (By kind permission of Professor W H Binnie.)

Systemic mycoses

Histoplasmosis or cryptococcosis can give rise to proliferative or ulcerative lesions.

Hairy leukoplakis

Hairy leukoplakia is highly characteristic of HIV infection (Ch. 15) (Figs 24.5 and 24.6).

Tumours

Nearly 50% of patients with AIDS have a malignant tumour at the time of presentation. By far the most frequent are Kaposi's sarcoma and non-Hodgkin lymphomas. Unlike non-AIDS patients, these tumours are particularly frequent in the head and neck region.

Among patients with AIDS, Kaposi's sarcoma is mainly seen in men who have sex with men, and in some areas of the US, for example, it has become the most common malignant tumour of the oral cavity. It is also very occasionally seen in HIV-negative immunosuppressed organ transplant patients.

Kaposi's sarcoma in the mouth, particularly in a young male who is not receiving immunosuppressive treatment, is virtually pathognomonic of AIDS. It is usually associated with a CD4 lymphocyte count of less than $200/\mu L$ and frequently associated with other effects of HIV infection such as candidosis, hairy leukoplakia or HIV-associated gingivitis. Though oral Kaposi's sarcoma may be the cause of early symptoms, the tumour is usually multifocal, with lesions affecting skin, lymph nodes and viscera. At autopsy most organs are frequently found to be involved.

The site may be oropharyngeal, cutaneous or in the cervical lymph nodes. Within the mouth the palate is the most frequent site and the tumour typically produces a flat or nodular purplish lesion. The clinical differential diagnosis is from oral purpura, bacillary angiomatosis and pyogenic granulomas, from which it can be distinguished by biopsy (Ch. 20).

Lymphomas

AIDS-related lymphomas can develop in intraoral sites or salivary glands far more frequently than in HIV-negative persons. Typical sites within the mouth are the palate or gingiva, where the tumours form soft painless swellings which ulcerate when traumatised.

Microscopically, most lymphomas in AIDS are high-grade B-cell lymphomas of large cell or immunoblastic type. EBV is associated in about 50%.

Burkitt's lymphoma is 1000 times more common than in HIV-negative persons in the Western world.

Lymphadenopathy

Lymphadenopathy is characteristic of AIDS and its prodromes. Cervical lymphadenopathy is probably the most common head and neck manifestation of HIV infection.

Microscopy. Typical findings are smaller numbers of T-helper cells in the paracortical region associated with greater numbers of T-suppressor cells there and in the follicles. Follicles may initially be hyperplastic but later undergo involution. The lymph nodes become virtually or entirely functionless.

Enlarged cervical lymph nodes can also be due to lymphomas.

Autoimmune disease

The most common autoimmune phenomenon in AIDS is thrombocytopenic purpura (Fig. 24.7). This can give rise to oral purple patches which may be mistaken for Kaposi's sarcoma, petechiae or blood blisters.

Other autoimmune diseases reported in AIDS are lupus erythematosus and a Sjögren-like salivary gland disease.

Gingivitis and periodontitis

HIV-related periodontal disease includes necrotising gingivitis and accelerated periodontitis (Ch. 5). Necrotising ulcerative

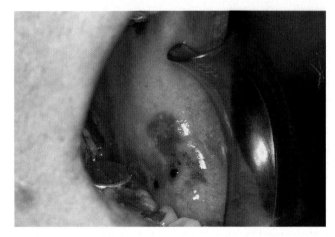

Fig. 24.7 Purpura. Patches such as these in AIDS can be mistaken for Kaposi's sarcoma.

periodontitis (NUP) indicates immunological deterioration and a poor prognosis (Fig. 24.8).

Salivary gland disease

Chronic parotitis, possibly due to Epstein–Barr virus or cytomegalovirus, appears to affect children with AIDS particularly.

A Sjögren-like syndrome with xerostomia, but lacking the characteristic autoantibodies (particularly SS-A and SS-B), can affect adults.

Parotid swellings due to lymphoepithelial lesions are frequently cystic, bilateral and identifiable by CT scanning or ultrasound.

Recognition of parotid cysts or microscopic diagnosis of Sjögren-like changes, particularly in a young adult male, are important indicators of HIV infection of which surgeons should be aware when dealing with a tumour-like lesion of salivary glands.

Miscellaneous oral lesions

Mucosal ulcers. Major aphthae (Fig. 24.9) can be troublesome, interfere with eating and accelerate deterioration of health. They become more frequent and severe with declining immune function. Necrotising oral ulceration of an ill-defined nature and aphthae-like ulcers are common oral signs (Fig. 24.10). In the floor of these ulcers, cytomegalovirus can sometimes be seen.

Oral ulcers associated with HIV infection should always be biopsied as they may be amenable to treatment if specific agents such as herpes virus, cytomegalovirus or mycobacteria

are identified. Major aphthae may respond dramatically to thalidomide but this should only be used when other causes have been excluded.

Oral hyperpigmentation. Occasionally, pigmentation may be secondary to Addison's disease due to fungal destruction of the adrenals. Alternatively, it may be a complication of treatment with zidovudine or due to unknown mechanisms.

Neurological disease

Orofacial effects include facial palsy and trigeminal neuropathy.

Risks of transmission of HIV infection to health care workers

All patients, even if not known to be HIV positive or receiving HAART, must be regarded as potentially infective and treated with full infection control as for hepatitis B. A few nurses and others have become infected as a result of needle-stick injuries

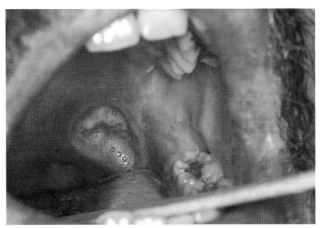

Fig. 24.9 HIV-associated aphthous stomatitis. Major aphthae typically become more frequent and severe as immune function deteriorates, and can add considerably to the patient's disabilitites.

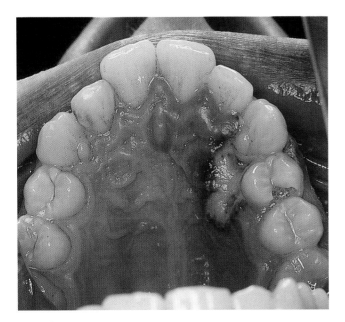

Fig. 24.8 HIV-associated necrotising periodontitis. Soft tissue and bone are lost virtually simultaneously and tissue destruction of the degree shown here can take only a few months. A low CD 4 count and a poor prognosis are typically associated. (By kind permission of Professor W H Binnie.)

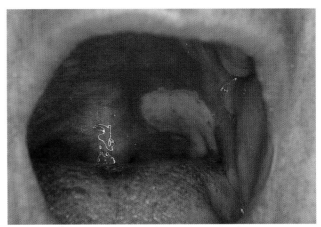

Fig. 24.10 Major aphthous ulcers are a complication of HIV infection and become more frequent and severe as immune function declines.

CHAPTER 24

causing accidental injection of a significant amount of infected blood. By contrast, many other needle-stick injuries where little blood has been transferred have failed to transmit the virus. Most health care workers who have developed AIDS have *not* acquired it as a result of their occupation.

As to the risk to general surgeons, at least two in the Western world are known to have died from the disease, acquired at operation. By contrast only one dental surgeon is known as yet to have acquired the disease occupationally. He was working in New York (by far the highest incidence area in the Western world), did not practice a high standard of infection control and had had many needle-stick injuries. No other dental surgeons, even in high incidence areas, are known to have acquired the disease occupationally.

Infection control, as discussed earlier, and awareness of the patient's low resistance to secondary infection are then major management considerations.

RESTRICTIONS ON TYPE OF WORK THAT MAY BE PERFORMED BY INFECTED DENTAL CLINICIANS

Current regulations require that dental clinicians who have become or think that they have become infected by HIV, hepatitis or other blood-borne viruses should seek counselling and appropriate medical supervision.

If infection is confirmed, changes to clinical practice may mean cessation of work involving exposure-prone procedures. The latter are those where there is a risk of exposing the patient's open tissues to the blood of the worker and include procedures where clinicians' gloved hands may come into contact with sharp instruments or tissues (spicules of bone or teeth) inside patients' open body cavities.

In practice this may mean that infected clinicians may be restricted to carrying out prosthetic dentistry. ?

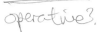

operative?

SUGGESTED FURTHER READING

Barrett A P 1986 Oral complications of bone marrow transplantation. Aust NZ J Med 16:239–240

Berkowitz R J, Strandford S, Jones P et al 1987 Stomatological complications of bone marrow transplantation in a pediatric population. Pediatr Dent 9:105–110

Carpenter C C J, Cooper D A, Fischl M et al 2000 Antiretrovial therapy in adults. Updated recommendations of the International AIDS Society — USA Panel. JAMA 283:381–389

Chaushu G, Itzkovitz-Chaushu S, Yefenof E et al 1995 A longitudinal follow-up of salivary secretion in bone marrow transplant patients. Oral Surg Oral Med Oral Pathol Oral Endod 79:164–169

Dahllof G, Heimdahl A, Modeer T et al 1989 Oral mucous membrane lesions in children treated with bone marrow transplantation. Scand J Dent Res 97:268–277

D'Aquila R, Walker B 1999 Exploring the benefits and limits of highly active antiretroviral therapy. JAMA 282:1668–1669

DeSimone J A, Pomerantz R J, Babinchak T J 2000 Inflammatory reactions in HIV-1 infected persons after initiation of highly active antiretroviral therapy. Ann Intern Med 133:447–454

Grabar S, Le Moing V, Goujard C et al 2000 Clinical outcome of patients with HIV-1 infection according to immunologic and virologic response after 6 months of highly active antiretroviral therapy. Ann Intern Med 133:401–413

Greenberg M S, Dubin G, Steward J C B et al 1995 Relationship of oral disease to the presence of cytomegalovirus DNA in the saliva of AIDS patients. Oral Surg Oral Pathol Oral Radiol Endod 79:175–179

Greenspan D, Greenspan J S 1996 HIV-related oral disease. Lancet 348:729–733

Kline M W 1996 Oral manifestations of pediatric human immunodeficiency virus infection: a review of the literature. Pediatrics 97:380–388

Lin R Y, Goodhart P 1993 The role of oral candidiasis in survival and hospitalization patterns: analysis of an inner city hospital human immunodeficiency virus/acquired immune deficiency registry. Am J Med Sci 305:345–353

Loder N 2000 Drug-resistant HIV shows a worrying increase in the UK. Nature 407:120

Rosen F S, Cooper M D, Wedgwood R J P 1995 The primary immunodeficiencies. N Engl J Med 333:434–440

Schwartzlander B, Garnett G, Walker N et al 2000 AIDS in a new millenium. Science 289:64–67

Scully C, Laskaris G, Pindborg J et al 1991 Oral manifestations of HIV infection and their management. Oral Surg Oral Med Oral Pathol 71:158–171

Silverman S 1996 *Color atlas of oral manifestations of AIDS*, 2nd Edn. Mosby, St Louis

Smaglik P 2000 Reservoirs dog AIDS therapy. Nature 405:270–272

Weinert M, Grimes R M, Lynch D P 1996 Oral manifestations of HIV infection. Ann Intern Med 125:485–496

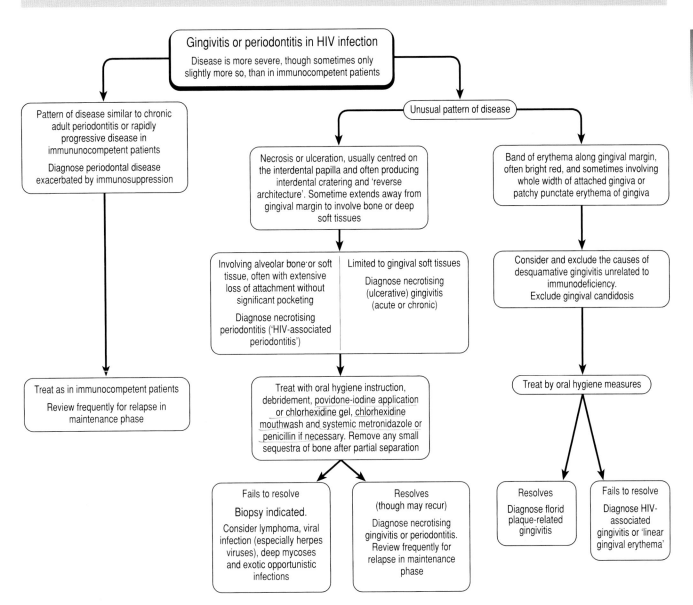

Summary 24.1 Types of gingivitis and periodontitis seen in HIV infection.

CHAPTER
25
Allergy and autoimmune disease

Many endocrine diseases are immunologically mediated and most of the immunologically-mediated diseases have some dental relevance (Table 25.1).

Table 25.1 Aspects of immunologically-mediated diseases affecting dental management

- Systemic effects affecting dental management
- Immunologically-mediated oral diseases
- Risks of abnormal reactions to drugs (e.g. penicillin anaphylaxis)

Immunologically-mediated diseases fall into two main groups (Table 25.2). By far the most common are atopic disease and contact dermatitis, which are abnormal reactions to *exogenous antigens*. The autoimmune diseases, by contrast, are mediated by *antibodies directed against host tissues*.

Table 25.2 Important immunologically-mediated diseases

- Atopic disease and related allergies (reactions to exogenous antigens)
    Asthma; eczema; hay fever; urticaria; food allergies
    Some drug reactions
    Anaphylaxis and acute allergic angio-oedema
    Contact dermatitis
- Autoimmune diseases (reactions to endogenous antigens causing autoantibody production)
- Connective tissue diseases
    Rheumatoid arthritis
    Sjögren's syndromes*
    Lupus erythematosus*
    Systemic sclerosis*
- Autoimmune diseases with specific autoantibodies
    Pernicious anaemia*
    Idiopathic and drug-associated thrombocytopenic purpura*
    Drug-associated leucopenia*
    Autoimmune haemolytic anaemia
    Addison's disease*
    Hypothyroidism (Hashimoto's thyroiditis)
    Hyperthyroidism
    Idiopathic hypoparathyroidism*
    Pemphigus vulgaris*
    Mucous membrane pemphigoid*

*Can give rise to characteristic oral changes

ATOPIC DISEASE

Atopic disease is the common type of allergy and affects approximately 10% of the population. It is mediated by IgE and susceptibility is genetically determined.

There are no oral manifestations of atopic disease itself, and there is no such entity as oral eczema. However, acute angio-oedema (sometimes a drug reaction) can indirectly involve the mouth by causing oedematous swelling of the floor of the mouth or lips as discussed below.

Acute severe asthma has a significant mortality and is a potential cause of an emergency in the dental surgery. Drugs (Table 25.3) used to treat it and other atopic diseases may complicate dental treatment.

Table 25.3 Effects of drugs used for atopic disease

- Antihistamines (for minor allergies)
    Drowsiness
    Potentiation of sedating drugs
    Dry mouth
- Corticosteroid inhalers
    Oropharyngeal thrush
- Systemic corticosteroids for severe asthma (see Table 31.7)

Contact dermatitis

Contact dermatitis resembles eczema clinically, but is a cell-mediated (type 4) reaction. There is no convincing evidence of any oral counterpart to contact dermatitis (Figs 25.1 and 25.2). Contact dermatitis of the hands to dental materials is a hazard to dentists and especially to laboratory technicians. Methyl methacrylate monomer, in particular, is a sensitising agent, but contact dermatitis to it is a surprisingly rare occupational hazard of dentistry.

Latex allergy

The necessity for gloving for all clinical work has resulted in a growing frequency of latex allergy. In one dental school the

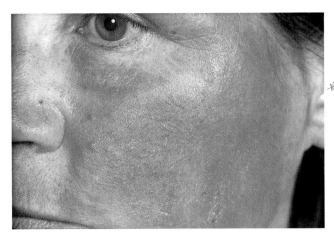

Fig. 25.1 Allergic rash triggered by impression material. There is generalised facial erythema and slight oedema.

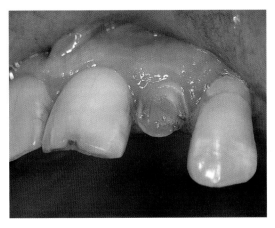

Fig. 25.2 Hypersensitivity to impression material. The same patient as in Figure 25.1, showing the site of the impression photographed at the same time. No allergic response is evident intraorally.

prevalence of latex allergy was 9%, while 22% complained of chronic glove dermatitis. For those with latex allergy, gloves made from other plastics are required, but as yet there is no completely satisfactory alternative.

Occasionally also patients may react to a dentist's gloves with a perioral rash.

Rarely, reactions to latex can be severe and anaphylactoid in character, and have been fatal.

HEREDITARY AND ALLERGIC ANGIO-OEDEMA

Hereditary angio-oedema is due to deficiency of C1 esterase inhibitor. Since C1 esterase inhibitor is an inactivator of the first complement component, its absence leads to uncontrolled activation of the classical pathway. In the process, C4 is consumed and its persistently low level in the serum during asymptomatic periods is a useful diagnostic test. Alternatively, serum C1 esterase inhibitor titration may be necessary for diagnosis of genetic variants.

As a result of stimuli such as minor injuries (including dental trauma), episodes of increased capillary permeability cause gross but localised oedematous swelling. Visceral angio-oedema can cause acute abdominal pain but, more important, oedema of the head and neck region can cause respiratory obstruction, and there is a significant mortality.

Management

Treatment of an acute attack is with purified C1 esterase inhibitor concentrate. Prophylaxis and maintenance treatment is with the synthetic androgen stanozolol which, if taken daily, maintains C1 esterase inhibitor at normal levels.

Allergic angio-oedema is an IgE-mediated acute hypersensitivity reaction to an allergen. It can cause gross swelling of the lips, face and neck and can then also threaten the airway. Patients may have a history of allergic disease and usually, raised IgE levels.

Intramuscular epinephrine should be given immediately, if the airway is threatened by an attack of allergic angio-oedema.

Mercury allergy and toxicity

The dangers of mercury are either from systemic absorption, particularly of organic mercury compounds such as methyl mercury, or from the development of hypersensitivity (contact dermatitis). Mercury intoxication is frequently confused with allergy by the public and the media.

Hypersensitivity to mercury or its salts causes an inflammatory and sometimes vesiculating reaction when contacting skin. This can readily be confirmed by patch testing, but even those with proven sensitivity can tolerate mercury amalgams in the mouth (Fig. 25.3). Nevertheless, in practical terms, it is

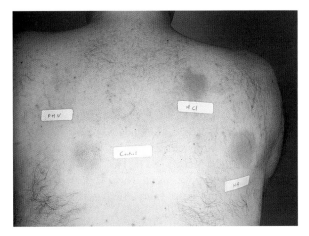

Fig. 25.3 Patch testing for dental materials. Four panels of 12 patches impregnated with different dental materials have been in contact with the skin for 48 hours. Erythema, oedema and a palpable nodule indicate reaction to mercury but amalgam restorations provoked no intraoral reaction.

usually simpler to use composite materials, to obviate the precautions necessary to prevent mercury coming into contact with their skin. If a dentist develops sensitivity, gloving and covering the arms (as required for infection control) should provide adequate protection during preparation and insertion of amalgams.

Systemic mercury toxicity is another possible occupational hazard of dentistry. Mercury, and particularly methyl mercury, are neurotoxic. To what extent the metal is converted to organic compounds in the body is unclear, but care should be taken in handling mercury and preventing it from being split or scattered in fine particles during amalgam mixing. Drilling out old amalgams also gives off traces of mercury vapour if the bur is poorly cooled. Serious pollution arises from spilling a substantial quantity of mercury, particularly on to carpeted or wooden flooring. Decontamination can then be difficult. Even worse is when (as has happened) a dental surgery assistant spills mercury behind an autoclave but fails to report the accident. As a result of the rapid evaporation, mercury absorption by the dental staff can then rise to alarming levels.

Nevertheless, many dentists have had decades of exposure to mercury and absorbed significant amounts, but do not appear to have been significantly harmed.

Though mercury, and particularly its organic compounds, are undoubtedly toxic, public anxiety about mercury-containing dental amalgams has been aroused by unscrupulous practitioners, scaremongers and others. It was conspicuous, for example, that the alleged dangers of mercury toxicity ('allergy') achieved sudden publicity when a new and expensive composite restorative material was introduced.

Minute traces of mercury can be absorbed through the oral mucosa from amalgams and may occasionally give rise to mucosal lichenoid reactions. Otherwise, there is no evidence that dental amalgams are toxic or the cause of vague symptoms such as poor memory, lassitude and depression from which most people seem to suffer from time to time. It has also been shown that patients who complain of vague symptoms from 'mercury allergy' tend also to suffer from a variety of complaints (such as irritable bowel syndrome) which have no clear organic basis. In one group of 20 patients complaining of amalgam-related symptoms, none was found to be hypersensitive to mercury. It also, incidentally, cannot be shown that alternative materials such as composites, of which there is much less experience, are necessarily safer. Some of them give off traces of formaldehyde, a suspected carcinogen.

A few patients with multiple sclerosis have been persuaded that their disease had been caused by their amalgam restorations and demanded their replacement. There is no medical justification for so doing, apart from offering the patient some temporary emotional comfort.

Despite the high risks of litigation in the US, the Council on Dental Therapeutics of the American Dental Association has stated that, 'there is insufficient evidence to justify claims that mercury from amalgam restorations has an adverse effect on the health of the patients'.

THE AUTOIMMUNE DISEASES

This blanket term is used for a variety of diseases due to defective modulation of immune responses and production of auto-antibodies which can damage host tissues. By no means all of their mechanisms are clearly understood. The autoimmune diseases have many features in common (Table 25.4). All of those listed in Table 25.2 are likely to show these features. Those with particular dental relevance have been discussed in other chapters and only the connective tissue diseases are described here.

Table 25.4 **Typical features of autoimmune disease**

- Significantly more common in women
- Onset often in middle age
- Family history frequenty positive
- Levels of immunoglobulins (autoantibodies) usually raised
- Circulating autoantibodies frequently also detectable in unaffected family members
- Circulating autoantibodies to several tissues but not all attacked (e.g. antithyroid antibodies are common in Sjögren's syndrome)
- Often an increased risk of developing other autoimmune diseases (e.g. greater risk of patients with thyroiditis developing pernicious anaemia)
- Immunoglobulin and/or complement often detectable at sites of tissue damage (e.g. pemphigus vulgaris)
- Often associated with HLA B8 and DR3
- Immunosuppressive treatment frequently limits tissue damage

---

The connective tissue diseases

The main connective tissue diseases are rheumatoid arthritis, lupus erythematosus, systemic sclerosis, primary biliary cirrhosis and Sjögren's syndrome. The last can be associated with any of them or develop in isolation.

A characteric feature is the multiplicity of autoantibodies, none of which is specific to the tissues under attack and which frequently also are not specific to the disease either. Thus in rheumatoid arthritis the most constantly found autoantibody (rheumatoid factor) is not directed against the joint tissues but against an immunoglobulin. Moreover, rheumatoid factor is frequently detectable in other diseases of this group in the absence of arthritis. The connective tissue diseases are probably mediated by immune complex (type 3) reactions causing inflammation and tissue damage.

Rheumatoid arthritis

Rheumatoid arthritis is by far the most common connective-tissue disorder and affects at least 3% of the population. Arthritis is the main feature but it is a multisystem disease. The temporomandibular joints are often involved in the more severe cases, but clinical effects are frequently insignificant (Ch. 11).

The chief importance of rheumatoid arthritis in dentistry is its association with Sjögren's syndrome. Drugs used for rheumatoid arthritis (particularly aspirin and other anti-inflammatory drugs, corticosteroids, antimalarials, gold and penicillamine) can also affect dental management or occasionally cause oral reactions. Many patients with rheumatoid arthritis are anaemic as a result of the disease itself, or as a result of gastric blood loss induced by analgesics.

Sjögren's syndromes (see Ch. 18)

Systemic lupus erythematosus (SLE)

Systemic lupus erythematous can affect almost any body system, which may affect dental management. Oral mucosal lesions are seen in about 20%.

The most important of the many autoantibodies seen in SLE are antinuclear factors. Only antibodies against double-stranded DNA (anti-dsDNA) are peculiar to SLE but many other antinuclear factors are found in other connective tissue diseases.

Clinically the features vary according to the main organ systems affected (Table 25.5).

Table 25.5 Organs and tissues affected in systemic lupus erythematosus

Organ/tissue	Clinical feature
Joints	Joint pains and arthritis
Skin	Rashes
Mouth	Stomatitis, Sjögren's syndrome
Serous membranes	Pleurisy, pericarditis
Heart	Endocarditis, myocarditis
Lungs	Pneumonitis
Kidneys	Nephritic syndrome
Central nervous system	Neuroses, psychoses, strokes, cranial nerve palsies
Eyes	Conjunctivitis, retinal damage
Gastrointestinal tract	Hepatomegaly, pancreatitis
Blood	Anaemia, purpura

Joint pains and rashes are the most commons manifestations but the 'classical' picture of a young woman with a butterfly rash across the mid-face is uncommon, and not peculiar to SLE. Corticosteroids and other immunosuppressives or antimalarials are the main forms of treatment.

Dental aspects. About 20% of patients with SLE develop oral lesions. These somewhat resemble lichen planus (Ch. 13). However, they are more difficult to treat and may not respond to the doses of systemic corticosteroids which control more major manifestations of the disease.

Antimalarials used in treatment can also cause oral lichen planus. Otherwise dental management may be affected according to the pattern of systemic involvement, but frequently the treatment is likely to affect dental management more than the disease itself. The chief dental considerations are summarised in Table 25.6.

Table 25.6 Features of lupus erythematosus affecting dental management

- Corticosteroid and other immunosuppressive drugs
- Painful oral lesions
- Sjögren's syndrome
- Bleeding tendencies (antiplatelet antibodies or anticoagulants)
- Anaemia
- Cardiac disease and risk of endocarditis

Discoid lupus erythematosus

Discoid LE mainly causes mucocutaneous lesions essentially similar to those of SLE but without the latter's serological changes and systemic disorders.

Systemic sclerosis (scleroderma)

Systemic sclerosis is rare but causes subcutaneous and visceral fibrosis. It has a poor prognosis. The pathogenesis of the progressive fibrosis and stiffening of the skin and often the gastrointestinal tract, lungs, heart and kidneys is unclear. Inflammatory changes are minimal. Circulating antinuclear antibodies are detectable in about 50% of patients but their role is also unclear.

Clinically the most common early sign is Raynaud's phenomenon and joint pains. Later the skin becomes thinned, stiff and pigmented and the facial features become smoothed-out and mask-like. Opening of the mouth may become limited (Ch. 11). Fibrosis of viscera is liable to cause dysphagia, dyspnoea and pulmonary hypertension. Later there may be renal involvement, hypertension and cardiac failure.

Immunosuppressive drugs appear to be ineffective and the 5-year survival rate is only about 50%. Oral features are summarised in Table 25.7.

Table 25.7 Possible oral features of systemic sclerosis

- Sjögren's syndrome
- Limited oral opening
- Widened periodontal ligament shadow in 7%
- Gross resorption of the jaws, rarely.
- Firm whitish-yellow fibrotic mucosal plaques, very rarely.

Localised scleroderma (morphoea)

Morphoea is characterised by localised fibrosis resembling that of scleroderma but without the latter's systemic involvement of serological changes. The face is frequently the chief site and the area of fibrosis resembles the scar from a sabre cut (coup de sabre). Childhood morphoea is a possible cause of facial hemiatrophy.

CHAPTER
25

SUGGESTED FURTHER READING

Black C 1994 Scleroderma (systemic sclerosis). Medicine UK
22:70–75

Hall F C, Walport M J 1994 Systemic lupus erythematosus. Medicine
UK 22:58–64

Herrström P, Högstrom B 1993 Clinical study of oral galvanism: no
evidence of toxic mercury exposure but anxiety disorder an
important background factor. Scand J Dent Res 101:232–237

Katelaris C H, Widmer R P, Lazarus R M 1996 Prevalence of latex
allergy in a dental school. Med J Aust 164:711–714

Mjör I A 1994 Side effects of dental materials. No evidence that
dental restorations are hazardous to health (editorial). Br Med J
309: 621–622

Sim T C, Grant J A 1990 Hereditary angioedema: its diagnostic and
management perspectives. Am J Med 88:656–665

Smart E R, Macleod R I, Lawrence C M 1992 Allergic reactions to
rubber gloves in dental patients: report of three cases. Br Dent J
172:443–445

Walls R S 1996 Latex allergy: a real problem (editorial). Med J Aust
164:707–708

CHAPTER 26

Cervical lymphadenopathy

Dental and periodontal infections are by far the most common causes of cervical lymphadenopathy (Fig. 26.1). However, other possible causes include life-threatening diseases such as carcinomatous metastases or lymphomas. In HIV infection, lymphadenopathy is one of its most common features. Cervical lymphadenopathy without an obvious local cause is therefore a warning sign that must not be ignored.

Important causes of cervical lymphadenopathy are summarised in Table 26.1 but many have been discussed in other chapters.

Investigation

The most common cause of persistent cervical lymphadenopathy is a recent viral illness. Various clinical features provide important guides as to the likely cause of lymphadenopathy (Table 26.2).

A soft lymph node in an otherwise healthy child is unlikely to be of great significance. It is usually due to a recent viral infection and typically resolves spontaneously after a month or so. Cervical lymphadenopathy associated with generalised lymphadenopathy in a child with a sore throat and fever is likely to be due to infectious mononucleosis as discussed below. By contrast, persistent lymphadenopathy associated with anaemia in a child is likely to be due to lymphocytic leukaemia. In the older patient with a hard lymph node, a carcinoma must be suspected. Rarely, such a metastasis can

Table 26.1 Important causes of cervical lymphadenopathy

Infections
- Bacterial
  Dental, tonsils, face or scalp infections
  Tuberculosis
  Syphilis
  Cat-scratch disease
  Lyme disease
- Viral
  Herpetic stomatitis
  Infectious mononucleosis
  HIV infection
- Parasitic
  Toxoplasmosis
- Possibly infective
  Mucocutaneous lymph node syndrome (Kawasaki's disease)

Neoplasms
- Primary
  Hodgkin's disease
  Non-Hodgkin lymphoma
  Leukaemia — especially lymphocytic
- Secondary
  Carcinoma — oral, salivary gland or nasopharyngeal
  Malignant melanoma
  Other mesenchymal tumours

Miscellaneous
  Sarcoidosis
  Drug reactions
  Connective tissue diseases

Table 26.2 Preliminary considerations

- Patient's age
- Localised or generalised lymphadenopathy
- Clinical characters of the nodes
- Duration of the swelling
- Associated signs or symptoms

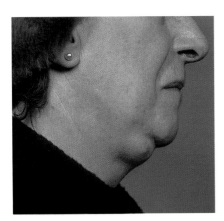

Fig. 26.1 Enlarged submandibular lymph node with incipient drainage to the skin.

form in the early stages of the disease when the primary is still small. Otherwise, a carcinoma in the anterior part of the mouth should be readily detectable by careful clinical examination. By contrast, a carcinoma of the posterior lateral border of the tongue may be difficult to visualise. Even more difficult to detect is a small primary in the nasopharynx. Various patterns of involvement of cervical lymph nodes can be produced by spread of carcinoma of the mouth (Ch. 17).

Investigations for cervical lymphadenopathy where the cause is not obvious are summarised in Table 26.3.

Table 26.3 **Investigation of cervical lymphadenopathy**

History
- Is there a history of a systemic illness?
- Has there been any contact with infectious disease (e.g. HIV or syphilis)?
- Has there been an animal scratch?
- Are there recurrent fever, lassitude, sweats or anaemia to suggest Hodgkin's disease?
- Do any symptoms (e.g. epistaxis or hoarseness) suggest a nasopharyngeal cause?
- Are any drugs (especially phenytoin) being taken?

Examination
- Check the temperature
- Identify the node and its drainage area.
- Check carefully for dental, other oral, pharyngeal or skin causes in the area
- If a possible primary cause is found (e.g. an oral ulcer) it should be biopsied
- If no local cause is found, consider ENT referral for a nasopharyngeal cause
- Examine the other side of the neck. Bilateral lymphadenopathy suggests a systemic cause

Special investigations (as appropriate)
- Blood picture (leukaemia? glandular fever?)
- Chest radiograph for mediastinal nodes (e.g. Hodgkin's disease, sarcoidosis)
- Serology (glandular fever, toxoplasmosis, HIV)
- Angiotensin-converting enzyme and calcium levels (sarcoid)
- Mantoux test (tuberculosis)
- Fine needle aspiration (primary or metastatic neoplasm, tuberculosis)
- Thyroid scan and function tests for unsuspected thyroid tumour
- Blind biopsy of nasopharynx and tonsils if needle biopsy of the node shows malignancy
- Biopsy of node itself is a last resort. Send fresh material for mycobacterial culture

---

In difficult cases, biopsy provides the most reliable diagnosis. Biopsy is only justified if all other investigations have proved inadequate. Removal or aspiration cytology of enlarged cervical lymph nodes is mandatory in any patient with a carcinoma, treated or untreated, even when there seems to be some other cause such as dental infection.

Similarly, in a patient with Sjögren's syndrome, enlargement of cervical lymph nodes may be due to infection secondary to the dry mouth, but may alternatively be due to the development of lymphoma — a recognized hazard of this disease.

If all else fails, lymph node biopsy should be carried out, but this must be done by an expert. If not, biopsy may spill infectious material or malignant cells into the neck as well as produce unsightly scarring.

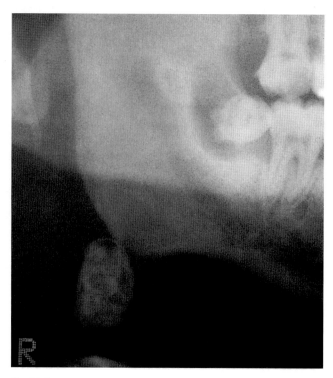

Fig. 26.2 Tuberculosis. Calcified cervical lymph node seen in a panoramic tomogram. Calcified nodes are often multiple and indicate past rather than active infection. (By kind permission of Mr E J Whaites.)

TUBERCULOUS CERVICAL LYMPHADENOPATHY

Tuberculous infection of the cervical lymph nodes is a primary infection which accounts for less than 10% of tuberculosis in Britain. *Mycobacterium tuberculosis* (human) accounts for over 90% of isolates. Patients are mostly adults, mainly immigrants of Asian or Afro-Caribbean origin. Non-tuberculous ('atypical') mycobacteria, particularly *M. avium intracellulare* or *M. scrofulaceum*, are now the major cause of cervical mycobacterial lymphadenitis in immunocompetent children. As discussed earlier, the incidence of mycobacterial infections is growing and multiply-resistant strains are becoming widespread.

Clinical features (Table 26.4)

Table 26.4 **Typical clinical features of tuberculous lymph nodes**

- Firm swelling, usually of a group of nodes
- Nodes typically become matted
- Abscess or sinus formation, if neglected
- Calcified nodes from past, healed disease (Fig. 26.2).

Pathology

Diagnosis depends on finding granulomas in which mycobacteria should be demonstrable by Ziehl–Neelsen staining or

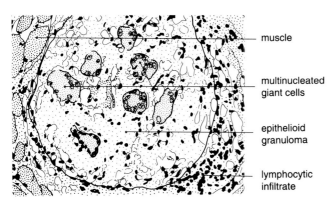

muscle

multinucleated
giant cells

epithelioid
granuloma

lymphocytic
infiltrate

Fig. 26.3 Tuberculosis. Numerous multinucleate Langhans giant cells are conspicuous in this granuloma.

by immunofluorescence using auramine-rhodamine. However, infection by non-tuberculous mycobacteria, even in immuno-competent children, is likely to give rise to poorly-defined or irregular granulomas without palisading, or to ill-defined aggregates of epithelioid histiocytes (Fig. 26.3). Caseation may be absent but there may be areas of necrosis with numerous neutrophils. Ziehl–Neelson staining is also negative.

Mycobacterial culture or detection of mycobacterial DNA is required. The tuberculin skin test should be positive, unless the patient is severely immunodeficient.

Management

The clinical picture is variable and the diagnosis is usually only made after fine needle aspiration or excision of a node. If a tuberculous ('cold') abscess and sinus form, incision is contra-indicated and affected nodes should be excised intact. A course of isoniazid should also be given.

SYPHILIS

The cervical lymph nodes are enlarged, soft and rubbery when the primary chancre is in the mouth or on the lip. They are also involved in the widespread lymphadenopathy of the secondary stage.

In the primary stage, diagnosis is by finding *Treponema pallidum* in a direct smear from the oral lesion. Later, diagnosis depends on the serological findings (Ch. 12).

Management

Antibiotic treatment, usually with penicillin, is required.

CAT-SCRATCH DISEASE

This infection is common in the US and, though uncommon, is

increasingly frequently found in Britain. Typical features are summarised in Table 26.5.

Table 26.5 Typical features of cat-scratch disease

- Children frequently affected
- Frequently a history of a scratch by a cat or other animal
- Formation of papule, which may suppurate, at the site of inoculation
- Mild fever, malaise and regional lymphadenitis 1–3 weeks after exposure
- Lymph nodes soften and typically suppurate
- Conjunctivitis may be associated. Encephalitis is a rare complication

Pathology

There is destruction of lymph node architecture, necrosis and lymphocytic infiltration, formation of histiocytic granulomas and central suppuration (Fig. 26.5).

These appearances can readily be mistaken for one of the systemic mycoses. However, it may be possible to show the usual causative organism. *Bartonella henselae*. It is a small Gram-negative bacillus demonstrable with a silver (Warthin–Starry) stain, but not with haematoxylin & eosin, at the site of inoculation or in the lymph nodes.

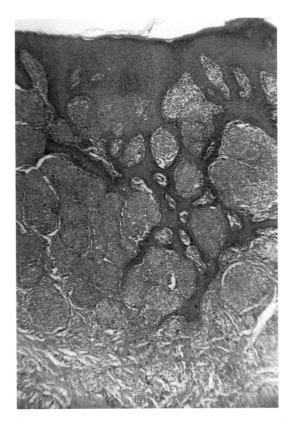

Fig. 26.4 Leprosy, another granulomatous disease. In the tuberculoid form, multiple compact non-caseating granulomas are present in the corium.

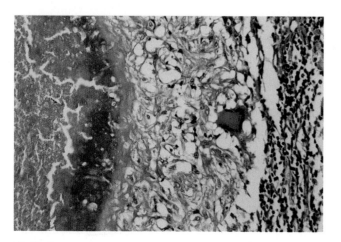

Fig. 26.5 Cat-scratch disease. There is necrosis in larger more irregular foci than tuberculosis, and giant cells.

Management

Diagnosis depends on a history of a scratch, particularly by a cat, clinical features and exclusion of other causes for lymphadenopathy. The histological findings are confirmatory if *B. henselae* can be identified.

The disease is typically mild and self-limiting but may lead to suppuration and sinus formation. The response to antibacterials is variable. Trimethoprim-sulphamethoxazole has been recommended but some cases resolve spontaneously.

LYME DISEASE

Lyme disease is caused by a spirochaete, *Borrelia burgdorferi*, which is transmitted by insects, particularly deer ticks. The disease is worldwide but far more common in the US than in Britain. Typical features are summarised in Table 26.6.

Table 26.6 Typical features of Lyme disease
• A rash spreading outwards from the insect bite
• Enlarged regional lymph nodes
• Fever and often other systemic symptoms
• Arthritis (the main chronic effect) particularly of the knees, rarely of the temporomandibular joints
• Neurological complications (in about 15% of patients) include facial palsy or other cranial nerve lesions

Management

Diagnosis is by the history and clinical picture. It is confirmed serologically or, sometimes, by demonstration of the spirochaete by silver staining of a skin biopsy.

The spirochaete is sensitive to penicillin or tetracycline which should be given as early as possible. However, joint pains may recur or destructive arthritis may develop later.

INFECTIOUS MONONUCLEOSIS

The Epstein–Barr virus (EBV) is the main cause of this self-limiting lymphoproliferative disease with polyclonal activation of B lymphocytes. Typical features are summarised in Table 26.7.

The clinical features are usually distinctive, but rarely there is more persistent lymphadenopathy which may mimic a lymphoma both clinically and histologically.

Table 26.7 Typical features of infectious mononucleosis
• In children especially
Generalised lymphadenopathy, typically with conspicuous enlargement of the cervical nodes
Sore throat
Fever
• In adolescents
Lymphadenopathy often less conspicuous
Vague illness with fever
• In the anginose type of disease
Sore throat, tonsillar exudate and pharyngeal oedema
Palatal petechiae (Fig. 26.6)

Management

The diagnosis is confirmed by a peripheral blood picture showing the atypical (monocyte-like) lymphocytes. A heterophil antibody (Paul–Bunnell) test and, if necessary, demonstration of a raised titre of EBV antibodies are confirmatory. If these tests are negative in an otherwise typical case, cytomegalovirus infection or toxoplasmosis should be considered. Acquisition of HIV infection frequently also gives rise to an illness resembling infectious mononucleosis.

There is no specific treatment but infection is usually self-limiting.

Ampicillin or amoxycillin should be avoided. They are prone to cause irritating macular rashes unrelated to penicillin allergy.

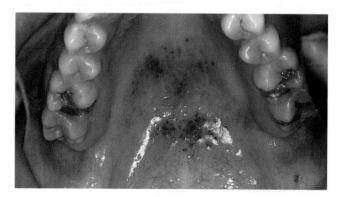

Fig. 26.6 Petechiae on the palate are frequently seen in infectious mononucleosis.

THE ACQUIRED IMMUNE DEFICIENCY SYNDROME

Lymphadenopathy is one of the most frequent manifestations of HIV infection (Ch. 22). Soon after infection there may be a transient glandular fever-like illness. Later there may be widespread and persistent lymphadenopathy (generalised lymphadenopathy syndrome: GLS), which is likely to progress to AIDS in over 50% within less than 4 years. Lymphadenopathy in AIDS may also be due to lymphomas.

TOXOPLASMOSIS

Toxoplasma gondii is a common intestinal parasite of many domestic animals, particularly cats. *T. gondii* is a low-grade pathogen but can affect previously healthy persons, particularly young women. Infection can be acquired by ingestion of oocytes and three main types of disease can result (Table 26.8).

Table 26.8 **Possible effects of toxoplasmal infection**

- Acute toxoplasmosis in normal children or adults
  Cervical lymphadenopathy in a disease resembling infectious mononucleosis
  Atypical lymphocytes present in the blood but heterophil antibody production is absent
  Infection usually self-limiting
- Toxoplasmosis in immunodeficient patients
  Disseminated disease, particularly encephalitis
- In pregnant women
  An important cause of fetal abnormalities
- Toxoplasmal chorioretinitis
  Impairment or loss of sight
  Usually due to congenital infection
  Rarely, results from severe infections in previously healthy adults

Management

The diagnosis is confirmed serologically by a high or rising titre of antibodies or by other immunological methods.

Antimicrobial treatment is required only for severe infections and is with pyrimethamine and a sulphonamide.

MUCOCUTANEOUS LYMPH NODE SYNDROME (KAWASAKI'S DISEASE)

Kawasaki's disease is endemic in Japan and there have been outbreaks in Hawaii and the United States, where it has surpassed rheumatic fever as the leading cause of childhood-acquired heart disease. In Britain, it has caused approximately 100 deaths per annum.

The distribution of cases suggests an infectious cause, but no agent has been identified with certainty.

Typical clinical features are summarised in Table 26.9.

The overall mortality is 1–3%, from heart failure secondary to coronary artery disease or dysrhythmias secondary to myocardial ischaemia.

Table 26.9 **Typical features of Kawasaki's disease**

- Children under 5 years old affected
- Fever persisting for more than 5 days
- Generalised, often morbilliform rash
  Palms and soles become red, swollen and indurated
- Erythematous stomatitis
  Swelling and cracking of the lips and pharyngitis
- Unilateral mass of cervical lymph nodes
- Abdominal symptoms frequently
- Deterioration of mood ('extreme misery')
- Heart disease in approximately 20%

Management

The diagnosis usually depends on the clinical and, particularly, electrocardiographic findings.

There is no specific treatment, but aspirin, despite the possible risk of Reye's syndrome, is frequently given to lessen vascular damage and thromboses. However, a single large dose of intravenous gamma globulin given with aspirin, in the early, acute stages appears to be the most effective means of reducing the risk of coronary artery damage.

LANGERHANS' CELL HISTIOCYTOSIS

Cervical lymph nodes can be enlarged, sometimes massively, in isolation or more frequently in association with multisystem disease (Ch. 9).

PHENYTOIN AND OTHER DRUG-ASSOCIATED LYMPHADENOPATHIES

Lymphadenopathy is an occasional toxic effect of long-term treatment with the antiepileptic drug phenytoin. Phenytoin lymphadenopathy (unlike that caused by many other drugs) is not usually associated with serum sickness-like symptoms of fever, rashes and joint pains. Moreover, the histopathology of phenytoin-associated lymphadenopathy can mimic a lymphoma.

Lymphadenopathy frequently first affects the neck but usually becomes widespread.

Management

Substitution of phenytoin with another anticonvulsant such as carbamazepine should allow the lymphadenopathy to subside and confirm the diagnosis.

Other drugs which can cause lymphadenopathy include penicillin (rarely), phenylbutazone (limited use), some other non-steroidal anti-inflammatory drugs, and some antimalarials. As mentioned earlier, lymphadenopathy with these drugs is typically associated with serum sickness-like features.

SUGGESTED FURTHER READING

Collip P J 1992 Cat-scratch disease: therapy with trimethoprim-sulphamethoxazole. Am J Dis Child 146:397–399

Eisenkraft B L, Som P M 1999 The spectrum of benign and malignant etiologies of cervical node calcification. NJR 172:1433–1437

Evans M J, Smith N M, Thornton C M et al 1998 Atypical mycobacterial lymphadenitis in childhood — a clinicopathological study of 17 cases. J Clin Pathol 51:925–927

Haberman T M, Steensma D P 2000 Lymphadenopathy. Mayo Clin Proc 75:723–732

Karcher A M, Zaman A, Brewis C et al 2000 Neck lumps: expect the unexpected. Lancet 355:1070

Mason W H, Takahashi M 1999 Kawasaki syndrome. Clin Infect Dis 28:169–187

Ogden G R, Kerr M 1989 Mucocutaneous lymph node syndrome (Kawasaki disease). Oral Surg Oral Med Oral Pathol 67:569–572

Pinder S E, Colville A 1992 Mycobacterial cervical lymphadenitis in children: can histological assessment help differentiate infections by nontuberculous mycobacteria from *Mycobacterium tuberculosis*. Histopathology 22:117–119

Ruef C 1999 Tuberculosis in Europe at the end of the second millenium. Infection 27:311–312

Sakai O, Curtin H D, Romo L V et al 2000 Lymph node pathology. Benign proliferative, lymphoma and metastatic disease. Radiol Clin N Am 38:979–998

Stansfeld A G, d'Ardenne A J, eds 1992 *Lymph node biopsy interpretation*, 2nd Edn. Churchill Livingstone, Edinburgh

Steiner M, Gould A, Wilkie W, Porter K 1994 Cat-scratch disease in the submandibular region: report of a case. J Oral Maxillofac Surg 52:614–618

Terezhalmy G T 1979 Mucocutaneous lymph node syndrome. Oral Surg Oral Med Oral Pathol 47:26–30

CHAPTER 27
Cardiovascular disease

Cardiovascular disease is common and many patients with heart disease require dental treatment. Heart disease becomes more frequent and severe in later life and is the most frequent single cause of death in Britain. Younger patients can also be affected. Infective endocarditis is one of the few ways in which dental treatment can lead to death of a patient, but only very rarely. As mentioned earlier (Ch. 5), surveys have suggested that dental disease may possibly also contribute to the development of atherosclerosis and myocardial infarction. Myocardial infarction is a cause of major emergencies in the dental surgery and initial measures by the dental surgeon may be life-saving (Ch. 36).

In terms of dental management, patients fall into two main groups (Table 27.1) but a few may fall into both, and drug treatment may create additional problems (Table 27.2). It must be appreciated therefore that the following management suggestions are generalisations and each case must be considered on its own merits.

Table 27.1   Dental management in major types of cardiac disease

- Valvular or related defects (congenital or due to past rheumatic fever) or who have a prosthetic replacement, susceptible to infective endocarditis
  Prophylactic antibiotic cover, particularly before extractions, is mandatory
- Ischaemic heart disease with or without severe hypertension and cardiac failure
  Routine dentistry presents little hazard but the risk of dangerous arrhythmias must be minimised
  Local anaesthetics in normal dosage have only theoretical dangers, but pain and anxiety must be minimised
  The main risk is from general anaesthesia

General aspects of management

Patients chiefly at risk are severe hypertensives and those who have angina or have had a myocardial infarct. Anxiety or pain can cause outpouring of adrenaline which can both greatly increase the load on the heart and also precipitate dangerous dysrhythmias.

There is some evidence that dental infections, particularly chronic periodontal disease, are possibly a risk factor for atherosclerotic coronary artery disease.

Table 27.2   Some dental implications of drugs used for heart disease

Drugs	Implications for dental management
Methyldopa, captopril	Stomatitis (Ch. 13)
Nifedipine (and analogues), diltiazem	Gingival hyperplasia (Fig. 27.1)
Anticoagulants	Risk of prolonged postoperative bleeding
Antihypertensives	Potentiated by general anaesthetics
Digoxin	Enhanced risk of dysrhythmias with halothane

To die of fright is not a figure of speech but it can sometimes result from severe dysrhythmia. The first essential for these patients is therefore to ensure painless dentistry and to alleviate anxiety.

Patients should be asked whether routine dental treatment under local anaesthesia is acceptable, and in any session of treatment as little or as much may be done as they feel able to tolerate.

Oral temazepam may be helpful (5 mg on the preceding night and again half an hour before treatment, and the patient accompanied by a responsible adult). If sedation is required, relative analgesia is safer because nitrous oxide has no cardio-respiratory depressant effects and is more controllable, but it should be administered by an expert.

Local anaesthesia for patients with cardiac disease

For local anaesthesia, an effective surface anaesthestic should be applied and the injection given very slowly to minimise pain. The most effective agent is 2% lidocaine with epinephrine and, after half a century of use, no local anaesthetic has been shown to be safer. The adrenaline (epinephrine) content can theoretically cause a hypertensive reaction in patients receiving beta-blocker antihypertensives, because of an unopposed alpha-adrenergic effect, but only if doses are considerably larger than used in dentistry.

Though patients with cardiovascular disease need to be treated with care, the risks of routine dental treatment under local anaesthesia (despite many statements to the contrary) and of significant adverse reactions are very low.

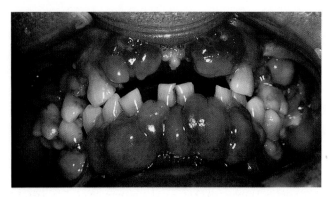

Fig. 27.1 Drug-induced gingival hyperplasia resulting from treatment of hypertension with nifedipine. These swellings are centred on the interdental papillae.

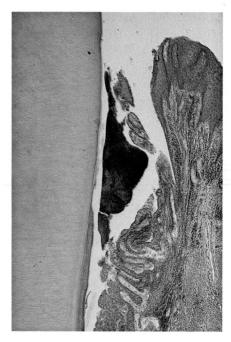

Fig. 27.2 Subgingival plaque. The area of pocket wall in contact with plaque is large and the tissue contains numerous thin-walled blood vessels near the surface. This illustration serves to remind how easily microrganisms may be transferred into the circulation.

In Britain, all three deaths associated with dental local anaesthesia during the 10 years 1980–1989 were related to the use of prilocaine. This does not, of course, mean that prilocaine is necessarily dangerous but it hardly suggests that it is safer than the more widely used lidocaine with adrenaline (epinephrine).

Local anaesthetics can undoubtedly cause mild dysrhythmias, but it is not always appreciated that more severe dysrhythmias can be triggered by anxiety *before* they have been given, or later during the operation.

However, doses of local anaesthetics should be kept to a minimum and no more than 2 or 3 cartridges should be given (or be necessary) for an acceptable session of treatment. If larger doses have to be given, for example for multiple extractions, then continuous cardiac monitoring is necessary.

If general anaesthesia is unavoidable it must be given by a specialist anaesthetist in hospital, especially as some of the drugs used for cardiovascular disease increase the risks. Cardiovascular disease is the chief cause of sudden death under anaesthesia.

Patients at risk from infective endocarditis

Normally, bacteria entering the bloodstream are rapidly cleared by circulating leucocytes, but if there is a cardiac defect which can be colonised, infective endocarditis can develop.

There are many sources of bacteraemias, such as cardiac surgery, intravenous catheterisation and intravenous drug addiction. Bacteraemias can also be detected in over 80% of persons after extractions and even after toothbrushing, but the numbers of bacteria released are often very small. Even in a patient with a heart lesion, infective endocarditis does not necessarily follow.

Relatively few bacteria inhabit the oral mucosa, and most are being constantly washed away by the saliva. By contrast, vast numbers of bacteria inhabit the gingival margins when oral hygiene is poor and even greater numbers occupy periodontal pockets. These bacteria are in close contact with dilated, thin-walled blood vessels (Fig. 27.2). Movement of teeth in their sockets repeatedly compresses and stretches or ruptures

these vessels, so that bacteria can be pumped into the bloodstream.

Fewer that 15% of cases of infective endocarditis can be related to dental operations but in these cases extractions have been the precipitating factor in over 95%. Viridans streptococci, such as those which colonise the teeth, are of low virulence but may be able to colonise heart valves because of attachment mechanisms (Ch. 3) which also enable them to cause dental disease.

Factors determining susceptibility to infective endocarditis are difficult to identify. For example, children with Down's syndrome — who are prone to severe periodontal disease, have multiple immune defects and, frequently, congenital cardiac defects — are not particularly susceptible to infective endocarditis.

Currently, advanced age, especially if there is periodontal sepsis, is the main risk factor (Fig. 27.3). Infective endocarditis is rare in children and the peak incidence and mortality is after the age of 60 years.

Once infective endocarditis develops, vegetations of bacteria and fibrin form on the valves, which are progressively destroyed (Fig. 27.4). Cardiac failure is the main cause of death but emboli and bacteria released into the bloodstream can also cause renal or cerebral damage.

Prevention is all-important. Patients who have valvular defects (congenital or due to past rheumatic fever) or some other congenital anomalies, such as septal defects, or who have prosthetic heart valves, should receive antibiotic prophylaxis (Appendix 27.1) before extractions (the highest risk), scaling and periodontal surgery. These are likely to release significant numbers of bacteria from the gingivae or, particularly, periodontal pockets.

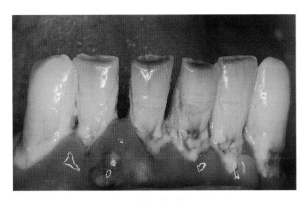

Fig. 27.3 Poor oral hygiene and severe pocketing such as this constitutes a risk to life, particularly in an elderly patient with a cardiac valve defect.

Other dental procedures such as fitting metal bands which extend deep to the gingival margins, though they may cause bacteraemias, have rarely been followed by infective endocarditis and antibiotic cover is not officially recommended. However, if the clinician considers the patient to fall into a high-risk group, then it may be prudent to give cover. Otherwise, orthodontic procedures in general are not recommended for antibiotic cover, particularly because most of these patients are children in whom infective endocarditis is rare.

Endodontic treatment rarely if ever leads to infective endocarditis and the risks of antibiotic prophylaxis exceed any benefits.

Infective endocarditis does not appear to be a risk after myocardial infarction or coronary artery bypasses, or for wearers of cardiac pacemakers, and antibiotic cover is not recommended for dental procedures.

It should be noted that the onset of infective endocarditis is typically very insidious. Even when antibiotic cover has been given, patients must be made to understand that they should report to the dentist if they develop any mild, unexplained, febrile illness within 3 months of the dental treatment. Delay in diagnosis is the main factor affecting survival in infective endocarditis.

While prevention of infective endocarditis is clearly mandatory there is growing doubt how best this can be achieved. Several surveys have shown that few cases of infective endocarditis can be reliably related to dental operations. Also, because spontaneous bacteraemias, due for example to mastication, are common, it is by no means certain that when infective endocarditis has followed a dental procedure, that the procedure was the actual cause. Moreover, it cannot be proved that the recommended prophylactic measures are effective or that the risks outweigh the benefits. One survey calculated that in the UK, in a year, no fewer than 670 000 at risk patients may be undergoing high risk dental procedure *without* antibiotic prophylaxis. Yet, there are fewer than 2500 cases of infective endocarditis, of which only a minority are related to dentistry, in the same period. Sceptics also point out the incidence of infective endocarditis has not fallen despite the introduction of scientifically-based prophylactic measures.

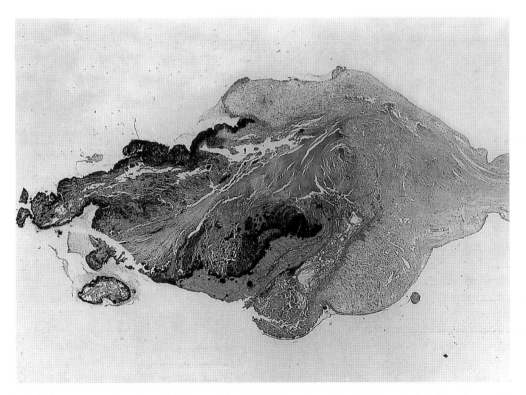

Fig. 27.4 Heart valve in subacute infective endocarditis. The free edge of the valve lies to the left of the picture and is covered by vegetations; centrally the valve is inflamed and thickened; and to the right the normal thickness of the valve at its attachment to the heart is seen.

On the one hand therefore, it cannot be denied that endocarditis can occasionally follow dental treatment. On the other hand, there is growing doubt whether this happens so frequently as to justify antibiotic prophylaxis or even whether the risks of antibiotic prophylaxis outweigh the benefits. Nevertheless, until these questions are answered, it is necessary to follow the current recommendations for at risk patients (Appendix 27.1). Also, by doing so the risk of medicolegal claims (of which there have been many) may be minimised.

For cardiac transplantation, patients are deeply immunosuppressed and might be considered to be at high risk of infective endocarditis after dental operations. However data is limited and there is no agreed protocol for such patients.

Cardiac pacemakers

Pacemakers provide a stimulus to cardiac contraction when the normal rhythm is disturbed by disease of the sinoatrial node or conducting tissues as a result, for example, of myocardial infarction.

Any ultrasonic scaler or electrosurgical equipment that interferes with pacemaker function should be avoided but pulp testers are safe.

Kawasaki's disease (mucocutaneous lymph node syndrome)

As noted earlier (Ch. 12), Kawasaki's disease is the only form of serious heart disease with specific orofacial manifestations, namely mucositis and cervical lymphadenopathy.

Cardiac damage is the result of vasculitis which may result in coronary artery aneurysm formation, myocardial infarction and a mortality of over 5%.

Aspirin (80–100 mg/kg daily) has been the standby of treatment but is more effective if supplemented with intravenous gammaglobulin.

Antibiotic prophylaxis of infective endocarditis for dental patients

Prophylaxis is recommended for dental extractions, scaling or periodontal surgery. Prophylaxis is not considered necessary for other procedures such as orthodontic manipulations unless there is likely to be significant damage to the gingival margins.

Under local or no anaesthesia

- Patients not allergic to the penicillins and who have not received penicillin more than once in the previous month

Amoxycillin

Adults 3 g single oral dose taken under supervision, 1 hour before dental procedure
Children 5–10 years Half adult dose
Children under 5 years Quarter adult dose

- Patients allergic to penicillins or who have received penicillin more than once in the previous month

Clindamycin

Adults 600 mg single oral dose taken under supervision, 1 hour before dental procedure
Children 5–10 years Half adult dose
Childern under 5 years Quarter adult dose

Under general anaesthesia

- Patient not allergic to the penicillins, who have not received penicillin more than once in the previous month and who are not special risk patients (see below)

Amoxycillin

Adults 1 g intravenously *or* 1 g in 2.5 ml 1% lidocaine hydrochloride intramuscularly *or* 3 g orally 4 hours before induction then 3 g orally as soon as possible after recovery
Children 5–10 years Half adult dose
Children under 5 years Quarter adult dose
or 3 g orally plus oral probenicid 1 g, 4 hours before procedure

---

Special risk patients who should be referred to hospital

---

1. Patients who have had a previous attack of infective endocarditis (whether or not general anaesthesia is to be given), and patients with prosthetic valves requiring a general anaesthetic but not allergic to penicillin.
   Adult amoxycillin 1 g i/v or i/m plus *gentamicin* 120 mg i/v or i/m at induction
   Children 5–10 years amoxycillin half adult dose plus gentamicin 2 mg/kg
   Children under 5 years amoxycillin quarter adult dose plus gentamicin 2 mg/kg

2. Similar patients who are allergic to penicillins
   either vancomycin i/v, 1 g given over at least 100 minutes, then i/v *gentamicin* 120 mg at induction or 15 minutes before dental procedure
   Children under 10 years vancomycin i/v 20 mg/kg, gentamicin 2 mg/kg

   or teicoplanin i/v, 400 mg plus *gentamicin* 120 mg at induction or 15 minutes before dental procedure.
   Children under 14 years teicoplanin 6 mg/kg, *gentamicin* 2 mg/kg.

   or clindamycin i/v, 300 mg given over at least 10 minutes, at induction or 15 minutes before dental procedure, then oral or i/v *clindamycin* 150 mg, 6 hours later
   Children 5–10 years. Half adult dose
   Children under 5 years. Quarter adult dose

Antibiotic prophylaxis may be supplemented with chlorhexidine gluconate gel 1% applied to the gingival margins.

Precautions

1. When clindamycin is used, periodontal or other multistage procedures should not be repeated at intervals of less than 2 weeks.

2. Whatever antibiotic cover has been given, patients must be instructed to report to the dentist any mild, unexplained, febrile illness developing within 3 months of the dental treatment.

SUGGESTED FURTHER READING

Aitken C, Cannell H, Sefton A M et al 1995 Comparative efficacy of oral doses of clindamycin and erythromycin in the prevention of bacteraemia. Br Dent J 178:418–422.

Blinder D, Shemesh J, Taicher S 1996 Electrocardiographic changes in cardiac patients undergoing dental extractions under local anaesthesia. J Oral Maxillofac Surg 54:162–165

Campbell J H, Huizinga P J, Rodriguez J P et al 1996 Incidence and significance of cardiac arrythmia in geriatric oral surgery patients. Oral Surg Oral Med Oral Pathol Oral Radiol Endod 82:42–46

Durack D T 1995 Prevention of infective endocarditis. N Engl J Med 332:38–45

Findler M, Galili D, Meidan Z et al 1993 Dental treatment in very high risk patients with active ischaemic heart disease. Oral Surg Oral Med Oral Pathol 76:298–300

Findler M, Mazor Z, Galili D, Garfunkel A A 1993 Dental treatment in a patient with malignant pheochromocytoma and severe uncontrolled high blood pressure. Oral Surg Oral Med Oral Pathol 75:290–291

Glick M 1995 Intravenous drug abusers: a consideration for infective endocarditis in dentistry? Oral Surg Oral Med Oral Pathol 80:125

Lockhart P B 1996 An analysis of bacteremias during dental extractions. Arch Int Med 156:513–520

Mattila K J, Valtonen V V, Neiminen M, Huttunen J K 1995 Dental infection and the risk of new coronary events: prospective study of patients with documented coronary artery disease. Clin Infect Dis 20:588–592

Rahn R, Schneider S, Diehl O et al 1995 Preventing post-treatment bacteremia. JADA 126:1145–1148

Smith A J, Adams D 1993 The dental status and attitudes of patients at risk from infective endocarditis. Br Dent J 174:59–64

Uyemura M C 1995 Antibiotic prophylaxis for medical and dental procedures. Postgrad Med 98:137–152

Van der Meer J T M, van Wilk W, Thompson J et al 1992 Awareness of need and actual use of prophylaxis: lack of patient compliance in the prevention of bacterial endocarditis. J Antimicrob Chemother 29:187–194

Working Party of the British Society for Antimicrobial Chemotherapy 1992 Antibiotic prophylaxis of infective endocarditis. Lancet 339:1292–1293

Respiratory tract disease

SINUSITIS

Nasal congestion, purulent nasal discharge, some fever and malaise usually follow an upper respiratory infection such as a cold. Pain and facial tenderness are felt over the involved antrum. However, pain may be felt in teeth with roots close to the antral floor. Several adjacent molars may then be tender, but there should be little difficulty in distinguishing sinusitis from periodontitis. In sinusitis, radiographs typically show absence of periodontitis but opacity of the antrum.

Sinusitis can also result from dental infection or damage to the antral floor. A radiographic survey has also shown antral disease to be twice as frequent in patients with periodontal disease as in matched controls.

Dental damage to the maxillary antrum

The floor of the antrum may be damaged during dental extractions which cause an oroantral fistula. If the antrum is opened during an extraction, a displaced root or bacteria from the mouth can introduce infection. There is also damage to the ciliated lining and loss of normal mucociliary transport which carries foreign material out of the cavity. If sinusitis becomes established and the fistula has not been closed, the walls of the passage may become epithelialised and the opening becomes permanent.

Displacement of a root or tooth into the maxillary antrum

A whole tooth can be driven into the antrum if the tooth is conical and considerable upward force has been used. More frequently, a root is driven into the antrum when an attempt is made to dig it out via the socket, particularly when a thin antral floor extends down into the alveolar ridge.

Clinical features

Displacement of a tooth or root into the antrum can give rise to signs (Table 28.1), partly depending on the size of the opening.

Management

The position of the root or tooth should be confirmed. Some-

Table 28.1 Signs suggesting a tooth or root displaced into the antrum

- The root or tooth suddenly disappears during the extraction
- Blowing the nose may force air into the mouth or cause frothing of blood from the socket
- The patient may notice air entering the mouth during swallowing, or fluid from the mouth escapes into the nose
- Bleeding from the nose on the affected side, occasionally
- Later, a salty taste or unpleasant discharge
- Facial pain if acute sinusitis develops
- Rarely, antral lining may prolapse into the mouth

times it is still within the alveolar process or outside the antrum and between its lining and bony floor.

A periapical radiograph should be supplemented with occlusal intraoral views. If the root has been displaced far, antral views should be taken with the head in two different positions to determine whether the tooth is mobile.

A root displaced into the antrum usually causes sinusitis, but it may cause no more than mucosal thickening. Severe sinusitis is less common. The root should be removed from the antrum and any oro-antral opening closed. Several measures are important (Table 28.2)

Table 28.2 Principles of management of a root displaced into the antrum

- Explain to the patient how the accident has happened, and give the necessary reassurance
- Do not to try to retrieve the lost root immediately by digging through the socket opening and damaging the antral floor and lining further
- If a root or tooth has been displaced into the antrum, it should be removed by elective surgery (see below)
- If the tip of a root causes a minimal antral reaction or lies between the bony floor and the mucosal lining, removal may not be essential but there is a risk of infection later

After any acute sinusitis has been treated, the surgical approach depends on the position of the root and whether there is a wide oroantral opening. The usual method is to reflect a mucoperiosteal flap in the labiobuccal sulcus, open the antrum in the canine fossa (Caldwell–Luc approach) and find the root by endoscopy. The tooth or fragment may then be removable on a sucker nozzle

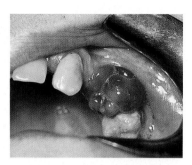

Fig. 28.1 Antral polyp. A polyp of inflamed antral mucosa has prolapsed through an oroantral fistula left untreated after the extraction of an upper first permanent molar.

small enough to prevent it from disappearing into the suction apparatus and being lost before confirmation of its removal.

Oroantral fistula

Rarely, the antrum may be accidentally opened during extractions if the antral floor is damaged. If the fistula is not obvious, its presence should be verified by telling the patient to blow gently while blocking the nose by pinching the nostrils together. Air (detectable with a tuft of cotton wool held in tweezers), blood, pus, or mucus will then be expelled from the opening into the mouth. Occasionally an opening may be blocked by prolapsed lining or antral polyp which is purplish red (Fig. 28.1), and, if the opening is large enough, it may sometimes be pushed gently back into the antrum, thus confirming its origin. Alternatively, a silver probe can be gently insinuated beside the mass into the antral cavity to detect the opening.

Usually, a large oroantral fistula gives adequate drainage, but a pinhole fistula blocks drainage and is often associated with recurrent attacks of sinusitis. If the patient is not seen until late after the accident, there is typically chronic antral infection, persistent discharge and proliferation of granulation tissue. The inflamed antral lining is usually much thickened, and polyps may fill part of the cavity. Principles of management are summarised in Table 28.3.

Table 28.3 Principles of management of an oroantral fistula

The 'fresh' fistula => Oroantral Communication
● Reflect a mucoperiosteal flap and suture it to give an air-tight seal over the opening

The established infected fistula
● Control chronic sinusitis by removal of any polyps, usually via a Caldwell–Luc approach, or through the oral opening if the fistula is sufficiently large
● Excise the entire epithelialised fistula
● Close the opening by reflecting a mucoperiosteal flap over it

Postoperatively
● Give penicillin for 5 days, and a 10-day course of decongestant nose drops and inhalations
● Warn the patient against blowing the nose

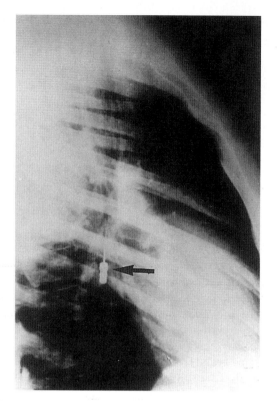

Fig. 28.2 Radiograph of the chest used to localise an inhaled reamer.

ASPIRATION OF A TOOTH, ROOT OR INSTRUMENT

A tooth or root can rarely slip from extraction forceps but is more frequently swallowed than inhaled. The patient should be reassured but should be sent for a chest radiograph and if necessary, bronchoscopy. Small instruments such as reamers can also occasionally be inhaled (Fig. 28.2).

If left, a tooth in a bronchus can cause collapse of the related lobe and a lung abscess.

COMMON VIRAL UPPER RESPIRATORY TRACT INFECTIONS ('COLDS')

Colds often precede sinusitis. They are a contraindication to general anaesthesia. Transmission to the dentist is also a hazard.

TUBERCULOSIS

Open pulmonary tuberculosis can occasionally cause lingual ulceration as a result of coughed-up mycobacteria in the sputum (Ch. 12).

Dentists are likely to be non-immune, and are at significant risk from acquiring tuberculosis from such patients. This can be particularly dangerous if the mycobacteria are multiply-resistant.

Rigorous infection control must therefore be maintained, particularly now that the incidence of tuberculosis is rising.

SARCOIDOSIS

Sarcoidosis is a chronic disease of unknown cause, in which granulomas form particularly in the lungs, lymph nodes (especially the hilar nodes), salivary glands and other sites such as the mouth (Fig. 28.3).

Oral lesions, usually painless swellings, may be seen. The most frequently affected sites are the gingivae (Fig. 28.4), lips, palate and buccal mucosa. In over 50% of patients with bilateral hilar lymphadenopathy, biopsy of a labial salivary gland shows typical granulomas and is a valuable diagnostic aid (Fig. 28.5).

Clinical involvement of major salivary glands is uncommon but can cause tumour-like swellings (Fig. 28.6). Parotid swelling due to sarcoidosis, with xerostomia, uveitis and, often, facial palsy is known as *Heerfordt's syndrome.* Many minor abnormalities of immune responses such as anergy to some antigens such as tuberculin and, frequently, hypergammaglobulinaemia, are detectable, but patients are not unusually susceptible to infection.

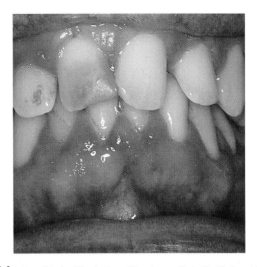

Fig. 28.4 Sarcoidosis. Gingival swelling is not clinically distinguishable from several other possible causes, but biopsy showed granuloma formation.

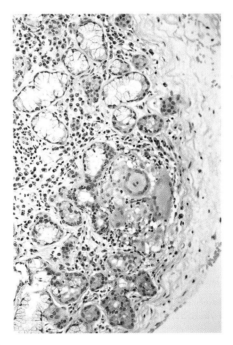

Fig. 28.5 Sarcoidosis of a salivary gland. There is a scattered lymphoplasmacytic infiltrate and granulomas are scattered through the tissue. The granuloma contains several large, multinucleate giant cells.

Pathology

Sarcoid granulomas are non-caseating, contain multinucleated giant cells and are surrounded by lymphocytes (Fig. 28.7). In an oral biopsy, sarcoid granulomas have to be distinguished from other granulomatous diseases (Table 28.4).

Management

Diagnosis depends on combined clinical and laboratory findings, particularly signs of pulmonary involvement and biopsy

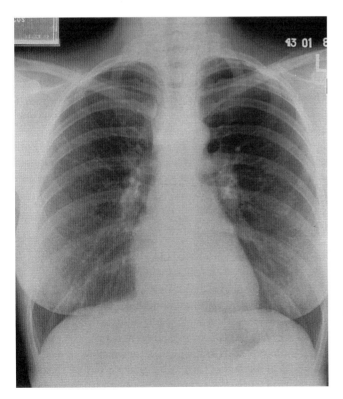

Fig. 28.3 Sarcoidosis. Prominent hilar lymphadenopathy is the main radiological finding, though granuloma formation may be widespread.

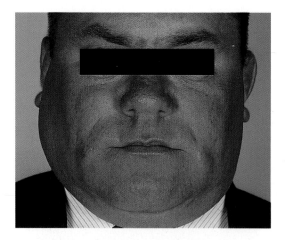

Fig. 28.6 Bilateral parotid swelling in a case of sarcoidosis.

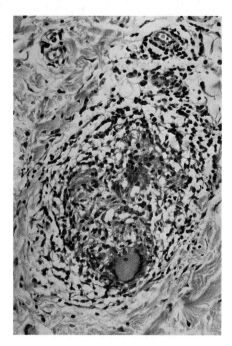

Fig. 28.7 Sarcoidosis. Microscopically the granulomas are compact with heavy peripheral lymphocytic infiltrate. However, they are not distinguishable by microscopy alone from other granulomatous diseases such as tuberculosis.

of affected tissue. Labial gland biopsy showing granulomas may greatly facilitate diagnosis. In the active stages of the disease, the plasma levels of angiotensin converting enzyme (ACE) are frequently raised. Also, as mentioned above, there is typically anergy to tuberculin. A strongly positive Mantoux reaction therefore virtually excludes sarcoidosis.

Treatment with systemic corticosteroids is indicated for pulmonary fibrosis, cerebral lesions, or hypercalcaemia.

CHRONIC OBSTRUCTIVE AIRWAYS DISEASE (COAD)

Chronic obstructive airways disease is typically caused by

Table 28.4 Important granulomatous diseases

- Infections
  Tuberculosis and non-tuberculous mycobacterioses
  Syphilis
  Systemic mycoses
  Cat-scratch disease
  Toxoplasmosis
- Reactive
  Foreign body reactions
- Unknown causes
  Sarcoidosis
  Crohn's disease
  Melkersson–Rosenthal syndrome
  Orofacial granulomatosis
  Wegener's granulomatosis

smoking and recurrent respiratory infections. Patients are hypoxic and may be cyanotic. COAD is a contraindication to intravenous sedation because of its respiratory depressant effect, and to general anaesthesia except in hospital.

ASTHMA

Asthma is a common, potentially lethal disease which accounts for at least 2500 deaths a year. Rarely, acute severe asthma precipitates an emergency in the dental surgery and calls for immediate attention (Ch. 36).

WEGENER'S GRANULOMATOSIS ('LETHAL MIDLINE GRANULOMA SYNDROME')

These formerly ill-defined diseases can cause variable degrees of destruction of the central facial tissues and a fatal outcome as their main features.

They start in the upper respiratory tract and are not clinically distinguishable in their early stages. They are now recognised to result from either Wegener's granulomatosis or a peripheral (nasopharyngeal) T- or NK-cell lymphoma (Ch. 22).

Wegener's granulomatosis

Wegener's granulomatosis is a potentially lethal but uncommon systemic vasculitis with features summarised in Table 28.5.

Clinically, granulomatous inflammation of the nasal tissues and discharge is typically the first sign and can result in destruction of the nasal septum and a saddle nose deformity.

Occasionally, a characteristic proliferative gingivitis appears first. The changes initially resemble pregnancy gingivitis but the gingivae become swollen with a granular surface and dusky or bright red ('strawberry gums' — Fig. 28.8). The changes can be widespread or patchy. Alternatively, mucosal ulceration may be widespread but appears at a later stage.

Table 28.5 Important features of Wegener's granulomatosis

● Granulomatous inflammation of nasal tract
● Cavitation of the lungs
● Potentially fatal glomerulonephritis
● Proliferative gingivitis occasionally
● Oral mucosal ulceration occasionally
● Antineutrophil cytoplasmic antibodies (ANCAs) typically present
● Histologically, granulomatous inflammation with giant cells and vasculitis

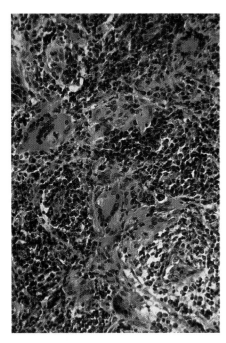

Fig. 28.10 Wegener's granulomatosis. Gingival biopsy showing clusters of giant cells.

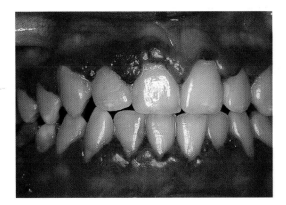

Fig. 28.8 Wegener's granulomatosis. There is irregular gingival hyperplasia affecting a few teeth and redness extending the full depth of the attached gingiva. The distribution is not related to plaque.

Pathology

Biopsy of affected gingivae typically shows a finely nodular surface, epithelial proliferation, a dense inflammatory infiltrate and collections of giant cells (Figs 28.9 and 28.10). In deeper tissues, vasculitis with destruction of small arteries is seen but granulomas are frequently inconspicuous.

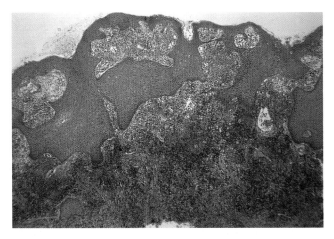

Fig. 28.9 Wegener's granulomatosis. There is epithelial hyperplasia with deeply penetrating irregular broad rete processes. In the connective tissue there is a dense mixed, inflammatory infiltrate in which eosinophils are prominent and there may be occasional scattered giant cells.

Management

The diagnosis must be established by biopsy at the earliest possible moment and may be possible as a result of the gingival changes. Detection of antineutrophil cytoplasmic antibodies (ANCA) is valuable. These show fine granular cytoplasmic fluorescence and are present in approximately 85%. Staining for classical antineutrophil cytoplasmic antibodies (cANCA) is more strongly positive in Wegener's granulomatosis than in other arteritides. They are valuable for distinguishing Wegener's granulomatosis from nasopharyngeal lymphoma when it presents a similar clinical picture and, frequently, arteritis-like changes histologically.

Examination of the nasopharynx, chest radiographs and renal function tests should also be carried out. Early cytotoxic treatment, usually with cyclophosphamide, may then be life-saving but haematuria suggests glomerulonephritis and a poor prognosis.

Nasopharyngeal T- and NK-cell lymphomas

These rare lymphomas start in the nasal cavity and can cause extensive destruction of the centre of the face. In their early stages they are typically clinically indistinguishable from Wegener's granulomatosis. However, they are ANCA negative. They have been discussed in Chapter 22.

CARCINOMA OF THE ANTRUM

Carcinoma of the antrum is rare. As with cancer of the mouth, pain is not an early symptom. Later, anaesthesia in the distri-

339

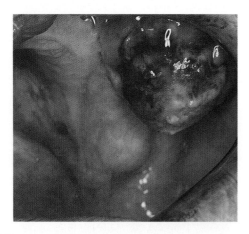

Fig. 28.11 Antral carcinoma. Occasionally an antral carcinoma will present intraorally, either after eroding the maxilla or through an extraction socket.

bution of any sensory nerves involved is almost as common as pain.

Oral and dental symptoms from carcinoma of the antrum result from involvement of its floor. This may cause pain in the teeth or under a denture. As the disease advances, teeth may become loose and a swelling becomes obvious (Fig. 28.11).

Radiographs should be taken for signs of destruction of the bony antral walls. It is a general rule that an opaque maxillary antrum in a person over 40 years of age without obvious underlying dental or nasal disease should have the antrum explored. If a mass is found, biopsy must be carried out.

MYCOPLASMAL (PRIMARY ATYPICAL) PNEUMONIA

Mycoplasmal pneumonia occasionally triggers bullous erythema multiforme (Ch. 13).

CYSTIC FIBROSIS (MUCOVISCIDOSIS)

In this disease, obstruction of the airways by the viscid sputum causes recurrent respiratory infections in childhood. Development and eruption of the teeth may be delayed and hypoplastic defects may be seen. Salivary gland swelling is another possible effect. Administration of tetracycline, for recurrent chest infections, during dental development may cause staining of teeth.

SLEEP APNOEA SYNDROME

In sleep apnoea syndrome there is recurrent spontaneous obstruction of the airway during sleep. In the middle-aged population approximately 2–4% are affected. Obese males, in particular, are affected and suffer daytime drowsiness and difficulty in concentrating (with a consequently raised risk of road traffic accidents), and impaired work performance. Depression and irritability may be associated. In the longer term there is a significantly raised risk of hypertension, ischaemic heart disease and stroke.

During sleep there are snoring and breathing pauses. The cause is recurrent occlusion at the back of the throat, partly due to relaxation of the palatoglossus and genioglossus, which, during wakefulness, maintain the patency of the airway. Because of the apnoea there is lowered oxygen saturation and risk of dysrhythmias.

Management

Avoiding evening alcohol and sedatives are important. In some, posteriorly set maxilla and mandible are contributory so that intraoral appliances to provide some degree of mandibular protrusion help to improve the airway. Long-term compliance is good and an oral appliance may be suitable treatment for mild obstructive sleep apnoea or for cases where surgery has failed. Orthognathic surgery may help by advancing the facial skeleton and hyoid bone to expand the airway. This may need to be combined with uvulopalatopharyngoplasty if there is both oro- and hypopharyngeal obstruction, but uvulopalato-pharyngoplasty alone is no longer considered to be effective. Yet another alternative is to perform a tracheostomy, but this can bring other complications. Trials have found that oral appliances are as effective for improving oxygenation as continuous positive airways pressure, delivered by a nasal mask, but only the latter has been shown to improve mortality in the long term.

BRONCHOGENIC CARCINOMA

Carcinoma of the lung is in most respects the most important disease of the respiratory tract. It is rising in frequency in women, who will soon achieve an unwanted equality with men as a result of their smoking habits. However, lung cancer has few implications for dentistry unless general anaesthesia has to be carried out. Respiratory obstruction and, sometimes, abnormal sensitivity to muscle relaxants may then make the procedure hazardous.

An uncommon oral manifestation of oral cancer is diffuse pigmentation of the soft palate. Also, metastases from the lung are sometimes deposited in the jaws or more rarely in the oral soft tissues.

SUGGESTED FURTHER READING

Abrahams J J, Glassberg R M 1996 Dental disease: a frequently unrecognised cause of dental sinus abnormalities? AJR 166:1219–1223

Bartlett J G A 1996 Antibiotic selection in sinusitis. Arch Otolaryngol Head Neck Surg 122:422–423

Benatar S R 1994 Sarcoidosis. Medicine Int 22:43–50

Brook I, Frazier E H, Gher M E 1996 Microbiology of periapical abscesses and associated maxillary sinusitis. J Periodontol 67:608–610

Calverley P M A 1995 Management of COPD. Medicine UK 23:308–312.

Cawson R A 1965 Gingival changes in Wegener's granulomatosis. Br Dent J 118:30–32

Davies K J, Herbert A-M, Westmoreland D, Bagg J 1994 Seroepidemiological study of respiratory virus infections among dental surgeons. Br Dent J 176:262–263

Davies P D O 1995 Tuberculosis. Medicine UK 23:325–332

Devaney K O, Travis W D, Hoffman G, Leavitt R, Lebovics R, Fauci A S 1990 Interpretation of head and neck biopsies in Wegener's granulomatosis. A pathologic study of 126 biopsies in 70 patients. Am J Surg Pathol 14:555–564

Eufinger H, Machtens E, Akuamoa-Boateng E 1992 Oral manifestations of Wegener's granulomatosis. Int J Oral Maxillofac Surg 21:50–53

Fernald G W, Roberts M W, Boat T F 1990 Cystic fibrosis: a current review. Pediatr Dent 12:72–78

Harrison B 1995 Acute severe asthma in adults. Medicine UK 23:298–301

Hoffman G S, Kerr G S, Leavitt R Y, Hallahan C W, Lebovics R S, Travis W D et al 1992 Wegener granulomatosis: an analysis of 158 patients. Ann Intern Med 116:488–498

John C J 1995 Pulmonary sarcoidosis. Medicine UK 23:405–408

Landau L 1995 Cystic fibrosis. Medicine UK 23:400–404

Mahaney M C 1986 Delayed dental development and pulmonary disease in children with cystic fibrosis. Arch Oral Biol 31:363–367

Nachbar F N, Classen V, Nachbar T et al 1996 Orificial tuberculosis detection by polymerase chain reaction. Br J Dermatol 135:106–109

Parsons E, Seymour R A, Macleod R I et al 1992 Wegener's granulomatosis. A distinct gingival lesion. J Clin Periodontol 19:64–66

Gastrointestinal and liver disease

Though the mouth is the entry to the gastrointestinal tract, few gastrointestinal diseases directly affect the oral cavity.

GASTRIC REGURGITATION

Chronic vomiting of gastric acid contents due to such causes as hypertrophic pyloric stenosis can lead to erosion of the palatal aspect of the anterior teeth particularly (Fig. 29.1). This type of dental erosion is an important diagnostic sign of self-induced vomiting in bulimia.

CROHN'S DISEASE

Crohn's disease is of unknown aetiology. It most frequently affects the ileocaecal region, causing thickening and ulceration. Effects include abdominal pain, variable constipation or diarrhoea and, sometimes, obstruction and malabsorption. Joint pain can also be troublesome.

Orofacial involvement (Table 29.1) may occasionally precede abdominal symptoms.

Table 29.1 **Typical orofacial features of Crohn's disease**

- Diffuse soft or tense swelling of the lips, or mucosal thickening
- Cobblestone thickening of the buccal mucosa, with fissuring and hyperplastic folds
- Gingivae may be erythematous and swollen
- Sometimes, painful mucosal ulcers, linear or resembling aphthae
- Mucosal tags in sulcuses sometimes present
- Glossitis due to iron, folate or vitamin B_{12} deficiency can result from malabsorption

Oral lesions such as these (Figs 29.2–29.4), particularly when associated with abdominal symptoms, can lead to the diagnosis of Crohn's disease. But sometimes oral symptoms precede gastrointestinal.

Histologically, the granulomas are typically small, loose and with few multinucleate giant cells. They are often deep in the corium and may be difficult to find. A biopsy may need to extend unusually deeply (Figs 29.5–29.7).

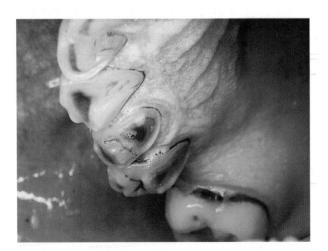

Fig. 29.1 Erosion of the palatal surfaces of the upper teeth due to repeated vomiting.

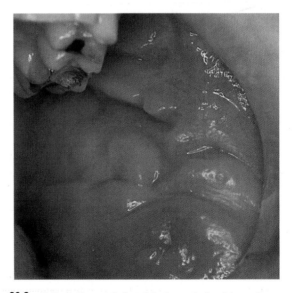

Fig. 29.2 Crohn's disease. Soft nodular hyperplasia of the oral mucosa is a typical feature and, in this case, was associated with facial swelling and intermittent diarrhoea.

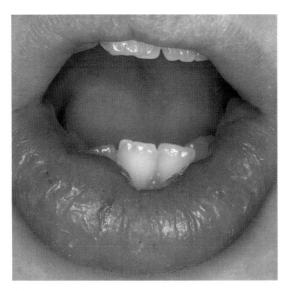

Fig. 29.3 Crohn's disease. Gross labial swelling and intraoral mucosal proliferation with typical histological changes led to the finding of extensive intestinal involvement.

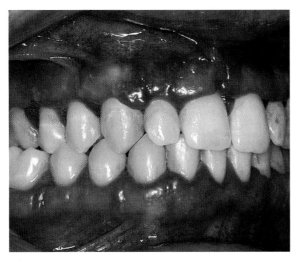

Fig. 29.4 Crohn's disease. The gingivae are hyperplastic and irregular and erythematous. These changes are obvious, but more subtle signs are easily missed. The appearances are identical to those in sarcoidosis in the gingivae.

Management

Oral symptoms may resolve when intestinal Crohn's disease is controlled with, for example corticosteroids, sulfasalazine or mesalazine. Alternatively, oral lesions may respond to oral sulfasalazine or to intralesional injections of a corticosteroid.

MALABSORPTION SYNDROMES

Malabsorption syndromes (Table 29.2) can cause haematological deficiencies which can contribute to development or exacerbation of recurrent aphthae, sore tongue or other symptoms.

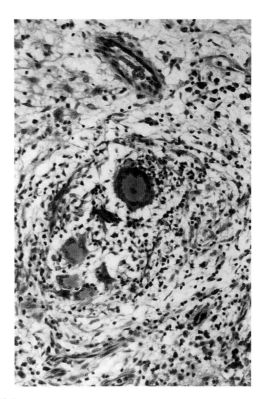

Fig. 29.5 Crohn's disease. The granulomas are frequently isolated and loose in texture with scanty peripheral lymphocytic infiltrate, as here.

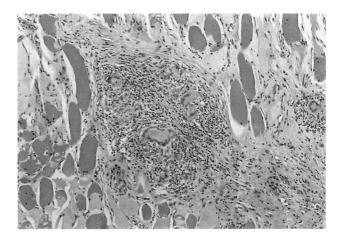

Fig. 29.6 Crohn's disease. The granulomas are frequently deep in the mucosa and widely dispersed. Here granulomas are present in muscle, showing the importance of adequate biopsy depth.

Table 29.2 Important causes of malabsorption syndrome

- Coeliac disease
- Crohn's disease
- Resection of stomach or ileum
- Pancreatic insufficiency
- Liver disease (failure of bile secretion into the gut)
- Some parasitic and other chronic gut infections

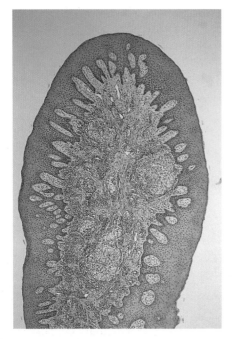

Fig. 29.7   Crohn's disease. A hyperplastic tag of gingiva contains several large round granulomas.

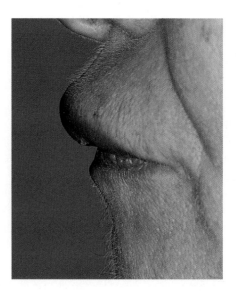

Fig. 29.8   Orofacial granulomatosis. There is conspicuous swelling of the upper lip with eversion of the vermilion border. The lip is thickened and tense.

OROFACIAL GRANULOMATOSIS

The term *orofacial granulomatosis* has been given to swellings of such sites as the gingivae or lips (Fig. 29.8) due to granulomatous reactions (Fig. 29.9) but none of the recognised diseases (Table 28.7) are involved. Some of these patients develop Crohn's disease or sarcoidosis later, but many others remain healthy.

In some, the granulomatous reaction appears to result from common food additives such as cinnamon or tartrazine. Such causes can only be confirmed by an exclusion diet which, if faithfully maintained, may greatly lessen the swellings.

When no cause can be found, regular follow-up should be maintained to ensure that any underlying condition such as Crohn's disease or sarcoidosis is recognised at an early stage.

The term 'orofacial granulomatosis' should not incidentally be confused with *midfacial granulomas* which are lethal diseases (Ch. 28).

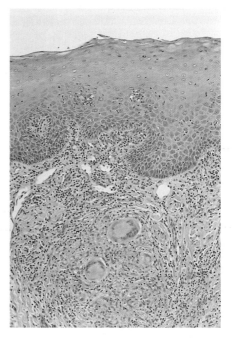

Fig. 29.9   Orofacial granulomatosis. Below the epithelium is a patchy inflammatory infiltrate and scattered granulomas containing large multinucleate giant cells.

PEUTZ–JEGHERS SYNDROME

In this disorder, pigmented macules, particularly oral, are markers for intestinal polyposis (see Fig. 21.5). Polyps may be present throughout the gastrointestinal tract, and in the small bowel can cause recurrent abdominal pain and minor intestinal obstruction. Cancer of the colon is a recognised complication but the risk for breast and gynaecological cancers is particularly high.

LIVER DISEASE

Common types of liver disease are infections (particularly viral hepatitis), obstructive jaundice, cirrhosis (often due to alcohol), and tumours. Rarely, liver disease has followed dental treatment when halothane has been given or as a result of transmission of hepatitis B, and there are other aspects of liver disease relevant to dentistry (Table 29.3).

Table 29.3 Important aspects of liver disease relevant to dentistry

- Haemorrhagic tendencies (Ch. 26)
- Impaired drug metabolism
- Transmission of hepatitis B, particularly
- Drug-dependent patients are frequently viral hepatitis carriers
- Rarely, a toxic effect of halothane

Impaired drug metabolism

Most drugs are metabolised in the liver, and no drugs should be given to patients with liver disease without first consulting the British National Formulary. Causes of parenchymal liver disease and liver failure are shown in Table 29.4. Cirrhosis is frequently the result of alcoholism but often of unknown cause. Halothane is a rare cause of severe liver damage and its use in dentistry has greatly declined.

Table 29.4 Important causes of liver failure

- Idiopathic cirrhosis
- Alcoholic cirrhosis
- Viral hepatitis
- Drugs, including halothane

VIRAL HEPATITIS

The main types of hepatitis, relevant here, are B, C and D. Hepatitis B is the chief risk to dental personnel but hepatitis C can also be transmitted during dentistry. The hepatitis B virus can also carry within it the delta agent which can cause a particularly virulent infection (hepatitis D).

Hepatitis B

Hepatitis B can be readily transmitted during dentistry and, despite the outbreak of AIDS, is currently the greatest infective hazard to dental staff (Table 29.5).

The risk of transmission of hepatitis B is emphasised by its previous name 'syringe jaundice'. In the past particularly, countless patients were infected via imperfectly sterilised syringes

Table 29.5 Special hazards to dental staff from hepatitis B

- The virus is widespread
- A chronic infective carrier state is common
- Minute traces of body fluids can transmit infection
- The virus survives well outside the body
- The virus is relatively resistant to disinfection
- Hepatitis B infection can cause serious complications (Table 29.6)

and needles. The effects of hepatitis B infection vary widely (Table 29.6).

Table 29.6 Possible results of hepatitis B infection

- Complete resolution
- Asymptomatic carrier state
- Acute hepatitis (rarely fatal)
- Chronic active hepatitis
- Cirrhosis
- Liver failure
- Liver cancer

Clinical aspects

The incubation period is at least 2–6 months. The majority of infections are subclinical (anicteric) but 5–10% of patients, particularly those who have had no overt illness, become persistent carriers and can transmit the infection. A minority develop acute hepatitis with loss of appetite, muscle pains, fever, jaundice and often a swollen, painful liver. The illness is often severe and debilitating but usually followed by complete recovery and long-lasting immunity. Overall mortality from clinical infection is probably about 1%. Occasionally it has been as high as 30%, probably as a result of co-infection by the delta agent.

Biochemical markers of infection are raised serum levels of liver transaminases, such as alanine aminotransferase (ALT), aspartate aminotransferase (AST) and gamma glutamyl transpeptidase (GGT), along with raised levels of bilirubin and often of alkaline phosphatase. However, confirmation of the diagnosis is by serology.

Serologically markers of hepatitis B

The hepatitis B virus (HBV) is a DNA virus termed the Dane particle. The Dane particle consists of a central core and an outer shell. The core contains DNA, an enzyme (DNA polymerase — DNA-P) and the hepatitis B core antigen (HBcAg). The protein shell contains the hepatitis B surface antigen (HBsAg).

The carrier state and complications

Most patients with acute hepatitis B recover completely within a few weeks. Approximately 5–10% fail to clear the virus within 6–9 months and become chronic carriers.

Chronic carriage of HBsAg but not HBeAg has a low risk of severe liver damage. Persistent carriage of both HBsAg and HBeAg is associated with chronic active (aggressive) hepatitis. These patients have biochemical evidence of liver damage. They are chronically ill and at special risk from cirrhosis and, possibly, carcinoma of the liver.

Chronic active hepatitis with persistent malaise, and sometimes mild jaundice, is particularly likely to develop in the very young or old, and HIV-positive patients. Cirrhosis can result and lead to liver failure or hepatocellular carcinoma.

Table 29.7 Serological markers of hepatitis B and their significance

Serological marker	Relation to infection	Significance
The surface antigen (HBsAg)	HBsAg particles detectable in late incubation period, and during acute and chronic infections	HBsAg carriage indicates past infection, but confers little risk of transmitting infection, unless HBeAg is also present
Antibody to HB surface antigen (HBsAb)	Begins to appear when recovery starts but HBsAg may briefly disappear before anti-HBs becomes detectable. Both serological tests then become negative	During recovery, anti-HBs usually appears and rises in titre; it usually implies persistent immunity. Anti-HBs also appears after hepatitis B immunisation
Hepatitis B core antigen (HBcAg)	Found only in liver cells, not serum	
Antibody to HB core antigen (HBcAb)	Anti-HBc appears at onset of disease. Quickly rises in titre and persists for many years	One of the most sensitive indicators of past infection
Hepatitis B e antigen (HbeAg)	Appears in the serum simultaneously with HBsAg but disappears earlier if there is full recovery	Indicator of high infectivity
Antibody to e antigen (anti-HBe, HBeAb)*	Usually appears in the serum soon after the e antigen and heralds recovery	Failure of development of anti-HBe indicates high infectivity
DNA polymerase (DNA-P)		Indicates high infectivity

*Carriers of both HBsAg and HBeAg but who lack anti-HBe are more likely to develop chronic active hepatitis and serious complications, and to transmit the infection.

Risks to dental staff

The carriage rate of hepatitis B virus in the general population of Britain is 0.1–0.2%. The rate in British dentists is probably double that in the general population.

In hot climates such as Asia and Africa, it may be 5–40%, and dental staff there are at high risk. There are also high-risk groups (Table 29.8) and the hazard of infection is highest in inner urban areas, particularly for oral surgeons and peri-odontists. In the USA, 20% of American oral surgeons have serological evidence of previous infection and one of the highest infection rates of all health workers.

Table 29.8 Patients with higher risk of being hepatitis B carriers

- Promiscuous male homosexuals and STD (VD) clinic patients
- Intravenous drug addicts
- Patients and staff of dialysis and transplant units
- Patients (especially with Down's syndrome) and staff of institutions for the handicapped
- Immunosuppressed or imnunodeficient patients
- Patients who have received unscreened blood or blood products
- Patients who have had acupuncture or tattooing, especially in tropical countries
- Consorts of patients with hepatitis B or of any of the above
- Certain associated diseases, particularly AIDS, some chronic liver diseases and polyarteritis nodosa
- Immigrants or travellers from high-risk areas, particularly tropical or subtropical countries

Transmission of HBV

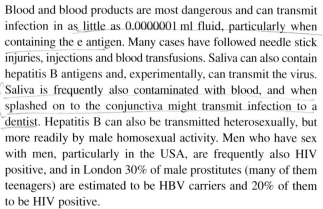

Blood and blood products are most dangerous and can transmit infection in as little as 0.0000001 ml fluid, particularly when containing the e antigen. Many cases have followed needle stick injuries, injections and blood transfusions. Saliva can also contain hepatitis B antigens and, experimentally, can transmit the virus. Saliva is frequently also contaminated with blood, and when splashed on to the conjunctiva might transmit infection to a dentist. Hepatitis B can also be transmitted heterosexually, but more readily by male homosexual activity. Men who have sex with men, particularly in the USA, are frequently also HIV positive, and in London 30% of male prostitutes (many of them teenagers) are estimated to be HBV carriers and 20% of them to be HIV positive.

As discussed earlier, the risk of infection is indicated by the serological markers. Infective carriers can only be suspected if they have a history of jaundice or are in a high-risk group. Nevertheless it must be emphasised that only 1 in 4 carriers gives a positive medical history. In statistical terms, therefore, if a dentist treats 20 patients a day, one hepatitis B carrier will be encountered every 7 working days. Many infectious patients, as in the case of HIV carriers, will therefore be treated unknowingly.

Dental staff who are carriers of or incubating hepatitis B can also transmit infection to patients, some of whom have died as a consequence. The dangers to dentists have been emphasised by the death from hepatitis B of an unvaccinated male nurse, after being bitten by a mentally handicapped carrier.

Prevention and management of hepatitis B

It is *essential* for dentists to have active immunisation. It is effective, safe and protects against both hepatitis B and delta infection. Three injections should be given at intervals into the deltoid muscle, but adequate protection may not develop until after 6 months. Side-effects are mild and rare, but a few (particularly the obese) do not produce adequate antibody levels after a normal course of vaccination and need it to be repeated. Booster doses are needed at 3–5-year intervals, or more frequently in persons in whom the half-life of the response is brief. Antibody levels should therefore be checked. Those who have not been immunised, but are wounded while treating a high-risk patient or known carrier, should have immediate active immunisation. Passive immunisation with hepatitis B immunoglobulin as well has also been advised. Treatment of chronic active hepatitis is with alpha-interferon which may prevent cirrhosis or other complications.

In addition to vaccination, strict infection control procedures should be maintained.

The delta agent: hepatitis D virus (HDV)

The delta agent is a defective RNA virus that can only replicate in the presence of HBsAg. Delta infection is mainly transmitted by blood or blood products. It is widespread among intravenous drug abusers and in endemic areas such as the Mediterranean region. Delta infection causes acute hepatitis. This usually resolves, but fulminant liver disease can follow and the mortality rate is high. A few dental patients have acquired delta hepatitis and some have died. Immunisation against hepatitis B also protects against the delta agent, and this strengthens the need for immunisation.

Hepatitis C

The hepatitis C virus (HCV) was the most common cause of post-transfusion hepatitis after hepatitis B, but donors are now screened for both hepatitis C and B. Before hepatitis C screening was available and blood products were inactivated, almost 100% of haemophiliacs became infected and remain carriers. Hepatitis C and B are similar in most respects but have some differences (Table 29.9).

Table 29.9 Important differences between hepatitis C and B

Hepatitis C:
- is less widespread
- is less readily transmitted by needle stick injuries
- is more vulnerable to antiseptics
- is rarely transmitted during dentistry
- acute hepatitis is uncommon and usually mild
But
- no protective vaccine is as yet available
- infections persists in 80% of individuals
- infection more frequently leads to chronic active hepatitis
- there is a higher risk of cirrhosis and liver cancer

In the USA, 2% of oral surgeons and 0.7% of general dentists were found to be anti-HCV positive in 1996. This compares with 21% of oral surgeons and 8% of general dentists who were anti-HBV positive in the same group.

Chronic active hepatitis C is treated with alpha-interferon plus ribavirin. Cirrhosis develops in approximately 20% of patients, 10% of whom may develop liver cancer. In one series of 131 patients with post-transfusion hepatitis C, 14.5% died of cirrhosis or hepatocellular carcinoma.

Control of transmission of viral hepatitis

Because of the ease of transmission of hepatitis the basic precautions are summarised in Table 29.10.

Table 29.10 Basic precautions against transmission of viral hepatitis

- Treat all patients as infectious ('universal precautions')
- Wear gloves for all clinical dental work
- Take special care to avoid needle stick injuries
- Wear goggles for eye protection
- Use disposable instruments and autoclave all others
- Be immunised against hepatitis B

Gloves, masks and eye shields provide only partial protection. Double gloving is necessary for surgeons at high risk from acquiring or transmitting these infections. Immunisation is therefore the single most important protective measure as it is virtually impossible completely to prevent transmission of hepatitis B by other means.

There is as yet no vaccine against hepatitis C and there are some strains of hepatitis B against which the current vaccine apparently confers no protection. Though the hazard from these is statistically small the risk from them emphasises the need to maintain rigorous infection control.

Sterilisation and disinfection for viral hepatitis

Hepatitis B virus is tougher than HCV but sterilisation and disinfection measures (Table 29.11) apply to both.

Dentists must ensure that infection control procedures are up to standard for their own protection. They are also a legal obligation under the Health and Safety at Work Act. Acquisition

Table 29.11 Sterilisation and disinfection for hepatitis B and C

Sterilisation
- Autoclaving at 134°C for 3 minutes *or*
- Hot air at 160°C for 1 hour (effective but automatic control necessary; not used in UK)
Disinfectants
- Sodium hypochlorite, 1% of freshly diluted stock solution (0.1% + detergent for surface disinfection) (HCV is also susceptible to solvent detergents)

of viral hepatitis as a consequence of dental treatment could result in substantial claims for compensation. Restrictions on dentists who are viral hepatitis carriers have been summarised on p. 316.

Hepatitis A

Hepatitis A is the common form of infectious hepatitis. It is frequently acquired from contaminated food during a holiday abroad in the sun. There is little evidence that hepatitis A is transmitted during dentistry.

SUGGESTED FURTHER READING

Bowden D S, Moaven L D, Locarnini S A 1996 New hepatitis viruses: are there enough letters in the alphabet? Med J Aust 164:87–89

De Mitri M S, Poussin K, Baccarini P et al 1995 HCV liver cancer without cirrhosis. Lancet 345:413–415

Gross J B, Persing D H 1995 Hepatitis C: advances in diagnosis. Mayo Clin Proc 70:296–297

Hosey M T, Gordon G, Kelly D A et al 1995 Oral findings in children with liver transplants. Int J Paediatr Dent 5:29–34

Porter S R, Lodi G 1996 Hepatitis C virus (HCV) — an occupational hazard to dentists. Br Dent J 180:473–474

Sanchez-Tapias J M, Rodes J 1995 Interferon in chronic hepatitis C. Lancet 346:s11

Shahara A I, Hunt C M, Hamilton J D 1996 Update. Hepatitis C. Ann Intern Med 125:658–668

Thomas D L, Gruninger S E, Siew C et al 1996 Occupational risk of hepatitis C infections among general dentists and oral surgeons in North America. Am J Med 100:41–45

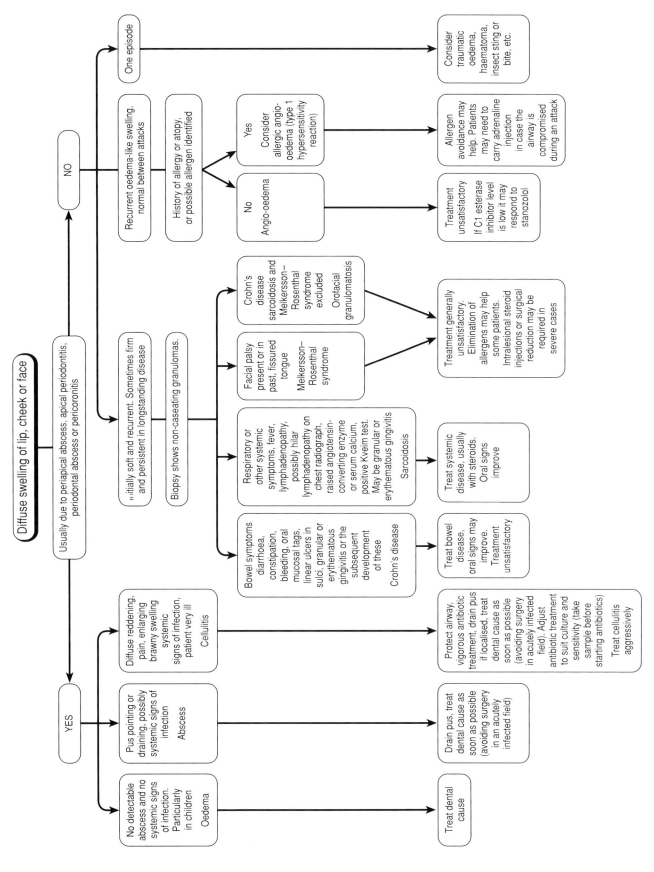

Summary 29.1 Causes and treatment of diffuse swelling of the lips and mucosa.

CHAPTER 30

Nutritional deficiencies

Patients with nutritional deficiencies are rarely seen in Britain. Susceptible patients are the elderly living on a scanty diet, food cranks and severe alcoholics living on a grossly unbalanced diet. Malabsorption syndromes (Ch. 29) are another cause.

Several oral conditions of doubtful cause, such as periodontal disease or glossitis, have been ascribed to vitamin deficiencies, though patients have been otherwise healthy and well-fed. In such cases, giving vitamin preparations brings benefit only to the multibillion pound vitamin industry. Vitamin deficiencies are not a contributory cause of dental caries.

Vitamin deficiencies

The effects of specific deficiencies are summarised in Table 30.1.

Vitamin A deficiency

In rats, vitamin A deficiency has severe effects on secretory epithelium. Columnar cells become squamous in type and keratinised. Dental development is severely affected and secretory cells of salivary glands also become squamous and keratinised. However, there is no evidence that vitamin A deficiency causes such changes in humans.

Successful treatment of keratotic plaques (leukoplakias) with retinoids (vitamin A derivatives) has been claimed but not confirmed. The toxic effects of these drugs are severe and they are teratogenic. Epidemiological studies have suggested an association between low vitamin A intake and oral and other cancers, but there is growing doubt whether beta-carotene is beneficial or harmful.

Riboflavin (B₂) deficiency

Riboflavin deficiency can occasionally result from a malabsorption syndrome. In severe cases there is typically angular stomatitis, with painful red fissures at the angles of the mouth, and shiny redness of the mucous membranes. The tongue is commonly sore. A peculiar form of glossitis in which the tongue becomes magenta in colour and granular or pebbly in appearance, due to flattening and mushrooming of the papillae, may be seen but is uncommon. The gingivae are not affected. Resolution follows within days when riboflavin (5 mg three times a day) is given.

Riboflavin is ineffective for the commonly seen cases of glossitis and angular stomatitis, which are rarely due to vitamin deficiency.

Table 30.1 Effects of specific vitamin deficiencies

Deficiency	Systemic effects	Oral effects
Vitamin A	Night-blindness, xerophthalmia	Unconfirmed contribution to leukoplakia and cancer
Thiamin (B₁)	Neuritis and cardiac failure	None
Riboflavin (B₂)	Dermatitis	Angular stomatitis and glossitis
Nicotinamide	Dermatitis, CNS disease, diarrhoea	Glossitis, stomatitis and gingivitis
Vitamin B₁₂	Pernicious anaemia	Glossitis, aphthae
Folic acid	Macrocytic anaemia	Glossitis, aphthae
Vitamin C	Scurvy (purpura, delayed wound healing, bone lesions in children)	Gingival swelling and bleeding
Vitamin D	Rickets	Hypocalcification of teeth (severe rickets only)

350

Nicotinamide deficiency (pellagra)

Pellagra, which affects the skin, gastrointestinal tract and nervous system, is rare in Britain but may occasionally result from malabsorption or alcoholism. Weakness, loss of appetite, and changes in mood or personality are followed by glossitis or stomatitis and dermatitis. The tip and lateral margins of the tongue become red, swollen and, in severe cases, deeply ulcerated. The dorsum of the tongue becomes coated with a thick, greyish fur which is often heavily infected. The gingival margins also become red, swollen and ulcerated, and generalised stomatitis may develop.

Vitamin B₁₂ deficiency

This disease, unlike the others described in this section, is primarily a defect of absorption (Ch. 25). It is exceptionally rare for it to be caused by dietary deficiencies (veganism).

Folic acid deficiency

Deficiency can result from malnutrition but is more often seen in pregnancy, or as a result of malabsorption or drug treatment (particularly with phenytoin) (Ch. 25). Women are advised to take folic acid supplements preconceptually with the aim of reducing the risk of neural tube defects. It also appears that multivitamin preparations containing folic acid may reduce the risk of orofacial clefts.

Vitamin C deficiency

Scurvy, once common among crews of sailing ships, is now exceedingly rare. In Britain, scurvy may very occasionally be seen among elderly people with an inadequate income, or in those devoted to eccentric diets. The main features of scurvy are dermatitis and purpura and, in advanced cases, anaemia, delayed healing of wounds and swollen bleeding gums may develop (Fig. 30.1). In children bone formation may be disturbed.

There is no evidence that deficiency of vitamin C plays any part in periodontal disease except in frank scurvy, and there is no correlation between low plasma ascorbic acid levels and gingivitis. There is no justification for giving ascorbic acid to healthy patients with periodontal disease.

Though it may be thought that scurvy is of historical interest only, a 24-year-old engineer was reported in 1983 to have the disease in classical form including swollen, bleeding gums. He had lived largely on peanut butter sandwiches, recalled having eaten an apple 4 years previously but could not recall ever having eaten an orange.

It has been suggested that massive doses of ascorbic acid prevent or ameliorate the common cold. This is unproven and the effect, if any, is marginal. Moreover, cessation of megadose intake of ascorbic acid can lead to rebound deficiency and scurvy. In one bizarre case, intravenous injection of no less than 80 g of ascorbic acid proved to be lethal. This really does seem to be carrying prevention too far.

Nevertheless, giving children vitamin C-rich fruit syrups is common. An incidental effect of this can be gross caries of the anterior teeth (Fig. 30.2).

Vitamin D deficiency

Deficiency of vitamin D during skeletal development causes rickets (Ch. 10).

A rich source of vitamin D is fish liver oils, but small amounts are also present in eggs and butter. In strong sunlight vitamin D can be synthesised in the skin. In Britain margarine is fortified with vitamin A and D, but requirements are small except during bone growth and pregnancy.

Rickets is now rare, but immigrants in the North of Britain are at risk. Contributory factors are lack of sunlight, a high-carbohydrate diet and possibly also the use of wholemeal flour (as in chupattis) containing factors which impair calcium absorption. However, there is no basis for the idea that dental caries is due to poor calcification of the teeth, and giving

Fig. 30.1 Scurvy. There is gross periodontal destruction with deep pocketing and mobility of several teeth resulting from the combination of poor oral hygiene and deficiency of vitamin C. (See also Ch. 10.)

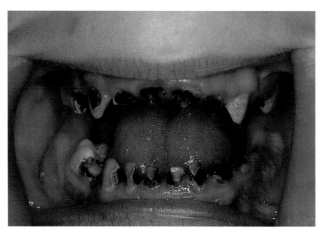

Fig. 30.2 Gross dental caries of the anterior teeth due to over-indulgence in sugar-rich vitamin C syrup.

vitamin D and calcium for dental caries is valueless. There are also dangers associated with raising children's intake of vitamin D. Some are sensitive to this potent drug and hyper-vitaminosis D causes hypercalcaemia and renal calcinosis. Dental defects (hypocalcification) are a feature only of exceptionally severe rickets (Ch. 2).

Anorexia nervosa and bulimia

Anorexia nervosa is, in simple terms, an eating disorder parti-cularly affecting young females, in which there is determined and persistent avoidance of food leading to emaciation and occasionally death. It is typically ascribed to fear of obesity and a distorted body image.

Bulimia is the term given to binge eating alternating with self-induced vomiting or purging to control excessive obesity but emaciation is not usually achieved. In a single eating binge up to 20 000 calories may be consumed and there may be addiction to drugs or alcohol also.

Oral and perioral effects of anorexia and bulimia are parotid swelling (sialadenosis) and dental erosion due to vomiting. Dentists may be able to identify such signs before medical intervention becomes imperative.

SUGGESTED FURTHER READING

Nowak R 1994 Beta-carotene: helpful or harmful? Science 294:500–501
Robb N D, Smith B G N 1996 Anorexia and bulimia nervosa (the eating disorders): conditions of interest to the dental practitioner. J Dentistry 24:7–16

Endocrine disorders and pregnancy

Endocrine disorders, apart from diabetes mellitus and thyroid disease, are uncommon. They are rare causes of oral disease but occasionally, oral changes can lead to their diagnosis. Patients with Addison's disease, diabetes mellitus and thyrotoxicosis, in particular, may also need special care for dental surgery.

PITUITARY HYPERFUNCTION — GIGANTISM AND ACROMEGALY

Overproduction of growth hormone by the anterior pituitary during the period of skeletal growth causes *gigantism*. Overgrowth of the skeleton and soft tissues causes the patient to become a giant. Acromegaly usually develops later.

After the epiphyses have fused, an adenoma of growth hormone cells causes *acromegaly*. There is renewed growth, particularly of the jaws, hands and feet. The condylar growth centre becomes active and the mandible becomes enlarged and protrusive (Fig. 31.1). Radiographically, the whole jaw is lengthened and the

angle becomes more oblique (Fig. 31.2). The jaw and other bones are also made thicker by subperiosteal bone deposition. The teeth become spaced, or, if the patient is edentulous, dentures cease to fit the growing jaw. The hands and feet become spade-like (Fig. 31.3). Overgrowth of soft tissues causes thickening and enlargement of the facial features, particularly the lips and nose.

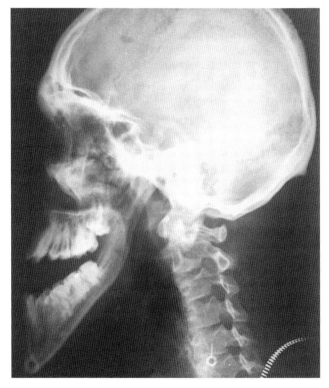

Fig. 31.2 Acromegaly. The mandible is enlarged with an elongated ramus and increased obliquity of the angle. The pituitary fossa is also enlarged due to the tumour causing the disease.

Headaches and visual disturbances due to the pituitary tumour are common. Later, weakness and, often, diabetes mellitus develop.

Rarely a growth hormone-producing pituitary tumour is part of type 1 multiple endocrine neoplasia syndrome (MEN1) as described below. In such patients gingival papules have also been described.

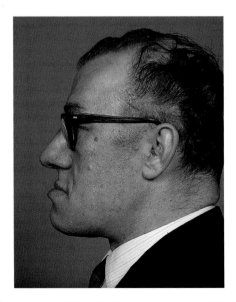

Fig. 31.1 Acromegaly. The typical facial appearance, resulting from excessive mandibular growth.

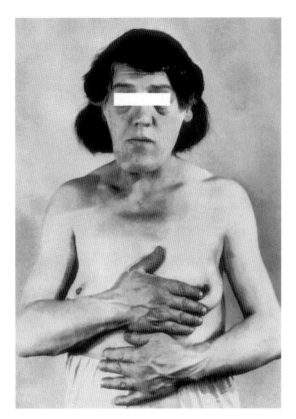

Fig. 31.3 Acromegaly. The jaw is enlarged and protrusive, the features thickened and the hands broad and spade-like. (Taken before the advent of colour photography.)

Irradiation or resection of the pituitary tumour may relieve the symptoms. Mandibular resection may be needed to improve the appearance.

THYROID DISEASE

Hyperthyroidism

Hyperthyroidism (Table 31.1) is most common in young adults, particularly women. Dental treatment of hyperthyroid patients may be affected by several factors (Table 31.2).

Table 31.1 Important features of hyperthyroidism

- Irritability and anxiety
- Loss of weight
- Exophthalmos (Fig. 31.4)
- Tachycardia
- Cardiovascular disease, particularly in untreated hyperthyroidism in older patients

Hyperthyroidism with excessive cardiac excitability is only a theoretical contraindication to lidocaine with adrenaline (epinephrine), and no other local anaesthetic has been shown to be safer.

Table 31.2 Dental management of hyperthyroid patients

- Control of nervousness and excitability
- If clinical signs are seen but the patient is not under treatment, refer to a physician
- Avoid general anaesthesia in patients with long-standing thyrotoxicosis, particularly older patients

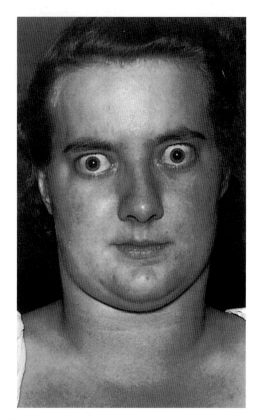

Fig. 31.4 Thyrotoxicosis. Exophthalmos is typical but the enlarged thyroid is not conspicuous. The patient had not then started to lose weight. (Taken before the advent of colour photography.)

Treatment of hyperthyroidism is by surgical removal of part of the gland, or by means of drugs such as thiouracil, carbimazole or I^{131}.

Hypothyroidism

Cretinism

Cretinism results from deficient thyroid activity at birth (Fig. 31.5). It is most common in areas of endemic goitre, but rare now that goitre is controlled with iodine. A cretin is occasionally the offspring of a normal mother. The main features (Table 31.3) are particularly dwarfism and mental defect.

Treatment with thyroid extract must be begun early to provide normal physical development and improvement in the mental defect.

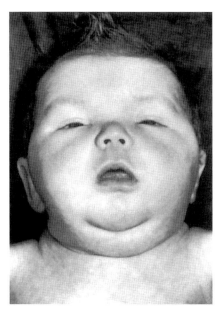

Fig. 31.5 Cretinism in a child. The facial expression, excessive broadening of the features and the protruding tongue are characteristic. (Taken before the advent of colour photography.)

Table 31.3 Typical features of cretinism

- Skeletal development and dental eruption greatly delayed
- Impaired mental development
- Broad, rather flat face partly due to defective growth of the skull and facial bones
- Overlarge, protrusive tongue
- Dull facial expression, dry thick skin
- Short stocky build and, often, umbilical hernia

Adult hypothyroidism

Hypothyroidism (Table 31.4) is frequently autoimmune but can follow removal of excessive thyroid tissue in the treatment of hyperthyroidism.

Table 31.4 Typical features of adult hypothyroidism

- Weight gain
- Slowed activity and thought
- Dry skin and hair loss
- Intolerance of cold
- Susceptibility to ischaemic heart disease

Aspects of dental management of hypothyroidism are summarised in Table 31.5.

Table 31.5 Dental management of hypothyroidism

- Avoid sedatives including diazepam, opioid analgesics and general anaesthetics because of the risk of myxoedema coma
- Anaemia or ischaemic heart disease may require dental treatment to be modified
- Local anaesthesia is always preferable
- Sjögren's syndrome is occasionally associated and requires to be treated

Lingual thyroid

Thyroid tissue is occasionally present in the tongue as a result of imperfect descent of the anlage into the neck. Clinically, it usually causes a purplish soft swelling and may not be recognised for thyroid tissue until after biopsy. Scanning of the neck to ensure the presence of a thyroid gland is therefore essential before the lingual gland is removed. However, this may have to be done anyway if it is causing significant obstruction. Life-long thyroid supplementation is then given.

PARATHYROID DISEASE

Hyperparathyroidism

This uncommon disease is usually caused by an adenoma of the parathyroids. Parathormone overproduction may cause decalcification of the skeleton and cyst-like areas of bone resorption (*osteitis fibrosa cystica* — Ch. 10). As discussed below, hyperparathyroidism is the presenting sign of the uncommon disease, type 1 multiple endocrine neoplasia syndrome (see p. 357).

Hypoparathyroidism

Post-surgical hypoparathyroidism. The most common cause of hypoparathyroidism is thyroidectomy. The resulting hypocalcaemia causes heightened neuromuscular excitability and tetany. These are controlled by giving the vitamin D analogue 1,25-dihydrocholecalciferol (DHCC) orally. Later, any residual parathyroid tissue undergoes compensatory hyperplasia.

Tetany. In mild cases, tetany is latent but can be triggered by tapping on the skin over the facial nerve; this causes the facial muscles to contract. In more severe cases, muscle cramps and tonic contractions of the muscles may progress to generalised convulsions. An early symptom of tetany is paraesthesiae of the lip and extremities. Tetany more frequently results from overbreathing, often neurotic in origin (*hyperventilation syndrome*).

Idiopathic hypoparathyroidism. Early onset hypoparathyroidism is rare. It sometimes forms part of the polyendocrinopathy syndrome with autoantibodies to a variety of glandular tissues and deficiency states (particularly Addison's disease) and frequently, mucocutaneous candidosis (see below). Otherwise the disease and its treatment are similar to postsurgical hypoparathyroidism.

Effects on calcified tissues are summarised in Table 31.6.

ADRENOCORTICAL DISEASES

Adrenocortical insufficiency is rarely primary (Addison's disease) and more frequently secondary to corticosteroid therapy.

Table 31.6 Effects of hypoparathyroidism on calcified tissues

- Retarded new bone formation and diminished resorption are usually in equilibrium so that skeletal changes are rare
- Aplasia or hypoplasia of developing enamel*, which becomes deeply grooved
- Dentine may be incompletely mineralised but lamina dura may be thickened
- Short roots to teeth (Ch. 2)

*Results from associated ectodermal defects.

Addison's disease

Addison's disease results from atrophy of the adrenal cortices and failure of secretion of cortisol and aldosterone. The result is a severe disorder of electrolyte and fluid balance and serious clinical effects (Table 31.7). The disease is usually autoimmune with organ-specific circulating autoantibodies. Tuberculous or fungal adrenal destruction are rare causes but can be secondary to HIV infection. Addison's disease is also the most frequent feature of the rare polyglandular autoimmune syndromes and is then associated with chronic mucocutaneous candidosis as described below.

Table 31.7 Typical clinical features of Addison's disease

- Lassitude, anorexia, weakness and fatigue
- Abnormal oral and cutaneous pigmentation
- Gastrointestinal disturbances
- Loss of weight
- Low blood pressure
- Susceptibility to hypotensive crises
- Associated with chronic mucocutaneous candidosis in polyendocrinopathy syndrome (p. 357)

Pigmentation is often an early sign and, in the mouth, is patchily distributed on gingivae, buccal mucosa and lips (Figs 31.6 and 31.7). It is brown or almost black. However, Addison's disease is an exceptionally uncommon cause of oral pigmentation. The skin pigmentation looks similar to suntan but with a sallow appearance due to underlying pallor. Exposed and normally pigmented areas are most severely affected.

Though Addison's disease is rare, it should be considered in a patient, other than a black individual, with pigmentation of the oral mucous membrane. A weak voice caused by general weakness and lassitude is also suggestive.

In an Addisonian crisis there is a rapid fall in blood pressure, circulatory collapse (shock) and vomiting. These crises, which may be fatal, are often precipitated by such causes as infections, injuries, surgery or anaesthesia. Immediate treatment with intravenous hydrocortisone (several 100 mg) and fluid replacement may be life-saving.

Long-term treatment of Addison's disease is usually by oral hydrocortisone which allows patients to live almost normal lives but with complications described below.

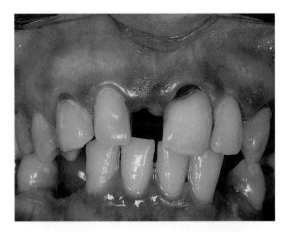

Fig. 31.6 Addison's disease. A close-up shows the characteristic distribution of pigment rather patchily along the attached gingivae. It is a brownish black in colour.

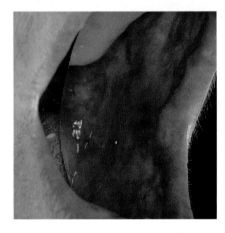

Fig. 31.7 Addison's disease. Deep pigmentation of the buccal mucosa.

Corticosteroid treatment

Corticosteroids can have physiological effects resembling those of Cushing's disease (Table 31.8). Thus there may be sodium and water retention, a raised blood sugar and impaired protein metabolism. Hypertension and diabetes are possible complications, and a characteristic moon-face appearance is produced.

Table 31.8 Important side-effects of long-term use of corticosteroids

- Depression of adrenocortical function and risk of circulatory collapse
- Depression of inflammatory and immune responses
- Opportunistic infections
- Depressed protein metabolism
- Impaired wound healing
- Moon face
- Raised blood sugar
- Sodium and water retention
- Mood changes

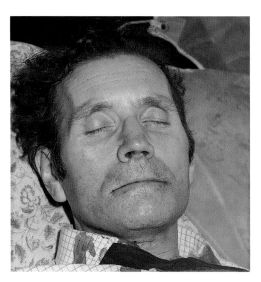

Fig. 31.8 Steroid collapse. This patient, taking only 5 mg prednisolone daily, was given brief sedation for an extraction. Adrenal suppression resulted in collapse and despite considerable doses of corticosteroid and fluid supplementation the patient did not recover fully for 48 hours.

Corticosteroids can also mask serious disease. The patient, for a time at least, can appear to be in perfect health with plump rosy cheeks and often a sense of well-being to match. Thus a young patient suffering from acute lymphocytic leukaemia taking corticosteroids can appear and feel well. However well a patient appears, the medical and drug history must therefore be carefully evaluated.

However, most important is the risk of circulatory collapse secondary to dental surgery or general anaesthesia (Fig. 31.8; Ch. 36).

Adrenocortical hyperfunction (Cushing's disease)

Cushing's disease is usually due to an adrenocorticotrophic hormone-secreting pituitary adenoma which causes adrenocortical hyperplasia. The effects (Table 31.9) are rarely dentally important.

Rarely, the moon-face of Cushing's disease has been mistaken for inflammatory swelling due to a dental infection.

Table 31.9 Important features of Cushing's disease

- Obesity of trunk and face
- Bruisability and haematomas after venepuncture
- Hirsutism
- Headaches
- Hypertension
- Osteoporosis, especially of the skull
- Glycosuria

POLYGLANDULAR AUTOIMMUNE ENDOCRINOPATHY SYNDROMES: TYPES I AND II

Addison's disease is an invariable feature of type 1 poly-

Table 31.10 Polyendocrinopathy syndromes

	Type 1	Type 2
Addison's disease	100%	100%
Hypoparathyroidism	76%	–
Chronic mucocutaneous candidosis	73%	–
Pernicious anaemia	13%	0.5%
Alopecia	32%	0.5%
Malabsorption syndromes	22%	–
Gonadal failure	17%	3.6%
Chronic active hepatitis	13%	–
Insulin-dependent diabetes	4%	52%
Autoimmune thyroiditis	11%	69%
Female:male ratio	1.5:1	1.8:1

glandular endocrinopathy syndrome. This uncommon disease features autoantibodies to a variety of glands (Table 31.10) as well as chronic mucocutaneous candidosis. The latter is not a feature of type 2 disease. In type 2 disease, Addison's disease is also an invariable feature, but not hypoparathyroidism. As discussed in Chapter 2, dental defects can also result from hypoparathyroidism in type 1 polyglandular endocrinopathy syndrome.

DISEASES OF THE ADRENAL MEDULLA

Phaeochromocytoma

Phaeochromocytoma is a catecholamine-producing tumour of the adrenal medulla. The main effect is potentially lethal hypertension and dysrhythmias. Occasionally it is part of the multiple endocrine adenoma syndrome type III, when it is associated with hyperparathyroidism, thyroid medullary carcinoma and oral mucosal neurofibromas. Alternatively, it may be associated with neurofibromatosis.

When an oral neurofibroma is found, the possibility of a phaeochromocytoma should be considered especially if the patient is hypertensive.

MULTIPLE ENDOCRINE NEOPLASIA SYNDROME

Multiple endocrine neoplasia syndromes (MEN) are autosomal dominant disorders with a prevalence of about one in 20 000.

The gene for MEN1 is on chromosome 11q13. In this disease hyperparathyroidism develops in 95%. Enteropancreatic tumours develop in over 40%, and pituitary tumours in over 30%. Also described are gingival papules.

In MEN2, the mutated gene is the RET proto-oncogene, located on chromosome 11q12. In this disease, medullary carcinoma of the thyroid is present in 95%, phaeochromocytoma in 50% and hyperparathyroidism in 15%. The oral feature of

MEN2 is mucosal neurofibromas, particularly along the lateral borders of the tongue. Screening for MEN2 is relatively readily carried out by identifying the RET mutation.

DIABETES MELLITUS

Diabetes mellitus is a common endocrine disease and results from relative or absolute deficiency of insulin, causing a persistently raised blood glucose. Approximately 2% of the population are affected but probably at least 50% of diabetics with mild or early disease pass unrecognised. There are two clinical types.

Juvenile onset (insulin-dependent) diabetes. Symptoms typically appear before the age of 25 and the disease is usually severe with thirst, polyuria, hunger, loss of weight and susceptibility to infection.

Maturity onset diabetes. Patients are typically over middle-age and obese. The onset is insidious, often with deterioration of vision or pruritus or, sometimes, thirst, polyuria and fatigue. However, many cases are asymptomatic. The disease can be controlled by dietary restriction and, if necessary, oral hypoglycaemic drugs.

In terms of dental management it is usually said that the greatest problems are with 'uncontrolled' diabetes. However, 'uncontrolled' applies to several diabetic states. At one extreme there is the mild, unrecognised, and therefore untreated, diabetic. At the other there is the treated diabetic whose disease is difficult to control ('brittle diabetes) or has been mismanaged. This last group is the one most likely to have oral complications and present difficulties in dental management (Table 31.11).

Table 31.11   Complications of diabetes mellitus that can affect dental management
● Susceptibility to infection, particularly candidosis ● Hypoglycaemic coma ● Diabetic coma ● Ischaemic heart disease ● Accleration of periodontal disease if control is poor ● Dry mouth secondary to polyuria and dehydration ● Oral lichenoid reactions due to oral hypoglycaemic drugs ● Sialadenosis

Rapidly destructive periodontal disease can result from severe untreated diabetes mellitus, but is rarely seen now. However, even treated diabetic children have slightly poorer periodontal health than controls. Diabetics also have higher DMFT levels (despite the sugar-free diet) and earlier loss of teeth than controls. Susceptibility to candidosis is another complication. The principles of dental management are summarised in Table 31.12.

Hypoglycaemic coma may be precipitated by dental treatment which delays a normal meal. Treatment should therefore be so timed as to avoid these risks – ideally, soon after the patient's breakfast.

Diabetic coma is a complication of poorly-controlled diabetes mellitus and much less likely to be seen.

Table 31.12   Principles of dental management of diabetics
● Time treatment to avoid disturbance of routine insulin administration or meals ● Use local anaesthesia for routine dentistry — the amount of adrenaline (epinephrine) in local anaesthetic solutions has no significant effect on the blood sugar ● Sedation can be given if required ● Dental operations under general anaesthesia should only be carried out in hospital under expert supervision ● Deal with any diabetic complications (Table 31.11) ● Manage hypoglycaemic coma as described in Chapter 36

PREGNANCY

Pregnancy (apart from other problems) can cause significant oral effects, and can affect dental management (Table 31.13). The chief oral effects are aggravation of gingivitis (Fig. 31.9) and possible development of a pregnancy epulis (Ch. 5). Occasionally, recurrent aphthae remit during pregnancy but may worsen due to iron or folate deficiency.

Table 31.13   Pregnancy: oral effects and management considerations

● Oral effects
  Aggravated gingivitis and epulis formation
  Variable effect on recurrent aphthae
● Management considerations
  Risk of hypotension when laid supine
  Possible hypertension of pregnancy
  Possible iron or folate deficiency
  Vomiting, especially with general anaesthesia

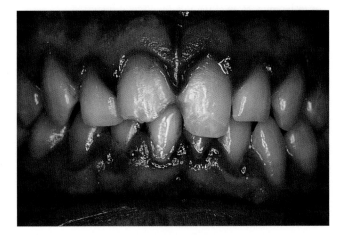

Fig. 31.9   Pregnancy gingivitis. Marginal gingivitis despite relatively good oral hygiene during the first trimester of pregnancy.

A few women in late pregnancy become hypotensive when laid supine, when the swollen uterus impedes venous return. They should be treated in a sitting position. Respiratory reserve is diminished and there is a risk of fetal hypoxia. Neonatal respiration is further depressed by drugs such as general anaesthetics and sedatives, especially barbiturates, diazepam and opioids, all of which cross the placenta. Local anaesthesia is generally safe. There are also other risks to the fetus (Table 31.14)

Table 31.14   Possible hazards to a fetus from dental procedures

- X-rays hazardous, especially in first trimester
- Respiratory depression due to sedatives, including benzodiazepines
- Dental pigmentation due to tetracycline
- Theoretical risk of depressed vitamin B_{12} metabolism by nitrous oxide
- Prilocaine may rarely cause methaemoglobinaemia
- Theoretical risk of uterine contraction caused by felypressin
- Teratogenic risks of thalidomide, retinoids, azathioprine and possibly other drugs
- Aspirin may cause neonatal haemorrhage

The main risks of fetal abnormalities are from drugs and radiation: the hazard is greatest during organogenesis in the first trimester. Few drugs are known to be teratogenic for humans, and in many cases the risk is no more than theoretical or results only from prolonged high dosage. For example, no teratogenic risk from metronidazole for humans has ever been substantiated. Non-steroidal anti-inflammatory drugs in high dosage may cause premature closure of the ductus arteriosus and fetal pulmonary hypertension. Aspirin may also increase the risk of neonatal haemorrhage and paracetamol is the preferred analgesic. Systemic corticosteroids can cause fetal adrenosuppression. However, the only drugs known to be teratogenic are thalidomide (used occasionally for major aphthae), etretinate (used experimentally for leukoplakia) and possibly azathioprine (used occasionally for Behçet's syndrome and sometimes for autoimmune diseases). For details of drug usage in pregnancy, see the current British National Formulary.

The risks from dental radiography are small but only essential radiographs should be taken, the minimal radiation exposure should be given, and the patient should wear a lead apron.

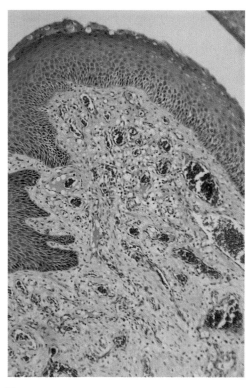

Fig. 31.10   Pregnancy epulis. When these lesions are not inflamed their vascular nature becomes obvious, as shown here.

SUGGESTED FURTHER READING

Cawson R A, Spector R G, Skelly A M 1995 *Basic pharmacology and clinical drug use in dentistry*, 6th edn. Churchill Livingstone, Edinburgh

Franklyn J A 1993 Hypothyroidism. Medicine (UK) 21:161–163

Franklyn J A 1993 Hyperthyroidism. Medicine (UK) 21:164–169

Learoyd D L, Delbridge L W, Robinson B G 2000 Multiple endocrine neoplasia. Aust NZ Med 30:675–682

Stephenson E, Haug R H, Murphy T A 1995 Management of the diabetic oral and maxillofacial surgery patient. J Oral Maxillofac Surg 53:175–182

Nathan D M 1993 Long-term complications of diabetes mellitus. N Engl J Med 328:1676–1685

Trainer P J, Howlett T, Besser E M 1993 Cushing's syndrome. Medicine Int 21:178–183

Trainer P J, Howlett T, Besser E M 1993 Addison's disease. Medicine Int 21:184–188

Williams J D, Slupchinsku O, Sclafani A P et al 1996 Evaluation and management of the lingual thyroid gland. Ann Otol Rhinol Laryngol 105:312–316

Renal disease

Renal disease has become important in dentistry because of the growing number of patients who, as a result of renal dialysis or transplantation, survive renal failure. Aspects of renal disease relevant to dentistry are summarised in Table 32.1.

Table 32.1 Aspects of renal disease affecting dental management

- Heparinisation before dialysis
- Possible hepatitis B or C carriage after chronic dialysis
- Permanent venous fistulae susceptible to infection
- Secondary hyperparathyroidism
- Immunosuppressive treatment for nephrotic or transplant patients
- Oral lesions due to drugs, particularly for immunosuppression
- Oral disease in chronic renal failure

Patients receiving regular dialysis remain otherwise in reasonably good general health. About 70% can return to full-time work. However, they are heparinised before dialysis and haemostasis is impaired for 6 to 12 hours.

These patients' permanent venous fistula for the dialysis lines is susceptible to infection, and antibiotic cover may be considered for dental surgical procedures. Drugs, including sedation, should not be given intravenously, because of the risk of damage to superficial veins which are patients' lifelines. Dialysis patients also have an greater incidence of cardiovascular and cerebrovascular disease.

Renal osteodystrophy and secondary hyperparathyroidism

Prolonged dialysis or renal failure are now more common causes of giant-cell lesions of bone than primary hyperparathyroidism. The jaws may be first affected (Ch. 10).

Renal transplant patients

Normal renal function and health can be restored by transplantation but it is associated with the complications of prolonged immunosuppressive treament, such as susceptibility to infections or lymphomas. While awaiting a compatible donor these patients have often also been on dialysis, with its attendant complications.

Ciclosporin, which is widely used to help control graft rejection, can cause persistent gingival hyperplasia with false pocketing which readily progesses to periodontal destruction in some patients. If a calcium channel blocker, such as nifedipine, is also being given for hypertension, gingival hyperplasia is virtually inevitable and uncontrollable.

Hairy leukoplakia may rarely develop in HIV-negative patients.

Complications of graft rejection such as bone lesions due to secondary hyperparathyroidism may be seen (see Fig. 10.20). It may be noted that graft rejection is frequently due to patients' non-compliance with immunosuppressive regimens.

Chronic renal failure

Some patients are unsuitable for, or unable to obtain, dialysis or a transplant. They can suffer a variety of oral effects (Table 32.2).

Table 32.2 Oral changes seen in renal failure

- Mucosal pallor (anaemia)
- Xerostomia
- Purpura
- Mucosal ulceration
- Thrush or bacterial plaques
- White epithelial plaques (Ch. 15)
- Giant-cell lesions of the jaws (secondary hyperparathyroidism)

Dental management of patients with renal disease, but particularly chronic renal failure, may be affected by many factors (Table 32.3).

Table 32.3 Factors potentially affecting dental management of patients with renal disease

- Corticosteroid and other immunosuppressive treatment
- Haemorrhagic tendencies
- Anaemia
- Impaired drug excretion
- Hypertension
- Hepatitis B or C carriage
- Underlying causes of renal failure (e.g. diabetes mellitus, hypertension, or connective-tissue disease)

CHAPTER 32

SUGGESTED FURTHER READING

Cove-Smith R 1995 Drugs and the kidney. Medicine Int 23:165–173

King G N, Fullinfaw R, Higgins T J et al 1993 Gingival hyperplasia in renal allograft patients receiving cyclosporin A and calcium antagonists. J Clin Periodontol 20:286–293

King G N, Healy C M, Glover M T et al 1994 Prevalence and risk factors associated with leukoplakia, hairy leukoplakia, erythematous candidiasis and gingival hyperplasia in renal transplant recipients. Oral Surg Oral Med Oral Pathol 78:718–726

Mallick N P 1995 Presenting features of renal disease. Medicine Int 23:91–96

Mallick N P 1995 Renal transplantation. Medicine Int 23:156–158

Ziccardi V B, Siani J, Demas P N, Braun T W 1992 Management of the oral and maxillofacial surgery patient with end-stage renal disease. J Oral Maxillofac Surg 50:1207–1212

Intellectual and physical disability

The terminology for disability is confusing, evolving and subject to the forces of political correctness. Health care professionals often demand clear-cut definitions of degrees of disability that can be used to plan dental services. Unfortunately, this approach over-simplifies the problems. People with disability see their needs in social terms rather than just the sum of their medical problems and, rightly, demand individualised care. The dentist must consider what each patient is prevented from doing, rather than concentrating on the physical or mental impairments themselves. This way of thinking illustrates the social and environmental aspects of disability, and highlights ways in which the individual's environment can be adapted to limit, or even abolish, handicap. Current terminology for disability is shown in Table 33.1.

Table 33.1 Current definitions of disability

Term	Definition
Impairment	Any loss or abnormality of physiological function or anatomical structure
Disability or limitation of activity	Restriction or lack of ability to perform a function considered normal
Handicap	The disadvantage for the individual, resulting from their disability, which prevents them from performing a normal role in society

Nowhere is terminology more difficult than in the case of intellectual impairment. The terms *mental retardation*, *subnormality*, *deficiency* or *handicap* are considered stigmatising and no longer acceptable. In practice, intellectual impairments cause a wide range of disability. Some patients are intelligent but cannot co-operate (e.g. cerebral palsy), others are intelligent but uncooperative (e.g. hyperactivity), yet others are intellectually impaired but easily treated (e.g. Down's syndrome). The specific diagnosis and its severity are much more helpful in planning treatment than non-specific labels such as learning difficulty or intellectual impairment.

The prevalence of disability is estimated at 1.5 to 2 per 1000 live births. Intellectual impairments account for approximately 0.9 per 1000 and major physical impairments for the remainder.

The prevalence is rising as a result of better medical care for adults and improved survival for babies with congenital disorders. Approximately 12 000 children with disabilities are registered with dental practitioners. The management of their dental care is affected by both the disability and parents' motivation and attitudes. However, mental or physical disability does not necessarily mean that dental care has to be compromised, though this may sometimes be inevitable.

Children and adults with disability present a wide variety of problems of dental management, but up to 90% of them can probably be managed by conventional means without sedation or general anaesthesia. Nevertheless, people with disability are a dentally neglected group, even though valiant attempts have been made to overcome this deficiency in recent years.

Preconceptions that 'the disabled' are necessarily grimacing, drooling and unco-operative are seriously misplaced. In fact, those who manage children with disability find the work more rewarding than dentistry in normal children. Such is the emptiness of some of these children's lives, particularly when institutionalised, that dental treatment, which involves both relatively prolonged personal attention and a change from other endless dreary days, can be a pleasure for them. One Down's syndrome child, for instance, though well looked after by affectionate parents, was in a state of mysteriously eager expectation for days at the prospect (it was later found) of having an x-ray. Dental treatment may therefore be a real source of pleasure for those so deprived.

There is a welcome concern about the dental care of *children* with disability but it should be remembered that disability persists for life. The transition from special school to community care can worsen dental disease because dental care must be provided in a less controlled setting and intensive prevention is more difficult to maintain. The elderly probably suffer more disabilities than children, because of the additional problems of declining health, but unfortunately are less likely to get sympathetic help.

Difficulties in the provision of dental care for people with disability are summarised in Table 33.2. Unless the disability is severe, most of these difficulties can be overcome with patience, training and experience. It should be remembered that when disability is viewed in its social context many difficulties become the responsibility of the dentist rather than being a

Table 33.2 Typical difficulties with dental care of patients with disability

- Co-operation with routine dental treatment
- Difficulties in performing routine home oral hygiene
- Associated systemic disease
- Difficulties with transport and access to the surgery
- Need for sedation or general anaesthesia
- Medications or diets promoting caries
- Dysphagia, drooling, bruxism
- Oral effects of medication
- Competence to give consent
- Financial problems for patients
- Discrimination or prejudice in health care

problem associated with the patient. For instance, if a patient cannot gain access to a surgery, this could be viewed as discrimination on the part of the dentist who has failed to ensure that all patients can receive care equally.

Mental illness often manifests itself as challenging behaviour and patients suffer many problems in common with people with disability, particularly discrimination and poor access to dental care. Those with personality defects can sometimes be totally unco-operative and their dental treatment may be severely compromised.

Epilepsy is often associated with other disabilities but with modern treatment should present no special difficulties. There may be problems with phenytoin-induced fibrous gingival hyperplasia (Ch. 5). It is also important to be able to recognise and manage a major fit, should it happen in the dental surgery (Ch. 36).

The importance of good prevention cannot be overemphasised. Many of the problems arising from treatment of people with disability would be solved by good preventive regimes.

Disabilities relevant to dentistry are summarised in Table 33.3.

Table 33.3 Common disabilities affecting dental management

- Intellectual impairment
  - Learning difficulty
  - Down's syndrome
  - Microcephaly and hydrocephalus
  - Metabolic disorders
  - Hypoxia at birth
  - Some syndromes
- Behavioural disorders
  - Autism
  - Attention deficit hyperactivity disorder
- Physical impairment
  - Cerebral palsy
  - Severe defects of the hands or arms
  - Muscular dystrophies
  - Spina bifida
  - Some syndromes
  - Communication problems: blindness and deafness
  - Cleft palate (Ch. 2)

Physical and intellectual impairment are frequently combined, as in Down's syndrome and some cases of cerebral palsy. Intellectual impairment (often associated with physical impairment) affects by far the largest group of children with disability needing dental care. All patients with Down's syndrome, many with cerebral palsy and some with epilepsy are also intellectually impaired. These four groups account for approximately 70–75% of children with disability. Conversely, many patients with cerebral palsy have normal intelligence but may be mislabelled as mentally impaired because of communication difficulties.

Heart disease, haemorrhagic disease (particularly haemophilia), diabetes mellitus and other systemic diseases are discussed in Chapters 26 to 32.

INTELLECTUAL IMPAIRMENT

Learning difficulty

Learning disability is an all-inclusive term to describe those with intellectual impairment whether caused by a specific disorder or of unknown cause. Down's syndrome, fragile X syndrome and hypoxia at birth are the more common causes and the specific features of these conditions are dealt with below. Learning difficulties may be unrelated to any physical disorder, or physical defects may be severe, as in some cases of cerebral palsy. A minority of patients with genetic syndromes have craniofacial anomalies associated with intellectual impairment.

Intellectual impairment is classified according to the level of learning difficulty and children are taught either in mainstream schools or special schools, according to the degree of impairment. Institutional care is avoided if possible. Unfortunately, the learning difficulty classification gives no more than a broad indication of probable problems with dental care because patients vary so widely.

Children with mild learning difficulty can usually be coaxed into accepting regular treatment and (if the parents are supportive) to maintain acceptable standards of oral hygiene. However, oral hygiene is usually suboptimal or poor when it depends on parents or carers. At the other extreme, all that may be possible, particularly for children with uncontrollable muscular activity such as jaw clenching, is first-aid dentistry under general anaesthesia. All intermediate grades exist, but the level of dental health that can be achieved depends greatly upon the level of the dentist's skill and devotion to the task (Fig. 33.1) and prevention by carers.

Down's syndrome

Down's syndrome is the most common clinically recognisable syndrome with severe learning difficulty. It is caused by trisomy of chromosome 21 giving a total complement of 47 chromosomes instead of 46. This is usually caused by failure of the chromo-

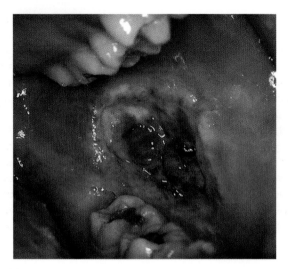

Fig. 33.1 Traumatic ulceration. This child with learning difficulties produced this deep and extensive ulcer after a local anaesthetic for dental treatment.

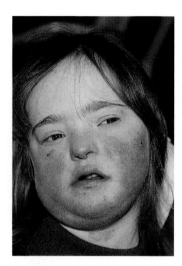

Fig. 33.2 Down's syndrome. This shows both the characteristic facial appearance and a cyanotic flush caused by associated congenital heart disease.

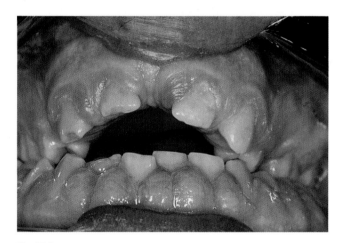

Fig. 33.3 Down's syndrome. This shows the characteristic anterior open bite together with gross gingival hyperplasia caused by phenytoin treatment for concomitant epilepsy.

somes to separate during meiosis in the ovum, a defect closely linked to maternal age. The overall incidence is 1 in 700 live births but the risk rises to 1 in 25 in mothers aged 45 years or over. Because the defect arises in the ovum, both parents are normal and the condition is not inherited.

In contrast, about 4% of Down's patients have the additional chromosome 21 genetic material translocated to another chromosome. The translocation is transmitted in a familial pattern but the parents are normal and the risk of an affected child is relatively low. In rare cases of mosaic Down's syndrome the trisomy arises during early development and the patients are a mosaic of cells with and without trisomy 21. In this type of Down's syndrome the features are very variable and intelligence may be normal despite the typical appearance.

General features

Down's children have a characteristic facial appearance (Fig. 33.2), abnormalities of the skull and frequently of the dentition, abnormal susceptibility to infection (particularly viral) due to multiple immune defects, and congenital cardiovascular disease in up to 50%.

The prominent medial epicanthic skin fold gives the eyes their readily recognisable appearance. There is hypoplasia of the mid-face, poorly developed paranasal sinuses and a malformed upper respiratory tract. Upper respiratory tract infections are common, and breathing is often snorting. Under-development of the maxillae is usually associated with a protrusive mandible and Class III malocclusion, with anterior open bite (Fig. 33.3, Table 33.4). The ears are often malformed and there is excess skin on the neck.

Upper lateral incisors are often absent and the teeth have short roots. Despite a higher than normal incidence of enamel hypoplasia, caries risk is low. The low caries activity has been ascribed to the form and spacing of the teeth and to the high

Table 33.4 Features of Down's syndrome relevant to dentistry

- Class III malocclusion with hypoplastic maxilla
- Protrusive, fissured and enlarged tongue (Fig. 33.4)
- Everted, thick, dry and crusted lips
- Oligodontia
- Delayed eruption of teeth
- Hypoplastic dental defects and short roots
- Low caries activity
- Gross plaque accumulation
- Rapidly progressive periodontal disease
- Large, protrusive tongue
- Bruxism
- Cleft palate in a minority
- Short stature with short limbs
- Poor muscle tone
- Generalised susceptibility to infection
- Cardiac anomalies in 40%
- Susceptibility to leukaemia
- Alzheimer-like dementia in later life

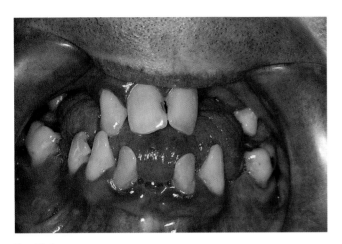

Fig. 33.4 Down's syndrome. As is frequently the case there are many missing teeth and in the gaps between them the over-large tongue is protruding.

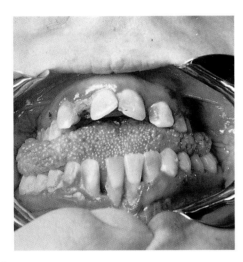

Fig. 33.5 Down's syndrome. Poor oral hygiene, periodontal destruction and malocclusion. (By kind permission of Professor C Scully.)

bicarbonate content and pH of the saliva. Despite the relative resistance, use of a sweetened dummy, poor diet or medications with sucrose can readily lead to caries.

Plaque accumulation and poor oral hygiene, due to the patient's disabilities and made worse by mouth breathing, together with the systemic predisposition to infection, contribute to the early onset of periodontal disease and early tooth loss (Fig. 33.5). Acute ulcerative gingivitis is also common and often recurs.

Management

All Down's children have learning difficulties, some severe, but they continue to learn throughout life and may develop many skills if supported by good educational programmes and occupational therapy. Some can maintain an independent life. Patients with Down's syndrome are often, but not invariably,

good-natured, co-operative within their ability, and affectionate and receptive to dental care. However, this stereotype ignores many who are frightened or more severely affected and completely unco-operative. The success of dental treatment mainly depends on the level of care provided. Those with milder learning disability can be treated normally in the dental chair, while the more severely affected, who are usually institutionalised, may require general anaesthesia.

Control of periodontal disease is usually difficult and success depends almost entirely on prevention by good oral hygiene. Teeth may be lost relatively early because of their short roots. Retention of teeth is important because dentures are usually poorly tolerated and retained because of the large protrusive tongue, poor muscle tone, and poor comprehension. The large tongue and muscle weakness cause problems with mastication and swallowing.

Other features of the syndrome may affect dental treatment. The unstable atlanto-occipital joint is at risk of dislocation with severe consequences if the head is manipulated, particularly during general anaesthesia or sedation. All Down's syndrome patients should have been screened for this anomaly during early childhood. Deafness and visual problems are common. With improved medical care life expectancy in Down's syndrome has lengthened and patients often live into their sixth decade. Unfortunately, almost half older Down's patients suffer an Alzheimer-like dementia which further compromises their independence.

Cardiac defects are present in 40% and half of these are severe enough to warrant surgical intervention. Atrial and ventricular septal defects, mitral and tricuspid valve defects, Fallot's tetralogy and patent ductus are common. These are repaired in childhood but in later life valvular regurgitation and prolapse may develop. Despite many contributory factors, the incidence of infective endocarditis does not appear to be particularly high, but prophylactic antibiotic cover must be given as for normal patients (Ch. 27).

Hydrocephalus

Hydrocephalus is caused by failure of drainage of cerebrospinal fluid and may be seen in isolation or associated with spina bifida. Compression of the cerebral tissue can cause severe intellectual impairment. Treatment is to relieve the intracranial pressure by insertion of a catheter and in the past this released the cerebrospinal fluid directly into the right atrium (Spitz–Holzer valve). This shunt is susceptible to infection, causing blockage rather than endocarditis. Although antibiotic prophylaxis is not of proven effectiveness, antibiotics are usually given as a precaution, using the same regime for infective endocarditis. Younger patients are more likely to have a shunt into the peritoneal cavity and this type does not require antibiotic prophylaxis. Severe hydrocephalus can also cause the skull to be so distended and heavy that the head has to be supported during treatment.

BEHAVIOURAL DISORDERS

Autism

Autism is a specific defect of mental development in which there is lack of emotional development, disordered use of language, defective communication and extreme 'aloneness'. The cause is unknown and both environmental and neuro-development causes are suspected. The condition is much more common in males. At one extreme there is severe learning disorder and repetitive behaviour so that it may be impossible to communicate with, or manage, autistic children without general anaesthesia. At the other, sympathy and patience may achieve all that is needed. Asperger's syndrome is the mildest form of autism.

Hyperactivity/attention deficit disorder

These conditions are often grouped together despite their different presentations. Attention deficit is characterised by day-dreaming, limited ability to concentrate and perform complex tasks. Hyperactivity is characterised by excessive movement, inability to concentrate on one task and, sometimes, repetitive movements. The number of children diagnosed with these conditions has risen dramatically since the advent of the drug methylphenidate (Ritalin) but there is no agreed dividing line between this disorder and normal child behaviour. Some cases seem to respond to dietary modification. It has been suggested that some children labelled as suffering hyperactivity/attention deficit are no more than mildly disruptive underachieving children. Such cases might be difficult dental patients but can be expected to respond to good behaviour management. Conversely, severe hyperactivity is profoundly disturbing and may be associated with self-mutilation. Extreme cases may require sedation or anaesthesia.

PHYSICAL IMPAIRMENT

Cerebral palsy

Cerebral palsy is common with an incidence of 1:1000 and can be one of the most severe disabilities. These children, in the past loosely referred to as spastics, suffer various types of neuromuscular dysfunction (Table 33.5).

Table 33.5 Types of cerebral palsy

- Spastic
- Athetotic
- Ataxic
- Hypotonic
- Mixed types

Neuromuscular dysfunction

Neuromuscular dysfunction can be so severe as to make speech unintelligible (dysarthria) and cause the children to appear intellectually impaired. Communication can sometimes be possible if dentists are prepared to spend time learning to comprehend them. Many cerebral palsy patients have visual speech-aids or computerised devices to help them communicate. Remarkably, some of these children, with otherwise incomprehensible speech, can understand one another.

Spasticity affects half the patients and causes fixed contraction of affected muscles and general stiffness. This may be so great that it may not even be possible to move an affected limb passively. Hemiplegia is the most common type: in such cases intellectual impairment is uncommon but other neurological disorders, such as epilepsy, are frequent. Quadriplegics, by contrast, are frequently intellectually impaired but less often epileptic. Athetosis refers to involuntary jerking movements, often of a wriggling character, sometimes accompanied by grimacing and is seen in almost half of patients.

Ataxia is least common and characterised by lack of balance, an unsteady gait and poor control over voluntary movements. In addition to variants of these three main types of disease, different parts of the body may be affected to a greater degree than others.

Dental aspects

Access to dental care for their wheelchairs is frequently difficult for those with cerebral palsy. Many have severe caries and often periodontal disease due to inability to maintain oral hygiene and their dental care is difficult, however willing they may be.

The first consideration is full assessment of the patient's capabilities. The child's ability to deal with dental disease can then be judged. If the child is uncontrollably anxious, sedation may help. If disabilities are not too severe, many of these children can be treated satisfactorily in the dental chair. The chief difficulty with athetotic children is their irregular movements. These may make it impossible to carry out good restorative work and also make it easy for the child to be injured with sharp dental instruments. The mildest cases may respond well to relaxation with inhalation sedation but some will need full sedation or general anaesthesia. It is always essential to use a mouth prop with conscious athetotic patients, as the jaws may suddenly clench. Epilepsy, falls and sudden uncontrolled movements also render them prone to dental injury. Bruxism and masseteric hypertrophy are frequent and drooling may result from the open mouth posture and defective swallowing. These latter complaints often most trouble these patients.

Many cerebral palsy patients suffer epilepsy and drug-induced gingival overgrowth. Key features are summarised in Table 33.6.

Spina bifida

Spina bifida is failure of fusion of the vertebral arches and may be inherited or environmental in aetiology. Approximately

Table 33.6 Key dental features of cerebral palsy

- Usually Class II malocclusion and anterior open bite
- Frequently severe caries and periodontal disease
- Bruxism and masseteric hypertrophy
- Impaired swallowing reflex but exaggerated gag reflex
- Dental erosion and gastric reflux
- Enamel hypoplasia
- Mouth breathing
- Dental trauma
- Delayed eruption
- Drooling

1:1000 children are affected. The mildest form (spina bifida occulta) is common but no more than a radiographic finding, sometimes with a tuft of hair overlying the defect. In the severe form (spina bifida cystica) there is a gross defect in the lower vertebral canal. The meninges and, often, nerve tissue protrude through it as a sac, which may be covered by skin. The consequences are paralysis and deformities of the lower limbs with loss of sensation and reflexes, incontinence and other complications. Meningitis is an obvious hazard and epilepsy is frequently associated. Hydrocephalus is associated in almost all cases.

Since the upper part of the body is normal, the main difficulty in dental management is getting a chair adapted to the child's disability. Associated epilepsy may also affect dental management.

Severe limb defects

These are rare but have been brought to public notice by the thalidomide tragedy. One of the striking effects of this drug is absence of the proximal part of a limb (phocomelia). Thus the hands, often also defective, are attached close to the shoulder.

These children can receive normal dental care, but are totally dependent on physical aids, parents or carers for tooth brushing. Again, preventive measures to minimise caries activity are important.

The muscular dystrophies

Muscular dystrophies, of which the Duchenne type is the most common (approximately 1 in 5000 male births), are the main crippling diseases of childhood. Weakness of the muscles leads to progressively severe disability and is frequently associated with cardiomyopathy and respiratory impairment.

There appear to be no specific dental problems other than that of stabilising a severely affected child in the chair. General anaesthesia is dangerous in the presence of cardiac disease or respiratory impairment.

THE ELDERLY

While the problems of looking after handicapped children centre largely on their physical and mental limitations, these are compounded in the elderly by the lack of parents or, often, carers to help them. Also, there is a great variety of oral complaints that they may suffer. In extreme cases for example, an elderly patient may be so intellectually impaired, deaf and depressed as to make communication excessively difficult but may also have oral cancer.

Communication is often the key problem in the management of the elderly. Factors which may exacerbate this problem are summarised in Table 33.7.

Table 33.7 Causes of disabilities in the elderly

Neurological and psychological disorders
- Intellectual deterioration
- Depression
- Dementia (particularly Alzheimer's disease)
- Confusional states
- Paranoia
- Dependence on hypnotics
- Parkinson's disease
- Strokes
- Deafness
- Impaired sight
- Trigeminal neuralgia (Ch. 34)

Mental deterioration is a common consequence of ageing and can affect all aspects of mental activity, such as intelligence, memory, emotional state and personality. These different functions tend to be affected to a variable and unpredictable extent. Thus the patient may seem bright enough but may immediately forget instructions, for example, about how to look after dentures. Other patients become confused, querulous, or even aggressive, behave in an irresponsible fashion, have delusions of persecution and are generally 'difficult'. Alzheimer's disease, the most common cause of dementia after middle age, can present in any of these ways.

In general, the older the patients, the less adaptable they are likely to be. While preservation of teeth for as long as possible may be desirable, it may create greater problems if extractions have to be postponed until late in life. The wearing of full dentures demands a remarkable feat of adaptation at any age, and older patients face greater difficulties. Also, some older patients may no longer care about appearance, may have few social contacts and may prefer a soft diet. Motivation, which plays so large a part in adaptation to denture wearing, may also therefore be diminished.

Difficulties with and complaints about dentures by elderly patients may therefore be as much due to mental deterioration as physical problems. Poor communication, often due to deafness, makes matters worse. Exasperating though such complaints may become, they must be treated with understanding and sympathy. This mental deterioration is something we all have to suffer if we live long enough; in the words of a physician '*insightless atrophy and ultimate obliteration of normal mental life ... is a remorseless enemy of the natural dignity of man*'.

Limitations on mobility

Conditions which may make it difficult for the elderly to attend for dental treatment are summarised in Table 33.8.

Table 33.8   Some causes of limitation of mobility in the elderly

- Ataxia
- Strokes
- Arthritis
- Heart disease

Systemic disease in the elderly

Systemic diseases which particularly affect the elderly are shown in Table 33.9.

A variety of drugs used for cardiovascular disease can also cause oral reactions (Ch. 15). As noted earlier, the elderly with heart lesions are at the highest risk for infective endocarditis and form the peak age group for this disease.

Malnutrition is particularly likely to affect the elderly. Poverty, poor mobility (which interferes with both cooking and shopping), and mental deterioration are some of the contributory factors. Poorly functioning dentures and impairment of taste sensation may make matters worse.

However, deficiency states, particularly scurvy and vitamin B group deficiencies, are remarkably rare nowadays, even in old age. It is important, nevertheless, that denture function should be the best possible in order not to worsen nutritional problems in older patients.

Pernicious anaemia due to impaired absorption of vitamin B_{12} is mainly seen after middle age. Iron deficiency often persists into later life or may be made worse by defects of absorption.

These conditions can cause oral signs and symptoms, particularly sore tongue (Ch. 14). Sore tongue or signs of atrophy of the mucosa should be investigated by haematological examination.

Some causes of systemic disease which particularly affect the elderly and may complicate dental management are summarized in Table 33.9.

Parkinson's disease

This common disease is characterised by rigidity, often most obvious as a mask-like fixity of facial expression, tremor sometimes affecting the lower jaw, and often dribbling as a result of impaired neuromuscular function.

Parkinson's disease, which affects the basal ganglia, may be associated (because of the age of affected patients) with, but is not a cause of, intellectual deterioration. However, the poverty of facial expression, which is easily mistaken for in-comprehension, and the defective speech often unjustly suggest impaired mental function. It is essential to take care therefore not to offend a patient with Parkinson's disease by making such an assumption.

Table 33.9   Important systemic diseases more common in the elderly

- Cardiovascular disease
  Hypertension and ischaemic heart disease (Ch. 20)
  Cardiac failure (any cause) (Ch. 20)
  Giant-cell (temporal) arteritis and polymyalgia rheumatica (Ch. 11)
- Respiratory disease
  Chronic bronchitis and emphysema
  Pneumonia
- Haematological
  Anaemia (especially pernicious anaemia) (Ch. 20)
  Chronic leukaemia (Ch. 20)
  Myeloma (Ch. 11)
- Neurological
  Parkinson's disease
  Trigeminal neuralgia
  Post-herpetic neuralgia
  Dementia
- Carcinomas (all sites)

Parkinson's disease can also cause difficulty with the management of dentures because of the loss of fine control of muscular movement. If there is also intellectual deterioration, the difficulties are proportionately increased.

The effects of Parkinson's disease can be diminished by giving anticholinergic drugs such as benzohexol (Artane), which tend to cause a dry mouth. But more effective are dopaminic agents such as levodopa.

Cardiovascular disease

It may be worthwhile to emphasise that the elderly are overall at the highest risk from infective endocarditis. A possible contribution to this is periodontal sepsis. In addition, drugs given for cardiovascular disease can be a cause of oral lesions (Ch. 27).

Oral disease in the elderly

To much greater extent than in the handicapped child, oral disease is likely to require considerably more attention. It comprises the categories in Table 33.10.

Table 33.10   Age changes in the mouth and jaws

- Wear and tear of teeth
- Periodontal sepsis and bone loss
- Possibly diminished salivary function
- Pain or difficulties with dentures
- Mucosal disease

All of these are important in varying degree, but the main dental need of most elderly patients is the provision of effective and comfortable dentures. Elderly patients tend to become even more infrequent visitors to the dentist than they once were, especially when dentures have been provided. As a consequence, cancer of the mouth, which both becomes more common as age advances and is insidious in development, is particularly likely to be missed in its earlier stages. The majority of cases of cancer of the mouth are at an advanced stage by the time they come for treatment.

The teeth

The teeth can undergo attrition, abrasion and, frequently, continued destruction by caries (Chs 3 and 4).

The roots gradually also become hypercalcified by progressive obliteration of the dentinal tubules. The roots may as a consequence become completely calcified and more brittle, so that they are more likely to fracture during extraction.

The periodontal tissues and jaws

In the edentulous elderly, progressive loss of denture-bearing bone brings with it the well-known difficulties, particularly retention and stabilisation of dentures. Later, as excessive amounts of bone become resorbed, pain can be caused by the dentures pressing upon anatomical structures, such as the mylohyoid ridge or genial tubercles, which become prominent after loss of overlying bone.

The temporomandibular joints

Though osteoarthritis of weight-bearing joints is a common and often disabling disease as age advances, osteoarthritis of the temporomandibular joints is not a significant problem. The condition is uncommon and only likely to be an incidental finding in radiographs and rarely causes pain (Ch. 11).

Pain or other symptoms from the temporomandibular joints in the elderly are remarkably uncommon. However, pain on mastication may be due to temporal arteritis and if so, requires urgent treatment, because of the risk of loss of sight (Ch. 11).

Salivary function

Evidence that salivary secretion diminishes with age has not been confirmed in all studies. However, depressed salivary flow is overall more common in the elderly as a result of such causes as Sjögren's syndrome or the use of drugs with antimuscarinic activity (Ch. 19).

Elderly patients who have a dry mouth must therefore be investigated accordingly.

Problems affecting denture-wearers

Between the ages of 55 and 64, the proportion of the population who are edentulous in the UK as a whole is 37%, but 53% in Northern England, and higher still in the lower socioeconomic groups.

Though mastication with dentures is less efficient than with healthy teeth, this seems to matter little, and most denture wearers suffer no more than discomfort or social embarrassment from time to time. Dietary deficiencies in the elderly are likely to be due to poverty or to inability to prepare an adequate diet.

Other troubles affecting the denture wearer may be due to faults in the denture itself or to some condition underlying it. Causes of discomfort or pain relating to dentures are summarised in Table 33.11, but cancer in particular must be excluded as it becomes increasingly common as age advances.

Table 33.11 Important causes of pain and other lesions under dentures

- Traumatic ulcers
- Denture hyperplasia
- Denture stomatitis
- Angular stomatitis
- Papillary palatal hyperplasia
- Frictional keratosis and other hyperkeratotic lesions
- Buried teeth, roots, or (rarely) odontomas
- Cysts, particularly residual and, less often, keratocysts
- Carcinoma
- Paget's disease
- Fracture of the jaws (uncommon but a possibility with a heavily resorbed mandible)

It must be emphasised therefore that the cause of progressive complaints about dentures must be looked for and not simply evaded by repeated 'eases' (see Ch. 34).

Mucosal diseases in the elderly

Some changes in the oral mucosa are directly related to age. Examples include Fordyce's granules, lingual varicosities and enlarged foliate papillae (Ch. 2). These are often causes of anxiety in the elderly who need to be reassured.

Mucosal diseases that may affect the elderly are summarised in Table 33.12 and discussed in more detail in Chapter 15.

It must be emphasised that recurrent aphthae are uncommon in older persons but when seen it is important to look for some underlying cause such as pernicious anaemia.

Table 33.12 Mucosal diseases in the elderly

- Lichen planus
- Mucous membrane pemphigoid
- Pemphigus vulgaris
- Herpes zoster
- Glossitis
- Burning mouth syndrome
- Carcinoma
- Leukoplakia

Radiation injury

Because of the rising frequency of carcinoma with advancing age, the elderly are more likely than the young to have had radiotherapy. They may therefore suffer from xerostomia or be at risk from osteoradionecrosis. Denture trauma can occasionally precipitate this complication, and experts in this field may not permit patients to wear lower dentures after radiotherapy (Ch. 22).

Factors affecting dental care of the elderly

Many factors limit the mobility of elderly patients who are frequently arthritic, may be unsteady on their feet, unwell for a variety of reasons or simply be unable to afford the cost of dental care or transportation. Arthritis of the hands may also make oral hygiene difficult or defective.

Illustrative of the dental problems of the elderly have been the findings in a survey of inhabitants of a residential home, 12% had denture stomatitis, 3% had oral ulcers, 19 of 1041 had red or white lesions, 250 had difficulty with eating, 206 had impaired taste, and 241 had difficulty caring for their mouths. Only 4% of dentate and 20% of edentulous persons had seen a dentist in the past 2 years. No systematic dental care was provided, or dental assessments made before admission. Domiciliary dental care of the elderly is even more inadequate.

SUGGESTED FURTHER READING

Cumming C G, Wight C, Blackwell C L et al 1989 Debenture stomatitis in the elderly. Oral Microbiol Immunol 5:82–85

Fiske J, Shafik H H 2001 Down's syndrome and oral care. Dental Update 2001 28:148–156

Flint S, Scully C 1988 Orofacial age changes and related disease. Dental Update 15:337–341

Hammond J 1996 Cerebral palsy. Medicine UK 24:82–84

Hildebolt O F 1997 Osteoporosis and oral bone loss. Dentomaxillofacial Radiol 26:3–15

Hollins S, Howlin P 1996 Learning disability and autism. Medicine UK 24:47–48

Ibbetson R J, Setchell D J 1989 Treatment of the worn dentition: 1 & 2. Dental Update 16:247–252, 300–304

Moore R S, Hobson P 1989 A classification of medically handicapping conditions and the health risks they present in the dental care of children. Part I — Cardiovascular, haematological and respiratory disorders. J Paediatr Dent 5:73–83

Moore R S, Hobson P 1989 A classification of medically handicapping conditions and the health risks they present in the dental care of children. Part II — Neoplastic, renal, endocrine, metabolic, hepatic, musculoskeletal, neuromuscular, central nervous system and skin disorders. J Paediatr Dent 6:1–14

Mouradian W E, Wehr E, Crall J J 2000 Disparities in children's oral health care and access to dental care. JAMA 284:2625–2631

Nunn J 2000 *Disability and oral care.* International Association for Disability and Oral Health/FDI World Dental Press, London

Sheiham A 1990 Dentistry for an ageing population: responsibilities and future trends. Dental Update 17:70–75

Simons D, Kidd E A M, Beighton D 2000 Oral health of elderly occupants in residential homes. Lancet 353:1761

Smith D G, Seymour R A 1988 Periodontal disease and treatment in the elderly. Dental Update 15:18–22

Walls A W G, Barnes I E 1988 Gerodontology: the problem? Dental Update 15:186–190

Walls A W G, Barnes I E 1989 Treatment planning for the ageing patient. Dental Update 16:438–443

Ward-Booth P 1988 Oral surgery for the older patient. Dental Update 15:410–414

Pain, anxiety and neurological disorders

'... within my private knowledge, two persons who had suffered alike from toothache and cancer, have pronounced the former to be on the scale of torture, by many degrees to be the worse'

Confessions of an English Opium Eater Thomas de Quincey 1821

Pain is the most common symptom for which patients seek help. Approximately 40% of the British population only visit a dentist for pain relief. Toothache can be so agonisingly severe that De Quincey, as well as quoting the opinions shown above, also claimed that it had made him dependent on opium. In the lay mind dentistry and pain are inseparable and there is the persistent belief that dental treatment is necessarily painful. This belief emphasises the important point that pain has strong emotional associations which, in turn, may be determined to a varying degree by patients' preconceptions. Emotional disturbance itself can also produce the symptom of physical pain.

There are many causes of oral or maxillofacial pain (Table 34.1). Pulpitis and periapical periodontitis as sequels of dental caries are by far the most common causes. The source of such pain is usually obvious on examination but some sources of dental pain can be exceedingly difficult to identify (Table 34.2).

These account for most causes of pain in this area. Disease of the teeth (usually the result of dental caries) and adjacent tissues must always be excluded in the investigation of pain.

Table 34.1 Causes of pain felt in the oral tissues

- Disease of teeth and/or supporting tissues
- Oral mucosal diseases
- Diseases of the jaw
- Pain in the edentulous patient
- Postoperative pain
- Pain triggered by mastication
- Referred pain
- Neurological diseases
- Psychogenic (atypical) facial pain

Table 34.2 Causes of pain from the teeth or supporting tissues

- Pulpitis
- Dentine hypersensitivity, cracked tooth or cracked cusp syndrome
- Periapical periodontitis
- Lateral (periodontal) abscess
- Acute necrotising ulcerative gingivitis
- HIV-associated periodontitis
- Pericoronitis

Pulpitis

Pulpitis is usually the cause when hot or cold food or drinks trigger the pain. It is also the main cause of spasmodic, poorly localised attacks of pain which may be mistaken for a variety of other possible causes. The pain of acute pulpitis is of a sharp lancinating character peculiar to itself, impossible to describe but unforgettable once experienced. Recurrent attacks of less severe, subacute or chronic pain, often apparently spontaneous, suggest a diseased and dying pulp.

Investigation of pulpitis has been discussed earlier (Ch. 4). The only non-dental condition that is indistinguishable from pulp pain by the patient is the pain of *herpes zoster* (Ch. 12). If no local cause can be found after the most careful search, it is important to look for early signs of the characteristic rash. Herpes zoster is an uncommon cause of toothache-like pain, but countless teeth have been extracted in patients with zoster under the mistaken impression that the pain was dental.

Acute periodontitis

Pain from acute periapical periodontitis should be readily identifiable as there is precisely localised tenderness of the tooth in its socket. Radiographs are of little value in the early stages but useful after sufficient destruction shows itself as loss of definition of the periapical lamina dura. In other cases, acute inflammation may supervene on chronic, and a rounded area of radiolucency is seen.

Acute maxillary sinusitis can rarely cause similar tenderness of a group of teeth, particularly upper molars, as discussed later.

Lateral, periodontal abscess

The tooth is tender in its socket, but is usually vital and there is deep localised pocketing (Ch. 6). Occasionally both a periodontal and periapical abscess may form together on a non-vital tooth with severe periodontal disease, or a periodontal abscess may be precipitated by endodontic treatment when a reamer perforates the side of the root.

Acute necrotising ulcerative gingivitis and HIV-associated necrotising periodontitis

Acute ulcerative gingivitis usually causes soreness, but when it extends deeply and rapidly, destroying the underlying bone, there may be severe aching pain. In such cases the diagnosis is usually obvious clinically. HIV-associated periodontitis presents a somewhat similar picture and is acutely painful.

Acute pericoronitis

Pericoronitis usually produces a characteristic clinical picture (Ch. 6).

Painful mucosal lesions

Ulcers generally cause soreness rather than pain, but deep ulceration may cause severe aching pain. Carcinoma in particular causes severe pain once nerve fibres become involved. It is important to emphasise again that early carcinoma is *painless*; pain is a late symptom. By the time that pain becomes troublesome the tumour is usually easily seen unless it is far back in the mouth.

As mentioned above, *Herpes zoster* causes severe aching pain, sometimes indistinguishable from toothache, because of involvement of cervical ganglia (Ch. 12).

Painful jaw diseases

The important feature of these conditions (Table 34.3) is that, as well as the history and clinical presentation, the provisional diagnosis depends on the radiographic findings. Fractures and osteomyelitis should be recognisable by such means. Other lesions of the jaws, by contrast, sometimes have less clearcut clinical and radiographic features, and the differentiation of (say) an infected cyst from a malignant tumour may be difficult.

Table 34.3 Painful jaw diseases

- Fractures
- Osteomyelitis
- Infected cysts
- Malignant neoplasms
- Sickle cell infarcts

With the exception of fractures and osteomyelitis, diagnosis then depends on biopsy and histological examination.

Pain in edentulous patients

These conditions (Table 34.4) differ from most others because dental causes can be excluded. The chief difficulty is to decide whether the pain is due to the dentures themselves, or to some condition of the mucosa or jaws on which a denture is pressing.

Table 34.4 Important causes of pain in edentulous patients

- Denture trauma
- Excessive vertical dimension
- Diseases (enumerated earlier) of the denture-bearing mucosa
- Diseases of the jaws (Table 34.3)
- Teeth or roots erupting under a denture

Traumatic ulcers, usually the consequence of over-extension, often cause trouble with a new denture. After the denture has been relieved, these ulcers heal within 24–48 hours. Persistent ulceration after adequate relief of the denture is likely to be due to some more serious cause, particularly a neoplasm. Biopsy is then essential. Later, dentures cause traumatic pain when the bone has become severely resorbed, allowing the denture to bear on the mylohyoid ridge or genial tubercles. These result from the patients' having worn the denture too long, and a well-designed replacement is necessary.

Lack of freeway space due to excessive vertical dimension of the dentures prevents the mandible and masticatory muscles from reaching their natural rest position. This causes the teeth to be held permanently in contact. Aching pain is usually felt in the fatigued masticatory muscles, but the excessive stress imposed on the denture-bearing area sometimes causes pain in this region. Very occasionally patients seem unable to tolerate dentures, however carefully they are constructed and complain of such symptoms as gripping, burning, or 'drawing' pain, particularly under the upper denture. These symptoms are not associated with any physical changes and are psychogenic.

It is usually straightforward to decide whether pain is caused by the dentures themselves or by some lesion under the dentures. Denture stomatitis is painless, but surprisingly few other mucosal diseases affect the denture-bearing area itself. Lichen planus can extend to the sulcus and impinge on the margin of the denture-bearing area. The most important condition to be excluded is *carcinoma*, either affecting the alveolar margin or in the labial or buccal sulcus, or floor of the mouth. Persistent lesions, whether ulcerated or not, developing beneath or at the margins of dentures, must be biopsied without hesitation, as it is in the edentulous age-group that the incidence of carcinoma is highest. A carcinoma can persist for a long time with minimal symptoms, and the patient may notice no more than the fact that the fit of the denture has deteriorated.

Jaw lesions causing pain in the edentulous patient may be associated with a swelling or an area of radiolucency and have been discussed above. A painful swelling of the jaw in the edentulous patient is probably most often due to an infected residual cyst. Malignant tumours are very much less common but must be considered, as they cannot be reliably distinguished from cysts and other benign conditions by radiography alone. Histological examination is therefore essential. Osteomyelitis of the jaws in edentulous patients must be considered virtually only in those who have had radiotherapy to this region. In such patients denture ulceration can allow infection to penetrate and set up persistent painful chronic osteomyelitis of the ischaemic bone.

Retained roots or, rarely, late eruption of buried teeth beneath a denture become painful as they reach the surface, causing the mucosa to be pinched between them and the denture. This trouble will be obvious on clinical or radiographic examination, as are the late effects of a healed malaligned fracture.

Postoperative pain

Important causes are summarised in Table 34.5. By far the most common cause of pain after dental extractions is *alveolar osteitis (dry socket)*, which can usually be recognised on clinical examination (Ch. 6). Fracture of the jaw following operative treatment is rare but can also be recognised from the history, and by clinical and radiographic examination. Forcible opening of the mouth under general anaesthesia, particularly for removing wisdom teeth, can damage the temporomandibular joint and lead to persistent pain on opening or during mastication. Postoperative osteomyelitis should be a thing of the past but could develop in an immunodeficient patient with, for example, unrecognised leukaemia.

Table 34.5 Postoperative pain

- Alveolar osteitis (dry socket)
- Fracture of the jaw
- Damage to the temporomandibular joint
- Osteomyelitis
- Damage to nerve trunks or involvement of nerves in scar tissue

---

Persistent postoperative pain is sometimes ascribed to damage to nerve fibres either as a result of operative trauma or by involvement in scar tissue. However, if there is no objective evidence of disturbed sensation there is little or nothing abnormal to be found. Operative intervention in the attempt to relieve such pain may do more harm than good. In some such cases there is complaint of persistent pain unresponsive to treatment but without any organic cause.

Rarely damaged nerve tissue may proliferate to form a traumatic neuroma, which is tender to pressure. Its excision should lead to relief of the pain. However, meticulous investigation of postoperative pain is important as it is a major cause of medicolegal claims.

Pain induced by mastication

The common dental cause for pain on mastication is apical periodontitis, but any conditions which causes the tooth to be

---

Table 34.6 Pain induced by mastication

- Diseases of teeth and supporting tissues
- Pain dysfunction syndrome
- Diseases of the temporomandibular joint
- Temporal arteritis
- Trigeminal neuralgia (rarely)
- Salivary calculi

---

tender in its socket, whether it be a lateral periodontal abscess or, occasionally, maxillary sinusitis, can cause this symptom (Table 34.6).

The *least* common cause of pain during eating is organic disease of the temporomandibular joint. Pain during eating comes much more frequently from the many other structures involved.

Fractures and dislocations of the temporomandibular joint are usually obvious from the history, their effects on the occlusion and the radiographic changes (Ch. 11).

Pain dysfunction syndrome usually causes dull, aching pain, often associated with clicking sounds from the joint, episodes of locking and some limitation of opening, in varying combinations. Young women are predominantly affected and there is typically a strong neurotic element.

The typical manifestation of temporal (giant-cell) arteritis is headache. However, it is also a cause of masticatory pain and should be considered particularly in patients over middle age with this symptom. The pain is due to ischaemia of the masticatory muscles, caused by the arteritis and is comparable to intermittent claudication (Ch. 11). Corticosteroids are effective in controlling the disease and relieving symptoms. They should be given when there is headache or masticatory pain associated with a tender scalp vessel and a high ESR.

The characteristic pain of trigeminal neuralgia is occasionally triggered by mastication. Trigeminal neuralgia may then be misdiagnosed as dental or due to pain dysfunction syndrome. However, the quality of these types of pain is quite different, as discussed later.

Calculi, particularly when obstructing the parotid duct, can cause pain when salivation is triggered by eating. Hence the history of the relationship of the pain to stimulation of salivation is distinctive.

Pain from extraoral disease

Extraoral causes of pain are summarised in Table 34.7.

Antral disease can cause pain felt in the upper teeth but a sinus radiograph should provide the diagnosis. Salivary gland and ear diseases typically cause preauricular pain. They may simulate temporomandibular joint symptoms but are rarely mistaken for dental problems.

Acute sinusitis is the most common paranasal disease that causes facial pain but antral carcinoma is rare (Ch. 28).

Mumps is a common cause of pain from, and swelling of, the parotid glands. In children the diagnosis is usually quickly

Table 34.7 Pain from extraoral disease

- Diseases of the maxillary antrum
  Acute sinusitis
  Carcinoma, particularly when it involves the antral floor
- Diseases of salivary glands
  Acute parotitis
  Salivary calculi (see above)
  Sjögren's syndrome
  Malignant neoplasms
- Diseases of the ears
  Otitis media
  Neoplasms in this region
- Myocardial infarction

made on clinical grounds. In adults the diagnosis may not be immediately suspected and, occasionally, these patients think they have dental disease.

Suppurative parotitis is uncommon but may be a complication of dry mouth. Acute parotitis may therefore be seen as a complication of Sjögren's syndrome or irradiation damage to the glands. Sjögren's syndrome itself can occasionally cause parotid pain and swelling of the glands (Ch. 18)

Swelling rather than pain is usually the first symptom of malignant tumours of salivary glands. Parotid gland tumours can also cause facial palsy and, finally, ulceration and fungation.

Myocardial infarction usually causes constricting or crushing pain substernally, but pain may radiate down the inside of the left arm or up into the neck or jaw. Rarely, cardiac pain is felt in the jaw alone. There is even a case on record where a dentist recognised the cardiac cause of jaw pain to the dismay of his patient, who was a cardiologist. This pain can come on at any time, at rest or during exercise. The clinical picture is variable, but in typical cases the patient is obviously anxious, pale and sweating with a rapid pulse and low blood pressure.

Intracranial and psychological disorders

Trigeminal neuralgia is one of the most important of these conditions (Table 34.8).

Table 34.8 Painful intracranial and psychological disorders

- Trigeminal neuralgia
- Multiple sclerosis
- Herpes zoster
- Postherpetic neuralgia
- Migrainous neuralgia
- Intracranial tumours
- Bell's palsy
- Psychogenic pain (atypical facial pain)

Trigeminal neuralgia

Typical features are summarised in Table 34.9. Elderly patients are affected, and though the pain is excruciatingly severe, there

is complete, or almost complete, relief between spasms. During an attack the patient's face is often distorted with anguish, while between attacks the patient may appear apprehensive at the thought of recurrence. The severity of the pain may also make the patient depressed.

Table 34.9 Typical features of trigeminal neuralgia

- Pain confined to the distribution of one or more divisions of the trigeminal nerve
- Pain is paroxysmal and very severe
- Trigger zones in the area
- Absence of objective sensory loss
- Absence of detectable organic cause

The pain is paroxysmal, i.e. severe, sharp and stabbing in character, but lasts only seconds or minutes and may be described as like lightning. However, attacks may sometimes be quickly recurrent at short intervals. Stimuli to an area (trigger zone) within the distribution of the trigeminal nerve can provoke an attack. Common stimuli are touching, draughts of cold air, or toothbrushing. Occasionally, masticatory effort induces the pain.

There are no objective signs. Either the second or third division of the trigeminal nerve is usually first affected, but pain soon involves both. The first division is rarely affected and pain does not spread to the opposite side. Less typical features of trigeminal neuralgia which make diagnosis difficult are more continuous, long-lasting, burning or aching pain, absence of trigger zones, and extension of the pain beyond the margins of the trigeminal area, though not to the opposite side.

Typically, the disease undergoes spontaneous remissions, with freedom from pain for weeks or months. These remissions may make it difficult to decide whether treatment has been effective.

Diagnosis

In typical cases the diagnosis should be readily made from the features described. In some patients multiple sclerosis should be excluded. A careful search should be made for diseased teeth, though pain of this severity is unlikely to be due to dental disease. An inflamed pulp can cause stabs of severe pain in its early stages, but the pain changes in character and soon becomes more prolonged. Pulpitis can usually also be identified as toothache by most patients and is felt to be different in character from pain in the face due to neuralgia. Any diseased teeth should of course be treated, though this does not affect the neuralgia. In the absence of disease, teeth should not be arbitrarily extracted, as this only adds to the patient's misfortunes. Pulp stones in particular, seen on a radiograph, are not a reason for extracting teeth.

Treatment

The most effective drugs are anticonvulsants, particularly carbamazepine and to a lesser extent phenytoin. Carbamazepine, with or without phenytoin, will usually relieve the pain, at least for a time. The action seems specific and other types of pain are not relieved. Abolition of the pain of trigeminal neuralgia by giving an anticonvulsant, such as carbamazepine, also helps to confirm the diagnosis. Carbamazepine (100 mg/day gradually raised if necessary to 800 mg/day) must be given long-term (essentially prophylactically) to reduce the frequency and severity of attacks. If a patient has trigeminal neuralgia which appears unresponsive to carbamazepine it sometimes transpires that instructions about continuous use have either not been given or not understood so that the drug has been used as if it were an analgesic. Up to 80% of patients are relieved of pain partly or completely by carbamazepine, but minor side-effects are common. Drowsiness, dryness of the mouth, giddiness, diarrhoea, and nausea are all to some extent dose-related. A small initial dose should therefore be given and gradually raised as necessary. In some patients tolerance to the side-effects may develop. Leucopenia is a rare toxic effect.

Surgical treatment. A few patients are unresponsive to carbamazepine or cannot tolerate the side-effects. If drug treatment fails, the final resort is surgery. The simplest option is cryotherapy to the trigeminal nerve or, if this fails, cryotherapy at the base of the skull. If these fail, microvascular decompression of the trigeminal ganglion may be required. This operation requires great skill and a mortality of 1% has been noted in some studies. In a series of over 1000 patients treated in this way in the US, the mortality was 0.2%, 30% had recurrences of pain and 11% underwent a second operation. Overall it was claimed that 70% of the patients were pain-free without medication 10 years postoperatively.

Glossopharyngeal neuralgia

This rare condition is characterised by pain similar to that of trigeminal neuralgia but felt in the base of the tongue and fauces on one side. It may also radiate deeply into the ear. The pain, which is sharp, lancinating and transient, is typically triggered by swallowing, chewing, or coughing. It may be so severe that patients may be terrified to swallow their saliva and try to keep the mouth and tongue as completely immobile as possible. Glossopharyngeal neuralgia sometimes responds to carbamazepine, but less often than trigeminal neuralgia. Once an organic cause has been excluded, surgical treatment may be needed. However, like trigeminal neuralgia, there can be spontaneous remissions, sometimes for years.

Postherpetic neuralgia

Up to 10% of patients who have had trigeminal herpes zoster, particularly if elderly, may develop persistent neuralgia. The pain is more variable in character and severity than trigeminal neuralgia. It is typically persistent rather than paroxysmal. The diagnosis is straightforward if there is a history of facial zoster or if scars from the rash are present.

Unfortunately, postherpetic neuralgia is remarkably resistant to treatment. Nerve or root section are ineffective and the response to drugs of any type, including carbamazepine, is poor. When pain is severe, large doses of analgesics can be given, and may give relief. Application of transcutaneous electrical stimulation to the affected area by the patient himself is sometimes effective. The instrument is applied hourly for 5–10 minutes every day, and persistent bombardment of the sensory pathways by the stimulator may prevent perception of pain centrally.

Multiple sclerosis

A minority of patients with multiple sclerosis have pain indistinguishable from trigeminal neuralgia, usually as a late symptom. Between 2% and 3% of patients with 'classical' symptoms of trigeminal neuralgia may have multiple sclerosis, but younger persons (under 50) are typically affected. In about 30%, pain, unlike trigeminal neuralgia, may be persistent and lack trigger zones, or may spread beyond the trigeminal area. Disturbances of sensation are capriciously distributed according to the sites of lesions in the brain. The lip may be affected and symptoms may range from paraesthesia to extreme hypersensitivity, whereby the patient will literally jump or scream with pain if the lip is touched.

The diagnosis usually depends on the presence of multiple deficits, particularly defects of vision, weakness of the limbs, and sensory losses. Disturbed sensation in the trigeminal area is likely only to be seen in patients with advanced disease and multiple paralyses. There is unlikely to be any doubt about the diagnosis as a consequence.

Carbamazepine is sometimes effective for trigeminal neuralgia-like pain, otherwise surgical treatment as for trigeminal neuralgia may be required.

Migrainous neuralgia (cluster headache)

Migrainous neuralgia is caused by vascular changes at the base of the skull and may occasionally be mistaken for trigeminal neuralgia. It is rarely seen in dental practice. Migrainous neuralgia has many features in common with classical migraine (hemicrania) and is due to oedema and dilatation of the wall of the internal carotid and probably also the external carotid arteries.

Cluster headache mainly affects men, usually young adults but up to the age of 50. Attacks may be precipitated by alcohol or vasodilators, or come on spontaneously one to three times a day. Attacks sometimes recur at precisely the same time each day or may disturb sleep. Pain is localised to the region of the orbit, or maxilla. The duration is 0.5–2 hours. Obvious vascular changes in the affected side of the face typically accompany the pain. The eye may become suffused and water, the nostrils may be blocked, the skin over the cheek may become red and there may be sweating on that side. After one to several months there is usually sudden and spontaneous complete remission and the patient remains completely free from pain for months, or even years. An uncommon variant of cluster headache is a chronic variety with attacks confined to the cheek or lower jaw, known as *lower half headache*.

Unlike migraine, there are neither visual symptoms nor nausea or vomiting. Cluster headache may respond to simple analgesics or to ergotamine. Ergotamine should be given an hour before the expected attack and is most effective by subcutaneous injection or by suppository. Alternatively, ergotamine powder can be inhaled from a spinhaler. Success depends on an accurate idea of the timing of the attacks, and two or three doses a day for the duration of the cluster of attacks may be necessary. Treatment should preferably be stopped for one day each week to see whether there has been spontaneous remission. Sumatriptan or indomethacin may be more effective.

In a double blind trial, intranasal lidocaine (4%) has been shown to provide rapid relief from the headache of classical migraine in approximately 55% of patients. The effectiveness of this treatment for migrainous neuralgia is not known but it is simple and safe, and worth a trial.

Intracranial tumours

Pain resembling trigeminal neuralgia can rarely be caused by intracranial tumours. Features suggesting an intracranial lesion are associated sensory loss especially if associated with cranial nerve palsies. Frequently, anatomically related nerves (especially III, IV and VI, causing disordered oculomotor function) are affected. Pain associated with neurological deficits in the area is known as trigeminal neuropathy.

Bell's palsy

As discussed later, facial paralysis is the predominant and most troublesome feature. In about 50% pain, usually in or near the ear but sometimes spreading down the jaw, either precedes or develops at the same time as the facial palsy. Rarely, a patient with early Bell's palsy seeks a dental opinion for the pain felt in the jaw, since this may precede paralysis by several days.

Psychogenic (atypical) facial pain

Pain is not a simple sensation, but has been described as the unpleasant experience felt 'when hurt in body or mind'. The psychological aspects of pain are often overwhelmingly important, and the patient's reaction is affected by such factors as mood, emotional characteristics, personality and cultural background. At one extreme a footballer may receive a relatively severe injury in the middle of a game without feeling it. At the other extreme there are patients who complain bitterly and persistently about trivial lesions. Pain causes emotional disturbance, and prolonged severe pain, as in rheumatoid arthritis, can cause depression. There are many patients whose facial pain is psychogenic rather than organic in nature.

It must be emphasised that the diagnosis of psychogenic facial pain is a diagnosis by exclusion, but it is important to try

Table 34.10 Features suggestive of psychogenic (atypical) facial pain

- Women of middle age or older mainly affected
- Absence of organic signs
- Pain often poorly localised
- Description of pain may be bizarre
- Delusional symptoms occasionally associated
- Lack of response to analgesics
- Unchanging pain persisting for many years
- Lack of any triggering factors
- Sometimes good response to antidepressive treatment

to recognise the condition, however limited diagnostic methods may be. The symptoms (Table 34.10) cause real enough suffering to the patient and should if possible be relieved. It is also important to avoid unnecessary surgery.

A common site for the pain is the maxillary region or in relation to the upper teeth, but localisation may not be precise or in a recognisable anatomical pattern. The description of the pain may be vague, bizarre ('drawing' or 'gripping') or exaggerated ('unbearable') but without obvious effect on the patient's health. It is often described as having been continuous, even unremitting and unchanging for several years.

Pain is usually not provoked by any recognisable stimulus such as hot or cold foods or by mastication. Despite the fact that the pain may be said to be continuous and unbearable, the patient's sleeping or even eating may be unaffected. Analgesics are often said to be completely ineffective, but some patients have not even tried them, despite the stated severity of the pain. Objective signs of disease are absent. Although teeth have often been extracted and diseased teeth may be present, none of these can be related to the pain. As a consequence, treatment of diseased teeth does not relieve the symptoms.

Other signs of emotional disturbance are highly variable. Some patients are more or less obviously depressed; some of them mention, in passing, difficulties they have had, for instance, at work with their colleagues. Others may complain how miserable the pain makes them. Others may complain of bizarre (delusional) symptoms such as 'slime' in the mouth or 'powder' coming out of the jaw.

Pain can be a symptom of depression. Since mental illness, even now, carries with it a stigma, patients frequently suppress the overt misery of depression. The patient may also fear (often rightly) that doctors or dentists are intolerant of what is regarded as their weakness in being unable to cope with their life situation.

This pain can be regarded as their cry for help. This is occasionally strikingly evident in a patient who appears emotionally in control but who, when given a chance to describe the complaint at length, suddenly loses control and starts to weep uncontrollably. At the other extreme, there are patients who so aggressively reject the idea of mental illness that they insist from the start that the pain is not 'due to their nerves' and typically refuse psychiatric help.

Occasionally, anxiety such as cancerophobia can give rise to atypical facial pain and may respond to reassurance.

Burning mouth syndrome

In this distressing and troublesome condition, symptoms may affect the whole mouth or only the tongue may be sore. This complaint has many features in common with atypical facial pain and may be a variant of it. Clinical features (Table 34.11) may suggest psychogenic factors.

Table 34.11   Features suggestive of 'burning mouth syndrome'

- Middle-aged or older women are mainly affected
- No visible abnormality or evidence of organic disease
- No haematological abnormality
- Pain typically described as 'burning'
- Persistent and unremitting soreness without aggravating or relieving factors, often of months or years duration; no response to analgesics.
- Bizarre patterns of pain radiation inconsistent with neurological or vascular anatomy
- Sometimes, bitter or metallic taste associated
- Associated depression, anxiety or stressful life situation
- Obsession with symptoms which may rule the patient's life
- Constant search for reassurance and treatment by different practitioners
- Occasionally, dramatic improvement with antidepressive treatment

---

These symptoms are seen in varying combination but psychological disturbance is frequently well disguised or suppressed. In practice, as with atypical facial pain, there are many patients who complain bitterly and persistently of sore tongue, in whom no organic disease can be found and who show no response to psychoactive drugs or any other form of treatment.

Management

The first essential is to exclude organic disease by a careful search for all possible sources of pain. Any potential sources of pain must be dealt with, but there should not be too much expectation of benefit. If no organic cause can be found and if sympathetic discussion suggests psychogenic factors, then it may help to explain to the patient in simple terms that depression and other emotional disturbances are just as much illnesses and cause as much suffering as physical diseases. It is also important to explain that emotional disturbances affect almost everyone to some degree. It may also help to point out that more common symptoms, particularly headache, are rarely due to organic disease. Patients should also be reassured that there is no dangerous disease and that frightening possibilities such as cancer can be confidently excluded. Such reassurance is sometimes remarkably effective.

While it is obviously reasonable gently to recommend psychiatric help, patients are often resentful of the idea and it is more tactful to refer to the psychiatrist as a 'pain expert'. Sometimes, antidepressant treatment with dothiepin, or one of the newer generation, antidepressive drugs, is strikingly effective.

Unfortunately, there is a hard core of patients who complain of persistent facial pain, have gone the round of specialists (including psychiatrists), have been treated with a wide range of drugs, but still continue to complain of severe pain. This problem may be a reflection of the limited range of treatment available, or perhaps such patients 'need' their pain for obscure emotional reasons.

It is essential also to appreciate that a few patients thought to have atypical facial pain are found later to have some disease such as an occult adenoid cystic carcinoma infiltrating nerve fibres.

Psychogenic dental pain (atypical odontalgia)

This is a less common variant of atypical facial pain. Pain is often precisely localised in one tooth or in a row of teeth, which are said either to ache or to be exquisitely sensitive to heat, cold, or pressure. If dental disease is found, treatment has no effect, or if, as a last resort, the tooth is removed, the pain moves to an adjacent tooth. Again, if no organic cause can be found and treatment is ineffective, psychiatric assessment is needed. Early diagnosis is essential to avoid overtreatment and serious dental morbidity.

PARAESTHESIA AND ANAESTHESIA OF THE LIP

Paraesthesia of the lip can be caused by osteomyelitis or fracture of the jaw. Very occasionally it results from neurological disease. The main causes of anaesthesia or paraesthesia of the lip are summarised in Table 34.12.

Table 34.12   Important causes of paraesthesia or anaesthesia of the lip

- Inferior dental blocks
- Trauma (fracture or operative damage)
- Acute osteomyelitis
- Malignant tumours of the mandible
- Exposed mental foramen
- Herpes zoster
- Multiple sclerosis
- Tetany

Prolonged anaesthesia or paraesthesia of the lip can occasionally follow *inferior dental blocks*, possibly as a result of damage to the nerve by the needle. Spontaneous recovery usually takes place.

Paraesthesia of the lip can be a complication of *fractures of the mandible* where the nerve has become stretched, particularly over the sharp edge of the canal. The effect is temporary but complete recovery may take some months. The inferior dental nerve may occasionally be damaged in *operations on the mandible* and there may be anaesthesia or paraesthesia lasting for many months. Complete loss of sensation is unusual but recovery may take a year or more.

The inferior dental nerve is rarely involved in *osteomyelitis* but, with effective treatment, recovery is the rule. Alternatively it may be compressed by a *neoplasm* or a tumour may infiltrate the nerve sheath. A jaw tumour causing pain or paraesthesia strongly suggests malignancy. In such cases, the prognosis is poor either because the tumour may be a secondary carcinoma or a primary but highly malignant tumour such as an osteosarcoma.

The mental foramen can become exposed by *excessive resorption of mandibular bone* in an edentulous patient. The denture can then press upon the nerve as it leaves the foramen. Though these changes are common, they rarely cause paraesthesia of the lip.

Herpes zoster affecting the trigeminal nerve can leave residual disturbances of sensation. The most severe and troublesome is postherpetic neuralgia but in other patients there may be persistent paraesthesia of the lip.

Disturbances of sensation of the face and other regions can be caused by *multiple sclerosis* as discussed earlier.

Tetany is the result of hypocalcaemic states and causes heightened neuromuscular excitability together with minor disorders of sensation such as paraesthesia of the lip. A significant cause of tetany is overbreathing, usually due to anxiety (*hyperventilation syndrome*).

FACIAL PALSY

Important causes of facial palsy, which include both upper and lower motor neurone lesions, are summarised in Table 34.13.

Table 34.13   Causes of facial palsy

- Extracranial causes
  - Bell's palsy
  - Malignant parotid neoplasms
  - Parotid surgery
  - Sarcoidosis (Heerfordt's syndrome)
  - Misplaced local anaesthetic
  - Melkersson–Rosenthal syndrome
- Intracranial causes
  - Strokes
  - Cerebral tumours and other neurological diseases
  - Multiple sclerosis
  - HIV infection
  - Lyme disease
  - Ramsay Hunt syndrome
  - Trauma to the base of the skull

Bell's palsy

Bell's palsy is a common cause of facial paralysis. It probably results from compression of the facial nerve in its canal as a result of inflammation and swelling. A viral infection, particularly *herpes simplex*, is suspected as the cause. Either sex may be affected, usually between the ages of 20 and 50. As mentioned earlier, pain in the jaw sometimes precedes the paralysis or there may be numbness in the side of the tongue. Though this disease is uncommon in dental practice, its recognition is important as early treatment may prevent permanent disability and disfigurement.

Function of the facial nerve is tested by asking the patient to perform facial movements. When asked to close the eyes, the lids on the affected side cannot be brought together but the

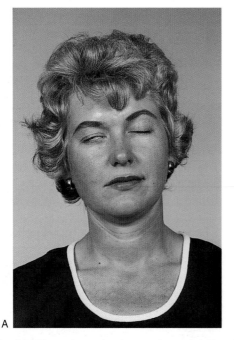
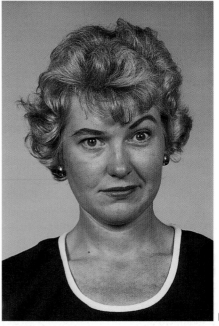

Fig. 34.1   Bell's palsy (**A**). When trying to shut the eyes, that on the affected (right) side fails to close completely but the eyeball rolls up normally (**B**). When trying to smile, the mouth fails to move on the affected side, which remains expressionless, having lost all natural skin folds. The difference is made more striking by covering each side of the picture in turn. This patient, incidentally, complained primarily of facial pain, though increasingly aware of the facial disability. The severely disfiguring effect of this disorder and the need for early treatment is obvious. In this case response was complete. (By kind permission of the patient.)

eyeball rolls up normally, since the oculomotor nerves are unaffected. When the patient is asked to smile, the corner of the mouth on the affected side is not pulled upwards and the normal lines of expression are absent (Fig. 34.1). The wrinkling round the eyes which accompanies smiling is also not seen on the affected side and the eye remains staring. This is a *lower motor neurone lesion* unlike the upper motor neurone lesion seen, for example, after a stroke, as discussed below.

The majority of patients recover fully or partially without treatment. At least 10% of patients with Bell's palsy are unhappy about the final outcome because of permanent disfigurement or other complications. A guide to the need for treatment is the severity of the paralysis when first seen. Full recovery is usual in patients with an incomplete palsy seen within a week of onset, but more than half of those with a complete lesion fail to recover completely. Electromyography and other electrodiagnostic techniques can be used to measure the degree of functional impairment as a guide to the need for treatment. Prednisolone, by mouth (20 mg four times a day) may be given for 5–10 days and then tapered off over the following 4 days, and may be effective if given within 24 hours of the onset. The addition of aciclovir appears to produce more reliable results and also suggests a role for a herpes virus.

If treatment fails or is not given, persistent facial weakness is disfiguring. The affected part of the face sometimes also contracts involuntarily in association with movement of another part. There may, for example, be twitching of the mouth when the patient blinks. More uncommon is unilateral lacrimation (crocodile tears) when eating. The majority of patients with persistent denervation develop contracture of the affected side of the face. Watering of the eye (epiphora) due to impaired drainage of tears, or occasionally to excessive and erratic lacrimal secretion, may remain particularly troublesome. Sagging of the affected side of the face may be limited by an intraoral prosthesis.

Melkersson–Rosenthal syndrome

Melkersson–Rosenthal syndrome in its rare complete form comprises unilateral recurrent facial paralysis which may become permanent, labial or facial swelling and fissured tongue. Recurrent, soft, painless facial swelling is more common, but may become persistent due to progressive fibrosis. The buccal mucosa may have a cobblestone pattern like that in Crohn's disease and histologically granulomas are found. Facial palsy is troublesome and disfiguring but there is no specific treatment.

Other causes of facial palsy

Cerebrovascular accidents (thrombosis or haemorrhage) are a common complication of hypertension in the elderly. Unilateral paralysis (hemiplegia) and often loss of speech (aphasia) are frequent in survivors of the acute episode. Unilateral facial palsy is common but differs from Bell's palsy in that it is an *upper motor neurone lesion*. The lower part of the face is mainly

affected and spontaneous emotional facial reactions may be retained.

As in the case of persistent paralysis in Bell's palsy, an intraoral prosthesis may limit sagging of the face. A stroke is occasionally the cause of an emergency in the dental surgery (Ch. 36). As mentioned earlier (Ch. 5), dental disease, particularly chronic periodontitis, may be significantly associated with the risk of strokes.

Facial palsy is an uncommon but characteristic manifestation of a *malignant parotid tumour*. Alternatively, a facial nerve may have been sacrified during resection of a malignant tumour, or is accidentally damaged during a parotidectomy. The variable course of the facial nerve within the parotid gland makes it particularly vulnerable to surgical injury and great skill is needed to trace its course.

Ramsay Hunt syndrome is severe facial palsy, together with pain, usually felt in the throat. Vesicles of herpes zoster may be seen in the external auditory meatus or throat.

Lyme disease is caused by *Borrelia burgdorferi* and transmitted by animal ticks. It is common in the USA but now seen in many other countries. Facial palsy or cervical lymphadenopathy are sometimes prominent but arthritis is the chief effect.

Heerfordt's syndrome is the rare combination of facial palsy, uveitis and parotid swelling caused by sarcoidosis of cranial nerves and salivary glands.

SUGGESTED FURTHER READING

Adour K K, Rubioyianes J M, von Doerstein P G et al 1996 Bell's palsy treatment with acyclovir and prednisone compared with prednisole alone: a double-blind, randomized, controlled trial. Ann Otol Rhinol Laryngol 105:371–378

Baringer J R 1996 Herpes simplex virus and Bell's palsy. Ann Intern Med 124:63–65

Barker F G, Jannetta P J, Bissonette D J et al 1996 The long-term outcome of microvascular decompression for trigeminal neuralgia. N Engl J Med 334:1077–1083

Bergdahl J, Anneroth G, Perris H 1995 Cognitive therapy in the treatment of patients with resistent burning mouth syndrome: a controlled study. J Oral Pathol Med 24:213–215

Devlen J 1994 Anxiety and depression in migraine. J Royal Soc Med 87:338–341

Fields H L 1996 Treatment of trigeminal neuralgia (editorial). N Engl J Med 334:1125–1126

Huong W, Rothe M J, Grant-Kels J M 1996 The burning mouth syndrome. J Am Acad Dermatol 34:91–98

Kost R G, Straus S E 1996 Postherpetic neuralgia — pathogenesis, treatment and prevention. N Engl J Med 335:32–42

Maizels M, Scott B, Cohen W, Chen W 1996 Intranasal lidocaine for treatment of migraine. J Am Med Assoc 276:319–321

Morgan M, Nathwain D 1992 Facial palsy and infection: the unfolding story. Clin Infect Dis 14:263–271

Ruboyianes J M, Trent C S, Adour K K et al 1996 Bell's palsy treatment with acyclovir and prednisone compared with prednisone alone: a double-blind, randomized, controlled trial. Ann Otol Rhinol Laryngol 105:371–378.

Shafshak T S, Essa A Y, Bakey F A 1994 The possible contributing factors for the success of steroid therapy in Bell's palsy: a clinical and electrophysiological study. J Larngol Otol 108:940–943

Whitley R J, Weiss H, Gnann J W 1996 Acyclovir with and without prednisone for the treatment of herpes zoster. A randomized, placebo-controlled trial. Ann Intern Med 125:376–383

Zakrzewska J M 1996 Assessment of a patient with orofacial pain. Primary Dent Care 3:57–60

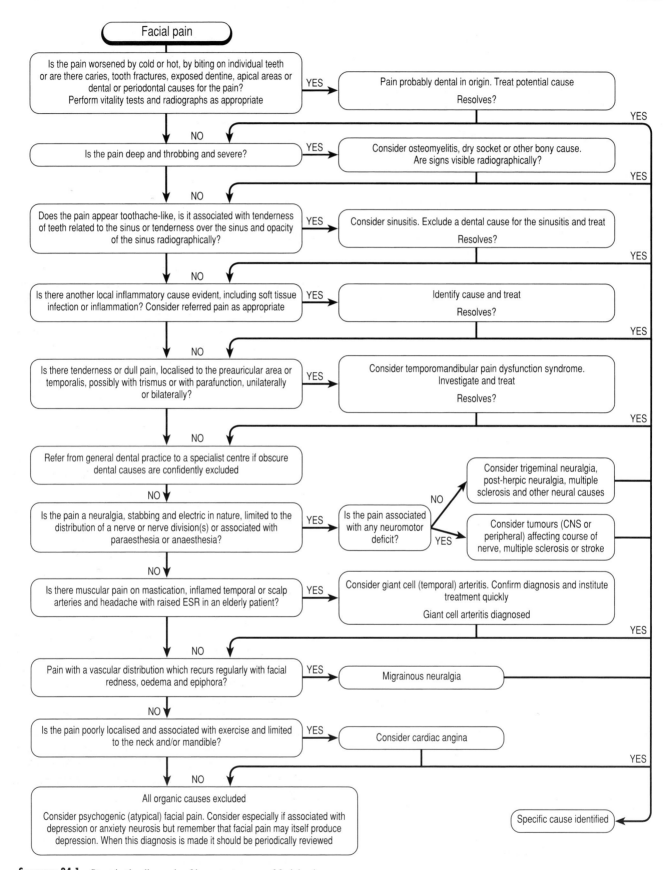

Summary 34.1 Steps in the diagnosis of important causes of facial pain.

Complications of systemic drug treatment

About 10% of ambulant outpatients may be having systemic drug treatment. Though not a common source of difficulties, some drugs can complicate dental management, occasionally catastrophically. Drug addicts are also a growing clinical problem. The effects of systemically administered drugs on dental management are varied (Table 35.1).

Table 35.1 Significance of drug treatment to dental management

- Drugs may complicate dental treatment itself (Table 35.2)
- Drugs may react with drugs given for dental purposes
- Drugs may cause stomatitis (Ch. 13) or have other oral effects

Oral reactions to drugs

Many drugs can occasionally cause oral reactions. They are varied in type but frequently lichenoid or ulcerative (Figs 35.3 and 35.4).

The mechanisms of reactions to drugs are often obscure but the various types are shown in Table 35.3.

Local reaction to drugs

Chemical burns. The best-known example is that of aspirin tablets held against the mucosa close to an aching tooth. This causes superficial necrosis and a white patch. When the irritant is removed, dead epithelium is shed and the mucosa heals. Other irritant chemicals are acid etchants, or phenol dropped on the mucosa.

Interference with the oral flora: superinfection. Prolonged topical use of antibiotics (particularly tetracycline) in the mouth kills off sensitive organisms and allows resistant ones, particularly *Candida albicans*, to proliferate, causing thrush. In susceptible patients, use of a topical antibiotic may precipitate candidal infection within 48 hours.

Systemically mediated reactions

Depression of marrow function. Few drugs significantly depress red cell production alone, though any drug which causes anaemia might give rise to oral signs. The main example is prolonged use of phenytoin (for epilepsy) which, in susceptible patients, can occasionally cause folate deficiency and macrocytic anaemia. This in turn can cause severe aphthous stomatitis. Response promptly follows administration of folate, and the blood picture returns to normal.

White cell production is depressed by a variety of drugs. Leucopenia may be severe enough to produce the clinical picture of agranulocytosis, with necrotising ulceration of the gingivae and throat which can go on to a severe prostrating illness and septicaemia if untreated. Drugs which may have this effect include antibacterials, particularly co-trimoxazole, chloramphenicol, analgesics, particularly amidopyrine (obsolete in the UK), phenothiazines and antithyroid agents. When the main effect is on granulocytes, low-grade oral pathogens, particularly of the gingival margins, are able to overcome local resistance and produce necrotising ulceration (Ch. 22).

Other drugs may affect haemostasis and cause oral purpura (Ch. 23). Drug-induced purpura is often also an early sign of aplastic anaemia caused by drugs such as chloramphenicol, which depress marrow function, as indicated above. Purpura can produce severe spontaneous gingival bleeding or blood blisters and widespread submucosal ecchymoses.

Depression of cell-mediated immunity. Immunosuppression by such drugs as corticosteroids is induced in patients having organ transplants or with immunologically-mediated diseases (see Fig. 24.1). Viral and fungal infections of the mouth are common in immunosuppressed patients and can be severe. Recurrences of childhood viral infections such as measles and chickenpox are also possible.

Lichenoid reactions. Several drugs, notably gold and antimalarials (both used in the treatment of rheumatoid arthritis or other collagen diseases), and the antihypertensive agent methyldopa can cause disease indistinguishable from lichen planus, both clinically and histologically (Ch. 13). The mechanism of such reactions is unknown.

Acute erythema multiforme. As discussed earlier, sulphonamides, barbiturates or other drugs are occasionally implicated, but the mechanisms are unknown and more frequently there is no evidence of a drug reaction.

Toxic epidermal necrolysis. This, which probably represents the extreme end of the spectrum of erythema multiforme, is one

Table 35.2 Examples of drugs having dentally relevant adverse effects

Type of drug	Dentally relevant adverse effects
Antibiotics	Superinfection (usually candidosis) Allergy (mainly penicillin) (Figs 35.1 and 35.2)
Anticoagulants	Risk of postoperative haemorrhage
Calcium channel blocker antihypertensives (e.g. nifedipine) and diltiazem (an antidysrhythmic)	Gingival hyperplasia
Phenytoin	Gingival hyperplasia Lymphadenopathy occasionally Folate deficiency occasionally
Aspirin	Potentiation of any haemorrhagic tendencies Avoid in children because of risk of Reye's syndrome
Other non-steroidal anti-inflammatory analgesics	Oral lichenoid reactions rarely
Hypnotics and sedatives[a]	Potentiation of general anaesthetics and other sedating drugs
Barbiturates	Risk of erythema multiforme
Phenothiazine antipsychotics ('major tranquillisers')	Dry mouth Tardive dyskinesia (uncontrollable facial movements) Parkinsonian tremor Postural hypotension Oral mucosal pigmentation
Metoclopramide	Clenching of jaw muscles
Tricyclic antidepressants (e.g. amitriptyline)[b]	Dry mouth
Monoamine oxidase inhibitors[b]	Dry mouth Dangerous interactions with opioids, particularly pethidine
Insulin	Risk of hypoglycaemic coma
Antihistamines	Dry mouth Drowsiness Potentiate sedatives
Corticosteroids	Opportunistic infections Risk of circulatory collapse (see also Table 31.8)
Other immunosuppressive and cytotoxic drugs	Oral ulceration (especially methotrexate) Opportunistic infections Cisplatin can cause grey gingival line Vincristine can cause jaw pain, and weakness of the facial muscles
Ciclosporin	Gingival hyperplasia

[a]Benzodiazepines ('minor tranquillisers') have few adverse effects apart from sedation, additive effects with other CNS depressants, and slight respiratory depression which is not significant in normal persons. However, they are addictive.
[b]*Do not* cause significant interactions with adrenaline (epinephrine) in local anaesthetics.

of the most dangerous and severe types of drug reaction. Mucosal involvement is common and causes widespread erosions due to epithelial destructions. Oral ulceration may precede the dermal changes, and cause the patient to seek treatment for the extreme soreness of the mouth. Early diagnosis and treatment is important as the reaction can be lethal. Metals such as gold salts are important causes but phenylbutazone, barbiturates and other drugs have also been implicated. Healing of oral lesions may leave a pattern of lichen planus.

Fixed drug eruptions. These consist of sharply circumscribed skin lesions recurring in the same site or sites each time the drug is given. Many drugs are capable of causing this reaction, but phenolphthalein, a widely use component of purgatives, is one of the more common causes. Involvement of the oral mucous membrane has been described but is exceedingly rare.

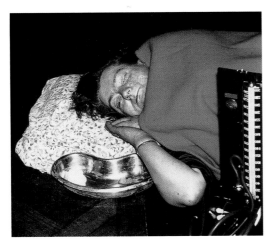

Fig. 35.1 Collapse caused by type I hypersensitivity to penicillin.

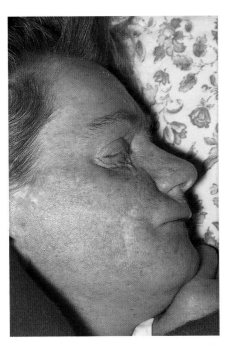

Fig. 35.2 Hypersensitivity to penicillin. There is a generalised slight oedema of the face, pallor and a macular rash.

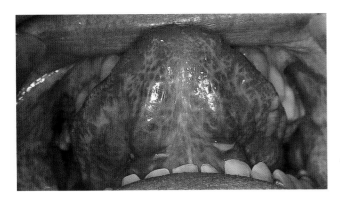

Fig. 35.3 Lichenoid reaction to captopril. In this milder reaction there are several small ulcers, but the main effect is the production of striae covering the whole ventral surface of the tongue.

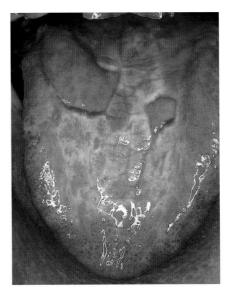

Fig. 35.4 Lichenoid reaction to gold treatment for rheumatoid arthritis. There is extensive ulceration of the dorsal tongue, atrophy and keratosis. Biopsy showed changes very similar to lichen planus.

Table 35.3 Important types of oral drug reactions
I.   Local reactions to drugs
● Chemical irritation
● Interference with the oral flora
II. Systematically mediated reactions
● Depression of marrow function
● Depression of cell-mediated immunity
● Lichenoid reactions
● Erythema multiforme (Stevens-Johnson syndrome)
● Fixed drug eruptions
● Toxic epidermal necrolysis
III. Other effects
● Gingival hyperplasia
● Pigmentation
● Dry mouth

Other drug effects (Table 35.3)

Gingival hyperplasia. Phenytoin and other drugs (Ch. 5) can cause fibrous hyperplasias, particularly concentrated at the interdental papillae.

Oral pigmentation. Heavy metals such as mercury, bismuth and lead can cause black or brown deposits in the gingival sulcus by interaction with bacterial products to form sulphides. The blue lead line may be particularly sharply defined and indicate the level of the floor of the pocket. These effects are rarely seen now that mercury and bismuth are no longer used in medicine and lead is no longer a major industrial hazard. However, cisplatin, a cytotoxic drug, can cause a blue line. Topical antibiotics and antiseptics may cause dark pigmentation, particularly of the dorsum of the tongue, due to overgrowth of pigment-forming bacteria.

Dry mouth is a relatively common side effect of drugs, particularly those with an atropine-like action, such as the tricyclic antidepressants which are widely used (Ch. 18).

Management considerations

Oral reactions to drugs are not overall common; nevertheless they may be important as an early sign of a dangerous or lethal reaction.

However, a drug being taken by a patient is not necessarily the cause of any oral symptoms. Coincidence is often difficult to exclude, particularly with common oral diseases such as lichen planus. The problem is made more difficult by multiple drug treatment. However it is essential to get a detailed history of drug treatment as this may affect other aspects of dental treatment.

Precautions

Though drugs only occasionally cause clinical difficulties, patients must always be asked whether they are under medical treatment. In such enquiries the word 'drugs' should be avoided as inevitably leading to misinterpretation. Patients should be asked whether they are taking 'medicines, tablets, injections, or any sort of medical treatment for *any* purpose' or have received any medications recently, or whether they have been given any sort of hospital card.

DRUG DEPENDENCE

Drug dependence, particularly addiction to intravenous drugs, is a major social problem, particularly in large cities. However, alcohol remains the most widely abused drug. There are few direct oral effects of drug dependence apart from maxillofacial injuries secondary to alcohol abuse particularly, but difficulties in management are more common (Table 35.4).

Addicts may manipulate dentists into prescribing drugs, particularly opioids, by complaining of pain. Multiple drug abuse is also common, and attempts may be made to obtain any drugs such as benzodiazepines or antihistamines which are mood-altering or sedative. Because of the risk of dependence, benzodiazepines should only be prescribed for short periods. Codeine

Table 35.4 Implications of drug dependence for dental management

- Stealing prescription pads
- Attempts to manipulate dentists into prescribing drugs
- Carriage of hepatitis viruses or HIV by intravenous addicts
- Maxillofacial injuries, particularly among alcoholics
- Impaired liver function secondary to alcoholism or hepatitis
- Lymphadenopathy secondary to drug injection in unusual sites
- Infective endocarditis secondary to dirty injections
- Severe infections such as osteomyelitis among alcoholics
- Increased risks from general anaesthesia
- Gross oral neglect and sometimes enhanced sensitivity to pain
- Rarely, ulceration of the palate secondary to cocaine-induced ischaemia of the nasal cavity
- Occasionally, parotid swelling in alcoholics.
- Interactions with other drugs

or dextropropoxyphene (in co-proxamol) are opioids and occasionally a cause of dependence.

Liver function damaged by alcoholism or hepatitis impairs drug metabolism. This makes general anaesthesia, in particular, hazardous, as does respiratory disease or covert use of the drug of abuse preoperatively. Once infective endocarditis has resulted from dirty injections, the damaged heart becomes vulnerable to endocarditis after some types of dental procedures (Ch. 27).

SUGGESTED FURTHER READING

Cawson R A, Spector R G, Skelly A M 1995 *Basic pharmacology and clinical drug use in dentistry*, 6th Edn. Churchill Livingstone, Edinburgh
Passeri L A, Ellis E, Sinn D P 1993 Relationship of substance abuse to complications with mandibular fractures. J Oral Maxillofac Surg 51:22–25
Robb N D, Smith B G N 1996 Chronic alcoholism: an important condition in the dentist–patient relationship. J Dentistry 24:17–24
Strang J 1995 Substance abuse: the size of the problem. Medicine Int 23:41–44
Vale A 1995 Alcohol intoxication and alcohol–drug interactions. Medicine Int 23:51–53

Emergencies in dental practice

Dentists must know how to recognise and manage medical emergencies, rare though they may be. Their professional skills and equipment should enable them occasionally to save patients' lives. Patients suffering life-threatening emergencies should be quickly transferred to hospital, but city traffic and the load on ambulance services are so heavy that the delay can be considerable. Under such circumstances, measures taken by the dentist may be critical.

Dentists are also required to ensure that all members of their staff are able to provide practical assistance in these circumstances.

Many types of emergencies may have to be faced (Table 36.1).

Table 36.1 Emergencies that may arise during dental procedures

- Sudden loss of consciousness (collapse)
  1. Fainting
  2. Acute hypoglycaemia
  3. Circulatory collapse secondary to corticosteroid therapy
  4. Anaphylactic shock
  5. Myocardial infarction
  6. Cardiac arrest
  7. Strokes
- Acute chest pain
  1. Angina
  2. Myocardial infarction
- Difficulty in breathing
  1. Asthma
  2. Anaphylactic shock
  3. Left ventricular failure
- Convulsions
  1. Epilepsy
  2. Any other cause of loss of consciousness, including fainting
- Other emergencies
  1. Haemorrhage
  2. Drug reactions and interactions
  3. Major maxillofacial injuries

the dental surgery. There are several predisposing factors (Table 36.2), but some patients are particularly prone to faint and frequently do so. Signs and symptoms are usually readily recognisable (Table 36.3).

Table 36.2 Factors predisposing to fainting

- Anxiety
- Pain
- Injections
- Fatigue
- Hunger

Table 36.3 Fainting: signs and symptoms

- Premonitory dizziness, weakness or nausea
- Pale, cold moist skin
- Initially slow and weak pulse becoming full and bounding
- Loss of consciousness

Sometimes consciousness is lost almost instantaneously. Minor convulsions or incontinence are occasionally associated. Principles of management are summarised in Table 36.4.

Table 36.4 Management of a fainting attack

- Lower the head, preferably by laying the patient flat*
- Loosen any tight clothing round the neck
- Give a sweetened drink when consciousness has been recovered
- If no recovery within a few minutes, consider other causes of loss of consciousness

*To keep the patient upright worsens cerebral hypoxia and is harmful.

SUDDEN LOSS OF CONSCIOUSNESS

Fainting

Fainting, caused by transient hypotension and cerebral ischaemia, is the most common cause of sudden loss of consciousness in

Prevention

Regular fainters are frequently helped by an anxiolytic, such as temazepam 5 mg orally, on the night before and again an hour before treatment, but must be accompanied by a responsible adult.

Acute hypoglycaemia

Hypoglycaemia affects diabetic patients after an overdose of insulin or if prevented from eating at the expected time by dental treatment (Table 36.5).

Table 36.5 Signs and symptoms of acute hypoglycaemia

- Premonitary signs are similar to those of a faint, but little response to laying the patient flat
- Unconsciousness steadily deepens

Management of hypoglycaemia is important (Table 36.6). If there is any doubt about the cause of loss of consciousness, insulin must *never* be given as it can be fatal to a hypoglycaemic patient.

Table 36.6 Management of hypoglycaemia

- Patients often aware of what is happening and able to warn the dentist
- Before consciousness is lost, give glucose tablets or powder, or sugar (at least four lumps) as a sweetened drink, repeated if symptoms not completely relieved
- Ideally, if consciousness is lost, give sterile intravenous glucose (up to 50 mL of a 50% solution)
- If sterile glucose not available give subcutaneous glucagon (1 mg) then give sugar by mouth during the brief recovery period.
- Hypostop, a gel containing glucose, may provide sufficient glucose absorbed through the oral mucosa to combat declining consciousness

---

Circulatory collapse in patients on corticosteroid treatment

The response of patients on long-term corticosteroid treatment to surgery is unpredictable, but near-fatal circulatory collapse can follow minor dental extractions under anaesthesia in a patient taking as little as 5 mg of prednisone a day. All patients who are taking or have been taking systemic corticosteroids are at risk. Adrenocortical function may possibly take up to 2 years to recover. Corticosteroid skin preparations used liberally, particularly for widespread eczema, can also lead to stress-related collapse.

Since large doses of corticosteroids given for a short period are safe and can be life-saving, management (Table 36.7) should lean towards being over-protective. Prevention is all important.

Causes and clinical features of corticosteroid-related collapse

General anaesthesia, surgical or other trauma, infections or other stress are the main causes (see Fig. 31.8).

Myocardial infarction

A patient typically has severe chest pain, but may suddenly lose consciousness as a result of a myocardial infarct (see below).

Table 36.7 Signs and management of corticosteroid-related collapse

Signs
- Pallor
- Rapid, weak or impalpable pulse
- Loss of consciousness
- Rapidly falling blood pressure

Management
- Lay the patient flat and raise the legs
- Give at least 200 mg hydrocortisone sodium succinate intravenously*
- Call an ambulance for immediate transfer to hospital
- Give oxygen and, if necessary, artificial ventilation
- Consider other possible reasons for loss of consciousness

*The intramuscular route can be used if a vein cannot be found but absorption is slower.

Anaphylactic reactions

Penicillin is the most common cause of these type I hypersensitivity reactions. Similar reactions due to direct histamine release by morphine or intravenous barbiturate anaesthetics are rare. Anaphylactic reactions can also be precipitated by insect stings, foods (nuts or shellfish particularly) and, exceptionally rarely, by aspirin.

In general, the quicker the onset the more severe the reaction. A severe reaction to penicillin may start within a minute of an injection but immediate loss of consciousness is more likely to be due to fainting. A reaction starting 30 minutes after an injection is unlikely to be dangerous. Acute reactions to oral penicillins are rare but can develop after half an hour or more because of slower absorption from the gut.

Collapse is due to widespread vasodilatation and increased capillary permeability causing potentially fatal hypotension (see Figs 35.1 and 35.2).

Signs and symptoms

The clinical picture is variable (Table 36.8).

Table 36.8 Typical features of acute anaphylaxis

- Initial facial flushing, itching, paraesthesiae or cold extremities
- Facial oedema or urticaria
- Bronchospasm (wheezing)
- Loss of consciousness
- Pallor going on to cyanosis
- Cold clammy skin
- Rapid weak or impalpable pulse
- Deep fall in blood pressure
- Death if treatment is delayed or inappropriate

Table 36.9 Management of anaphylactic collapse

- Lay the patient flat. Raise the legs to improve cerebral blood flow
- Give 0.5–1 mL of 1:1000 adrenaline (epinephrine) by intramuscular injection. Repeat every 15 minutes if necessary, until the patient responds
- Give 10–20 mg chlorpheniramine (diluted in the syringe with 10 mL of blood) slowly intravenously
- Give 200 mg of hydrocortisone sodium succinate intravenously
- Give oxygen and, if necessary, assisted ventilation
- Call an ambulance

Management

Adrenaline (epinephrine) is the mainstay of treatment (Table 36.9). It raises cardiac output, combats excessive capillary permeability and bronchospasm, and also inhibits release of mediators from mast cells.

Circulatory collapse is probably largely due to histamine release which is combated by parenteral chlorpheniramine. Hydrocortisone is slow to take effect but maintains the blood pressure for some hours and combats the continued effect of the antigen–antibody reaction.

Rapid transfer to hospital is necessary to provide circulatory support by intravenous fluids and other measures. The patient must also be given a card warning against the use of the causative drug.

Minor anaphylactic reactions such as urticaria can be treated with oral or intramuscular chlorpheniramine.

Cardiac arrest

Cardiac arrest can follow myocardial infarction, or the acute hypotension of an anaphylactic reaction or of corticosteroid insufficiency. Otherwise, it may be the result of an anaesthetic accident and due to hypoxia, anaesthetic overdose or severe hypotension.

Dentists should be aware of and alert to the possibility of cardiac arrest and be able to recognise it (Table 36.10) and manage it (Table 36.11) when it happens. Speed of response is essential and there is a legal obligation that the dental team should be trained in cardiopulmonary resuscitation and be able to carry it out immediately.

Table 36.10 Signs and symptoms of cardiac arrest

- Sudden loss of consciousness
- Absence of arterial pulses (the carotid artery, anterior to sternomastoid should be felt)

Respiratory arrest and eventual cyanosis, pupil dilatation and loss of reaction to light, and absence of measurable blood pressure are other signs but resuscitation must be started before they develop.

Table 36.11 Management of cardiac arrest

- Summon help. Telephone for an ambulance and state that there has been a cardiac arrest
- Put the patient on a firm flat surface, i.e. the floor, if possible[a]
- Clear the airway and keep it clear by extending the neck and holding the jaw forward
- Start external cardiac compression immediately. Kneel (or stand) beside the patient and put one hand over the other on the patient's lower sternum. Forcefully depress the sternum about 1.5–2 inches (4–5 cm) at about 80 times a minute
- The assistant should inflate the lungs between each 5 compressions of the sternum either as a mouth-to-mouth procedure or with a self-inflating bag with oxygen supplementation as described below[b]
- Persist until expert help arrives or there are signs of restoration of blood pressure with disappearance of facial pallor, and a good spontaneous pulse. Other signs of success are contraction of the pupils, return of reflex activity such as the blink reflex and reaction of the pupils to light, lightening of unconsciousness and purposeful spontaneous movements — not twitching or convulsions
- Transfer the patient to hospital for advanced life support

[a]If the patient is too heavy to lift out of a dental chair but can be laid supine there, resuscitation can be carried out by the operator and assistant standing beside the chair. An operator's stool can be placed under the headrest to stabilise the chair.
[b]If there is no assistant, the ratio of chest compressions to lung inflations should be 15:4.

The optimal pressure for chest compression is about 40 or 50 kg (the weight of the upper part of the body applied through stiffly extended arms). External cardiac massage is tiring and another person should preferably take over as soon as the first operator becomes fatigued. If no signs of life appear within 15 minutes (timed by the clock) recovery is unlikely.

Unless the operator is skilled in its use, time should not be wasted in trying to pass an endotracheal tube. However, a self-inflating bag with an oxygen supply should be available to provide positive pressure ventilation. A plastic airway should be put in the patient's mouth and the mask applied firmly over the nose and mouth with the resuscitation bag attached. The patient's lungs should be inflated with oxygen by squeezing the bag, so that the chest is visibly expanded at each respiration. Passive recoil of the chest wall causes spontaneous inspiration as soon as the pressure is removed.

If a self-inflating bag is not available, mouth-to-mouth ventilation can be given, preferably with an intervening Laerdal pocket mask.

During artificial ventilation the patient's nose must be closed. Deep inflations are given by the operator and time allowed for passive recoil of the chest. If there is no airway adjunct available, direct mouth-to-mouth resuscitation, with the nose occluded, must be given. Causes of failure are summarised in Table 36.12.

Strokes (Table 36.13)

Patients are usually hypertensive and middle-aged or elderly. The clinical picture varies with the size and site of brain

Table 36.12 Causes of failure of cardiopulmonary resuscitation

- Giving external cardiac compression without artificial ventilation
- Giving artificial ventilation without cardiac compression
- Failing to clear the airway or to keep it open by failing to hyperextend the head adequately
- Failing to close the nose during mouth-to-mouth ventilation
- Failing to fit the mask closely onto the patient's face when using an inflating bag
- Failing to make sure that ventilation is adequate, as shown by movement of the chest
- Timidity in applying external cardiac compression, and using insufficient force to compress the heart. The risk of cracking a rib should be disregarded
- Failing to release pressure on the chest completely between compressions and thus preventing cardiac filling
- Compressing the chest too rapidly to allow the heart to fill between compressions
- Putting the hands in incorrect positions
- Failing to act sufficiently quickly and fretting about details rather than getting on with the essentials of external cardiac compression and artificial ventilation.

Table 36.13 Signs and management of a stroke

Signs
- Loss of consciousness
- Weakness of an arm and leg on one side
- Drooping of the side of the face
- Often stertorous breathing

Management
- Maintain the airway
- Call an ambulance for transfer to hospital

damage. Subarachnoid haemorrhage from a ruptured berry aneurysm on the circle of Willis is the main cause of stroke in a younger person. It typically causes intense headache followed by coma without localising signs.

CHEST PAIN

Angina pectoris (Table 36.14)

A patient with coronary atheroma might have a first anginal attack as a consequence of an emotional response to dental treatment. However, more patients have already had attacks and carry medication. Acute chest pain due to myocardial ischaemia is the only symptom.

Myocardial infarction

Myocardial infarction is a common cause of death and must be recognised (Table 36.15), as the patient's fate may be decided by the first few minutes' treatment. Several aspects of dentistry, particularly apprehension, pain or the effect of drugs, might contribute to make this accident more likely in a susceptible patient.

Table 36.14 Management of angina

- Give the patient his anti-anginal drug (usually 0.5 mg of glyceryl trinitrate sublingually) *or*
- Glyceryl trinitrate spray* (400 mg) gives rapid relief
- If there is no relief within 3 minutes the patient has probably had a myocardial infarct (see below)

*Glyceryl trinitrate spray has a better shelf-life for the emergency kit.

Table 36.15 Typical signs and symptoms of myocardial infarction

- Severe crushing retrosternal pain
- Shallow breathing
- Vomiting
- Weak or irregular pulse

Some patients die within a few minutes after the start of the attack and it is rash to try over-ambitious treatment. Drugs, apart from those described below, should not be used as, without continuous monitoring, they may do more harm than good.

Pain can radiate to the left shoulder or down the left arm but very occasionally is felt only in the left jaw. Vomiting is common and there is sometimes shock or loss of consciousness. Principles of management are summarised in Table 36.16.

Aspirin is a valuable antiplatelet drug but it is only feasible to give a fibrinolytic drug such as streptokinase in hospital where lidocaine or other antidysrhythmic drugs can be given as appropriate.

There is concern about dentists giving aspirin under these circumstances in case there has been a misdiagnosis and the pain is due to a perforated peptic ulcer or dissecting aneurysm. However, the danger of giving a single tablet of aspirin in such conditions is unlikely to be significant.

DYSPNOEA

Status asthmaticus (Table 36.17)

Causes

Loss of or forgetting to bring a salbutamol inhaler, anxiety, infection or exposure to a specific allergen are possible causes.

Left ventricular failure

Extreme breathlessness is a typical sign of left ventricular failure. This is most likely to be a consequence of a myocardial infarct (see above) but can occasionally result from a severe dysrhythmia, particularly in a patient who has had a previous

Table 36.16 Management of myocardial infarction

- Put the patient in a comfortable position that allows easy breathing. Do not lay flat if there is left ventricular failure and pulmonary oedema
- Send an assistant to telephone for an Intensive Care ambulance.
- Give 50/50 nitroux oxide and oxygen from a general anaesthetic or relative analgesia machine, to relieve pain and anxiety
- Constantly reassure the patient
- Give oxygen if necessary
- Give aspirin 150 mg by mouth as soon as more urgent measures have been carried out
- Check for possible cardiac arrest

Table 36.17 Signs and management of status asthmaticus

Signs
- Breathlessness.
- Inability to talk
- Expiratory wheezing (may be disguised as rapid shallow breathing)
- Rapid pulse (usually over 110 per minute). Progress to bradycardia is a danger sign
- Accessory muscles of respiration start to come into action
- Cyanosis

Management
- Call an ambulance for transfer to hospital
- Reassure the patient.
- Do *not* lay the patient flat.
- Give normally used anti-asthmatic drugs (such as salbutamol) by inhaler or better, by nebuliser.
- Give hydrocortisone sodium succinate 200 mg intravenously
- Give oxygen
- If no response within 2–3 minutes, ideally, give salbutamol 250 micrograms by slow IV injection
- If IV salbutamol not available and patient continues to deteriorate, give adrenaline (epinephrine) as for anaphylaxis

Table 36.18 Signs and management of a tonic-clonic epileptic attack

Signs
- Sometimes a brief warning cry as the chest muscles contract and air is forced through a closed larynx
- Consciousness lost immediately
- The body becomes rigid (tonic phase) and cyanosis appears
- Widespread jerking movements start (clonic phase)
- Sometimes incontinence or frothing of the mouth
- Flaccidity sometimes follows after a few minutes
- Consciousness regained after a variable period. Confusion or drowsiness may persist

Management
- Put the patient prone in the coma ('recovery') position as soon as possible
- Prevent patients from injuring themselves
- Do not try to put anything in the mouth in the attempt to prevent the patient biting the tongue
- Make sure the airway is clear after convulsions have subsided
- Do not give any medication but await recovery
- Reassure patients as soon as consciousness returns
- Only allow patients to return home when fully recovered and accompanied by a responsible adult

Table 36.19 Management of status epilepticus

- Give 10 mg intravenous diazepam to an adult patient
- If venous access cannot be obtained give 5 mg of intramuscular midazolam* (absorption of intramuscular diazepam is slow and erratic)
- Repeat diazepam or midazolam if no recovery within 5 minutes
- Maintain the airway and give oxygen
- Call an ambulance and transfer to hospital

*Not officially approved for this purpose but can be life-saving.

myocardial infarct. Apart from measures for an infarct and sitting the patient upright, little can be done in the dental surgery apart from immediately calling an Intensive Care ambulance.

CONVULSIONS

Epilepsy (Table 36.18)

Hunger, menstruation and some drugs such as methohexitone, tricyclic antidepressants, alcohol or frequently flashing lights (*not* merely turning the operating lamp on and off) may sometimes precipitate a fit.

Status epilepticus (Table 36.19)

If convulsions do not stop within 15 minutes, or are rapidly repeated, the patient is in status epilepticus and can die from anoxia.

OTHER EMERGENCIES

Haemorrhage

Prolonged bleeding is usually due to traumatic extractions. A major vessel is unlikely to be opened during dental surgery and patients are unlikely to lose any dangerous amount of blood if promptly managed (Table 36.20). Post-extraction bleeding is usually only an emergency in the sense that the dentist may be woken up at 3 o'clock in the morning by a frightened patient.

Occasionally, bleeding is due to unsuspected haemophilia or other haemorrhagic disorders.

Drug reactions and interactions

Apart from anaphylactic reactions discussed earlier, very few other drug reactions or interactions endangering life are likely to be seen in the dental surgery.

Table 36.20   **Management of prolonged dental haemorrhage**

- Reassure the patient
- Coax excited relatives out of the surgery
- Clean the mouth with swabs and locate the source of bleeding
- Give adrenaline (epinephrine)-containing local anaesthetic, remove ragged tissue, squeeze up the socket edges and suture it
- When bleeding has been controlled, ask about the history and especially any family history of prolonged bleeding
- If bleeding continues despite suturing or if the patient is obviously anaemic or debilitated, transfer to hospital for investigation and management of any haemorrhagic defect
- Meanwhile, limit bleeding as much as possible with a pressure pad over the socket and by supporting the patient's jaw with a firm barrel bandage
- Ideally, tranexamic acid (500 mg in 5 mL, by slow intravenous injection) should be given and may be effective in a mild haemophilic while awaiting transfer to hospital

Local anaesthetics with vasoconstrictors

Noradrenaline (norepinephrine) (1:20 000), used as a vaso-constrictor in local anaesthetic solutions, has caused deaths from acute hypertension or cerebral haemorrhage. Such reactions can be combatted by an alpha-blocker such as phentolamine. Quite apart from its dangers, noradrenaline (norepinephrine) has no advantages and is no longer available.

Adrenaline (epinephrine). There is no evidence of hypertensive reactions to adrenaline (epinephrine) used in normal concentration and quantity.

Interactions with beta blockers. Adrenaline (epinephrine), in *large* doses, can interact with drugs such as propranolol to raise the blood pressure. It causes constriction of skin and visceral vessels (alpha effect) but dilatation of muscle arterioles (beta effect).

Dilatation of muscle vessels by adrenaline (epinephrine) is opposed by the beta-blocker but the alpha effect on skin and visceral vessels is unopposed. The consequent constriction of both muscle and skin vessels raises the peripheral resistance and blood pressure.

Clinically, occasional cases of hypertensive interactions between adrenaline (epinephrine) and propranolol have been reported in patients receiving large amounts of adrenaline (epinephrine) in local analgesics for plastic surgery. In 1995, a dentist was convicted of manslaughter after causing the death of a patient on beta-blockers by giving her 16 cartridges of lidocaine with adrenaline (epinephrine) though it appears overdose of lidocaine was the cause. Though healthy adults can tolerate large amounts of lidocaine with adrenaline (epinephrine) the dose should be limited to 5 cartridges given over the space of an hour unless cardiac monitoring is available.

Otherwise, in all three deaths associated with dental local anaesthetics in the 10-year period 1980–1989, prilocaine had been given.

Monoamine oxidase inhibitors

Monoamine oxidase inhibitors (MAOIs) can cause severe reactions with opioids. The onset can be very sudden and, with pethidine, can be fatal. Monoamine oxidase inhibitors also interact with indirectly-acting sympathomimetic drugs (such as ephedrine used as a nasal decongestant) to cause acute severe hypertension. The treatment is to give an alpha-blocker such as phentolamine. Adrenaline (epinephrine) or noradrenaline (norepinephrine) in local anaesthetics do not cause hypertensive reactions with MAOIs.

General anaesthetics

General anaesthetics, particularly intravenous barbiturates, have been the main cause of fatalities in the dental surgery.

Corticosteroids

As already described, patients on long-term corticosteroid treatment when exposed to stress can suffer circulatory collapse as a result of adrenal suppression.

SUGGESTED FURTHER READING

Cawson R A, Spector R G, Skelly M 1995 *Basic pharmacology and clinical drug use in dentistry*, 6th Edn. Churchill Livingstone, Edinburgh

Edmondson H D, Frame J W, Malins A F 1989 Medical emergencies in dental practice: an update on drugs and the management of acute airway obstruction. Dental Uptake August:254–256

European Resuscitation Council Basic Life Support Working Group 1993 Guidelines for basic life support. BMJ 306:1587–1589

European Resuscitation Council Working Party 1993 Adult advanced cardiac life support; The European Resuscitation Council guidelines 1992 (abridged). BMJ 306:1589–1593

Fisher M 1992 Treating anaphylaxis with sympathomimetic drugs. In severe anaphylaxis adrenaline by any route is better than none (editorial). BMJ 305:1107–1108

Gallagher E J, Lombardi G, Gennis P 1995 Effectiveness of bystandard cardiopulmonary resuscitation and survival following out-of-hospital cardiac arrest. JAMA 274:1922–1925

Pennycook A, Makower R, Brewer A et al 1993 The management of dental problems presenting to an accident and emergency department. J Roy Soc Med 86:702–703

Sanders B J, Weddell J A, Dodge N N 1995 Managing patients who have seizure disorders: dental and medical issues. J Am Dent Assoc 126:1641–1647

Index